VETERINARY ANAESTHESIA

Veterinary Anaesthesia

NINTH EDITION

L. W. HALL

MA, BSc, PhD, DVA, Dr (HonsCausa) Utrecht, HonDipACVA, MRCVS
Reader in Comparative Anaesthesia, University of Cambridge;
Fellow of Girton College, Cambridge

K. W. CLARKE

MA, VetMB, DVA, DVetMed, MRCVS
Senior Lecturer in Anaesthesia, Royal Veterinary College,
University of London

W B Saunders Company Ltd
London · Philadelphia · Toronto · Sydney · Tokyo

W. B. Saunders
Company Ltd

24–28 Oval Road
London NW1 7DX, England

The Curtis Center,
Independence Square West,
Philadelphia, PA 19106–3399, USA

Harcourt Brace & Company
55 Horner Avenue
Toronto, Ontario M8Z 4X6 Canada

Harcourt Brace & Company, Australia
30–52 Smidmore Street
Marrickville, NSW 2204, Australia

Harcourt Brace & Company, Japan
Ichibancho Central building
22–1 Ichibancho
Chiyoda-ku, Tokoyo 102, Japan

First edition 1941 by J. G. Wright
Second edition 1947 by J. G. Wright
Third edition 1948 by J. G. Wright
Fourth edition 1957 by J. G. Wright
Fifth edition 1961 by J. G. Wright and L. W. Hall
Sixth edition 1966 by L. W. Hall
Seventh edition 1971 by L. W. Hall reprinted 1974 and 1976
Eighth edition 1983 by L. W. Hall and K. W. Clarke
Reprinted 1985 and 1989
Ninth edition 1991 by L. W. Hall and K. W. Clarke
Fourth printing 1996

Spanish edition (Acribia Zaragoza) 1970
English Language Book Society edition 1983

British Library Cataloguing in Publication Data
Wright, John George
  Veterinary anaesthesia. — 9th ed.
  1. Anaesthesia in veterinary surgery.
  I. Title II. Hall, L. W. III. Clarke, K. W.
  636.089′7′96 SF914

ISBN 0–7020–1421–4

Typeset by J&L Composition Ltd, Filey, North Yorkshire
Printed in Great Britain by The Bath Press, Avon

CONTENTS

PART I   PRINCIPLES AND PROCEDURES

PART II   ANAESTHESIA OF THE SPECIES

PART III SPECIAL ANAESTHESIA

APPENDICES

PREFACE TO THE NINTH EDITION

Although all the chapters have been extensively revised, the general concepts of this edition remain the same as those of the preceding ones. The aim is still to provide a text for students and a reference work for veterinarians in general practice together with a comprehensive and stimulating introduction to the subject for those wishing to specialize in veterinary anaesthesia through examinations such as those of the Royal College of Veterinary Surgeons and the American College of Veterinary Anesthesiologists.

For these purposes the first part of the book covers generalities and basic principles; the second part is concerned with clinical anaesthesia in the various species of animal. No attempt has been made to include a comprehensive bibliography but we believe the greatly increased number of references should provide a useful introduction to the literature. We have removed much of the now out-of-date material in order to keep the text roughly the same length as that of the eighth edition and we have been mindful of the resurgence of interest in intravenous anaesthesia so that more consideration is now given to this topic. Because we believe that clinical anaesthesia encompasses much more than an exercise in applied pharmacology, emphasis is still on the effects of clinically useful doses of drugs and of techniques in animal patients, rather than on pharmacological effects demonstrated in healthy experimental animals in laboratories.

We wish to express our appreciation of all the many authors and publishers who have kindly allowed their work to be quoted and reproduced in this edition and to others who have contributed to the text. Special thanks are due to Mr. A. R. W. Porter, CBE, MA, HonAssocRCVS for updating Appendix I (Duties of an anaesthetist), Dr Sue Dyson for bringing the anatomical nomenclature up to date, Dr Sherry Faye for providing details of animal cholinesterases, Dr Peter Jackson for details of porcine sedation, Richard Kock for Table 17.2, Dr Guy Watney for Appendix III, Dr Alistair Webb for details of elephant anaesthesia and Dr Simon Young for assistance with computer-generated diagrams of breathing circuits.

Finally, our warmest thanks are due to Elisabeth Hall for invaluable assistance with typing of the manuscript, as well as to David Gunn, ABIPP, Charlotte Hall, GradDipApplSci and David Johns, LBIPP for expert photographic help.

L. W. Hall.   K. W. Clarke.
January 1991

PART I

PRINCIPLES AND PROCEDURES

CHAPTER 1

GENERAL CONSIDERATIONS

INTRODUCTION

The clinical discipline concerned with the reversible production of insensibility to pain is known as 'anaesthesia', a term introduced by Oliver Wendell Holmes in 1846 in an attempt to describe in a single word what was then a new phenomenon. It is essentially a practical subject and although becoming increasingly based on science it still retains some of the attributes of an art.

Veterinary anaesthesia has to satisfy the two requirements of humane handling of animals and of technical efficiency. Humanitarian considerations dictate that gentle handling and minimal restraint should always be employed; these minimize apprehension and protect the struggling animal from possible injury. In Britain veterinary anaesthesia is, in addition, regulated by the legal obligations imposed by the Protection of Animals (Anaesthetics) Act of 1964 and its subsequent Amendments which together specify the very few operations that can be performed legally on certain species of animal without any anaesthetic — such as the castration of calves, sheep, goats and pigs, docking of tails, removal of dewclaws and disbudding of calves below specified age limits. All veterinarians in the UK must be familiar with the provisions of this Act.

Technical efficiency is not restricted to facilitation of the procedure to be carried out on the animal, it must also take into account the protection of personnel from bites, scratches or kicks as well as the risks of accidental or deliberate self-injection with dangerous or addictive drugs. Moreover, today it is considered that personnel need protection from the possible harmful effects of breathing air contaminated with very low concentrations of inhalation anaesthetic agents.

For over 100 years anaesthetists have been conditioned to accept the concept of 'depth' of anaesthesia but this concept can have no real meaning and the search for some method to measure anaesthetic depth has delayed understanding of the phenomenon used daily to render animals insensitive to the trauma of surgery [1]. While the term 'anaesthesia' has precisely the same meaning today as when it was first coined, i.e. the state in which an animal is insensible to the trauma of surgery, it is now used much more widely and can be compared to terms such as 'illness' and 'shock' which are too non-specific to be of real value. Starting with the premise that 'pain is the conscious perception of a noxious stimulus' it is possible to give some definitions of terms as commonly used today [1]:

Anaesthesia is a state of unconsciousness produced by a process of controlled, reversible drug-induced intoxication of the central nervous system in which the patient neither perceives nor recalls noxious stimuli.

This definition is entirely consistent with the original concept of anaesthesia and is in accord with our present-day usage of the word. From this it follows that anaesthesia is an all-or-none state and there cannot be degrees of anaesthesia nor variable depths of anaesthesia. All the other attributes of drugs which produce the state of anaesthesia should be classed as alternative pharmacological properties of the drugs and not as *components* of anaesthesia.

Hypnosis is synonymous with anaesthesia as it implies drug-induced sleep. The philosophical question which arises from this is whether it is possible to distinguish between hypnosis and amnesia as components of anaesthesia since human patients who were apparently in a state of anaesthesia have been made to recall when hypnotized [2, 3]. Recall may thus imply failure to anaesthetize [4]. Confusion has arisen unnecessarily because hypnosis was proposed as a component of anaesthesia [5] together with analgesia and muscle relaxation.

Analgesia implies diminished or abolished perception of pain in an otherwise conscious subject. Given in a sufficient dose, opioid analgesics can produce a state indistinguishable from that induced by intravenous or inhalation anaesthetics but unlike the latter agents anaesthesia can only be produced by doses of opioids which cause total suppression of central respiratory drive (although combinations of opioids

3

with other drugs can produce a state of anaesthesia without this complication). There are several ways of achieving a state of anaesthesia regardless of whether the ultimate mechanism is unitary or non-unitary but there is no need to confuse pharmacological effects with the state of anaesthesia and as yet this 'anaesthetic' state produced by opioids cannot be linked to specific analgesic properties mediated at specific opioid receptors [6].

Muscle relaxation was, before the advent of neuromuscular blocking drugs, commonly achieved by increasing the inhaled concentration of volatile anaesthetics or giving more of the intravenous agents. It was, therefore, not unreasonable at that time to regard this dose-dependent pharmacological effect of the drugs which produced anaesthesia as a component of anaesthesia [1]. However, muscle relaxation induced by neuromuscular blocking drugs *cannot* be regarded as a component of the state of anaesthesia. Muscle relaxation, however achieved, is often necessary to satisfy the requirements of the surgeon for surgical access but it is not an alternative to inadequate anaesthesia.

The anaesthetist aims to prevent awareness of pain, provide immobility and, whenever this is needed, relaxation of the skeletal muscles. These aims must be achieved in such a way that the safety of the patient is not jeopardized during the perianaesthetic period.

Many animals fear and resist the restraint necessary for the administration of anaesthetics thereby increasing not only the technical difficulties of administration but also the dangers inseparable from their use. A fully conscious animal forced to breathe a strange and possibly pungent vapour struggles to escape and the sympathoadrenal stimulation produced greatly increases the risks associated with the induction of anaesthesia. For this reason, veterinary anaesthetists often employ sedative drugs to facilitate the completion of general anaesthesia as well as to overcome the natural fear of restraint inherent in animals and control any tendency to move suddenly during operations under local analgesia. In addition, the anaesthetist must recognize that not only does the response of each species of animal to the various anaesthetics differ due to anatomical and physiological differences, but that there is often a marked variation in response between breeds within each particular species. Another factor which must be considered is that many veterinarians have to carry out tasks without highly skilled assistance and, when employing general anaesthesia, after inducing it themselves, have to depute its maintenance to a nurse or even a lay attendant. For all these reasons the continued development in recent years of safe, simple, easily applied techniques of general anaesthesia and regional analgesia is particularly welcome.

TYPES OF ANAESTHESIA

Broadly speaking, two distinct types of substances are used in anaesthesia. The first have selective, transient paralytic actions on sensory nerves and nerve endings. They are applied in aqueous or oily solution by topical application to mucous or abraded surfaces; by intradermal, subdermal or submucous infiltration; and by peripheral, paravertebral or spinal perineural injection. The anaesthesia, or analgesia as it is better described (for unconsciousness is not featured), is classified as local or regional. In veterinary practice, lignocaine hydrochloride is probably the drug most often used for these purposes.

The second type of substance has a depressant, and ultimately paralytic, action on the central nervous system, producing progressive loss of consciousness and voluntary motor function. In the main these substances fall into two distinct groups: volatile or gaseous agents, typified by enflurane, halothane, isoflurane and nitrous oxide, which are given by inhalation; and non-volatile agents such as propofol, etomidate, metomidate and the barbiturates, which are usually administered by intravenous injection.

Thus, the subdivisions of the subject of anaesthesia are:

1. *Local analgesia*
   (a) by surface application
   (b) by intra- and subdermal infiltration
   (c) field analgesia: the blocking of an area by linear infiltration of its margins
2. *Regional analgesia*
   (a) by perineural injection
   (b) spinal block
      (i) by epidural injection
      (ii) by intrathecal injection
3. *Sedation*
   (a) in combination with local analgesia
   (b) as an adjunct to general anaesthesia
4. *General anaesthesia*
   (a) by inhalation
   (b) by the intravenous administration of non-volatile or non-gaseous anaesthetics (some may be given by intraperitoneal, intramuscular or other routes)
   (c) by a combination of the above two with or without premedication.

ANAESTHETIC RISK

Anaesthesia is not a naturally occurring state and its induction with drugs which are never completely devoid of toxicity must constitute a threat to the life of the patient. This can be a major or trivial threat depending on the circumstances, but no owner must ever be told that anaesthesia does not constitute such a risk. When the owner raises the question of the risk involved the veterinarian, before replying, needs to consider:

1. *The state of health of the animal.* Animals presented for anaesthesia may be fit and healthy or suffering from disease; they may be presented for 'cold' surgery or as emergency cases needing immediate attention for obstetrical crises, intractable haemorrhage or thoracic injuries. In the USA the American Society of Anesthesiologists has adopted a classification of physical status into categories, an 'E' being added after the number when the case is an emergency:
   Category 1 — normal healthy patient with no detectable disease.
   Category 2 — slight or moderate systemic disease causing no obvious incapacity.
   Category 3 — slight to moderate systemic disease causing mild symptoms (e.g. moderate pyrexia, anaemia or hypovolaemia).
   Category 4 — extreme systemic disease constituting a threat to life (e.g. toxaemia, uraemia, severe hypovolaemia, cardiac failure).

   Category 5 — moribund or dying patients.
   This is a useful classification but it is most important to appreciate that it refers only to the physical status of the patient and is *not necessarily a classification of risk* because additional factors such as its species, breed and temperament contribute to the risk involved for any particular animal.
2. *The influence of the surgeon.* Inexperienced surgeons may take much longer to perform an operation and by rough technique produce intense and extensive trauma to tissues thereby causing a greater metabolic disturbance. Increased danger can also arise when the surgeon is working in the mouth or pharynx in such a way as to make the maintenance of a clear airway difficult, or is working on structures such as the eye or larynx and provoking autonomic reflexes.
3. *The influence of available facilities.* Crises rising during anaesthesia are usually more easily overcome in a well-equipped veterinary hospital than under the primitive conditions which may be encountered on farms.
4. *The influence of the anaesthetist.* The competence, experience and judgement of the anaesthetist have a profound bearing on the degree of risk to which the patient is exposed. Familiarity with anaesthetic techniques leads to greater efficiency and the art of anaesthetic administration is developed only with experience.

GENERAL CONSIDERATIONS IN THE SELECTION OF THE ANAESTHETIC METHOD

The first consideration will be the nature of the operation to be performed; its magnitude, site and duration. In general the use of local infiltration analgesia will suffice for simple operations such as the incision of superficial abscesses, the excision of small neoplasms and the castration of immature animals. Nevertheless, what seems to be a simple interference may have special anaesthetic requirements. The equine capped elbow is an example, for with this lesion the degree of subdermal fibrosis is often such as to make local infiltration impossible to effect. Again, the site of operation, consequent on the complexity of the structures in its vicinity, may render operation under local analgesia dangerous because of possible movement by the conscious animal, e.g. operations in the vicinity of the eyes.

When adopting general anaesthesia the likely duration of the procedure to be carried out will influence the selection of the anaesthetic. Minor, short procedures may be performed quite satisfactorily after the intravenous injection of a small dose of an agent such as propofol or thiopentone sodium. For longer operations a longer-acting agent supplemented by local analgesia may be chosen, or it may be decided to induce general anaesthesia with an ultrashort-acting agent and maintain it with an inhalation anaesthetic with or without tracheal intubation. For most major operations under general anaesthesia, preanaesthetic medication ('premedication') will need to be considered, particularly when they are of long duration and the animal must remain quiet for several hours after the procedure. Undesirable effects of certain anaesthetics such as the provocation of salivation may also be controlled by suitable premedication. Although sedative premedication may significantly reduce the amount of general anaesthetic required it may also increase the duration of recovery from anaesthesia. Premedication may be omitted for outpatients when a rapid return to full awareness is desirable.

The species of animal involved is, of course, a pre-eminent consideration in the selection of the anaesthetic method. The anaesthetist will be influenced not only by size and temperament but also by any anatomical and physiological features peculiar to a particular species or breed. In general it may be taken that the larger an animal is, the greater are the difficulties and dangers associated with the induction and continuation of general anaesthesia. Methods which are safe and satisfactory for the dog and cat may be quite unsuitable for the horse or the ox. In heavy and vigorous creatures like horses the mere upset of locomotor coordination may entail risks, as also may prolonged recumbency.

The horse

In horses, the need for adequate restraint, even for quite simple operations, may necessitate recumbency of the animal to ensure the safety of the surgeon and of the patient. The old-fashioned process of casting the fully conscious animal with ropes and tackle is not only frightening to the animal but exposes it to injury unless the assistance of an experienced casting team is available. Such assistance is most unlikely to be generally available today but, by way of compensation, we now have very effentive sedatives available to facilitate horse management. It was sometimes claimed that the use of muscle-paralysing drugs as the means of casting the conscious animal entailed less risk, was more convenient and no more distressing to the animal than forcible casting with ropes and tackle. However, most veterinarians (including the authors) reject this view and consider that the use of muscle-paralysing drugs for this purpose is both more dangerous for the animal and inhumane. The recent introduction of drugs which induce very transient periods of unconsciousness enable this problem to be resolved in a way which cannot be challenged on either of these grounds. The facility with which certain of the peripheral sensory nerves can be 'blocked' in horses should always be borne in mind.

An important consideration when selecting a general anaesthetic for the horse, particularly when it is proposed to use one of the intravenous agents to be administered in the standing position, is that induction shall be unassociated with excitement. Moreover, when using agents from which recovery is relatively slow it is important that this period too shall be free from excitement and that the horse shall be able to rise to its feet relatively soon after the completion of the operation. When it does so, locomotor power and coordination must have been regained to a degree whereby the animal is able to retain the standing position without floundering or falling. These

requirements preclude the use of some intravenous anaesthetics and sedatives.

Cattle, sheep and goats

Cattle, sheep and goats are unsuitable subjects for inhalation anaesthesia unless endotracheal intubation is practised. For work in the field, general anaesthesia by intravenous injection without abolition of the swallowing and belching reflexes gives satisfactory results, especially if combined with some form of local analgesia. It is in these animals that regional analgesia has attained its greatest development. For major abdominal operations, paravertebral or lumbar epidural injections are most satisfactory; for obstetrics, caudal epidural block is extensively employed; for dehorning, perineural block is suitable; for surgery on digits, intravenous regional analgesia (IVRA) can be ideal.

Pigs

The continuous squealing and struggling provoked by restraint makes most veterinarians disposed to adopt general anaesthesia for all but the most rapidly performed operations. Fortunately the pig is a good subject for general anaesthesia provided its airway can be kept patent by maintaining its head normally flexed on the neck with the lower jaw pushed forward. Where this is not possible endotracheal intubation is mandatory and the pig is probably the most difficult of the domestic animals to intubate. In the little pig most operations can be satisfactorily carried out under heavy sedation combined with local infiltration analgesia and some of the recently introduced sedative drugs now enable this to be done with the minimum of trouble.

Dogs

In dogs anaesthetic methods have now attained a degree of perfection so that general anaesthesia is used not only for practically all surgical operations but in many instances for examination procedures also. It must be borne in mind that breeds having a markedly brachycephalic type of skull with depression of the nasal bones — the bulldog, the Pekingese, etc. — are bad subjects for general anaesthesia without endotracheal intubation because relaxation of the jaw muscles may cause obstruction of the airway and particular care will always be required when using agents which give rise to a slow recovery from anaesthesia. Some of the more recently introduced sedative and opioid drugs can be combined to produce profound sedation and in a busy practice there is the temptation to use them to control dogs undergoing procedures such as radiography when a veterinarian is not present. While this may be safe in healthy, fit young animals, older dogs with cardio-pulmonary disorders are likely to be far safer when general anaesthesia with a guaranteed clear airway and oxygen administration is employed.

Cats

The cat is often a difficult subject to anaesthetize quietly and smoothly, for restraint may provoke violent struggling and sometimes frenzy. Cats should always be handled gently, using the minimum of restraint, and when this is done the most satisfactory method of inducing general anaesthesia is by intravenous injection. For young cats, inhalation anaesthesia without the use of an intravenous induction agent, but with forcible restraint, was often used in the past and although it proved to be quite safe it cannot be denied that it was very distressing for the animal. Today, there are agents which can be given by intramuscular injection to produce a quiet, trouble-free onset of unconsciousness and there is little excuse for subjecting a fully conscious cat to the unpleasant experience of induction with an inhalation anaesthetic.

The variable reaction of the different species of animals, and of individuals, to the various anaesthetic agents will also influence the choice of anaesthetic.

Sometimes the barbiturates, when used in subanaesthetic doses in an attempt to sedate horses, provoke marked excitement, whilst a cat under the influence of large doses of opioids may become maniacal if stimulated. Factors causing increased susceptibility to the toxic actions of anaesthetic agents must also be borne in mind. These include:

1. *Prolonged fasting.* This, by depleting the glycogen reserves of the liver, greatly reduces its detoxicating power and, when using parenterally administered agents in computed doses, allowance must be made for an increased susceptibility to them.
2. *Diseased conditions.* Toxaemia causes degenerative changes in parenchymatous organs, particularly the liver and heart, and great care must be taken in giving computed doses of agents to toxaemic subjects. Quite often it is found that a toxaemic animal requires very much less than the 'normal' dose. Toxaemia may also be associated with a slowing of the circulation and unless this is recognized it may lead to gross overdosing of intravenous anaesthetics. In those diseases associated with wasting there is often tachycardia and a soft, friable myocardium; animals suffering from such diseases are, in consequence, liable to develop cardiac failure when subjected to the stress of anaesthesia. It is most important that the presence of a diseased condition is detected before anaesthesia is induced.

EXAMINATION OF THE PATIENT BEFORE ANAESTHESIA

It is probable that most veterinary operations are performed on normal, healthy animals. The subjects are generally young and represent good 'anaesthetic risks'. Nevertheless, enquiry should be made to ensure that they are normal — bright, vigorous and of hearty appetite. Should there be any doubt, operation is best delayed until there is assurance on this point. Many a reputation has been damaged by performing operations such as castration or spaying on young animals which are in the early stages of some acute infectious disease.

When an operation is to be performed for the relief of disease, considerable care must be exercised in assessing the factors which may influence the choice or course of the anaesthetic. Once these are recognized the appropriate type of anaesthesia can be chosen and other measures enforced preoperatively and postoperatively to diminish or, where possible, prevent complications. The commonest conditions affecting the course of anaesthesia are those involving the cardiovascular and respiratory systems, but the state of the liver and kidneys cannot be ignored.

History

The owner or attendant should always be asked whether the animal has a cough. A soft, moist cough is associated with the presence of airway secretions and these may give rise to respiratory obstruction and lung collapse when the cough reflex is suppressed by anaesthesia. Severe cardiovascular disease may be totally asymptomatic and the object of taking the history is to gauge the level of functional incapacity and to indicate the underlying pathophysiology. Enquiry should be made to determine whether the animal suffers from undue breathlessness (respiratory distress) after exertion, or indeed appears unwilling to take exercise, since these signs may precede other signs of cardiac and respiratory failure by many months or even years. Dyspnoea on exercise is generally the first sign of left ventricular failure.

A history of excessive thirst may indicate the existence of advanced renal disease, diabetes mellitus or diabetes insipidus.

Examination

The actual examination may be restricted to one which is informative yet will not consume too much time nor unduly disturb the animal. While a more complete examination may sometimes be necessary, attention should always be paid to the pulse, the position of the apex beat, the presence of cardiac thrills, the heart sounds, the jugular venous pressure and any signs arising from the respiratory system. Examination of urine for the presence of albumin and reducing substances is also valuable.

Tachycardia is to be expected in all febrile and in many wasting diseases and under these circumstances is indicative of some degree of myocardial weakness. It can, however, also be due to nervousness and where this is so it is often associated with rather cold ears and/or feet. Bradycardia may be physiological or it may indicate complete atrioventricular block. In horses, atrioventricular block that disappears with exercise is probably of no significance. Careful inspection of the external jugular vein is a most helpful guide towards making the diagnosis. If the head is lowered to a position where jugular vein pulsation can be seen, it will be observed that, whilst with physiological bradycardia the usual three waves appear in a regular sequence (Fig. 1.1), in cases of complete atrioventricular block two kinds of waves occur. The first is the largest and obvious pulsation caused by:

1. The distension of the atrioventricular valves as they close producing a shock wave back in the jugular veins
2. The pulse in the underlying carotid artery

The second kind of wave occurs at a regular but different rhythm and is due to contractions of the

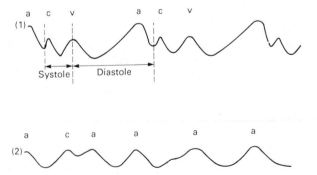

Fig. 1.1 Pressure tracings of (1) the normal jugular venous pulse and (2) of the jugular pulse in a horse suffering from complete atrioventricular block: a = atrial contraction preceding the carotid pulse, v = rise in atrial pressure due to continuous venous filling whilst the tricuspid valve is closed, c = inconstant wave due to arterial pulsation and/or deformation of the atrium with bulging of the tricuspid valve during early systole.

atria. In small animal patients, or where the jugular vein pulsation cannot be seen, an electrocardiogram may be the only way of determining whether bradycardia is physiological or is due to heart block. The jugular venous pressure is also important. When the animal is standing and the head is held up so that the neck is at an angle of about 45° to the horizontal, distension of the jugular veins should, in normal animals, be just visible at the base of the neck. When the venous distension rises above this level, even in the absence of other signs, it indicates an obstruction to the anterior vena cava or a rise in the right atrial or ventricular pressures. The commonest cause of a rise in pressure in these two chambers of the heart is probably right ventricular hypertrophy associated with chronic lung disease although congenital conditions such as atrial septal defects may also be indicated by this sign and it should be remembered that cattle suffering from constrictive pericarditis, or bacterial endocarditis, may have a marked increase in venous pressure.

The presence of a thrill over the region of the heart is always a sign of cardiovascular disease and suggests an increased risk of complications arising during anaesthesia. More detailed cardiological examination is warranted when a cardiac thrill is detected during the preoperative examination.

Auscultation of the heart should never be omitted but the findings are perhaps of only limited interest to the anaesthetist. The timing of any murmurs should be ascertained by palpation of the pulse while listening to the murmur. Diastolic murmurs are always indicative of heart disease and, while they may be of little importance in relation to cardiac function during anaesthesia, it is unwise to come to this conclusion unless other signs, such as displacement of the apex beat, are absent. Systolic murmurs may or may not indicate the presence of heart disease, but if other signs are absent they are probably of no significance.

Accurate location of the apex beat is possibly the most important single observation in assessing the state of the cardiovascular and respiratory systems. It is displaced in most abnormal conditions affecting the lungs (e.g. pleural effusion, pneumothorax, lung collapse) and in the presence of enlargement of the left ventricle. In the absence of any pulmonary disorder a displaced apex beat indicates cardiac hypertrophy or dilatation.

Oedema in cardiac failure has multiple causes which are not fully understood but include a failing right ventricle and an impaired renal blood flow that gives rise to secondary aldosteronism and excessive reabsorption of salt and water by the renal tubules. The tissue fluid appears to accumulate in different regions in different species — in horses in the limbs and along the ventral body surface, in cattle it is seen in the brisket region and in dogs and cats the fluid tends to accumulate in the abdominal cavity. The differential diagnosis of peripheral oedema includes renal disease, liver disease and impaired lymphatic drainage.

Pulmonary disorders provide particular hazards for an animal undergoing operation or anaesthesia and any examination, no matter how brief, must be designed to disclose their presence or absence. On auscultation, attention should be directed towards the length of the expiratory sounds and the discovery of any rhonchi or crepitations. If rhonchi or crepitations are heard, excessive sputum is present, and the animal is either suffering from, or has recently suffered, a pulmonary infection. Prolongation of the expiratory sounds, especially when accompanied by high-pitched rhonchi, indicates the existence of narrowed airways or bronchospasm. Respiratory sounds may be absent in animals with pneumothorax, extensive lung consolidation, or severe emphysema; they are usually faint in moribund animals. Uneven movement between the two sides of the chest is a reliable sign of pulmonary disease and one which is easily and quickly observed. The animal should be positioned squarely while the examiner stands first directly in front of it and then directly behind it. In small animals uneven movement of the two sides of the chest is often better appreciated by palpation rather than by inspection.

The mouth should be examined for evidence of anaemia denoted by paleness of the mucous membranes, and the presence of loose teeth which might become dislodged during anaesthesia and inhaled into the tracheobronchial tree.

Urine testing is particularly important in dogs, for in these animals renal disease is common. In dogs suffering from chronic nephritis, curtailment of water intake associated with general anaesthesia and operation may provoke a uraemic crisis. Urine testing may also uncover previously undiagnosed diabetes mellitus.

Haematological examinations and scanning of biochemical data may be of value in some cases but their routine use is debatable, for in the vast majority of cases they constitute an unnecessary expense.

Provided a brief examination such as that described is carried out thoroughly, and that the examiner has sufficient skill to realize the significance or lack of significance of the findings, most of the conditions which have a bearing on the well-being of an animal during and after anaesthesia will be brought to light so that appropriate measures can be taken to protect it from harm.

SIGNIFICANCE OF CONDITIONS FOUND BY PREANAESTHETIC EXAMINATION

During the course of even a brief examination the examiner will form some opinion of the animal's temperament. Animals which are unduly nervous or aggressive need special care in the immediate preoperative period and many of them may be difficult to handle or nurse postoperatively. The appropriate choice of sedative and analgesic medication can do much to facilitate the handling of such subjects. An impression of the 'real' age of an animal as opposed to its chronological age will also have been gained. This is most valuable for the young animal which looks, for example, several years older than its chronological age is liable under stress to behave as an older animal might be expected to.

Heart disease

A knowledge of the exact nature of the cardiac lesion is less important in anaesthesia than a knowledge of the effective function of the heart. A broad division into congenital and acquired heart disease is, however, of some value. In animals, acquired disease is more commonly encountered than is congenital disease, for animals suffering from congenital disease usually die or are killed in early life. Acquired disease is of more serious import since, unlike congenital disease, it tends to affect both the myocardium and the valves so that even in its earliest stages the heart muscle is weakened. Fitness for anaesthesia must be assessed from a knowledge of what the heart can do both at rest and at exercise set against such factors as the importance and urgency of operation coupled with experience of how animals similarly affected have behaved in like circumstances. It is rarely possible to state that an animal will not tolerate anaesthesia because of heart disease. Of course, major operations on large animals suffering from heart disease can seldom be justified on economic grounds, but in small animal practice such considerations may not apply. Provided that the anaesthetist is aware of the existence of a heart lesion and exercises care in the administration of the anaesthetic, these small animal patients will usually tolerate anaesthesia and the operation well.

A feature of complete atrioventricular block is the occurrence of syncope due to ventricular asystole, the so-called 'Stokes-Adams attack'. In these attacks the animal loses consciousness, lies limp, still and pulseless, with fixed dilated pupils; breathing, however, continues. As a rule, ventricular contractions are resumed and recovery occurs quite spontaneously, but sometimes ventricular fibrillation supervenes.

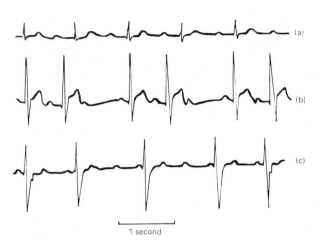

Fig. 1.2 Electrocardiogram (ECG) tracings from dogs showing first-degree heart block (a), second-degree block (b) and complete block (c). In (a) there is an increased P-R interval, in (b) some impulses are transmitted whilst others are not and in (c) none of the P waves are transmitted to the ventricles. If the P-R interval lengthens progressively until a P wave occurs without a QRS complex this is known as a Mobitz type-I block and is benign. Sudden failure of atrioventricular conduction without previous lengthening of the P-R interval is known as a Mobitz type-II block; this has a very different connotation because sudden asystole is a very real hazard and the majority of cases have widespread fibrosis of the conducting tissues.

Episodes may occur under anaesthesia and may not be noticed unless an electrocardiogram is being recorded or a very careful watch is being kept on the pulse. Sudden asystole is also a feature of aortic stenosis and in this condition it may occur at any time, even when the animal is apparently at rest. It is uncertain whether such animals are more liable to sudden death when under anaesthesia than they are at any other time, but many have survived carefully administered anaesthetics without incident. In these cases survival depends on the force of ventricular contraction and agents such as thiopentone sodium, which is known to decrease this, must be used with caution. Physiological bradycardia is associated with a marked ability to increase the cardiac output to meet extra demands but, except in horses, where it is physiological at rest, the presence of heart block implies an inability to produce more than a fractional increase in output. Thus, whereas animals with physiological bradycardia are well able to withstand the stresses of anaesthesia, animals (other than horses) with heart block are liable to develop circulatory failure when exposed to such strains as the vasodilatation induced by anaesthetic agents and hypovolaemia due to haemorrhage. Except in emergencies drugs have no place in the modern management of bradyarrhythmias.

Other important, common causes of fixed low cardiac output are constrictive pericarditis and mitral stenosis.

Respiratory disease

Hypoxaemia results from many pulmonary conditions. Horses afflicted with the syndrome which is commonly referred to as 'broken wind' where there is marked hypoxaemia, hypercapnia and polycythaemia and other animals suffering from conditions such as chronic bronchiolitis, asthma and alveolar emphysema may be difficult to keep well oxygenated during anaesthesia unless high concentrations of oxygen are administered. Pneumonitis, or lung collapse such as may occur with space-occupying lesions of the thorax or ruptures of the diaphragm, disturbs the ventilation–perfusion relationships within the lungs, and alveoli which are perfused with blood but not ventilated act as venous-arterial shunts. Significant desaturation of the arterial blood can result from this, even if cyanosis is not readily apparent.

Anaemia

All the various conditions of the heart and lungs which have been mentioned, and one other factor — the haemoglobin content of the blood — clearly affect the rate at which oxygen can be made available to the tissues of the body. Nunn and Freeman [7] drew attention to the fact that this rate is equal to the product of the cardiac output and the oxygen content of the arterial blood. Since the arterial oxygen content approximates to the product of the oxygen saturation and the quantity of oxygen which can be carried by the haemoglobin (about 1.36 ml/g of haemoglobin), the oxygen made available to the body can be expressed by a simple equation:

Available oxygen (ml/min) =
Cardiac output (ml/min) × Arterial saturation (%) ×
Haemoglobin (g/ml) × 1.36

This equation, of course, makes no allowance for the small quantity of oxygen which is carried in physical solution in the plasma, but it serves to illustrate the way in which the three variables combine to produce an effect which is often greater than is commonly supposed.

If any one of the three determining variables on the right-hand side of the equation is changed, the rate at which oxygen is made available to the tissues of the body is altered proportionately. Thus, if the cardiac output is halved, the available oxygen is also halved. If two determinants are lowered simultaneously while the third remains constant, the effect of the available oxygen is the product of the individual changes. For example, if the cardiac output and the haemoglobin concentration are both halved while the arterial oxygen saturation remains at about the normal 95%, only one-quarter of the normal amount of oxygen is made available to the body tissues. If all three variables are reduced the effect is, of course, even more dramatic.

The full significance of these facts can, perhaps, be best illustrated by considering a hypothetical case. If a 500 kg horse has a cardiac output of 30 l/min, a haemoglobin level of 15 g/dl of blood, and the arterial blood is 95% saturated, then the oxygen made available to the tissues of the animal is equal to

$$30\,000 \times \frac{95}{100} \times \frac{15}{100} \times 1.36 \text{ ml/min}$$

i.e. approximately 5700 ml/min. Thus, the oxygen made available to the horse would be adequate for its needs, since at rest its oxygen consumption is of the order of 1400 ml/min, corresponding to an arterio-venous oxygen difference of 5 ml/dl of blood, and a mixed venous blood saturation of about 75%. (Because different organs extract widely differing amounts of oxygen from the blood, a mixed venous saturation of about 20% is the minimum that can be tolerated by the body: some organs and especially the heart already extract most of the oxygen from their arterial supply.)

If this hypothetical horse is now assumed to become anaemic so that its haemoglobin concentration falls by one-third to 10 g/dl of blood, and is anaesthetized by an agent which reduces the cardiac output by one-third to 20 l/min, and the arterial oxygen saturation decreases to 64%, then the oxygen made available to the tissue equals

$$20\,000 \times \frac{64}{100} \times \frac{10}{100} \times 1.36 \text{ ml/min}$$

i.e. approximately 1700 ml/min. Since the oxygen consumption is unchanged, making oxygen available at this rate would lead to the haemoglobin in the mixed venous blood being almost completely desaturated — a condition which is incompatible with life. It is important to note that none of the values substituted on the right-hand side of the equation would, individually, cause alarm. A reduction of one-third in the cardiac output is often encountered in anaesthesia, oxygen saturation of 64% may occur without obvious cyanosis and haemoglobin levels of 10 g/dl are commonplace. Nevertheless, these three apparently mild departures from normal can, in combination, be lethal.

In most cases, especially when it is limited by disease, little can be done to increase the cardiac output, and this is the factor which determines the lowest permissible levels of the other two variables. The haemoglobin level, however, is capable of being raised and in a critical situation every effort must be made to do this. The concentration is often low preoperatively and may be further reduced by transfusion of plasma or plasma volume expanders. Pulmonary conditions which are likely to interfere with blood oxygenation should, if possible, be treated before anaesthesia to reduce the severity of their effect. When this cannot be done the administration of high concentrations of oxygen during anaesthesia may be life saving.

Hypoproteinaemia

Most drugs are carried in the bloodstream partly bound, usually by electrostatic bonds, to the proteins of the plasma, albumin being by far the most important for the majority of agents. Light or moderate protein binding has relatively little effect on drug pharmacokinetics and pharmacodynamics. Heavy protein binding with drugs such as thiopentone results in a low free-plasma concentration of the drug which may become progressively augmented as the available binding sites become saturated. The bound drug is, of course, in dynamic equilibrium with free (active) drug in the plasma water.

Anaemia is often associated with hypoproteinaemia and this can have marked effects in anaesthesia. In conditions where there is anaemia and hypoalbuminaemia, a greater fraction of a given dose of a drug will be unbound and this will be even greater if other bound drugs have already occupied many of the binding sites. This can result in an increased peak activity of the drug. Liver disease giving rise to hypoalbuminaemia can result in reduced binding of drugs such as morphine so that smaller than normal doses of this analgesic will be effective when pain relief is needed. A rapid intravenous injection of an albumin-bound drug may also lead to increased pharmacological activity because the binding capacity of the albumin in the limited volume of blood with which the drug initially mixes is exceeded and more free (active) drug is presented to the receptor sites. Plasma protein binding enhances alimentary absorption of drugs by lowering the free plasma concentration and thereby increasing the concentration gradient for diffusion from the gut lumen.

An apparent exception to the increased activity of drugs in hypoproteinaemic animals is the resistance to tubocurarine seen in cases of liver disease. This is explained by the fact that tubocurarine binds to γ-globulin rather than albumin [8]); dose requirements are related to globulin and reversed albumin/globulin ratios are common in hepatic diseases [9, 10].

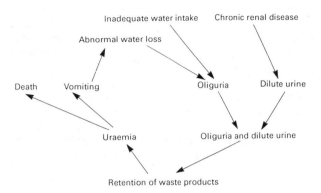

Fig. 1.3 Illustration of how curtailment of water intake may give rise to uraemia in dogs suffering from chronic nephritis.

Renal disease

Chronic renal disease is common in dogs, and affected animals cannot produce concentrated urine. Dehydration from any cause deprives the kidneys of sufficient water for excretory purposes, so that urea and other waste products are retained, giving rise to uraemia. Curtailment of water intake for a day when a general anaesthetic is administered may easily be responsible for uraemia in dogs suffering from chronic nephritis. Uraemia precipitates a vicious circle as it causes malaise and vomiting which not only themselves limit the water intake, but also produce further water depletion (Fig. 1.3). To guarantee that these animals receive an adequate fluid intake it may be necessary

to administer fluid by intravenous infusion if the length of anaesthesia and/or the recovery period is prolonged. A uraemic circle can also be set up in animals suffering from chronic renal disease if the arterial blood pressure falls as a result of anaesthetic overdose or haemorrhage and renal ischaemia ensues (Fig. 1.4). The replacement of blood as it is shed is very important in these animals.

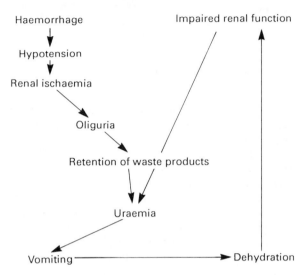

Fig. 1.4 Illustration of the development of uraemia when an animal suffering from chronic nephritis is subjected to haemorrhage.

PREPARATION OF THE PATIENT

Certain operations are performed in emergency when it is imperative that there shall be no delay, and little preparation of the patient is possible. Among these operations are those for repair of thoracic injuries, the control of severe, persistent haemorrhage, and certain obstetrical interferences where the delivery of a live baby animal is of paramount importance. For all other operations, time and care spent in pre-operative preparation are well worthwhile since proper preparation not only improves the patient's chances of survival, but also prevents the complications which might otherwise occur during and after operation. When operations are to be performed on normal, healthy animals, only the minimum of preparation is required before the administration of a general anaesthetic, but operations on dehydrated, anaemic, hypovolaemic or toxic patients should only be undertaken after careful preparation.

Food and water

Food should be withheld from the animal on the day it is to undergo an elective operation under general

anaesthesia. A distended stomach may interfere with the free movement of the diaphragm and hinder breathing. In dogs, cats and pigs, a full stomach predisposes to vomiting under anaesthesia and exposes the animal to the danger of inhaling vomitus. A full or distended stomach may rupture when a horse is forcibly cast or falls to the ground as unconsciousness is induced. In ruminants, a few hours of starvation will not result in any appreciable reduction in the volume of the fluid content of the rumen, but it seems to reduce the rate of fermentation within this organ, thus delaying the development of tympany when eructation is suppressed by general anaesthesia. Excessive fasting exposes the patient to risks almost as great as those associated with lack of preparation and should not be adopted. Any fasting of birds and many small mammals is actually life threatening. Many clinicians are of the opinion that prolonged fasting in horses predisposes to postanaesthetic colic by encouraging gut stasis. In non-ruminants, free access to water should be allowed right up to the time when premedication is given, but in ruminants there is some advantage in withholding water for about

6 hours before abdominal operations because this appears to result in a slowing of fermentation in the rumen.

Fluid and electrolytes

The water and electrolyte balance of an animal is a most important factor in determining the uncomplicated recovery or otherwise after operation. The repair of existing deficits of body fluid, or of one or more of its components, is complex because of the inter-relations between the different electrolytes, and the difficulties imposed by the effects of severe sodium depletion on the circulation and renal function. Fortunately, the majority of animal patients suffer only minor and recent upsets of fluid balance so that treatment by intravenous infusion with isotonic saline, Hartmann's solution or 5% dextrose, depending on whether sodium depletion or water depletion is the more predominant, is all that is required. An anaesthetic should not be administered to an animal which has a decreased circulating blood volume, for the vasodilatation caused by anaesthetic agents may lead to acute circulatory failure, and every effort should be made to repair this deficit by the infusion of blood, plasma or plasma volume expander before anaesthesia is induced. In many instances, anaesthesia and operation may be safely postponed until the total fluid deficit is made good and an adequate renal output is achieved but, in cases of intestinal obstruction, operation should be carried out as soon as the blood volume has been restored. Attempts to restore all the extracellular deficit before the intestinal obstruction is relieved result in further loss of fluid into the lumen of the obstructed bowel and make subsequent operation more difficult, especially in horses. When in doubt about the nature and volume of fluid to be administered, it is as well to remember that, with the exception of toxaemic conditions and where severe hypotension due to hypovolaemia is present, an animal's condition should not deteriorate further if sufficient fluid is being given to cover current losses. These current losses include the inevitable loss of water through the skin and respiratory tract (approximately 20–60 ml/kg/day depending on age and species of animal), the urinary and faecal loss, and any abnormal loss such as vomit.

Haemoglobin level

As already mentioned on p. 10 anaemia may be treated to raise the haemoglobin concentration to more reasonable levels before any major premeditated surgery is performed. When operation can be delayed for 2 or more weeks, the oral or parenteral administration of iron may raise the haemoglobin to a satisfactory concentration, but when such a delay is inadvisable the transfusion of red blood cells is indicated.

Treatment of diabetes mellitus

It is sometimes necessary to anaesthetize a dog or cat suffering from diabetes mellitus and if the condition is already under control no serious problems are likely to be encountered. However, if the normal dose of insulin is given, starvation before surgery and inappetence afterwards may give rise to hypoglycaemia. There are over 30 commercially available preparations of insulin and they have different durations of action. Short-acting insulins (e.g. soluble insulin) have a peak effect at 2–4 hours and their effects last for 8–12 hours. Medium-acting insulins (e.g. semilente) have a peak effect at 6–10 hours and activity for up to 24 hours. Long-acting insulins (e.g. lente, protamine-zinc) have a peak effect at 12–15 hours and one dose lasts for at least 36 hours. For this reason it is advisable to switch to purely short-acting insulin a few days prior to elective surgery. By doing this, there is effectively no active long-acting insulin preparation left on the day of operation and it becomes much easier to control the blood sugar around the perioperative period.

If an emergency operation has to be performed on an uncontrolled diabetic then the condition of the animal requires careful assessment and treatment. Ketonuria is an indication for treatment with glucose and soluble insulin, whilst overbreathing is a sign of severe metabolic acidosis. This must be treated by the infusion of sodium bicarbonate solution but the amount of bicarbonate needed in any particular case can only be calculated when the acid–base status is known from laboratory examination of an anaerobically drawn arterial blood sample. In veterinary general practice, facilities for such examination of arterial blood samples are unusual and metabolic acidosis has to be treated by infusing 2.5% sodium bicarbonate solution until the animal ceases to overbreathe. Because of the presence of an osmotic diuresis, many uncontrolled diabetics also require treatment for dehydration. The object of management is not to try to correct all disturbances as quickly as possible so achieving in an hour or two what normally should take 2–3 days. Doing this can produce swings in serum osmolarity which may be responsible for the development of cerebral oedema. All that is necessary prior to emergency surgery is to correct any hypovolaemia and ensure that the blood glucose level is declining.

INFLUENCE OF PRE-EXISTING DRUG THERAPY

Modern therapeutic agents are often of considerable pharmacological potency and animals presented for anaesthesia may have been exposed to one or more of these. Some may have been given as part of the preoperative management of the animal but whatever the reason for their administration they may modify the animal's response to anaesthetic agents, to surgery and to drugs given during and following operation. In some cases drug interactions are predictable and these may form the basis of many of the combinations used in modern anaesthesia, but effects which are unexpected may be dangerous.

In an ideal situation a drug action would occur only at a desired site to produce the sought-after effect. In practice most drugs are much less selective and are prone to produce 'side-effects' which have to be anticipated and taken into account whenever the drug is administered. (A side-effect may be defined as a response not required clinically, but which occurs when a drug is used within its therapeutic range.) Apart from these unavoidable side-effects which are inherent, adverse reactions to drugs may occur in many different ways which are of importance to the anaesthetist. These include:

1. *Overdosage.* For some drugs exact dosing may be difficult. Overdosage may be absolute, as when an amount greater than the intended dose is given in error, or because the nature of the preparation differs from one manufacturer to another (e.g. thyroxine) in spite of apparently strict pharmaceutical specifications, so that bioavailability is inconstant. Drugs may also be given by an inappropriate route — e.g. a normal intramuscular dose may constitute a gross overdose if given by accidental intravenous injection. Relative overdosage may be due to an abnormality of the animal; for example an abnormal sensitivity to digitalis is found in hypokalaemic animals, and newborn animals are sensitive to non-depolarizing relaxants. The use in dogs and cats of flea collars containing organophosphorus compounds may reduce the plasma cholinesterase to low levels and prolong the action of a normal dose of the relaxant drug suxamethonium.

   Overdose manifestations vary from acute to chronic and may produce toxicity by a quantitatively enhanced action which can be an extension of the therapeutic action, e.g. neostigmine in excess in the antagonism of competitive neuromuscular block resulting in a depolarizing block. They may also be due to side-effects (e.g. morphine producing respiratory depression).

2. *Idiosyncrasy.* Some animals may have a genetically determined response to a drug which is qualitatively different to that of normal individuals, e.g. the porcine hyperpyrexia syndrome ('porcine malignant hyperthermia').

3. *Intolerance.* An intolerant animal exhibits a qualitatively normal response but to an abnormally low or high dose. This is usually simply explained by the Gaussian distribution of variation in response to drugs seen in any animal population. The normal distribution curve includes responses in individuals unusually sensitive to the drug as well as responses in resistant animals.

4. *Allergy.* Allergic responses are, in general, not dose related and the allergy may be due to the drug itself or to one of its metabolites or even the vehicle in which it is presented (e.g. Cremophor in preparations of steroid anaesthetics). Most drugs which produce allergic responses do so because they are small molecules which act as haptens combining with a body protein to form the antigen against which immunological activity is directed and which in turn produces antibodies and/or antigen-reactive T cells. These latter then react with any antigen remaining or subsequently formed (by further administration of the same or related compound) to elicit one of the characteristic allergic responses. The reaction may take a number of forms: anaphylactic shock, asthma or bronchospasm, hepatic congestion from hepatic vein constriction, blood disorders, rashes or pyrexia. Usually there is a history of previous exposure to the drug or to a related compound but there are exceptions to this general rule.

5. *Drug interactions.* Despite the importance of drug interactions there is little information in the veterinary literature on this subject and for this reason only the general principles can be reviewed here. Drug interactions can occur outside the body as when two drugs are mixed in a syringe before they are administered or inside the body after administration by the same or a different route. It is generally unwise to mix products or vehicles in the same syringe or to administer a drug into an intravenous infusion for this may result in the precipitation of one or both drugs or even possibly the formation of new potentially toxic or inactive compounds.

   The result of the interaction between two drugs inside the body may be an increased or decreased action of one or both or even an effect completely different from the normal action of either drug. The result of interaction may be simply the sum of the actions of the two drugs $(1 + 1 = 2)$, or greater $(1 + 1 > 2)$ when it is known as 'synergism'. When one agent has no appreciable effect but exaggerates the response to the other $(0 + 1 > 1)$ the term 'potentiation' is used to describe the action of the first on the effect of the second. An agent may also antagonize the effects of another and the antagonism may be 'chemical' if they form an inactive complex, 'physiological' if they have directly opposing actions though at different sites, or 'competitive' if they compete for the same receptors. Non-competitive antagonism may result from modification by one drug of the transport, biotransformation or excretion of the other. In the liver the non-specific process of oxidation and conjugation are implicated in the metabolic degradation of many drugs and many different agents have the ability to cause an increase in the activity of these systems — 'enzyme induction' — whilst a few decrease the activity — 'enzyme inhibition'. In experimental animals, enzyme induction has been reported to double the size of the liver but this does not seem to have been recorded in clinical cases.

The barbiturates, some other anticonvulsants, chloral hydrate and analgesics such as phenylbutazone cause enzyme induction and can produce a great increase in the rate of metabolism of substrates. For example, barbiturate treatment of epilepsy may almost halve the half-life of dexamethasone with a consequent marked deterioration in the therapeutic effect of this steroidal substance.

Most drugs are carried to their sites of action and elimination by the blood stream and are present in the blood either in simple solution or, as mentioned on p. 11, partly bound to proteins of the erythrocytes or plasma. The degree of binding varies widely with different drugs and the veterinary anaesthetist needs to be aware that competition for binding sites and the displacement of one drug from the bound to the unbound (active) form may lead to increased toxicity. For example, warfarin (which is sometimes used in the management of navicular disease in horses) is displaced by several agents, including the analgesic drug phenylbutazone, with a resulting risk of haemorrhage.

USE AND ABUSE OF DRUGS IN ANAESTHESIA

While the rationale behind the concept of modern anaesthesia is undoubtedly sound, there has been a regrettable tendency towards ever-increasing complexity in the number of drugs given to anaesthetized animals. If potentiation can occur in respect to desirable drug actions it may, as already indicated, also occur in relation to toxic effects. It is, therefore, likely that some of the difficulties encountered in anaesthesia today are produced by the anaesthetist in the sense that they are aggravated, if not caused, by the misuse of sedative, anaesthetic and analgesic drugs and their pharmacological antidotes. In the hands of the inexperienced or careless anaesthetist the apparently rational use of a combination of drugs, each employed for a specific purpose, can easily degenerate into polypharmacy in which the advantages become lost by the development of complications, the origin of which is promptly made more obscure by the administration of antidotes that often introduce further complications. This is not to say, however, that anaesthetists should revert to deep general anaesthesia to produce satisfactory operating conditions, or avoid the use of muscle relaxants, for this would be a very retrograde step, but the number of agents used in any one case should be kept to a minimum. The skilled anaesthetist, keeping to this minimum, using each agent for a specific purpose and bearing in mind the pharmacokinetics of the agents used as well as their principal pharmacological actions, can easily demonstrate that the advantages can outweigh the alleged safety of the old, simple depression techniques.

REFERENCES

1. Prys-Roberts, C. (1987) *British Journal of Anaesthesia* **59**, 1341.
2. Levinson, B. W. (1965) *British Journal of Anaesthesia* **37**, 544.
3. Cherkin, A. and Harroun, P. (1971) *Anesthesiology* **34**, 469.
4. Eich, E., Reeves, J. L. and Katz, R. L. (1985) *Anesthesia and Analgesia* **64**, 1143.
5. Gray, T. C. and Rees, C. J. (1952) *British Medical Journal* **ii**, 891.
6. Dodson, B. A. and Miller, K. W. (1985) *Anesthesiology* **62**, 615.
7. Nunn, J. F. and Freeman, J. (1964) *Anaesthesia* **19**, 120.
8. Stovner, J., Theodorsen, L. and Bjrlke, E. (1971) *British Journal of Anaesthesia* **43**, 385
9. Sherlock, S. (1958) *Diseases of the Liver and Biliary System*, 2nd edn. Oxford: Blackwell Scientific.
10. Ford, E. J. H. and Ritchie, H. E. (1968) *Journal of Comparative Pathology* **78**, 207

CHAPTER 2

PATIENT MONITORING AND CLINICAL MEASUREMENT

From the earliest days of anaesthesia the anaesthetist has monitored the patient's pulse rate, pattern of breathing and general condition. In the last 10 years advances in electronic technology have made reasonably reliable, easily attached, non-invasive monitoring devices available for clinical practice. The impact of electronic surveillance during anaesthesia has been great and there can be no doubt that its application has yielded accurate information relating to hitherto suspected, but unmeasured, physiological disturbances. However, there have been no controlled trials to determine whether such surveillance has produced a significant improvement in anaesthetic-related mortality or morbidity in veterinary patients. It would seem that much of the current enthusiasm for monitoring physiological processes in patients arises from laudable scientific curiosity and from the pressures generated by medicolegal activity — especially in human medicine in the USA — rather than any proven improvement in patient care resulting from its use. It is most important to note that in situations similar to those reported by Kellagher and Watney [1] the monitoring apparatus in use may fail to give warning of impending disaster. Nevertheless, common sense suggests that measurement of certain parameters, particularly if made before, during and after surgery, should provide important data to support the clinical assessment of the animal's condition and improve the chances of survival of the very ill by indicating what treatment is needed, as well as the response to treatment already given. Moreover, many of those who have used patient monitors very extensively have experienced crises in which a monitor has enabled treatment to be made on a rational basis after the crisis has arisen.

It is necessary to know what to measure as well as how to measure it and over the years a wide range of views has been expressed as to the value of monitoring equipment. At the one extreme there are those who hold the view that a finger on the pulse will tell all, while at the opposite extreme Schreiber and Schreiber [2] consider elaborate equipment desirable and attempt to rate the importance of the various devices and indicators available to the anaesthetist. There can be little doubt that to introduce the full panoply of monitoring equipment for short bloodless procedures on healthy animals turns a simple exercise into a needlessly complex one, inundating the anaesthetist with a mass of information, most of which is of little use, when concentration on the maintenance of a clear airway is all that is really needed. This situation would be especially undesirable for the inexperienced trainee. However, for major surgery, especially in valuable horses, and for anaesthesia and surgery of poor-risk patients, it would be difficult to defend the failure to use such apparatus if it were available.

Most measurements relate to the efficiency of the respiratory and cardiovascular systems but, ideally, safety in anaesthesia depends on monitoring the performance of the anaesthetist, the function of the apparatus used for the administration of the anaesthetic, the animal's response to anaesthesia and surgery, and the performance of any monitoring apparatus used. At the present moment, for a variety of reasons, monitoring falls far short of this ideal [3].

MONITORING THE PERFORMANCE OF THE ANAESTHETIST

It is now widely recognized that the most effective monitor is the constant presence of a skilled, attentive anaesthetist. The Harvard group of hospitals in Boston, USA, and the American Society of Anesthesiologists have acknowledged this by according it the first position in their published standards for minimum monitoring [4, 5]. Thus, no matter what else may or may not be monitored it is essential for the anaesthetist to monitor his or her own performance. In medical practice it is commonly believed that the major source of anaesthetic morbidity and mortality is human error. The majority of complications associated with anaesthesia result from inadequate training or experience of the anaesthetist [6–9] while some are caused by tiredness or boredom and others by lack of attention. There is no reason to suppose that similar considerations do not apply in veterinary anaesthesia. Knowledge and experience are a function of the nature of the training received and the years of practice, but proper vigilance at all times can only be generated by self-motivation [3].

Routines should be developed to ensure that each aspect of apparatus function is checked before use. Failure to follow a simple check list in every case is probably the greatest single cause of anaesthetic disasters. Similar check lists ought to be applied to the execution of common procedures such as the setting up of intravenous infusions or endotracheal intubation. The anaesthetist should also follow the animal's progress after operation, for a record of the incidence of postoperative vomiting, coughing, bruising at injection sites and of analgesic requirements provides a good corrective to clumsy, inappropriate practice.

GENERAL CONSIDERATIONS RELATING TO MONITORING

Most devices used for electronic surveillance of the patient have less than optimal reliability because of the problems associated with the patient–transducer interface and poor rejection of artefacts which can confuse the interpretation of their signals. This lack of reliability discourages many anaesthetists from using them and can actually create a hazard for the patient because an anaesthetist trying to ascertain the cause of a monitor failure is likely to be paying less than proper attention to complete patient care. Should equipment develop a fault, it must 'fail safe' and warn the anaesthetist that a problem exists rather than simply cease to function. Too frequent alarms arising from malfunction of the equipment may, however, lead the anaesthetist to presume equipment failure when, for example, it may be correctly indicating that the patient has suffered cardiac arrest. If more than one monitor is in use several alarm messages may be generated at the same time; they can arrive in an unorganized pattern and the condition giving rise to the alarm message is sometimes difficult to locate. The usual reaction of an anaesthetist is to silence the alarm while the source of the indicated adverse condition is sought and there is the danger that the alarm may be inadvertently left in the silenced condition when the problem has been diagnosed and rectified so that should the problem recur later on the device will fail to issue an alarm message.

Proficiency with methods of electronic surveillance must be acquired during minor procedures so that they can be applied properly in circumstances where their use is mandatory (e.g. during induced hypotension or hypothermia). Unfortunately, the greatest factor inhibiting this acquisition of skill is often the time taken to attach sensors or electrodes to an animal. Electrodes designed for use in man may not be suitable for direct application to animals' skin unless the hair is clipped or the area shaved and it is often difficult to explain to an owner the reason for the resulting bald patches when the animal has

undergone only a minor, perhaps non-surgical, procedure. Needle electrodes have become popular in veterinary practice because they are quickly applied after disinfection of the skin and overlying hair but unless disposable after each case they may give rise to problems. The more complex, time-consuming measurements must always be carried out by other personnel if the anaesthetist's attention is not to be seriously distracted from the care of the anaesthetized animal and these helpers also require practice in making the measurements if their observations are to be reliable.

Electrical monitoring apparatus must be well maintained and compatible for use with other electrical equipment, particularly diathermy, which may also be in use during an operation. Whenever electrical apparatus is connected to the patient there is a danger of ventricular fibrillation should any fault allow current to pass through the heart. The current required is around 80 mA if the electrodes are on the skin, but only 150–400 µA where there is an internal electrode in or near the heart. Mains frequencies are more likely to give rise to trouble than currents with higher or lower frequencies. The traditional method of earthing the patient does not necessarily provide for safety because it may allow a fatal current to pass through the patient to earth if the equipment used becomes faulty. In veterinary practice it is unlikely that very expensive integrated monitors will be common and usually there will be several stand-alone monitors each with its own earth; two or more of these earths may be at different potentials, allowing a small current to pass through the patient when the apparatus is switched off. Isolated systems, using isolation transformers, have been introduced in order to provide protection of patients from such electrical hazards. Many monitors require, as a standard practice or by common sense, a battery back-up to overcome a temporary or prolonged failure in the main electricity supply. This introduces the additional problems of the maintenance and replacement of batteries and safeguarding against their unauthorized removal. Intra-arterial and intravenous lines for the measurement of pressures should be filled with 5% dextrose and not saline, for salt solutions are good conductors of electricity. Asepsis is essential when invasive techniques are used and care must be taken to avoid all unnecessary damage to blood vessels.

The times when monitors are used is most important. Current practice is to establish monitoring only after the animal has been anaesthetized and placed on the operating table. The logic of this practice is questionable for many anaesthetic disasters occur during induction or recovery from anaesthesia or when the animal is being moved from one place to another. Monitoring, therefore, needs to be portable and high-risk cases may need to be anaesthetized in the operating theatre after attachment of the monitors.

Used uncritically, monitoring may be at worst a bane and at best a mixed blessing. Appropriate use can be a boon for both the safety and control of anaesthesia and consists of the rational use of devices that, throughout the period of risk, supplement or enhance clinical skills rather than encourage them to wither [10].

CLINICAL ASSESSMENT OF THE PATIENT

The extent to which a patient's condition can be monitored by simple means without electronic surveillance has been set out by Lillehei [11]. The pulse volume reflects cardiac output; urine output parallels visceral perfusion; skin temperature indicates peripheral resistance. If, in addition, central venous pressure is monitored, the adequacy of the circulatory volume can be demonstrated. Pulse volume and skin temperature may be assessed by palpation; measurement of urinary output requires only the timed collection of urine voided or obtained by catheterization of the urinary bladder; measurement of the central venous pressure has been greatly simplified by the introduction of disposable, sterile packs prepared for transfusions. All these procedures can be carried out on the conscious animal prior to anaesthesia; their value during operation and in the immediate postoperative period cannot be overestimated, and all are well within the capability of veterinarians working with the minimum of assistance outside of large hospitals. The direct determination of arterial blood pressure cannot always be carried out on conscious animals but is reasonably easy when they are unconscious or anaesthetized. Indirect measurement, using a cuff

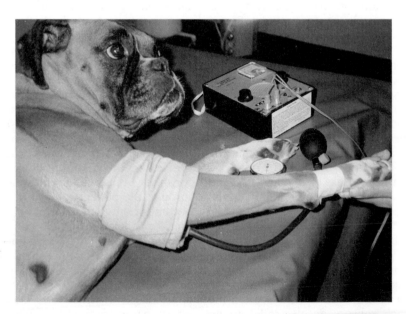

Fig. 2.1 Indirect measurement of the arterial blood pressure in a conscious dog using an inflatable cuff and a flow detector. It is important that the cuff does not slip down the limb as it is inflated, that there is no air gap between the detector and the skin and that the detector is not strapped to the limb so tightly that it occludes the underlying artery. Most animals do not react to inflation of the cuff unless grossly excessive pressures are created by overinflation.

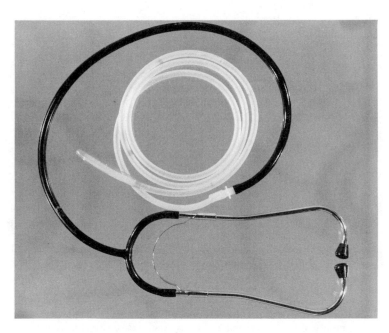

Fig. 2.2 The oesophageal stethoscope. It may be used with a single earpiece or with a conventional stethoscope headpiece. Many claim this to be one of the simplest, most inexpensive yet effective monitoring devices for heart beat and respiratory activity.

and flow detector (Fig. 2.1), is nearly always possible in conscious animals.

The sound from the simple bell stethoscope placed over the region of the apex beat of the heart may be amplified by suitable electronic means to give a signal audible throughout a room, but most useful for monitoring during anaesthesia is the oesophageal stethoscope, where the sounds can be heard only by the anaesthetist. This instrument consists of a blind-ended, plastic or rubber tube with side holes over an area 1–3 cm from the blind end (Fig. 2.2) covered by a thin rubber or plastic sleeve to prevent fluid from entering the tube. The instrument is passed into the oesophagus of the anaesthetized animal until the blind end lies over the heart and the open end is attached either to an ordinary stethoscope headpiece, or to a single earpiece which can be worn continuously by the anaesthetist. Oesophageal stethoscopes suitable for dogs and cats are commercially available and ones for large animals can be constructed from stomach tubes. It might well be claimed that the instrument provides one of the simplest, most inexpensive yet effective monitors of the heart beat and respiration. There are some situations in which it is safer to use an oesophageal stethoscope rather than a vast array of more complicated devices but, unfortunately, the prolonged use of a binaural stethoscope is uncomfortable and repeated use of a monaural moulded earpiece may lead to the anaesthetist developing otitis externa.

The sounds can, of course, also be amplified by electronic means and made generally audible to other personnel by a loudspeaker.

Determination of the central venous pressure can be made quite rapidly (see p. 30), but the circumstances of anaesthesia can profoundly affect it. If it is allowed to rise unduly, the difficulty of certain operations can be greatly increased. It rises in the presence of respiratory obstruction or raised mean intrathoracic pressure, and a close correlation between the central venous pressure and the degree of bleeding at the site of operation is easily demonstrable.

While such observations are simple to make, their interpretation may not be so easy. Palpation of the pulse allows knowledge of its rate, rhythm and volume as well as giving an indication of cardiac output and of the adequacy of the circulation to the region of the body where the pulse is being monitored. Difficulty in feeling the pulse in a major artery suggests severe vasoconstriction and/or hypotension.

In normal subjects standing quietly the central venous pressure varies from animal to animal and, at the moment, the variations of normal resting central venous pressure seem to be as inexplicable as the normal variations of normal resting arterial pressure. In the dog and cat the value is relatively constant between 3 and 7.5 cmH$_2$O (0.3 and 0.75 kPa), no matter what the position of the animal's body; but in normal horses in lateral recumbency it is usually

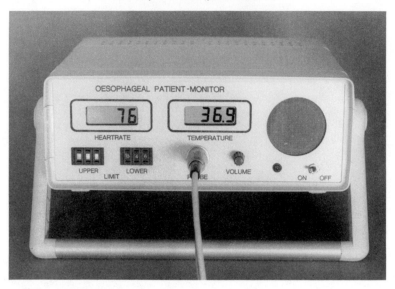

Fig. 2.3 The Aacomonitor monitors core body temperature, heart sounds, respiratory sounds and cardiac frequency from one oesphageal probe. A standard ECG
monitor can be connected to the rear panel. (Aacofarma b.v., the Netherlands,
courtesy of P. Gootjes and Y. Moens, State University of Utrecht.)

recorded as being between 25 and 35 cm H_2O (2.5
and 3.5 kPa), whilst in dorsal recumbency the reading
may fall below the reference level [12]. A single
central venous pressure reading may indicate that all
is not well but it is the change in pressure during the
intravenous administration of fluid which is most
informative. When the administration of fluid improves
the animal's condition (improved pulse volume,
increase in skin temperature and urine production),
therapy should be continued until the central venous
pressure remains steady in the normal range. Excessive administration of fluid with overloading of the
heart is extremely unlikely to occur if the central
venous pressure is not allowed to exceed the upper
limit of normality. If the apparent beneficial effects of
fluid administration are short lived and the central
venous pressure falls quickly after an initial rise, it is
likely that the blood is pooling in dilated peripheral
vessels, i.e. the abnormality present is an increase in
the vascular bed, and more fluids should be given. If
an infusion or transfusion increases the central venous
pressure without improving the animal's condition,
then the cardiac pump mechanism is at fault.

The colour of the mucous membranes can be a very
deceptive guide to the state of the patient, for while
pink membranes suggest adequate oxygenation of the
blood, a brighter pink or red colour may indicate
hypercapnia. White coloration may be due to anaemia,
peripheral vasoconstriction, or lack of circulating
fluid. Cyanosis can only be seen where there is
adequate blood flow to carry the deoxygenated
haemoglobin to the mucous membranes and, in

practice, except when α_2-adrenoceptor agonists are
used, is it rarely observed during anaesthesia unless
there is a marked oxygen lack due to severe lung
disease or failure of the oxygen supply to the breathing
circuit. The more usual causes of inadequate oxygenation such as respiratory obstruction, or respiratory
depression induced by overdose of anaesthetic drugs,
often result in concurrent circulatory failure so that
the mucous membranes appear white. Abnormal
coloration of the mucous membranes is also seen in
dehydrated animals, in animals with a raised venous
pressure and from the presence of fetal haemoglobin
in young animals.

Capillary refill time (the time taken for the colour
to return to the skin or mucous membrane in an area
which has been blanched by pressure) is also a
deceptive observation as capillaries may refill from
engorged veins as well as from the arterial side and it
is sometimes possible to obtain a reasonable refill
time shortly after the death of the patient.

Respiratory efficiency is particularly difficult to
judge from clinical observation. Chest movement
indicates the rate of breathing but gives no indication
of tidal volume and, in fact, where severe respiratory
obstruction exists the patient may make violent
respiratory efforts which result in no movement of air
into and out of the lungs. With anaesthetic breathing
circuits that include a reservoir bag the volume
change in the bag produced by the respiratory efforts
of the patient is a good guide to tidal volume but
where a reservoir bag is not included it is almost
impossible to be certain that tidal volume is adequate.

Colour of the mucous membranes may give a guide to the respiratory efficiency but, as already mentioned, the various factors influencing this colour often makes it difficult.

Assessment of the depth of unconsciousness is based mainly on reflex suppression, both somatic and autonomic, and the reflex suppression which occurs at different depths is discussed in another chapter, but this does not form more than a rough guide. Variations occur depending on the species of animal concerned and the drugs used, while it must also be remembered that the level of unconsciousness depends not only on the amount of drugs administered but also on the level of stimulation at the moment when the observation is made. Evoked reflex responses may be difficult to elicit because of lack of ready access to the patient, and may be modified by drugs (e.g. analgesics) which have been administered. Even the respiratory response to painful stimulation applied to the body may be difficult to assess and, while during general anaesthesia increasing depth of central nervous depression usually results in a decreased respiratory minute volume, this is often due to a decreased tidal volume and the rate may be increased or decreased. Hypercapnia, whether due to faulty equipment or respiratory depression from overdose of anaesthetic agent, causes increased muscle tone and may even result in muscular twitches which can lead to the erroneous assumption that the depth of anaesthesia is insufficient. When neuromuscular blocking agents are used, all reflexes involving somatic muscle are abolished and judgement of the depth of unconsciousness becomes more difficult still (see Chapter 7).

METHODS OF ELECTRONIC SURVEILLANCE

While the human element represented by the anaesthetist is without any doubt the most important factor in patient management, the relatively rare occurrence of what may be termed 'critical incidents' may reduce his or her vigilance. Electronic monitoring devices may be regarded as extensions of the anaesthetist's six senses and their vigilance is constant because machines are not subject to such human variables as mental and physical tiredness, emotional disturbances or environmental interruptions.

Monitoring the circulation

There are numerous monitoring devices available which continuously detect the presence or absence of vital signs relating to the adequacy of the circulation. Care must be taken in their use as many of them fail to give warning of the development of serious problems until it is too late to be of much help.

Heart rate monitors

Several monitors for veterinary patients are now available from commercial sources. All work by detection of the electrical signal of the electrocardiogram (ECG), the signal being processed in various ways to give a digital read-out of heart rate, an audible signal ('bleep') and/or a flash of light with each heart beat, or to sound a warning alarm when the heart rate ceases to lie within certain preset limits. At least one monitor allows the actual form of the ECG to be displayed, thus enabling abnormalities of rhythm as well as of rate to be observed. Although potentially useful, all such monitors suffer from various disadvantages in clinical use. The greatest problem encountered is that of electrical noise, for whilst this is easily identified when the signal is displayed on an oscilloscope or on a written trace, rate meters tend to incorporate it with the signal and give a false reading. In addition, unless the electrodes are correctly placed, some counters may be triggered by both the R and T waves of the electrocardiogram and display double the true heart rate. For their proper use there must be good contact between the leads and patient, and this is not always easy to maintain throughout surgery. Some instruments are incapable of handling the wide range of heart rates encountered in veterinary practice; instruments designed for use in man and small animals may 'double count' when receiving the greater amplitude signal from the hearts of large animals. All these problems are well recognized and newer instruments are often claimed to incorporate features to over-come them but in practice not all such claims are justified.

The most serious disadvantage associated with the use of heart rate monitors is that their use may engender a false sense of security in the surgical team. Derivation from the ECG means they only indicate a measure of electrical activity in the heart and the presence of such activity certainly does not guarantee that the heart is functioning adequately as a pump.

Electrocardiography

The use of an electrocardiograph during anaesthesia provides considerably more information than the heart rate monitors do and an electrocardiograph may not cost very much more to purchase. For monitoring purposes, display of the electrocardiograph signal, the ECG, on an oscilloscope screen is preferable to a pen write-out, for the pen may be damaged by interference from the high frequencies of surgical diathermy and the continuous consumption of recording paper is expensive. Versatile machines are available in which an oscilloscope is provided for monitoring purposes, but a pen recorder is available if the record is needed for diagnostic inspection of any abnormality seen in the oscilloscope display.

For monitoring during anaesthesia it is quite unnecessary to use the standard Eindhoven limb leads in which the right hind-leg lead is earthed. For safety when other electrical apparatus is connected to the patient, modern ECG machines do not require the patient to be earthed, so that all that is required is two leads spanning the heart and in positions where they do not interfere with the operation site. In the dog and cat the maximal signal is obtained if the 'right-arm' lead is placed on the brisket and the 'left-arm lead' between the xiphisternum and the umbilicus. In horses and ruminants leads placed as in dogs and cats give an inverted appearance to the ECG complex. Thus, to obtain a 'normal' ECG tracing it is necessary to reverse the lead positions. The difference between the lead positions needed in different species of animal is most significant if a heart rate monitor which counts deflections is included because if the deflection is in the reverse direction to 'normal' the machine may ignore it.

The artefacts in the ECG commonly encountered during anaesthesia have been reviewed by Purchase [13], and Sykes *et al.* [14] have described in detail the methods by which some of the problems may be overcome. In practice, the majority of avoidable 50 Hz electrical interference results from poor electrode contact with the patient. For monitoring purposes, needle electrodes may be inserted subcutaneously or intramuscularly; equally satisfactory is the use of crocodile clips with electrode jelly to ensure good contact with the skin. This jelly may need to be renewed during the course of a long operation. Many substances, including surgical spirit [15], have been recommended as alternatives to electrode jelly, but most dry or evaporate too rapidly to be useful for long-term monitoring.

Ideally, electrodes should be silver plated to eliminate polarization and electrochemical currents, but stainless steel is an acceptable although imperfect alternative. Artefacts in the ECG occur through movement of the leads by the patient or by the surgeon and with heart movement due to respiration. Although many modern electrocardiographs are reputed not to be affected by diathermy, with most instruments the ECG is completely obliterated when this surgical apparatus is in use. Other electrical equipment or mains power lines in close proximity to the patient may also be sources of interference.

The value of the information obtained from the

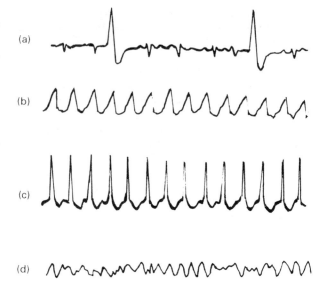

Fig. 2.4 Typical records of ventricular extrasystoles (a), ventricular tachycardia (b), supraventricular tachycardia (c) and ventricular fibrillation (d).

ECG increases with the anaesthetist's ability to interpret the tracing obtained. Changes in rate and rhythm of the heart are most easily recognized.

Sinus tachycardia is frequently encountered during anaesthesia and is usually observed after the administration of atropine. An increase in heart rate may also result from surgical stimulation in an inadequately anaesthetized animal, or from sympathoadrenal stimulation due to carbon dioxide retention. Sinus bradycardia is a normal consequence of some types of anaesthesia, but extreme bradycardia which cannot be overcome by the administration of atropine is usually only seen just before death.

Nodal rhythm is not of great significance and atrioventricular block is uncommon during anaesthesia. Ventricular extrasystoles, on the other hand, are common. They may be isolated or occur alternately with sinus beats as in bigeminal rhythm; they may be unifocal or multifocal in origin. Ventricular extrasystoles are seen most commonly in animals anaesthetized with agents that sensitize the heart to the effects of adrenaline, which may be exogenous in origin (e.g. injected with local analgesic solutions), or endogenous due to reflex sympathoadrenal activity. Sympathoadrenal stimulation occurs during hypercapnia and hypoxia and thus is usually due to respiratory inadequacy.

Frequently in dogs the pulse and heart rates may differ considerably. If an extrasystole occurs during a period when the heart is empty (ventricular bigeminy — ventricular premature depolarization coupled to the preceding sinus beat), no peripheral pulse will be produced. Thus, the heart rate is twice that of the pulse and this will not be diagnosed by palpation of the peripheral pulse. Single extrasystoles are of no significance, and bigeminy is only important in that it may precede more serious events. Ventricular tachycardia is usually considered to be the immediate precursor of ventricular fibrillation and its occurrence must be regarded as a serious portent. Because these changes frequently result from sympathetic activity on the sensitized myocardium, they often disappear if the depth of anaesthesia is reduced and adequate alveolar ventilation restored.

Changes in amplitude of the ECG are more difficult to interpret, as they may be significant or simply due to changing electrical conditions such as an alteration in the impedance of the skin–electrode contact. However, the anaesthetist should note that whilst S-T segment depression or elevation is considered by some to be normal in dogs, changes of more than a few millimetres are indicative of myocardial hypoxia and must not, therefore, be ignored. Changes in the amplitude in certain components of the ECG trace may be due to changes in blood electrolyte levels (especially of potassium) but considerable experience is required before interpretation of these changes can be made easily.

Asystole and ventricular fibrillation indicate extreme myocardial changes rendering the heart incapable of acting as a pump. On occasion, QRS deflections, which may appear to be almost normal, are recorded from animals long after the onset of circulatory arrest. These terminal signs of electrical activity are not associated with mechanical activity (Fig. 2.5).

Pulse monitors

An efficient monitor of a peripheral pulse would be invaluable to the anaesthetist as it would demonstrate the presence of a peripheral circulation and, if capable of measuring pulse volume, would also give some guide as to the cardiac output. Unfortunately, as yet, no such perfect monitor exists and there is no adequate substitute for the anaesthetist's finger on the pulse. It is, however, difficult to palpate the pulse continuously for long periods. Pulse monitors involving carbon microphone detectors were tested in dogs [16] but artefacts, particularly those due to movement of the limbs, caused problems. The xylol bead technique described by Glen [17], who employed it to detect the pulse for the measurement of arterial blood pressure, is not easy to use and has not become popular in veterinary practice because it is fragile and too subject to movement artefacts. Ultrasonic monitors based on detection of blood flow by the Doppler-shift principle (e.g. Model 811, Parks Medical Electronics, Oregon, USA) are now being successfully used in

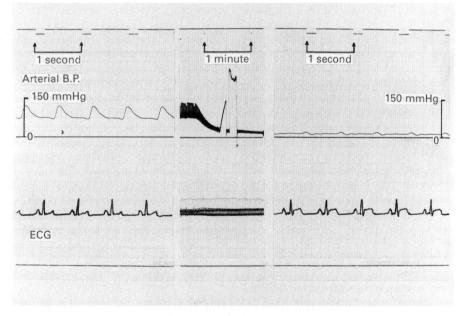

Fig. 2.5 Top: pressure trace from a dog's femoral artery. Bottom: Lead II electrocardiogram. Circulatory failure from an overdose of pentobarbitone. Note that while the pressure trace shows the circulation to be ineffective, the ECG trace is little different from normal — heart rate monitors relying on the QRS complex for detection of the heart beat would, under these circumstances, show an unchanged heart rate and in the absence of a blood pressure record encourage the erroneous belief that all was well with the circulatory system.

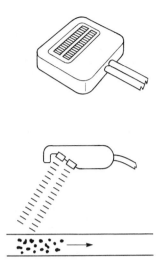

Fig. 2.6 Doppler-shift pulse detector. One piezoelectric crystal emits incident ultrasound signal whilst the other receives the reflected signal from the moving blood cells. The frequency shift between the incident and reflected sound is used to measure the velocity of the blood flow in the vessel. This is the best flow detector for the indirect measurement of arterial blood pressure (Parks Electronics, Oregon, USA).

animals. The flow detector consists of two crystals. One sends a beam of ultrasound energy into the skin through an aqueous gel applied to the skin. The other crystal receives the reflected waves from underlying tissue and the moving red blood cells (Fig. 2.6). Since the underlying tissue is stationary, the frequency of the reflected waves is exactly the same as the frequency of the transmitted waves. However, the reflected waves from anything in motion, in this situation the red blood cells, are of a different frequency, due to the Doppler effect (Fig. 2.5). The frequency difference is made audible by the monitor and the sound heard is this frequency difference between the transmitted and reflected sound waves. Because the red blood cells are moving at different (random) velocities, the sound is not a pure one but is best described as a hissing noise, the pitch being proportional to the velocity of the moving blood. The Doppler probe is fixed to the tail or to a limb (usually after clipping of the hair) over a palpable pulse, with an air-free coupling medium between it and the skin, and its position optimized to give the loudest blood flow signal — a pulsing, hissing noise. The transducer is taped in place, remembering that the sound beam is only about 1 cm wide and loose skin can shift it off the artery. These ultrasonic flow detectors do not suffer from problems due to movement of the extremity to which they are attached (Fig. 2.1); they will detect blood flow when the arterial pressure is as low as 40 mmHg (5.3 kPa) and the vessel constricted.

Regrettably, all pulse monitors, including even the

anaesthetist's finger, fail to detect the pulse when the arterial blood pressure falls below a certain level.

Pulse oximetry

The recent development of pulse oximeters, which both monitor the pulse rate and provide a continuous measurement of arterial oxygen saturation, represents a tremendous advance in monitoring. These devices may be placed on an animal's tongue or nasal septum and differ from all previous oximeters in that they are able to eliminate the background absorption attributable to tissue by measuring the light absorption at two different wavelengths at frequent intervals during each pulse. It is thus possible to derive an absolute measure of oxygen saturation of the arterial blood without precalibration. However, they are a very expensive way of measuring pulse *rate*; they are very sensitive to movement artefacts and may give inaccurate oxygen saturation readings when the pulse volume is reduced by blood loss or severe vasoconstriction. They may also be affected by the presence of excessive environmental lighting, bilirubinaemia or marked venous pulsations.

Measurement of arterial blood pressure

Measurement of arterial blood pressure has been routine in human medical practice for many years but in veterinary practice it is only recently that methods have become available for its easy determination. It can provide useful information in routine anaesthesia and is mandatory in surgical procedures which are likely to precipitate sudden dramatic changes in pressure, or when induced hypotension is employed. For routine monitoring, indirect methods of measurement which are non-invasive are clearly preferable. Direct measurement requires cannulation of an artery and is, therefore, more hazardous and troublesome in clinical practice. Whether direct or indirect methods of measurement are used, the value obtained depends on the reference point taken to represent zero pressure. Probably the best reference point is the mean right atrial pressure, but for all practical purposes the most appropriate appears to be the sternal manubrium, because this is easily located and seems to be relatively constantly related to the position of the right atrium in most animals, irrespective of body position.

Indirect measurement of arterial blood pressure (sphygmomanometry). All indirect methods of measuring arterial blood pressure are modifications of the Riva–Rocci technique, involving occlusion of an artery by an inflatable cuff and detection of returning blood flow distal to the occlusion site as the pressure in the cuff is reduced. The detection of returning blood flow distal to the cuff presents especial difficulties in animals due to the relatively thick skin and small size of easily accessible arteries. The auscultatory technique of sphygmomanometry is the most widely used method of indirect measurement in man and determines both systolic and diastolic pressures. A stethoscope is placed over a limb artery distal to the occluding cuff which encircles the limb. The cuff is inflated to a pressure greater than the systolic pressure and then slowly deflated. When the first Korotkoff sound is heard through the stethoscope the cuff pressure is assumed to equal the systolic blood pressure and when the Korotkoff sounds either become muffled or disappear the cuff pressure is taken to be equal to the diastolic pressure. The detection of the Korotkoff sounds in animals is eased by the use of microphone detectors [18–21], but today in veterinary practice the ultrasonic Doppler technique for the demonstration of blood flow in the artery is usually employed, thus avoiding all difficulties in sound detection. The cuff pressure at which the first, tapping, audible sound is produced is taken as the systolic pressure and the pressure at which the sound first becomes a continuous hissing noise is related to the diastolic pressure. Determination of the systolic pressure is relatively easy and reproducible from one observer to another but the diastolic point is very observer subjective. It is, however, probable that only the systolic pressure is important for Cullen [22] found that inferences made from the diastolic or pulse pressure measurements on the state of the circulation, particularly the total peripheral resistance and stroke volume, are misleading and do not add to knowledge gained from measurement of the systolic pressure alone. The Doppler-shift methods do not require cumbersome apparatus, have been shown to correlate well with simultaneous direct intra-arterial measurements [23, 24] and to be accurate down to pressures of 40 mmHg [25].

Both the length and width of the inflatable bladder in the occluding cuff are critical for accurate measurement of blood pressure. The optimum size of cuff for each species of animal remains controversial, although it has been suggested that a bladder which fully encircles the extremity compensates for any disproportion between bladder width and extremity circumference [26]. The effect of varying the cuff width can be explained on the basis of efficiency of the transmission of the cuff pressure to the artery and the resistance which the cuff offers to the pulse travelling underneath it [27]. Pressure is transmitted more efficiently as the cuff width is increased but after an optimum width is reached the frictional resistance offered to blood flow reduces the energy of the pulse and the occluding pressure has to be lowered excessively to allow blood flow through the compressed segment of artery and the pulse to become detectable in the distal region of the extremity. Combination of these two factors means that when the cuff width is below optimum for a given animal, readings will be erroneously high, and when the cuff width is too great the readings will be below the true value. Glen [17] found good correlation between indirect and direct systolic pressure measurements even with cuffs of different widths and commented that indirect methods were adequate for routine anaesthetic work where changes in pressure are usually of greater importance than absolute values.

Horses. Auscultation of the Korotkoff sounds has been used in horses, the occluding cuff being placed above the hock of the anaesthetized animal [28] or on the tail (Fig. 2.7). For accuracy the cuff should be at the same level as the heart, which is not possible in conscious animals. The method may be made more sensitive if the Korotkoff sounds are amplified and displayed on a printer or oscilloscope from a microphone mounted inside the occluding cuff. The necessary amplifying apparatus is cumbersome and often the procedure yields inaccurate results during hypotension. A less satisfactory technique is to detect the pulse by palpation because this is relatively insensitive and yields values which are lower than those obtained by the other methods. The occluding cuff itself can be used as a pulse detector because oscillations develop in the cuff pressure as it is lowered and the level at which the greatest oscillations occur corresponds well with the mean arterial pressure [29]. This oscillation technique is combined with an instrument which automatically provides a digital read-out of the pressure

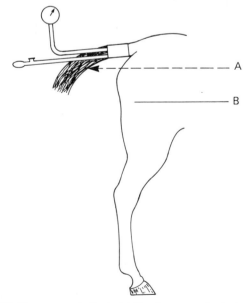

Fig. 2.7 Measurement of arterial blood pressure in the horse.

at the point of maximum pressure oscillation in the 'Dinamap' (Critikon). Instruments such as the Dinamap are particularly suited to long-term intermittent determination of the mean arterial blood pressure during anaesthesia but they are expensive instruments. Probably the most satisfactory, relatively inexpensive method for horses utilizes an ultrasonic Doppler-shift flow detector (e.g. Parks Model 811; Parks Electronics Laboratory, Oregon, USA) for sensing the pulse distal to the occluding cuff. Although continuous readings cannot be obtained, with practice the systolic pressure can easily be measured with accuracy every 30–60 seconds.

Cattle. Indirect blood pressure measurements are seldom made in cattle but they can be obtained from the coccygeal artery by very similar ways to those used in horses. In general, the tail circumference is less than in a horse of comparable weight so that a narrower occluding cuff is adequate and because the middle coccygeal artery is protected to some extent by the ventral spinous processes the cuff needs to be applied in an intervertebral region in order to ensure compression of the artery.

Sheep and goats. In sheep and goats the occluding cuff may be placed above the elbow and an ultrasonic Doppler-shift flow detector just below the carpus or, alternatively, the occluding cuff may be sited around the tibia just proximal to the hock joint and the flow detector over the perforating metatarsal artery.

Pigs. In clinical practice there is seldom any call to measure the arterial pressure in pigs. However, for experimental purposes the occluding cuff may be wrapped around the limb above the elbow and the pulse detected on the medial aspect of the limb just above the first phalanx. If the head end of the animal is not accessible to the anaesthetist the cuff may be applied just above the hock and the sensor over the anterior metatarsal artery.

Dogs. Methods for the indirect determination of arterial pressure have proved more difficult to apply in smaller animals. Many methods have been tried to detect the returning blood flow distal to the occluding cuff. Romagnoli [30] attempted to use oscillometric methods but with these techniques the systolic and diastolic end-points are not always clear. The 'Newcastle sphygmomanometer' with a xylol pulse detector [31] has been used in dogs [17], but has never become popular in small animal practice.

The development of the ultrasonic Doppler-shift pulse detector has enabled systolic blood pressure readings, sufficiently accurate for all clinical purposes, to be readily made in all dogs by the use of an inflatable

occluding cuff and associated pressure manometer. A 2.5 cm wide cuff is used for dogs up to about 15 kg bodyweight, and one 3.75 cm wide for those above this weight, but it is essential that the cuff is always long enough to completely encircle the limb and so they need to be 20–25 cm in length. For the best correlation with directly measured arterial pressures the cuff should be placed around the median artery above the elbow and it is usually convenient to site the detector over the subcarpal arch just below the stopper pad. It is most important to ensure an air-free contact between the detector and skin by clipping the hair and using adequate amounts of coupling gel while the detector is moved around to establish the clearest possible signal.

Direct measurement of arterial blood pressure. The direct continuous measurement of arterial blood pressure is a technique which is popular in veterinary anaesthesia, for until the advent of the Doppler-shift flow detector it was generally more reliable and satisfactory than indirect measurement. The mean arterial pressure can be measured with simple inexpensive apparatus but for accurate determination of the systolic and diastolic pressures more expensive pressure transducers and electronic amplifiers are necessary. Although direct measurement is invasive, it provides continuous monitoring for use in routine surgery, during the immediate postoperative period and for research purposes. It may be used in any animal where a suitable superficial artery is available for cannulation.

Cannulation is most simply performed percutaneously and stringent aseptic precautions must be observed. After cleansing of the skin and, if the animal is conscious, following local infiltration analgesia of the site, a small nick with a pointed scalpel blade is made in the skin just over the proposed site of arterial puncture. A plastic over-the-needle type of catheter is introduced through the nick in the skin into the lumen of the artery. As soon as the catheter enters the arterial lumen the needle is partially withdrawn and the catheter introduced fully into the vessel. Next, after complete withdrawal of the needle part, a sterile stopcock is attached to the hub of the catheter and the system flushed with previously prepared heparin–saline solution (2 units/ml). The catheter is fixed is fixed in position by suturing it to the skin. Loss of blood during the withdrawal of the needle part can usually be prevented by applying pressure over the artery proximal to the tip of the catheter until the stopcock is secured. Obviously, the length and type of catheter to be used in any particular case will vary with the size and depth of the artery from the skin surface, as well as the personal preference of the person concerned, but for ease of cannulation a fairly rigid one is necessary to enable the plastic outer component to be pushed through the thick arterial wall and advanced up the vessel.

The main objection to the use of this technique is the technical difficulty of arterial cannulation and doubt as to its safety. The skill necessary to become proficient at arterial cannulation can be acquired with practice. There is little evidence of any serious complications arising afterwards. The most common complication is haematoma formation following with-drawal of the catheter, but this can be minimized by applying firm digital pressure to the puncture site for 3 minutes (by the clock) after removal of the catheter. To date, over 4000 arterial catheterizations have been performed in horses, cattle, sheep and dogs at the Royal Veterinary College and the Cambridge Veterinary School with no complications other than occasional haematoma formation from accidental, not immediately recognized, dislodgement of the catheter.

The apparatus for measuring the mean arterial blood pressure is shown in Fig. 2.8. A number of variations are possible but the basic pattern [32] is as shown. A standard type of anaeroid manometer has connected to it a 6 or 8 cm length of plastic drip tubing ending in a male Luer connection. This assembly may be sterilized with ethylene oxide and kept in a covered container.

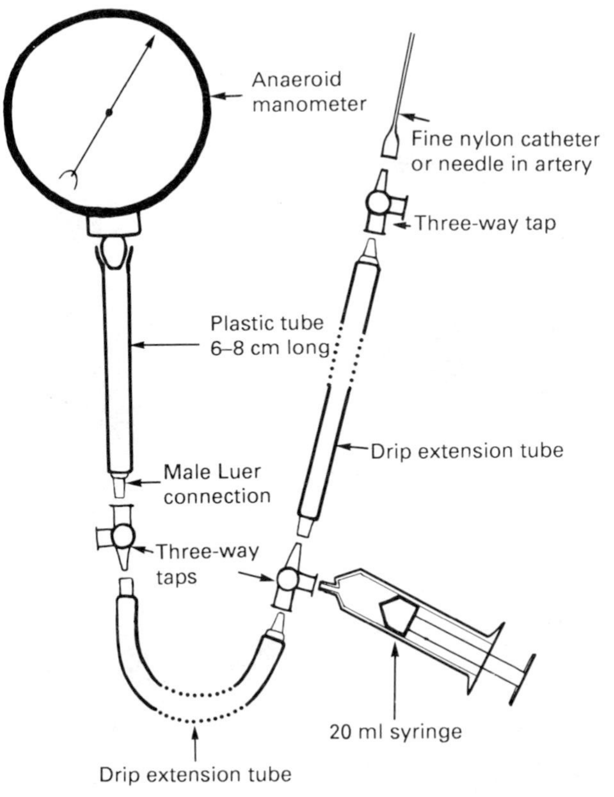

The remainder of the apparatus (two lengths of extension drip tubing or two manometer lines and two disposable stopcocks) is available as presterilized and disposable items. After assembly the tubing is filled with heparin–saline solution until the meniscus lies 10–12 cm below the manometer. The solution can be introduced into both lengths of tubing by opening the appropriate ports on the stopcocks and injecting the solution from a 20 ml syringe through the stop-cock. Both stopcocks have their side arms closed and the lower tubing is connected to the stopcock on the arterial catheter. This stopcock is opened and pressure readings should be obtained. There is an initial flow of blood into the lower tube as the air in the upper tube and manometer is compressed. This blood is flushed back into the animal by injection of heparin–saline solution through the middle stopcock. After this, flushing is only needed at infrequent intervals. The stopcock on the arterial catheter can be used for obtaining arterial blood samples and adds greatly to the convenience of setting up the apparatus and during transport of the animal from place to place.

The longer the air column between the meniscus of the heparin–saline solution and the manometer, the greater the damping, but care should always be taken to ensure that the manometer does not become contaminated by heparin–saline solution because the air column is too short. An air column of about 8 cm seems to be the optimum, and this can be adjusted by attaching a syringe full of air to the upper stopcock and introducing or removing air as required. The manometer must be attached to a suitable support so that the meniscus is at heart level. The air column can be replaced by a commercially available pressure transfer unit, in which a latex diaphragm inside a saline-filled barrel transmits the pressure from the saline column to the anaeroid manometer with minimal damping and prevents any fluid from entering the manometer ('Pressurveil'). The reduced damping in the system is a distinct advantage when the pressures to be measured are low. Another useful modification incorporates a continuous infusion valve which regu-lates a pressure infusion to keep the catheter flushed continuously with heparin–saline solution to prevent clots from forming (Fig. 2.9).

A pressure transducer may be used instead of the anaeroid manometer so that systolic and diastolic pressures may be determined. The pressure trans-ducer is connected to a recorder and/or an oscilloscope to give a continuous display of the pressure waveform.

Placing a reliable intra-arterial catheter that is to remain in position for a considerable period is a more difficult procedure than collecting an arterial blood

Fig. 2.8 Improvised apparatus for the direct measurement of mean arterial blood pressure. (After Zorab [32].)

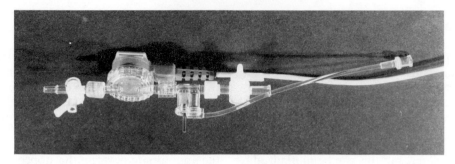

Fig. 2.9 Continuous infusion valve fitted to a pressure transducer. A pressurized bag of intravenous fluid is connected to the plastic tube to give a continuous infusion of 3 ml per hour. With this particular version, rapid flushing of the manometer line is achieved by pulling the rubber tag seen at the top of the valve.

sample. In dogs, the most easily cannulated vessel is the femoral artery. Percutaneous puncture of the femoral artery is facilitated by extending the hind-leg and rotating it slightly outwards (Fig. 2.10). It is essential to use a catheter at least 4 inches (10 cm) long in dogs otherwise movement of the skin over the underlying vessel when the position of the hind-limb is altered will pull the catheter out of the artery. Percutaneous catheterization of the metatarsal artery is a preferable alternative in many dogs. This artery is small but the catheter is less easily dislodged by skin movement when the position of the limb is altered. A small (21 or even 23 gauge) catheter can be used and haemorrhage after its removal does not tend to be

gross even if effective pressure is not applied to the puncture site.

The cat's temperament means that arterial cannulation in the conscious animal is extremely difficult, and unless the patient is moribund, this procedure is usually carried out after surgical exposure of the artery under general anaesthesia. The most suitable vessel is again the superficial musculocutaneous branch of the femoral artery, which is fairly prominent in cats. However, owing to its small size it is often

Catheter over needle

Leg in full extension

20° rotation

Femoral artery

Fig. 2.10 Position for catheterization of the femoral artery in the dog. The hind limb is extended and rotated about 20° outwards. This tenses the artery and provides the maximum length for cannulation. The catheter should be of the 'over needle' variety and long enough for several cms to be introduced into the vessel. Short catheters, no matter how well fixed to the skin, tend to pull out of the vessel when the relative positions of the skin and artery change with alteration in position of the limb.

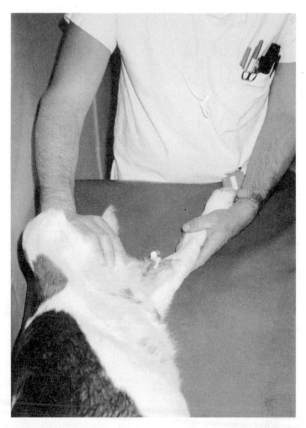

Fig. 2.11 Catheter in position in the femoral artery of a dog.

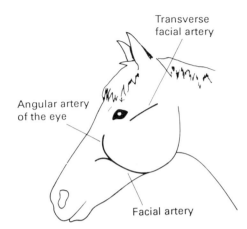

Transverse
facial artery

Angular artery
of the eye

Facial artery

Fig. 2.12 Sites for arterial puncture or catheterization about the horse's head. There is little to choose between the facial artery and the transverse facial artery; both are easily located by palpation and their position relative to the overlying skin is reasonably constant.

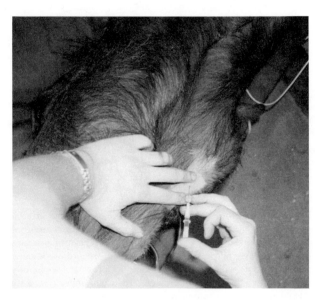

Fig. 2.13 Introduction of a catheter into the facial artery of the horse as the artery rounds the ventral border of the mandible; the artery is relatively fixed in position at this point but may be confused with the parotid duct.

missed and the main femoral artery cannulated by mistake. If this happens, care must be taken to maintain adequate pressure on the site for a sufficient time after withdrawal of the catheter, as haemorrhage can otherwise be profuse. The catheter must not be too large nor must the main femoral artery be tied off, for serious ischaemic problems may follow if the blood supply to the cat's hind-limb is compromised for any length of time.

In horses there are many large superficial arteries which may be easily cannulated for arterial pressure measurement. Among those which have been recommended are the facial artery and its branches, the great metatarsal artery, and the common digital arteries. The branches of the facial artery are shown in Fig. 2.12. It may be palpated where it ascends the face in front of the masseter muscle. Cannulation at this point has the advantage that the artery may be stabilized against the bone and, as the vein no longer lies directly alongside it, accidental venepuncture is unlikely. The artery may also be cannulated where it passes over the ventral border of the mandible. It is larger here and so is easier to penetrate, but accidental cannulation of the adjacent vein or parotid duct is not uncommon. In thin-skinned horses probably the best site for cannulation of this vessel is much higher up towards the medial canthus of the eye but in thicker-skinned animals it is often impossible to palpate the pulse in this region accurately enough to locate the artery. Cannulation of the facial artery can often be carried out under local analgesia in the quiet conscious horse and this vessel is accessible to the anaesthetist in all but head and neck surgery. Although complications could, theoretically, include damage to

the facial nerve or parotid duct, no reports of such complications are to be found in the literature. The transverse facial artery may also be used [33] and, at the Cambridge and London Veterinary Schools, several hundred horses have had their facial or transverse facial arteries cannulated with no ill effects. Use of the great metatarsal artery has been described [34] and this is a useful site when access to the head is denied. The digital arteries are also easily accessible but if complications should occur at this site they may have more serious consequences. Puncture of the carotid artery has often been advocated for arterial blood sampling but is not to be encouraged as it is impossible to maintain adequate pressure on the puncture site after withdrawal of the needle or cannula and massive haematoma formation inside the carotid sheath involving the vagus, recurrent laryngeal and sympathetic nerves may occur, with danger of subsequent infection.

In cattle, pressures may be recorded from the middle coccygeal or median auricular arteries. Cannulation of the middle coccygeal artery under caudal epidural block is not difficult in most conscious animals and complications arising after its use are most unlikely to have serious consequences. Cannulation of the median auricular artery with an 18 or 20 gauge indwelling catheter has been recorded by Trim

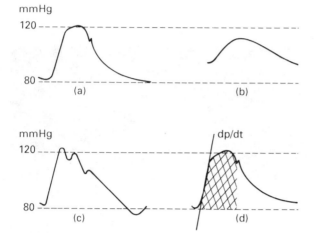

Fig. 2.14 Waveforms from direct measurement of the arterial pressure: (a), good trace; (b), recording of the same pressures but with excessive damping, systolic pressure low, diastolic pressure high, mean arterial pressure unchanged; (c), recording of same pressures but with resonance, systolic pressure apparently increased while diastolic pressure reduced, mean pressure unchanged; (d), illustration of how left ventricular contractility may be estimated from the rate of rise of pressure during early systole (dP/dt) while the shaded area gives an index of stroke volume.

[35] who has observed no subsequent complications but, if they do occur, it is possible that a large portion of the ear pinna may slough.

Sheep and goats are not often subjected to clinical procedures where direct arterial pressure monitoring is needed but it may be required for experimental surgery and in these circumstances it is usual to cut down on and cannulate an artery which is conveniently near the main operation site. The median auricular artery, although a small vessel, may be large enough to be used in some of these animals.

Direct measurement of arterial pressures is difficult in pigs and surgical cannulation of a vessel is usually necessary, although in some animals the median auricular artery can be cannulated percutaneously.

Measurement of the central venous pressure

Disposable venous manometer sets are available, but the complete apparatus for the measurement of central venous pressure can be made more cheaply from plastic three-way stopcocks, disposable giving sets and extension tubes (Fig. 2.15). A catheter of sufficient length is introduced into the jugular vein and advanced until its tip lies in the anterior vena cava. The distance the catheter tip has to be introduced is, initially, estimated by measurement of length, but once the catheter is connected to the manometer its position may be adjusted until the

level of fluid in the manometer tube moves in time with the animal's respiratory movements. In dogs and cats the introduction of a catheter into the jugular vein is often greatly facilitated by laying the animal on its side and extending its head and neck over a pillow or sandbag. If the catheter is to be left in position for a long time it is kept patent with a drip infusion through a three-way stopcock or the catheter is kept filled with heparin–saline solution (10 units/ml) between measurements. Readings may be taken at any time. If an intravenous drip is used it is turned full on and the stopcock manipulated first to fill the manometer tube from the fluid reservoir and then to connect the manometer tube to the catheter. The fall of fluid in the manometer is observed and should be 'step-like' in response to respiratory pressure changes. The central venous pressure is read off when fluid fall ceases.

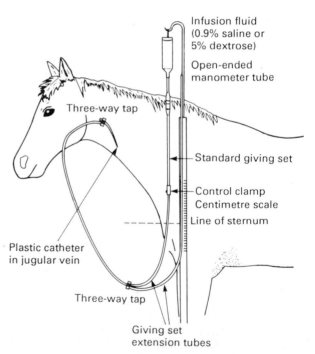

Fig. 2.15. Apparatus for the measurement of central venous pressure.

The central venous pressure may also be measured in the way previously described for arterial pressure if a suitably sensitive anaeroid manometer is used, but because low pressures are to be measured this system is only satisfactory when the damping is kept to a minimum by the use of commercially available pressure transfer units (e.g. 'Pressurveil', Fig. 2.16).

Venous pressures being low, the margin of error introduced by inaccuracies in obtaining a suitable reference point to represent zero pressure may be

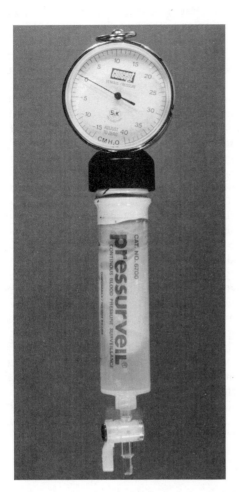

Fig. 2.16. Pressure transfer unit in which a latex diaphragm isolates the anaeroid manometer from the fluid-filled catheter line. These units are presterilized and disposable ('Pressurveil').

clinically significant. Whatever apparatus is used the zero of the scale should be carefully located, preferably by using a spirit level to ensure accuracy. The actual reading obtained obviously depends on the reference point taken to represent zero pressure. Probably the ideal reference point is the mean pressure in the right atrium but for practical purposes the most appropriate appears to the sternal manubrium, because this is easily located and seems to be most constantly related to the position of the right atrium in all animals, irrespective of body position.

Measurement of left atrial pressure (pulmonary wedge pressure)

Since measurement of the central venous pressure reflects the filling pressure of the right side of the heart, it is possible that left heart failure could precede that of the right side and precipitate pul-

monary oedema without a rise in central venous pressure. For this reason the pulmonary wedge pressure is used as a measure of the left atrial filling pressure. Swan *et al.* [36] introduced the flow-directed balloon-tip catheter for this purpose in critically ill human patients and the technique has been used in veterinary anaesthesia. It is not a difficult technique because soft catheters can easily be floated in the bloodstream from the jugular vein through the right side of the heart into the pulmonary artery and advanced until they wedge; balloon catheters and/or radiological control are not essential. The measurement is made using the same apparatus as is used for the measurement of central venous pressure but care must be taken to ensure that vessel occlusion is not maintained between measurements or pulmonary infarction may occur. If a balloon catheter is used the balloon should only be inflated while measurements are made and if a simple catheter is used it should be slightly withdrawn from the wedged position between measurements.

Measurement of cardiac output

Dye or thermal dilution are used for accurate measurement of cardiac output but both these methods are invasive. Another method which may be regarded as almost non-invasive and has been used during anaesthesia is aortic velography using an oesophageal ultrasound probe [37]. A probe on which piezoelectric crystals are mounted is introduced into the thoracic oesophagus and rotated until the maximum signal strength is obtained. Its use during clinical canine anaesthesia has been described by Stolk [38] and it has also been used in horses. Aortic velography is not claimed to give an accurate measurement of cardiac output but the technique yields a quantitative measurement of blood velocity in the aorta and, with certain assumptions, changes in both cardiac output and the inotropic state of the myocardium can be assessed.

All three methods of measuring cardiac output requires expensive equipment and are outside the scope of routine monitoring during veterinary anaesthesia but in some hospitals their use is now providing data which is of great value in the management of anaesthesia for ill animals and others undergoing major surgery.

Monitoring respiration

Respiratory function is particularly difficult to monitor by simple clinical observation of the animal and instruments capable of providing reliable information relating to respiratory activity are welcomed by the anaesthetist.

Rate monitors and apnoea alarms

Most rate monitors and apnoea alarms use a thermistor placed in the airway to detect temperature differences between the inspired and exhaled gases. The signal derived from the thermistor is used to drive a digital rate meter, to make a noise which varies in intensity or pitch in time with the animal's breathing, or to sound an alarm if a constant gas temperature is detected. A simple monitor of this type was described as long ago as 1973 [39]. It must be emphasized that these devices do not give an indication of tidal volume and may not, therefore, give warning of partial respiratory obstruction.

The oesophageal stethoscope (p. 19) not only enables cardiac action to be monitored but also serves as a particularly useful simple monitor for the presence of respiration, its character and the degree, if any, of obstruction. Its main disadvantage is that unless the sounds are amplified electronically, the freedom of movement of the anaesthetist is restricted.

Tidal and minute volume monitors

Measurement of the total minute volume of lung ventilation is relatively simple, but the strictly relevant part of this volume — the part which ventilates the alveoli — is much more difficult to estimate. It can be guessed as being a fixed proportion of the minute volume since the physiological dead-space, although increased during general anaesthesia, remains a reasonably constant fraction of the tidal volume. Unfortunately this fraction varies from species to species of animal and from individual to individual.

Tidal and minute volumes can be measured in small animals by introducing a Wright's respirometer [40] into the breathing circuit. This instrument gives useful information as to the adequacy of tidal volume and readings taken before the administration of muscle relaxants are valuable guides when spontaneous respiration is being restored after their use. It has a dead-space of 25 ml, a low resistance to breathing, and is reasonably accurate over volumes ranging from 4 to 15 l/min [41]. It under-reads below 4 l/min and is said to be fail-safe.

For horses and cattle the dry gas meter maybe used to measure tidal and minute volumes but this instrument is unlikely to be available for routine clinical monitoring unless it is built into a circle absorber circuit.

Measurement of arterial blood gas tensions

The most effective way of monitoring respiratory efficiency is to measure the levels of oxygen and carbon dioxide in the arterial blood and these blood gas measurements also give the anaesthetist valuable information as to the acid–base status of the animal. This information is essential if a veterinary surgeon wishes to perform complicated cardiac surgery, or to operate on very sick patients (e.g. equine 'colic' cases). Unfortunately, the equipment needed for these measurements is expensive, and is unlikely to be directly available in most veterinary practices, but every attempt should be made to locate a nearby laboratory which is willing to carry out blood gas analysis when this is urgently required. Arterial blood samples for blood gas analysis may be taken from any superficial artery used for blood pressure measurement (p. 26) and should be collected slowly over several respiratory cycles. The blood should be collected in glass syringes, as although disposable plastic syringes may be adequate if analysis is to be carried out immediately, the gas tensions may change if analysis is delayed. The dead-space of the hub of the syringe (and needle, if used) should be filled with heparin solution before collection of the sample and any gas bubbles in the syringe afterwards should be expelled before sealing the hub with a cap. After inverting the syringe several times to mix the blood with the heparin it should be kept immersed in a mixture of ice and water until analysis is performed. Analysis should be undertaken as soon as possible but, with these precautions, worthwhile values should still be obtained after several hours of storage.

Capnography

In animals with healthy lungs, the level of carbon dioxide contained in the air which is last expired (end-tidal air) approximates to that of the arterial blood. Infrared carbon dioxide analysers can be used to sample gas in the endotracheal tube and give a continuous record of carbon dioxide levels at this site throughout the respiratory cycle. Infrared analysers suffer from having a relatively slow response time so they are not satisfactory when respiratory rates are high. Collision broadening is produced by nitrous oxide but, provided the nitrous oxide concentration remains stable and the instrument is calibrated with mixtures of gases containing nitrous oxide in appropriate concentrations, the carbon dioxide measurement can be relied upon [42]. The loss of the sample volume (which may, with some instruments, be up to 500 ml/min) may seriously affect the dynamics of low-flow circle systems.

End-tidal carbon dioxide monitoring is in widespread use in the USA and on the Continent of Europe, mainly because it provides incontrovertible evidence of the endotracheal tube being correctly placed in the trachea, that carbon dioxide is being transported to the lungs and that it is being moved by ventilation to the sampling site [43].

Continuous measurement of carbon dioxide concentrations is a useful monitor for pulmonary embolism and may warn of changes in cardiac output. An acute reduction in the end-tidal carbon dioxide concentration occurs when there is a sudden decrease in cardiac output or a large pulmonary embolus of air or blood clot.

There is often a large and variable arterial to end-tidal carbon dioxide tension difference during anaesthesia so that it is necessary to carry out blood gas analysis to check the relationship from time to time during long operations. However, even when this is done it has been reported that the mean error of estimates of arterial carbon dioxide tension can be ± 6 mmHg (± 0.9 kPa), whilst maximum errors may be as high as ± 12 mmHg (± 1.8 kPa) [44].

An interesting account of capnography in equine anaesthesia has been given by Moens and De Moor [45] but the necessary apparatus is expensive.

Monitoring body temperature

General anaesthesia interferes with an animal's ability to control its body temperature and it may become hypothermic or hyperthermic, depending on environmental conditions. A rise in temperature during anaesthesia may signal the onset of malignant hyperpyrexia. In the past, insufficient attention has been paid to body temperature in veterinary anaesthesia but there are now clear indications that it cannot be ignored. The standard mercury-in-glass thermometer may be used to obtain a reading of rectal temperature but under anaesthesia the reading obtained from this site is often artificially low because of the presence of faeces and/or ballooning of the rectum precludes good contact with the thermometer. Simple electronic thermometers with thermistor probes are now available for application at various sites in the body. Body core temperature is best measured in the lower oesophagus at heart level because upper oesophageal temperature may be influenced by the temperature of the respired gases. Peripheral body temperature correlates well with blood lactate levels and cardiac output and may be measured from the skin. The peripheral to core temperature gradient may be a good index of cardiac output and is often claimed to be an invaluable simple measurement of the adequacy of tissue perfusion.

Monitoring urinary output

The urinary output depends on the renal blood flow which, in turn, depends on cardiac output and circulating blood volume, and thus it is a relatively sensitive indicator of the circulatory state during anaesthesia and at other times. Catheterization of the urinary bladder is a simple operation in most domestic animals and the urine may be drained into a plastic bag for collection and subsequent measurement. Repeated catheterization not only disturbs sick or badly injured animals but also multiplies the risk of introducing infection into the bladder and traumatization of the urethra, so that either self-retaining catheters should be used or, once inserted, the catheter should be fixed in place with a suture or adhesive plaster. In restless animals where continuous draining is difficult, the open end of the indwelling catheter may be clamped, the clamp being released every hour to drain the accumulated urine.

Monitoring metabolic changes

The degree of monitoring of metabolic changes through laboratory analysis of blood samples that is required in any case obviously depends on the condition of the patient and the surgery to be performed. Arterial blood gas measurements have already been discussed (p. 32) but estimation of the acid–base status of the animal provides a useful guide on which further treatment can be based in a rational manner. Venous blood samples suffice for other measurements such as those of serum sodium and potassium concentrations.

In the diabetic patient, blood glucose estimations may be necessary before, during and, perhaps most important, after surgery. Major chances in the level of certain blood electrolytes, in particular sodium, potassium and chloride, may occur in gastrointestinal disturbances, and accurate measurements of these ionic concentrations may be essential if therapy is to be appropriate. Blood urea measurement and liver function tests may be useful prior to anaesthesia in order to enable the fitness of the patient to be assessed, and sometime after surgery to ascertain what, if any, damage has been done to the liver and kidneys, but they do not yield any useful information during anaesthesia.

Monitoring of neuromuscular blockade

The mechanical response to nerve stimulation (i.e. muscular contraction) may be observed following the application of supramaximal single, tetanic or 'train-of-four' electrical stimuli to a suitable peripheral motor nerve. During general anaesthesia the response obtained may be influenced by the anaesthetic agents and any neuromuscular blocking drugs which have been used. Observation of the muscle contraction to a tetanic stimulus will give a crude indication of the state of any neuromuscular blockade. The long-lasting block due to a non-depolarizing muscle relaxant is characterized by a non-sustained response (fade) and post-tetanic facilitation. A pure depolarizing block shows no fade or post-tetanic facilitation. The train-of-four technique is useful,both experimentally and clinically. Four single 'twitch' stimuli are applied to the nerve at 0.5 second intervals. This rate of stimulation produces a depletion of acetylcholine at the nerve endings during stimulation but, at the same time, the 'tetanus' does not cause post-tetanic facilitation. Comparison between the first and fourth twitch response gives an index of the extent of the neuromuscular blockade. Following non-depolarizing block satisfactory relaxation for abdominal surgery is achieved at 95% suppression, i.e. when the fourth twitch is 25% of the first of the train-of-four. The technical problems of recording these evoked mechanical responses have been discussed by Cullen *et al.* [46] and are considered in more detail in Chapter 7.

Monitoring of equipment

Before any anaesthetic is administered all equipment likely to be used should be carefully checked. It is essential to ensure that the oxygen supply will be adequate, the circuit is free from leaks and that the correct volatile anaesthetic is in the vaporizer. If soda lime is to be used its freshness should be checked by blowing carbon dioxide through a small portion and testing to see whether this causes it to get hot. The colour indicator incorporated in many brands of soda lime cannot be relied upon to indicate freshness.

Interruption in the supply of oxygen to the patient is one of the most serious events which can occur during anaesthesia and many anaesthetic machines incorporate warning devices which sound alarms if the oxygen supply fails. However, when a rebreathing circuit is being used, the delivery of oxygen in the fresh gas supply does not always ensure that the inspired gases will contain sufficient oxygen to support life. Dilution of the oxygen in the rebreathing circuit is particularly likely to occur in the early stages of anaesthesia when denitrogenation of the patient is taking place, or when nitrous oxide is used with low total flow rates of fresh gas. Oxygen measurement devices are available which can be used to sample the inspired gases and to demonstrate to the anaesthetist that the patient is receiving an adequate concentration of oxygen. The oxygen fuel cell is one such instrument which is cheap, compact, portable and sufficiently accurate for clinical use. The long life and robustness of fuel cells should mean that in future they will be fitted to all anaesthetic machines. However, there are limitations to the use of inspired oxygen monitoring as a guide to the adequacy of fresh gas flow into a circle system. First, there is usually a cyclical variation in inspired oxygen concentration as a result of the mixing of fresh gas with the intermittent flow of expired gas, a steady inspired oxygen concentration only being found if the system is one in which fresh and expired gas are mixed in the reservoir bag before coming to the inspiratory tube. Thus, the use of a slow-response analyser such as a fuel cell may yield an inaccurate result. Secondly, there will be little difference between fresh gas and inspired oxygen concentration if the fresh gas is merely oxygen itself. For these reasons, inspired oxygen monitoring can provide a useful warning of the delivery of hypoxic gas mixtures to the patient but is of limited use in detecting an inadequate fresh gas flow into most circle absorption systems. With other breathing systems (e.g. Magill, Lack or Bain) there is a to-and-fro movement of gases which makes it very difficult to obtain a truly representative sample of inspired gas. Thus, the only infallible monitor of the composition and adequacy of the fresh gas supply is alveolar gas analysis [3]. This presents technical problems, for at the moment the only rapid-response oxygen analyser capable of giving breath by breath measurements that is commercially available is the mass spectrometer — an expensive, bulky apparatus which requires skilled servicing at regular intervals. Rapid-response polarographic and paramagnetic analysers are now becoming available but experience with their use is very limited.

Measurement of the end-tidal concentrations of volatile anaesthetics by sampling from the endotracheal tube could give an indication of the concentration in the arterial blood and the concentration of halothane at this site can be monitored continuously with an ultraviolet absorption meter. Expired concentrations of all the halogenated volatile anaesthetics can also be monitored by infrared analysers (e.g. Normac, Datex). One halothane analyser (Narkotent, North American Drager) which works on the principle of relaxation of silicone rubber bands in the presence of halothane vapour can be used with other volatile agents after appropriate calibration. All the halogenated hydrocarbon anaesthetic vapours can be measured by the Engstrom Multigas Monitor for Anaesthesia (EMMA) which utilizes a quartz crystal detector. The detector comprises a quartz crystal coated with a layer of silicone oil, whose frequency of oscillation alters as a result of increases in mass of the organic layer in the presence of anaesthetic vapours. The change in oscillation frequency is proportional to the vapour concentration and an electrical signal is generated in such a way that its magnitude is linearly related to the vapour concentration. The instrument is said to have minimal zero drift, sufficient sensitivity and a response which is rapid and accurate enough to permit continuous monitoring. It is, however, inaccurate in the presence of water vapour so that samples of expired gas must be dried before entering the detector and for this reason most anaesthetists only use it to measure concentrations of anaesthetics delivered to non-rebreathing circuits. Like many other monitors it does not give accurate results in herbivores for it also responds to other constituents of their expired air.

It must be remembered that it is unlikely that analysis of the end-tidal vapour concentration can be safely used as a guide to the depth of unconsciousness because the minimum alveolar concentration (MAC) is defined as the minimum concentration which will

prevent movement in response to surgical stimulation in 50% of subjects [47] — a condition which is not surgically acceptable! Even if the concept is expanded to relate to the log of the end-tidal concentration to the probit of the motor response [48] there is still a large variation in response to a stimulus at any given alveolar concentration. There are several reasons for this including the variable relationship between end-tidal and arterial concentrations due to shunting of blood in the lungs and variations in dead-space, age and the effect other agents administered (e.g. opiates, nitrous oxide) have on volatile anaesthetic MAC [49].

FINAL COMMENTS ON PATIENT MONITORING

In human medicine Kennedy and colleagues [50] noted that the primary intraoperative objectives of the anaesthetist were to observe the patient, observe monitoring equipment and review continuously the management of anaesthesia. A recent time and motion study of the anaesthetist's intraoperative time, by McDonald and Dzwonczyk [51], has produced some very interesting results in that in this study, while the anaesthetists performed 13 different tasks, only four were patient observation activities that made use of their specialist training. In addition the anaesthetists spent only 26% of the intraoperative time on these activities, the remaining 64% being spent on activities which required only various manual skills. It is likely that a similar situation

pertains in veterinary medicine and it seems that monitoring equipment need to be redesigned. The most immediate need is for automated or semi-automated systems for generating the intraoperative anaesthetic record, for in McDonald and Dzwonczyk's study some 12% of the anaesthetist's time was spent completing such records manually. 'There is also a need for integrated monitoring systems that not only monitor, display and record all important physiological data and drugs administered, but also detect abnormal values and combine data to indicate that adverse events may occur' [51].

It must be noted that most of the technology for such systems exists at the present time and it is to be hoped that its price will not make such monitoring impossible in veterinary medicine.

REFERENCES

1. Kellagher, R. B. and Watney G. C. G. (1986) *Veterinary Record* 119, 347
2. Schreiber, P. S. and Schreiber, J. M. (1986) *North American Draeger Seminar, Safety in Anaesthesia*, London and Birmingham.
3. Sykes, (1987) *British Journal of Anaesthesia* 59, 901.
4. American Society of Anesthesiologists (1986) *Annual Directory of the ASA*, p. 565. Philadelphia: Lippincott.
5. Eichhorn, J. H., Cooper, J. B., Cullen, D. J., Maier, W. R. Philip, J. H. and Seeman, R. G. (1986) *Journal of the American Medical Association* 256, 1017.
6. Cooper, J. B., Newbower, R. S., Long, C. D. and McPeek, B. (1978) *Anesthesiology* 49, 399.
7. Craig, J. and Wilson, M. E. (1981) *Anaesthesia* 36, 933.
8. Lunn, J. N. and Mushin, W. W. (1982) *Mortality Associated with Anaesthesia*. London: Nuffield Provincial Hospitals Trust.
9. Cooper, J. B., Newbower, R.S. and Kitz, R. J. (1984) *Anesthesiology* 60, 34.
10. Hanning, C. D. (1985) *British Journal of Anaesthesia* 57, 359
11. Lillehei, R. C. (1964) *Surgery, St. Louis* 56, 182.
12. Hall, L. W. and Nigam, J. M. (1975) *Veterinary Record* 97, 66.
13. Purchase, I. F. H. (1963) *Veterinary Record* 75, 326.
14. Sykes, M. K., Vickers, M. D. and Hull, C. J. (1981) *Principles of Clinical Measurement*, p. 48. London: Blackwell Scientific.
15. Ettinger, S. J. and Suter, P. F. (1970) *Canine Cardiology*. Philadelphia: W. B. Saunders.
16. Campbell, J. R., Lawson, D. D. and Sanford, J. (1964) *Journal of Small Animal Practice* 5, 255.
17. Glen, J. B. (1970) *Veterinary Record* 87, 349.
18. Engelhard, W. von and Hampel, K. H. (1962) *Tierarztliche Umschau* 117, 117.
19. Klemm, V. R. and Hembrough, F. B. (1966) *Journal of the American Veterinary Association* 149, 1297.
20. Prioli, N. A. and Winbury, M. M. (1960) *Journal of Applied Physiology* 15, 323
21. Ellis, P. M. (1975) *Equine Veterinary Journal* 7, 22.
22. Cullen, D. J. (1974) *Anesthesiology* 40, 6.
23. Johnson, J. H., Garner, H. E. and Hutcheson, D. P. (1976) *Equine Veterinary Journal* 8, 55.
24. Kvart, C. (1979) *Journal of Equine Medicine and Surgery* 3, 16.
25. Latshaw, H., Fessler, J. F., Whistler, S. J. and Geddes, L. A. (1979) *Equine Veterinary Journal* 11, 191.
26. Van Montfrans, G. A., Van Der Hoeven, G. M. A.,

Karemaker, J. M., Wieling, W. and Dunning, A. J. (1987) *British Medical Journal* **295**, 354

27. Schaffer, A. I. (1955) *American Journal of Diseases of Children* **89**, 204
28. Geddes, L. A., Chaffee, V., Whistler, J., Bourland, J. D. and Tacker, W. A. (1977) *American Journal of Veterinary Research* **38**, 2055.
29. Smith, M. (1969) *Equine Veterinary Journal* **4**, 204.
30. Romagnoli, A. (1953) *Cornell Veterinarian* **43**, 161
31. Ashworth, A. M., Neligan, G. A. and Rogers, J. E. (1959) *Lancet* **i**, 801
32. Zorab, J. S. M. (1969) *Anaesthesia* **24**, 431.
33. Taylor, P. M. (1981) *Equine Veterinary Journal* **13**, 271.
34. Manley, S. V. (1981) *Veterinary Clinics of North America, Equine Anaesthesia* (ed. E. P. Steffey). Philadelphia: W. B. Saunders.
35. Trim, C. M. (1980) *Veterinary Record* **109**, 265.
36. Swan, H. J. C. Ganz, W., Forrester, J., Marcus, H., Diamond, G. and Chonette, D. (1970) *New England Journal of Medicine* **283**, 447.
37. Tomlin, P. J. and Duck, F. A. (1975) *Canadian Anaesthetists Society Journal* **22**, 561.
38. Stolk, P. W. Th. (1978) *Proceedings Association of Veterinary Anaesthetists of Great Britain and Ireland* **7**, 21.
39. Hall, L. W. and Massey, G. M. (1973) *Veterinary Record* **93**, 225.
40. Wright, B. M. (1955) *Journal of Physiology (London)* **127**, 25.
41. Nunn, J. F. and Ez-Ashi, T. I. (1962) *British Journal of Anaesthesia* **34**, 422
42. Burton, G. W. (1969) *British Journal of Anaesthesia* **41**, 723.
43. Birmingham, P. K., Cheney, F. W. and Ward, R. J. (1968) *Anesthesia and Analgesia* **65**, 886.
44. Raemer, D. B., Francis, D., Philip, J. H. and Gabel, R. A. (1983) *Anesthesia and Analgesia* **621**, 1065.
45. Moens, Y. and De Moor, A. (1981) *Equine Veterinary Journal* **13**, 229.
46. Cullen, L. K., Jones, R. S. and Snowdon, S. L. (1980) *British Veterinary Journal* **136**, 154.
47. Eger, E. I., Saidman, L. J. and Brandstater, B. (1965) *Anesthesiology,* **261**, 756.
48. de Jong, R. H. and Eger, E. I. (1975) *Anesthesiology* **42**, 384.
49. Quasha, A. L., Eger, E. I. and Tinker, J. H. (1980) *Anesthesiology* **531**, 315.
50. Kennedy, P. J., Feingold, A., Wiener, E. L. and Hosek, R. S. (1976) *Anesthesia and Analgesia* **55**, 374.
51. McDonald, J. S. and Dzwonczyk, R. R. (1988) *British Journal of Anaesthesia* **61**, 738.

CHAPTER 3

INTRODUCTION TO GENERAL ANAESTHESIA

General anaesthesia is a state of unconsciousness produced by a process of controlled, reversible intoxication of the central nervous system whereby the patient neither perceives nor recalls noxious stimuli. Thus, an anaesthetic agent may be defined as a substance which produces loss of consciousness in a controllable manner. It may be a volatile or gaseous substance inhaled into the lungs, or a non-volatile compound usually administered by intravenous injection but which may be given by mouth, per rectum or by intra-peritoneal or intramuscular injection. Intravenous injection presents certain advantages over other methods but unless the actions of the agents administered in this way are fully appreciated these advantages may be more than offset by hazards peculiar to this technique. Intravenous agents are popular in veterinary anaesthesia for all species of animal and this is undoubtedly partly due to the speed and pleasantness with which they produce unconsciousness. However, undue emphasis is often placed on this aspect and it must be appreciated that a well-administered inhalation induction of anaesthesia can be more pleasant for the patient than innumerable unsuccessful attempts at venepuncture. Moreover, many intravenous anaesthetics are irritant to the tissues and the deposition of small amounts of these substances at various places in all four limbs and around the jugular veins, together with haematomata, is too great a price to pay for the rapid loss of consciousness which most intravenous anaesthetics should guarantee.

Drugs injected into a vein are distributed directly in the bloodstream to the brain and the other tissues of the body, while those given by the alimentary route (by mouth or into the rectum) must first be absorbed into the blood, they then pass through the liver before reaching the central nervous system. Their elimination from the body is not a reversal of the process of absorption; they are broken down, mostly in the liver, and are then excreted mainly by the kidneys. Volatile and gaseous anaesthetic agents introduced into the upper respiratory tract have to be transported in the blood to the brain before they will produce loss of consciousness and there are three steps involved in this process, each occupying an appreciable period of time. The first step is the transference of the gas or vapour from the upper respiratory tract to the lung alveoli, and free external respiration is necessary for this. The gases inhaled will contain a certain proportion of the anaesthetic agent, but it is important to note that the volume of that inspiration, the 'tidal volume' (Fig. 3.1), is only a small fraction of the volume of air contained within the lungs and air passages so that a considerable dilution of the anaesthetic agent will take place. Only after several breaths will the concentration of anaesthetic vapour or gas in the alveoli approximate to that in the inspired mixture. The actual depth of respiration or volume of the tidal air is an important factor in this process and deep breathing is more effective than shallow breathing. For, example, in a dog where the tidal volume is 300 ml and the respiratory anatomical dead-space volume (volume of the conducting airways) is 100 ml the effective alveolar ventilation will be 300 ml minus 100 ml, i.e. 200 ml. If, in this dog, the tidal volume is reduced to 200 ml the effective alveolar ventilation becomes 200 ml minus the same 100 ml dead-space volume, i.e. 100 ml, so that in this dog a decrease of one-third in the tidal volume halves the alveolar ventilation. From this it might be concluded that when the tidal volume is decreased so that it equals the volume of the conducting airways, the alveolar ventilation becomes zero. However, this does not happen because the gases travel through the airways not as a block with a square front, but rather with a spike or cone front. For this reason some inspired gas does reach the alveoli even when the tidal volume is less than the volume of the anatomical dead-space. It has been shown that a small fraction of the inspired gas penetrates into the alveoli when the tidal volume is as little as half the volume of the conducting airways. Thus, the type of calculation given above is not strictly valid, especially when the tidal volume is extremely low, but it serves to illustrate the effectiveness of deep breathing. Sedative drugs given to an animal as premedication before the administration of an inhalation anaesthetic usually cause a decrease in the tidal volume, and so interfere with the transport of the gas or vapour to the alveoli.

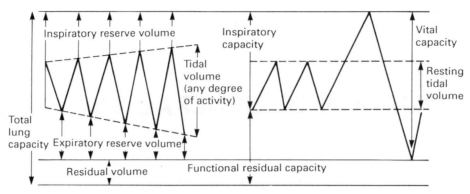

Fig. 3.1 Divisions of lung capacity. Only the tidal volume is readily measurable in animals but the functional residual capacity (FRC) can be measured in suitably equipped laboratories.

The second step, the absorption of the anaesthetic gas or vapour from the alveoli of the lung into the blood, depends on laws which govern the diffusion of gases through membranes. The flat cells of the alveoli epithelium and the endothelial cells of the capillaries constitute the membrane through which the anaesthetic agents will pass until they attain the same partial pressure on each side. The process of blood saturation is also influenced by the rate of blood flow through the lungs. For example, anaesthetic-induced reduction of cardiac output will delay induction of anaesthesia.

Another factor to be considered is that the respiratory dead-space comprises more than the volume of the conducting passages. That portion of the inspired gases which traverses the conducting passages and enters the alveoli is always called the alveolar ventilation but not all of this alveolar ventilation is equally effective in arterializing the mixed venous blood, or in adding or subtracting anaesthetic agents to this blood. There may be areas of the lung which are ventilated but have no blood flowing through their capillary network. The inspired gases that enter these areas are wasted; the animal must expend energy to move this gas back and forth, but this achieves no respiratory function. This condition may also vary in degree — some alveoli may have blood flowing through them but have ventilation far in excess of that necessary for the equilibration of the blood, so that a proportion of the ventilation which enters these alveoli is also wasted. The total wasted gas is called *alveolar dead-space* gas. The volume of this alveolar dead-space gas, however, is not the total volume of all the alveoli which either have no blood flow or excessive ventilation but only the volume of the inspired gas which is *wasted* in these alveoli on each breath. It therefore fills no physical or anatomical space as does the gas in the conducting passages and cannot be included in the anatomical dead-space. Together with the anatomical dead-space it is known as the *physiological dead-space*. Clearly, the physiological dead-space will be increased in pathological conditions of the lung and the presence of such conditions will interfere with the passage of gases and vapours to and from the blood.

Gas exchange within the alveoli also depends on the rate at which the gases are delivered to them or removed from them by the pulmonary circulation. Pulmonary capillary blood flow is pulsatile and this allows more time for equilibration between the blood and alveolar gas but it varies with the heartbeat and the degree of inflation of the lungs. It is restricted by increased vascular resistance in the pulmonary circulation as may occur when the chest is open, with varying degrees of vascular occlusion (embolism), venous to arterial shunts, cardiac failure or anaesthetic-induced cardiac depression, shock and lesions such as pulmonary fibrosis.

The final step in the process, circulation by the blood and diffusion into the tissues, results in the distribution of the anaesthetic agent throughout the body. Neither this distribution nor the rate of absorption by the cells is uniform; they vary with the differences in the blood supply and lipid content of the respective tissues. The brain is very vascular and has a high lipoid content and soon acquires a concentration of the anaesthetic equal to that in the blood. Cerebral function is thus depressed early in the process of induction of anaesthesia. If the anaesthetic is administered for only a short time, recovery of consciousness will be accelerated by the distribution of the drug from the brain to the other tissues of the body. On the other hand, if the administration is continued until the whole body is saturated with the drug, recovery of consciousness will be slower because of the absence of a tension gradient between the brain and the other tissues.

Because of their irritant nature or pungency the vapours of most of the volatile liquid anaesthetics can only be inhaled when given in low concentrations so

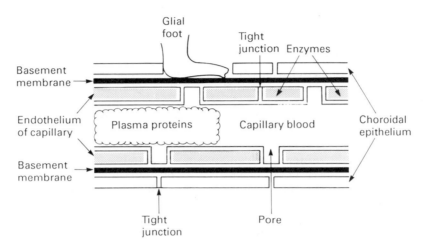

Fig. 3.2 Diagramatic illustration of the blood–brain barrier.

that the three phases of transference from the alveolar air to the tissues occupies an appreciable time. Gases such as nitrous oxide are not irritant to the respiratory tract; they can be administered in high concentrations so that their partial pressures in the lung alveoli soon become high and diffusion into the blood and body tissues is rapid.

Elimination of inhalation anaesthetics from the body takes place largely by a reversal of this process. The partial pressure of the anaesthetic in the alveoli falls below that in the blood so that the tension gradient is reversed and the agent passes from the tissues to the blood, from the blood to the alveolar air and from there, by exhalation, to the atmosphere. During anaesthesia a small quantity of the anaesthetic is lost from the body through the skin and from any operation wound. Limited metabolism also occurs.

Most drugs at some stage have to cross a capillary wall. Lipid-soluble drugs pass almost instantaneously across the whole surface of the capillary endothelium. Poorly lipid-soluble agents can cross through 'pores' in the membrane which have a variable size and pass between the endothelial cells; they then transit the enclosing basement membrane. Thus, for almost all drugs the only factor which significantly delays absorption from the bloodstream is plasma protein binding. Since the capillary wall does not represent a significant barrier to the passage of any drug (the blood–brain barrier being a notable exception) the factors which limit intravascular absorption from a subcutaneous or intramuscular site are local tissue binding, aqueous solubility and capillary blood flow. 'Depot' preparations, designed to slow absorption

from an injection site, are produced by the pharmaceutical incorporation of lipid-soluble factors. Also, the larger the particle size the less the surface area per unit volume and the slower the absorption.

Anaesthetic drugs have to reach the brain by crossing the blood–brain barrier (Fig. 3.2), which is both anatomical and enzymatic. The anatomical barrier arises because the capillaries in the central nervous system are unusual in possessing either close ('tight') junctions between their endothelial cells, an investment of neuroglial tissue ('glial feet') or, in the case of the choroid plexuses, an overlying modified ependymal layer — the choroidal epithelium — which has tight junctions. Lipid-soluble drugs penetrate this barrier by simple diffusion into the neuraxis and cerebrospinal fluid. Access by highly charged molecules is prevented unless the protective membranes have been disrupted by pathological conditions. The enzymatic barrier is due to the presence of enzymes in the cells lining the brain capillaries — for example, acetyl- and butyrylcholinesterases which preclude the entry of substances inactivated by either of these enzymes from entering the cerebrospinal tissue in significant concentrations. The ependyma lining the ventricles is not limited by either tight junctions or by glial feet so that drugs given experimentally into the cerebrospinal fluid do not encounter a blood–brain barrier. In addition, the blood–brain barrier does not seem to prevent drug access to either the chemoreceptor trigger zone of the vomiting centre or the anterior hypothalamic centres associated with temperature regulation.

MODE OF ACTION OF ANAESTHETIC DRUGS

The mechanism by which drugs produce anaesthesia is unknown and is likely to remain so until numerous questions are answered by research workers. The two main questions are obvious — how do anaesthetic agents work at cellular or subcellular levels and how do such actions produce the familiar clinical manifestations of general anaesthesia? When attempts are made to answer these questions many more problems are encountered because of the present inadequate understanding of fundamental aspects of biochemistry and neurophysiology. The relevance of research in these fields to clinical situations is often not appreciated because it is carried out in many diverse subjects and the results are often published in specialist journals using language which is difficult, if not impossible, for the average clinician to understand. This research can be given only brief consideration here: excellent reviews include those of Halsey [1, 2].

There is an excellent correlation between anaesthetic potency and hydrophobic solubility. Meyer in 1899 [3] and Overton in 1901 [4] postulated that the molar concentration of anaesthetic at the hydrophobic site of action was independent of any particular agent and could be represented by a constant, K. According to Halsey [2] this constant is equal to the minimal alveolar concentration (MAC) times the hydrophobic solubility and he has calculated that the mean value of K is 0.05 mol of anaesthetic per litre of hydrophobic membrane (range 0.03–0.1 mol/L). This relationship holds good for anaesthetics ranging from methoxyflurane to nitrous oxide and the implication of this hydrophobic solubility correlation is that the molecular sites of all anaesthetics are between the hydrophobic areas of membrane lipids or inside protein hydrophobic clefts of the neuronal membranes. This theory explains why anaesthetic potency increases when an animal's core temperature falls, since hydrophobic solubility increases and hence the required MAC decreases in order to maintain the same concentration, K, at the site of action. Agreement on molecular mechanisms of anaesthesia begins and ends at this point.

Suitable hydrophobic sites are found in both the protein and lipid regions of nerve cell membranes. The proteins are believed to control the membrane functions such as ion fluxes, transmitter release and receptor interactions, while the physical states of the surrounding lipids affect the activity in the proteins. The lipids are thought by some workers to be in a constant state of fluidity and as temperature rises a phase transition is said to take place between a gel state and a liquid crystalline phase. This phase transition is assumed to be altered by anaesthetics in such a way that the lipids become more fluid, in turn upsetting the functions of the neuronal membrane proteins. Opponents of this view point out that the changes in fluidity are very small when anaesthetics are present in anaesthetic concentrations, while the effect of changing temperature should be much greater than has been observed. It is possible that these conflicting views arise from the fact that to date only idealized membrane systems have been studied in any detail.

The alternative site of action for anaesthetics is in the different proteins in the cell membrane and several studies have made it clear that anaesthetics in clinical concentrations can bind to hydrophobic sites within proteins. A full review of the evidence for lipid and protein sites of action has been given by Dluzewski and coworkers [5]. Techniques for investigating anaesthetic–protein interactions are becoming more delicate and it should soon be possible to decide if the direct interactions are the critical factors in mechanisms of anaesthesia. At the moment it would seem likely that *both* lipids and proteins are concerned with anaesthetic interactions and the relative importance of the different membrane components depends on the particular anaesthetic agent.

Pressure reversal of some of the effects of anaesthetics has been observed in man and other animals, i.e. subjects anaesthetized with a wide range of agents apparently wake up despite the continued presence of the anaesthetic agent when the environmental pressure is raised to between 10 and 100 atm. An early explanation for this [6] was that anaesthesia occurs when the volume of a hydrophobic region was expanded beyond a certain critical volume by the absorption of molecules of the anaesthetic agent and that if the volume of this hydrophobic region could be restored by the application of pressure or temperature then anaesthesia would cease. This hypothesis assumed that all anaesthetics acted on the same molecular site, but later studies with a wide range of agents have suggested this to be an oversimplification. As a result of these studies Halsey and his coworkers [7] postulated that the *in vivo* sites of anaesthetic action do not behave as a simple bulk solvent but have limited capacities and molecular sites which are not the same for all anaesthetics — the so-called 'multisite expansion hypothesis'. The *in vivo* concept is consistent with *in vitro* actions of anaesthetics on both lipids and different proteins in the nerve cell membranes.

For many years it has been accepted that general anaesthetics depress synaptic transmission of nerve impulses and, unlike local analgesics, leave axonal conduction of nerve impulses unimpeded [8]. The most sensitive component of synaptic transmission is either the release of neurotransmitters from their synaptic vesicles along the synaptic cleft or the subsequent interaction between these and the receptor proteins. Different anaesthetics have either pre- or postsynaptic actions *in vitro* depending on which of the two functions are affected. It is not yet known whether the affected neurotransmitters have excitatory or inhibitory actions. They could depress excitatory synaptic transmission or enhance inhibitory transmission or act to disturb the balance between the two components.

The identification of specific opioid receptors and enkephalins has inspired much research and given rise to new interpretations of the analgesic properties of many drugs. As surmised by Goldstein [9]: 'It may be that general anaesthetic agents release enkephalin (or other endorphins) at opioid receptor sites in the pain pathways and it is even possible that the analgesic component of general anaesthesia is due to this enkephalin release. There is no reason to think, however, that the other phenomena characteristic of general anaesthesia are due to the release of endogenous opioid peptides.' The discovery of other substance-specific receptors in the central nervous system has suggested how combinations of drugs which do not themselves produce general anaesthesia (e.g. opioids and benzodiazepines) may induce a state very similar to it. In addition, the recent demonstration that phencyclidine and ketamine may, by occupying specific receptor sites, actually damage cells in rats' brains indicates that some drug side-effects, such as ketamine-induced hallucinations in human patients, may be due to such damage in addition to activity at opioid σ receptors.

In order to explain how these various actions produce anaesthesia it is now postulated that they occur in one region in the central nervous system which by its inter-relations with other systems brings about a general effect. The one region is, in the main, in the brain stem reticular information and its thalamic extensions ('the sensorimotor modulation system'), fed by the spinoreticular tracts [10]. This system projects to the mesencephalon and thence to the thalamic and subthalamic nuclei and receives downward projections from all the primary sensory cortical areas, the wealth of afferent and efferent connections indicating a correlational activity for the system. Anaesthetics may act by switching off excitatory systems and turning on inhibitory ones so that impulses from the periphery to the brain are blocked mainly at the ventrobasal thalamic level, whilst a similar action on the fusimotor system may explain the loss of motor control associated with general anaesthesia.

ELECTRICAL ACTIVITY OF THE BRAIN

Throughout all animal species when aggregates of neurones are organized into functional units by mutual intercommunication, they produce rhythmical electrical activity that oscillates within fairly narrow frequency limits. The study of such activity of the brain constitutes the field of electroencephalography. The dimensions of the electrical activity of the brain reflect the metabolic state of the millions of neurones of which it is comprised. Analysis of the records of such activity (electroencephalograms or EEGs) during an operation may, therefore, reveal to the anaesthetist not only the extent to which the patient's cerebral metabolism is specifically modified by the anaesthetic agents, but also the degree to which this pharmacological action is being influenced by the variations in circulatory, respiratory and general biochemical functions of the individual animal that arise during the course of surgical procedures [11].

In clinical practice, cerebral electrical activity is recorded from electrodes held in contact with the scalp and arranged in relation to the underlying anatomical regions of the brain. The techniques of electroencephalography (like those of anaesthesia) cannot be learnt from books; adequate skill can only be acquired by practical experience gained under the supervision of a properly qualified teacher. While a detailed analysis of the sequence of electroencephalographic changes associated with anaesthesia in man is available, little information relating to animals has been reported and, therefore, the value of electroencephalography in veterinary anaesthesia is largely unexplored.

The brain waves that are recorded from the surface of the head by clinical electroencephalography are oscillations of electrical potential generated in the cerebral cortex and modified by the resistance of the tissues (meninges, skull and scalp) through which they pass. Each component wave is the integrated envelope of the synchronous discharges of a large number of cortical units. The potential oscillations are generated mainly in the dendrites of the cortical neurones and the degree of synchronization between different cortical units varies from time to time and with alterations in the prevailing environmental circumstances. Furthermore, the synchronization of these cortical dendritic potentials is regulated from neurones located in the brain stem, from which axons ascend into the cerebral cortex to synapse with the cortical neurones.

Although changes in the EEG obtained from various electrode configurations give a crude index of cerebral activity it is difficult to display the signals in such a way as to be of use to the anaesthetist. The difficulty has been overcome to some extent by a device which filters a bipolar EEG to exclude frequencies other than 2–15 Hz — the so-called *cerebral monitor*. In this device appropriate rectification, amplification and display on a slow-moving paper chart yield what has been termed the 'integrated EEG'. The width of the trace indicates the character of the cerebral activity and the height from the baseline is a measure of the quantity of electrical activity. Integrated EEG assessment may be of use in routine anaesthesia but its value in veterinary practice has still to be determined.

Both inhalation and intravenous anaesthetics produce a dose-related depression of amplitude and a dose-related increase in latency of cortical evoked responses [12]. Latency is defined as the time from the stimulus until the first major negative peak occurs in the EEG (conventionally an upward peak). The amplitude of the evoked response is defined as the size of the response from the negative peak to the succeeding positive valley. Evoked responses are claimed to overcome many of the objections to monitoring the EEG as a measure of anaesthetic effects but this type of monitoring is not continuous and there is as yet little experience of its use in veterinary anaesthesia.

'SIGNS AND STAGES' OF ANAESTHESIA

In the past it was customary to divide the transition from consciousness to complete surgical anaesthesia into a number of 'stages' or 'levels'. The so-called 'classical signs' of anaesthesia, such as have been tabulated in earlier editions of this book and in most of the older textbooks on anaesthesia, were provided by the presence or absence of reflex responses in the anaesthetized subject to stimuli provided by the anaesthetist or surgeon. Particular clinical signs of anaesthesia were, therefore, equated with particular anatomical 'levels' or 'planes' of depression of the central nervous system. These signs were often likened to a series of landmarks used to assess the progress made on a journey. Such empirical, traditional methods of assessing the progress of anaesthesia and the anatomical implications that went with these methods incorporated a fallacy, because they took no account of time — and the changing function in any biological system can only be assessed scientifically in terms of magnitude and time. A depth of unconsciousness is really a particular moment in a continuous temporal stream of neurological phenomena to be interpreted by the magnitude and quality of these phenomena that obtain at that moment. Thus, there can be no such thing as the 'maintenance of an even plane of anaesthesia over a period of time', and the anaesthetist must appreciate that the whole idea of levels of anaesthesia is a purely neurological conception born towards the end of last century. This may once have had the virtue of simplicity but it bears no relation to the realities of physiology and pharmacology as they are now understood in the latter part of the twentieth century [11].

As applied to general anaesthesia the hierarchical model of neurological organization assumed that the cerebral cortex, being the most recently acquired portion of the central nervous system and, therefore, responsible for the maintenance of consciousness,

was the first part of the brain to be affected during the induction of anaesthesia. When its function was abolished, consciousness was lost and the 'lower' parts of the brain were released from the normal inhibiting influence of the cerebral cortex to become more active. Then, as unconsciousness deepened, various hypothetical centres were thought to be depressed in sequence from above down until only the neurones in the medulla and spinal cord continued to function and maintain life. The advances of neurology, particularly in the last 20 years, have made this concept quite untenable.

Starting with the definition given on p. 37 it is clear that the threshold event is *the loss of consciousness*. This being so, it follows that anaesthesia is an all-or-none phenomenon and there *cannot* be degrees of anaesthesia nor can there be variable depths of anaesthesia. All the other attributes of anaesthetics, the drugs used to produce the state of anaesthesia, can be classed as alternative pharmacological properties of the drugs and not as *components* of anaesthesia. There can, however, be degrees or depths of *unconsciousness* and these are commonly assessed by seeking signs of autonomic nervous system activity such as arterial hypertension, tachycardia, sweating, lacrimation, facial muscle movements and other muscle activity — reflex signs termed by Sherrington 'pseudaffective' reflexes. These reflexes occur simultaneously with the *perception* of unpleasant sensory experiences [13, 14] and are particularly prominent when evoked by stimulation of abdominal or thoracic viscera. The continuation of noxious stimulation into the postanaesthetic period also provokes a metabolic and endocrine response [15] but there are of little value to the anaesthetist in assessing depth of unconsciousness during surgical anaesthesia.

Use of the term 'depth of anaesthesia' is now so ingrained in common usage that it must be accepted since it probably cannot be eradicated. It is important, however, to realize that it commonly refers to depression of brain function beyond that necessary for the production of *anaesthesia*, i.e. unawareness of surroundings and absence of recall of events.

In general, the volatile anaesthetic agents halothane, enflurane and isoflurane produce a dose-dependent decrease in arterial blood pressure and many veterinary anaesthetists use this depression to assess the depth of anaesthesia. The effect is not so marked during anaesthetic techniques involving the administration of opioid analgesics and nitrous oxide. If the depth of unconsciousness is adequate, surgical stimulation does not cause any change in arterial blood pressure. There are, however, many other factors which influence the arterial blood pressure during surgery such as the circulating blood volume, cardiac output and the influence of drug therapy before anaesthesia. If ketamine or high doses of opioids are given, arterial blood pressure may change very little if the depth of unconsciousness is increased by the administration of higher concentrations of inhalation anaesthetics.

Changes in heart rate alone are a poor guide to changes in the depth of unconsciousness. The heart rate may increase under isoflurane and enflurane anaesthesia due to their direct effect on the myocardium. Arrhythmias are common during light levels of unconsciousness induced by halothane when they are usually due to increased sympathetic activity. In general, however, tachycardia in the absence of any other cause may be taken to represent inadequate anaesthesia for the procedure being undertaken.

All anaesthetic agents cause a dose-related reduction in muscle tone. Overdosage produces complete respiratory muscle paralysis. In the absence of neuromuscular blocking drugs the degree of muscle relaxation may, therefore, usually be used as a measure of the depth of anaesthetic-induced unconsciousness. With the use of neuromuscular blocking drugs, muscle relaxation usually gives no useful information of the depth of anaesthesia although even in the presence of apparently adequate doses of neuromuscular blockers it is not uncommon to observe movements of facial muscles, swallowing or chewing movements in response to surgical stimulation if the depth of unconsciousness becomes inadequate.

Anaesthetic agents affect respiration in a dose-dependent manner and this was responsible for the original classification of the 'depth of anaesthesia'. In deeply anaesthetized animals, tidal and minute volumes are decreased and eventually respiration ceases. Inadequate anaesthesia is often indicated by an increase in the rate and/or depth of breathing. Unfortunately, respiratory rate is also often increased during deep levels of unconsciousness and the unwary may be tempted to administer more anaesthetic agent in the mistaken impression that awareness is imminent. Laryngeal spasm, coughing or breath holding can indicate excessive airway stimulation or inadequate depth of unconsciousness. Needless to say, the neuromuscular blocking agents rob the anaesthetist of the signs of respiration as a guide to the depth of unconsciousness.

Sweating (in those animals which do) and lacrimation may both occur if surgical stimulation is intense while the depth of unconsciousness is too light. Autonomic stimulation commonly leads to sweating in horses and drugs that modify autonomic effects may also modify sweating responses.

It must be clearly recognized, however, that muscle relaxation and suppression of autonomic activity are not *components* of anaesthesia. Rather they must be considered as desirable supplements to the state of anaesthesia as a means to enable surgery to be performed [16]. Any reliable indicator that the level of unconsciousness is adequate to ensure lack of awareness in the presence of muscle relaxant drugs is highly desirable but, unfortunately, it seems that it does not exist. At the moment, all that can be done is to utilize doses of anaesthetics which, from past experience, have been found to prevent signs of awareness from appearing in similar animals breathing spontaneously during operations when relaxant drugs have not been used.

When animals are breathing spontaneously there are several signs which are generally recognized as indicating that the depth of unconsciousness is adequate for the performance of painful procedures, i.e. the animal is unaware of the environment and of the infliction of pain — it is anaesthetized. Unfortunately, there are many differences between the various species of animal in the signs which are usually used. One fairly reliable sign is that of eyeball movement, especially in horses and cattle. Fortunately for the animal this test involves inspection only and no touching of the delicate cornea and conjunctiva although it may be necessary to separate the eyelids because these are usually closed. Very slow nystagmus in both horses and cattle and downward inclination of the eyeballs in pigs and dogs indicates a satisfactory level of unconsciousness and, at this level, breathing should be smooth although its rate and depth may alter depending on the prevailing severity of the surgical stimulation. Nystagmus is also seen in horses just before death from hypoxaemia. Absence of the lash or palpebral reflex (closure of the eyelids in response to light stroking of the eyelashes) is another reasonably reliable guide to satisfactory anaesthesia. In dogs and cats it is safe to assume that if the mouth can be opened without provoking yawning or curling of the tongue, central depression is adequate. In all animals, salivation and excessive lacrimation usually indicate a returning awareness. Disappearance of head shaking or whisker twitching in response to gentle scratching of the inside of the ear pinna is a good sign of unawareness in pigs, cats, rabbits and guinea pigs. Pupil size is a most unreliable guide to unawareness because a dose of an opioid tends to cause constriction of the pupils while atropine causes dilation. The pupils do, however, dilate when an overdose of an anaesthetic has been given or when awareness is imminent.

The experienced anaesthetist relies most of the time on an animal's response to stimuli produced by the surgeon or procedure to indicate that the depth of unconsciousness is adequate. Effective anaesthesia is that which just obliterates the animal's response to pain and/or discomfort without depressing respiratory and circulatory function.

MINIMUM ALVEOLAR CONCENTRATION (MAC) AND MINIMUM INFUSION RATE (MIR)

Recognition of the problems in establishing that the patient is unconscious at any given moment together with the difficulty of reproducing the same degree of central nervous depression on another occasion led Merkel and Eger in 1963 [17] to propose the concept of the minimal alveolar anaesthetic concentration (MAC). In animals or in man, MAC is defined as the alveolar concentration of an anaesthetic that prevents muscular movement in response to a painful stimulus in 50% of test subjects. If adequate time is allowed for the anaesthetic in the brain to equilibrate with the anaesthetic in the blood, the alveolar partial pressure of the anaesthetic (which can be measured) is a reasonably accurate expression of the anaesthetic state. The stimulus, standardized as far as possible, usually consists of tail clamping in animals or surgical incision in man.

The measurement of MAC enables the relative potencies of anaesthetics to be compared, and with the MAC defined as 1.0, the level of central nervous depression can be stated as the ratio of the alveolar concentration to the MAC. This reproducible method may be contrasted with the difficulty in using physiological parameters as an indication, or the EEG which varies according to the agent used.

Other methods are possible and depression of synaptic transmission has been used for the same purpose [18]. Any well-defined response to a standard stimulus should be equally satisfactory provided the alveolar or arterial blood anaesthetic concentration is accurately measured. For example, in man (but not in animals such as dogs) oesophageal motility has been advocated as an indicator of depth of unconsciousness [19].

Although the MAC value represents the anaesthetizing dose for only 50% of subjects the anaesthetist can be reasonably certain that increasing the dose to 1.1 or 1.15 times MAC will ensure satisfactory anaesthesia in the vast majority of individuals because the dose–response curve will be relatively steep. In veterinary practice it is also important to note that, according to Eger [20], the variability of MAC is remarkably low between species and is quite constant from animal to animal. Unfortunately, measurement of the concentration of anaesthetic in the end-tidal gas requires expensive apparatus (see p. 34) and until such a time as this becomes readily available the concept of MAC is only likely to be of much practical value to veterinary anaesthetists using non-rebreathing systems incorporating accurate vaporizers for volatile anaesthetics.

The accurate control of depth of unconsciousness is even more difficult to achieve with intravenous anaesthetic agents than it is with inhalational agents. To obtain unconsciousness they must be administered at a rate which produces a concentration of drug in the bloodstream sufficient to result in the required depth of depression of the central nervous system [21]. The concept of minimum infusion rate (MIR) was introduced by Sear and Prys-Roberts in 1979 [22] to define the median effective dose (ED_{50}) of an intravenous anaesthetic agent which would prevent movement in response to surgical incision. Unlike the minimal alveolar concentration (MAC) of an inhalation anaesthetic, however, the MIR does not necessarily equate with the concentration of the anaesthetic in the blood [23]. In veterinary anaesthesia there is a paucity of information relating to the MIR and since there is no way of estimating the concentration of the agent in the blood sufficiently rapidly to enable the anaesthetist to adjust the rate of administration during any operation in the light of the analytical result, its usefulness in clinical anaesthesia is questionable. It may, of course, be of value in setting infusion rates in computer-controlled intravenous anaesthesia but the advent of such techniques in veterinary anaesthesia has yet to arrive.

INTRAVENOUS VERSUS INHALATION ANAESTHESIA

Although ether and chloroform had been shown to produce anaesthesia in animals by 1847, the conditions under which veterinarians so often had to operate prevented the development of inhalation anaesthesia. Injectable substances proved more convenient and the introduction of the hypodermic syringe and hollow needle enabled Humbert to describe the use of chloral hydrate in horses in 1875 [24]. The 1930s saw the development of barbiturate anaesthesia and by the middle of this century veterinary anaesthesia in most parts of the world involved little more than the administration of intravenous agents. However, the limitations of the available drugs were becoming recognized and, following the introduction of balanced anaesthetic techniques into small animal practice [25], the use of inhalation agents started to gain in popularity. The development of inhalation anaesthesia was boosted by the advent of halothane, first used in veterinary

anaesthesia in 1956 [26], and today probably most anaesthetics given to veterinary patients involve the use of inhalation techniques of some type. Atmospheric pollution results from spillage of gases and vapours into the air and attention was later drawn to possible hazards which might arise from this. Potential hazards to operating theatre personnel (p. 393) coupled with the synthesis of new intravenous agents are once again focusing attention on intravenous anaesthesia.

Intravenous anaesthetics are particularly useful for the induction of anaesthesia which is to be maintained by an inhalation technique, or where the operation to be performed is of relatively short duration and the induction dose can be relied on to give full anaesthesia for an adequate time. At the moment, however, there appears to be no intravenous agent which is really suitable for the maintenance of anaesthesia over prolonged periods.

EFFECTS OF GENERAL ANAESTHESIA UPON THE BODY

The distribution of anaesthetics throughout the tissues means that they will have widespread effects in the body but these effects are not entirely due to their local actions. Many organs are under nervous control and since the central nervous system is the principal site at which anaesthetics act it is obvious that any depression or stimulation of centres in this target area may have secondary effects elsewhere in the body. Clearly, the safe, rational administration of an anaesthetic is only possible if these local and secondary effects are understood.

Effects on respiration

The breathing pattern of a spontaneously breathing anaesthetized animal differs from normal in several respects. First, the expiratory muscles become active and inspiratory muscle tone ceases abruptly at the end of inspiration so that the expiratory waveform approximates to an exponential decay [27]. Secondly, the regularity of breathing may be disturbed. Irregular breathing patterns can often be correlated with varying intensity of surgical stimulation but some animals, particularly horses, often develop 'periodic breathing' where two, three or four breaths are followed by cessation of breathing for many seconds. The cause of 'periodic breathing' is not known.

Depression of the carbon dioxide/ventilation response by anaesthetics is well known, as is the progressive loss of the intercostal component of breathing with deepening anaesthesia, but only

recently have these two been connected. It has been demonstrated that the normal ventilatory response to carbon dioxide is largely achieved by increase in intercostal activity and loss of the contribution of intercostal muscles accounts for much of the reduction in response to carbon dioxide observed during anaesthesia [28].

Until quite recently, anaesthetists were reassured by the teaching that anaesthetics had little if any effect on the hypoxic drive to breathing. Unfortunately, at least in man, this comfortable doctrine has now been shown to be untrue, for the hypoxic drive is not so much depressed as abolished by halothane [29]. Thus, it seems likely that far from being a rugged protective reflex, the hypoxic drive to ventilation may be sensitive to anaesthesia and affected even at subanaesthetic concentrations of inhalation anaesthetics. The horse seems to be an exception, for it is not difficult to demonstrate a hypoxic respiratory drive in an anaesthetized horse. The clinical implications are important. First, an anaesthetized animal, other than a horse, may not respond to hypoxia by hyperventilation and no reliance should be placed on this as a monitor of hypoxia. Secondly, it can be expected that anaesthesia will arrest the breathing of many animals which have lost their sensitivity to carbon dioxide (e.g. bronchitic dogs). Thirdly, there is an obvious hazard in anaesthetizing an animal at high altitude where the partial pressure of oxygen is low [30].

It is often assumed that general anaesthesia is

associated with a reduction in oxygen consumption but there seems to be no real evidence that values under anaesthesia differ from those in well-rested or sedated animals. The respiratory quotient is probably unaltered by anaesthesia except for animals given intravenous glucose where the respiratory quotient is usually unity. Hypothermia reduces, and hyperthermia increases, oxygen consumption and consumption is also greatly increased by shivering occurring in the recovery period.

Pulmonary ventilation can vary between very wide limits in anaesthetized animals and during spontaneous breathing the minute volume is governed by the balance between the depressant effects of the anaesthetic drugs and the stimulation of surgery. Measurement of the ventilation during anaesthesia is often made in the absence of surgical stimulation and hence the results of many research studies must be viewed with caution since they tend to emphasize the very low levels of ventilation which may occur under these circumstances.

Endotracheal intubation both bypasses a large part of the animal's respiratory dead-space and results in the imposition of a smaller external dead-space than if a face mask is used. In general, however, the reduction in dead-space by endotracheal intubation is offset by the increase caused by anaesthesia. Much of this increase may be due to the use of atropine which can increase anatomical dead-space by 20–50% depending on the state of vagal tone and the dose of atropine given. The dead-space/tidal volume ratio is usually larger because of the reduction in tidal volume caused by anaesthesia and the approximation of the dead-space volume towards a normal value means that often well over half the tidal volume may

be wasted as far as alveolar ventilation is concerned. What is a normal respiratory minute volume in the awake animal may, therefore, produce severe hypoventilation under anaesthesia. Animals left to breathe spontaneously during anaesthesia with nitrous oxide supplemented by volatile agents such as halothane, or intravenous drugs such as opioid, tend to develop hypercapnia. It is normal British practice to tolerate arterial carbon dioxide tensions (P_aCO_2) of up to 8 kPa (60 mmHg) in anaesthetized spontaneously breathing animals and there is no evidence to suggest that healthy animals suffer as a consequence. In the USA and elsewhere any degree of hypoventilation is often regarded with great concern and it is customary in many centres to assist ventilation in such a way as to keep the P_aCO_2 at around normal (conscious) levels, but there is no evidence that the P_aCO_2 level found in a normal conscious animal is the optimum level for that animal when anaesthetized. Preoccupation with the maintenance of near-normal (conscious) levels of P_aCO_2 may, moreover, lead to the effects of intermittent positive pressure lung ventilation on the circulation (see p. 140) being overlooked.

A consistent feature of all types of general anaesthesia is a reduction in functional residual capacity (FRC), the magnitude of which is related to the posture of the anaesthetized animal. In many cases the reduction is sufficiently great to bring the lung volume close to residual volume and below that at which airways tend to close. This results in regions of the lung with greatly diminished or absent ventilation but unchanged vascular perfusion. Following equilibration of gas trapped by airway closure with pulmonary artery blood, circulation through these areas will

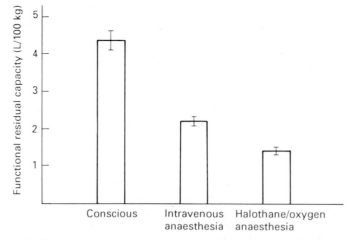

Fig. 3.3 Effect of anaesthesia on lung volume in the horse. Mean values with SEM from three ponies positioned in left decubitus after fasting for 18 hours. (From McDonell, 'The effect of anaesthesia on pulmonary gas exchange and arterial oxygenation in the horse', Ph.D. Thesis, University of Cambridge.)

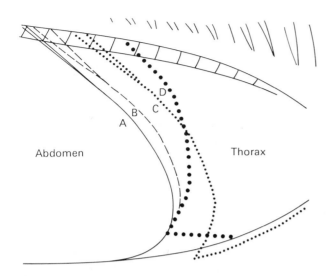

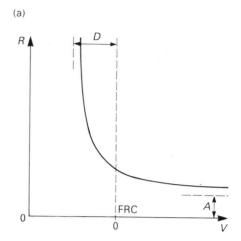

Fig. 3.4 Composite line drawing illustrating changes in the diaphragmatic outline with anaesthesia and positional changes: A, conscious and standing; B, anaesthetized, sternal recumbency; C, anaesthetized, supine; D, anaesthetized, left decubitus. (Redrawn from data presented by McDonell *et al.* (1979) *Equine Veterinary Journal* **11**, 24).

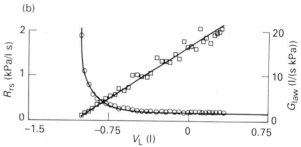

Fig. 3.5 (a) Airway resistance (*R*) is a hyperbolic function of lung volume (V), rising sharply as the lung volume decreases below functional residual capacity (FRC). Induction of anaesthesia, by decreasing lung volume, generally increases airway resistance. (After Jordan *et al.* (1981) *Journal of Applied Physiology: Respiratory, Environmental and Exercise Physiology* **52**, 715.) (b) Computer-generated plot of total respiratory resistance (R_{rs}, ○) and lower-airway conductance (G_{law}, □) against lung volume from FRC in a dog. (From Watney *et al.* (1988) *British Journal of Anaesthesia* **61**, 407).

constitute a shunt through which mixed venous blood flows to the arterial side of the circulation. There can be little doubt that this phenomenon is a factor in the increased alveolar–arterial oxygen tension differences encountered during anaesthesia, especially in horses.

The reduction in FRC would appear to be due, at least partly, to a change in the end-expiratory position of the diaphragm, for radiographic studies have shown the diaphragm to be displaced anteriorly into the chest following the induction of anaesthesia. The reason why induction of anaesthesia should cause the end-expiratory position of the diaphragm to change is not at all clear. Another factor responsible for the reduction of FRC from that found in the standing animal is probably loss of tone in the serratus ventralis muscles. The standing animal's body is normally slung between the scapulae by the serratus ventralis muscles which tend to pull the chest wall outwards but this pull is lost when the animal becomes recumbent and serratus muscle tone is lost.

Airway resistance is a hyperbolic function of lung volume, rising sharply in a hyperbolic manner as the lung volume decreases below FRC (Fig. 3.5) and hence the reduction of FRC consequent upon the induction of anaesthesia is associated with an increase in airway resistance. However, this effect may be counteracted by the bronchodilator effect of agents such as halothane. To a large extent these effects cancel each other out but small changes may be observed in either direction [30]. Pulmonary compliance is, like airway resistance, related to lung

volume and, unfortunately, most compliance measurements made in anaesthetized animals have not been related to lung volume so that the effects of anaesthesia on compliance are unknown for most species of animal. As a general rule, the compliance of the lungs can be expected to be reduced during anaesthesia when compared to the conscious state.

Available evidence suggests that the disturbance of the normal relationships between ventilation and perfusion encountered during general anaesthesia result from both anaesthesia and postural changes [31, 32]. For any given degree of mismatching of ventilation and perfusion within the lungs the alveolar–arterial oxygen tension difference is a function of the inspired oxygen tension and it is probable that in the majority of animal species a satisfactory $P_{a}O_2$ can only be obtained by keeping the oxygen content of the inspired gases above 30%. In particular, it would appear to be unwise to allow horses recovering from anaesthesia to breathe air which is not enriched with oxygen until they are sitting up or standing, but the problems involved in administering oxygen at this time are not always easy to solve.

Effects on the circulation

Many of the changes seen in cardiovascular function during anaesthesia may be directly related to the anaesthetic agents themselves but some are secondary to effects produced by these agents on pulmonary ventilation and on activity in the autonomic nervous system. The observed changes result from integration of these effects and differ according to the agents employed. It is, therefore, very difficult to ascribe any changes in cardiovascular function to anaesthesia itself.

The effect of some procedures used during anaesthesia is more readily understandable. For example, cardiac output depends on the venous return which itself depends on the existence of a pressure gradient from the peripheral to the great veins. Thus, if other factors remain constant any rise in the mean intrathoracic pressure causes a reduction in venous return to the right side of the heart and a fall in cardiac output. From this it is clear that the application of positive end-expiratory pressure (PEEP) to the airway in an attempt to minimize the reduction in FRC due to anaesthesia can, by simply raising the mean intrathoracic pressure, result in a severe fall in cardiac output (33). The use of inappropriate pressure waveforms during intermittent positive pressure ventilation of the lungs (IPPV) in animals with intact chest walls may also have a similar effect on venous return to the heart and cardiac output.

In supine anaesthetized animals with open chests, factors such as gravity, muscle pumps and the thoracic pump no longer contribute to the venous return and hence the sole remaining force for circulation of the blood must be in the heart itself — *viz à tergo* and *vis à fronte*. General anaesthetics, with the possible exception of certain agents such as ketamine, decrease myocardial contractility and hence this driving force. The completely supine posture should be avoided in grossly obese, heavily pregnant or herbivorous animals because the heavy abdominal contents may compress the posterior cava against the sublumbar muscles and seriously interfere with venous return from the hind end of the body.

Up to a certain rate the tachycardia produced by some general anaesthetics, or drugs such as atropine, may slightly increase the cardiac output but above this rate cardiac output decreases due to the relative change in durations of systole and diastole. An increase in rate usually shortens diastole whilst the period of systole remains constant but this shortening of diastole has little effect on ventricular filling until a critical rate is reached. Above this rate further increases encroach on the period of rapid ventricular filling and result in decreased end-diastolic volume which, in accordance with Starling's law, reduces stroke volume.

Effects on renal function

In general it can be said that anaesthesia produces a transient decrease in both renal blood flow and glomerular filtration rate, the degree of decrease depending on the dose of the agent in use. Renal vascular resistance is usually decreased and the filtration fraction increased. Autoregulation may or may not be abolished under general anaesthesia but it is known that it still occurs in isolated perfused kidneys subjected to the influence of halothane [34]. The renin–angiotensin mechanism may be involved in the reduction of renal blood flow and the increased vascular resistance because a high sodium intake may stop these from occurring in anaesthetized dogs [35].

Hypotensive anaesthesia causes a decrease in glomerular filtration rate for as long as the arterial pressure is low but the renal blood flow which shows an initial decline tends to return to near-normal values, presumably as further dilatation occurs in the renal vessels.

General anaesthesia is associated with an increased secretion of antidiuretic hormone, leading to a tendency towards water retention in the body for 24 hours or even longer after recovery from anaesthesia.

Effects on hepatic function

Adverse changes in liver function probably follow most surgical operations and it is difficult to establish whether these are due to anaesthesia or to surgery. Hepatic vasomotor control is minimal and a decrease in liver blood flow may be due to a decrease in either the portal vein or hepatic artery pressures. This can, in turn, be due to either increased splanchnic resistance, reduced systemic arterial or increased hepatic venous pressures.

In routine anaesthetic practice hypercapnia, hypocapnia, hyperoxia and hypoxia may be seen and knowledge of their effects is limited and sometimes contradictory. In one of the most recent studies [36] on intact greyhounds anaesthetized with pentobarbitone (which is claimed to have little effect on cardiovascular or hepatic haemodynamics) it was found the hyperoxia had no effect on hepatic blood flow, hypocapnia reduced it and that hypercapnia appeared to be beneficial in that it increased blood flow without increasing hepatic oxygen consumption. When the inspired oxygen level was reduced to produce hypoxia there was a small fall in portal venous flow and a larger decrease in hepatic arterial flow but these returned to normal values within 10 minutes. Although these effects are brief, hypoxia could be important in exacerbating hepatic injuries due to other agents.

USE OF OXYGEN IN VETERINARY PRACTICE

During air breathing extreme hyperventilation may raise the P_aO_2 to about 120 mmHg (16 kPa) and higher levels can only be obtained by oxygen enrichment of the inspired gas or by elevation of the ambient pressure. Although this will produce very great increases in P_aO_2 the increase in arterial oxygen content is, in normal subjects, quite small, since the effect is mainly confined to increasing the fraction in physical solution. Because of the shape of the oxyhaemoglobin dissociation curve the venous blood (which is in equilibrium with the tissues) will not become fully saturated until the ambient pressure is raised to more than 2 atm. It follows that the tissue oxygen tension is not raised to anything like P_aO_2 levels during the administration of oxygen at normal barometric pressures.

There are a number of indications for the oxygen enrichment of inspired gas at normal barometric pressure:

1. *The relief of tissue hypoxia.* Stagnant and anaemic hypoxia can be relieved by the inhalation of oxygen. The increase in P_aO_2 may be impressive but the content change is small and, therefore, the improvement in oxygen flux can only be minimal. Nevertheless, even a small improvement in oxygen flux may be worthwhile. Freeman [37] was able to show a reduced mortality in critically bled dogs following the administration of oxygen.
2. *Clearance of gas loculi in the body.* The principle here depends on reduction of the total tension of dissolved gases in the venous blood so that blood draining the tissues has a surplus capacity for carrying gas away from loculi. In normal animals breathing air the total gas tensions in venous blood are always about 53 mmHg (7 kPa) less than in arterial blood because the fall in oxygen tension between the arterial and venous blood is always about 10 times greater than the rise in carbon dioxide tension. This means that there is always a capacity to dissolve gas away from a loculus and ensures that all potential spaces (e.g. the pleural cavity) remain empty and can even sustain a pressure below atmospheric. When an animal breathes 100% oxygen the difference between the total gas tensions of the arterial and venous blood becomes even greater, the total tension in the venous blood becomes markedly subatmospheric and the venous blood has a greatly increased capacity to dissolve gas from loculi.

The use of oxygen to remove gas is indicated after air embolism and to reduce intestinal gas pressure in horses suffering from intestinal obstruction as well as to aid absorption of pneumothoraces.

3. *Carbon monoxide poisoning.* This is a well-recognized indication for oxygen therapy because it not only improves the oxygen content of arterial blood but also increases the clearance rate of carboxyhaemoglobin.

Oxygen toxicity

It seems extraordinary that oxygen, which is essential for the efficient synthesis of ATP required by all higher animals is, nevertheless, universally toxic. Toxicity is dependent on the partial pressure and the duration of exposure and is thus more likely to be encountered in hyperbaric oxygen than when oxygen is given at 1 atm pressure. For this reason, in veterinary practice oxygen toxicity is never likely to be a hazard of anaesthesia. Very high hyperbaric pressures of oxygen cause damage rapidly but the damage produced is not necessarily the same as that caused under normobaric conditions.

Research in oxygen toxicity is made difficult by the enormous species variation in susceptibility and wide intraspecies variation. In general, small animals are more susceptible than larger ones; the administration of 100% oxygen at 1 atm pressure kills mice in 1 or 2 days, dogs in 2–3 days and monkeys in approximately 2 weeks. Early respiratory distress is followed by severe dyspnoea, coughing and cyanosis, gasping respiration in the terminal stages and death in apnoea. This represents acute oxygen toxicity and is characterized by type-1 alveolar epithelial cell necrosis, endothelial cell damage, hyaline membrane formation, interstitial perivascular and intra-alveolar oedema and alveolar collapse. Lower doses of oxygen (e.g. exposure to 0.5–0.8 atm) are associated with the development of chronic oxygen toxicity in which the characteristic pathological changes are septal thickening and hyperplasia of type-2 alveolar epithelial cells. The acute and chronic changes probably merely represent a spectrum of response and the two types of lesion may coexist. Almost complete resolution of these changes can occur.

Mucociliary propulsion in the bronchioles and

trachea has been shown to be decreased in dogs breathing 100% oxygen [38] and the survival time of mice infected with influenza virus [39] is shortened by this treatment. Surfactant activity is also depressed, probably due to changes such as exudative oedema and its actual production may also be decreased. Central nervous oxygen toxicity, in the form of convulsions, only occurs at pressures above 2.5 atm and appears to be a function of P_aO_2 and not the arterial oxygen content.

The mode of action of oxygen toxicity is not understood and it is not clear how far it is due to oxygen itself and how far free radicals are involved. (Molecular oxygen contains two unpaired orbital electrons and, therefore, may be considered as a free radical.) Oxygen toxicity and the effects of irradiation have many common features and it is tempting to suppose that free radicals play a part in both processes [40].

In veterinary practice exposure of animals to high concentrations of oxygen at atmospheric pressures for long periods is seldom encountered and hyperbaric oxygen therapy is rarely practised, so toxicity is very unlikely to present problems. The main risk associated with the use of oxygen which veterinarians are likely to meet is that of fire. Fire risk is enormously increased when flammable material is exposed to an atmosphere of oxygen.

REFERENCES

1. Halsey, M. J. (1984) *British Journal of Anaesthesia* **56**, 98.
2. Halsey, M. J. (1986) *British Journal of Hospital Medicine*, December, p. 445.
3. Meyer, H. H. (1899) *Archiv Experimentell Pathologisch Pharmakologie* **421**, 109.
4. Overton, E. (1901) *Studien uber die Narkose*. Jena: G. Fischer.
5. Dluzewski, A. R., Halsey, M. J. and Simmonds, A. C. (1985) In *Molecular Aspects of Medicine* (eds H. Baum, J. Gergely and B. L. Fanburg), vol. 6, p. 459, Oxford: Pergamon Press.
6. Lever, M. J., Miller, K. V., Paton, W. D. M. and Smith, E. B. (1971) *Nature* **231**, 368.
7. Halsey, M. J., Wardley-Smith, B. and Green, C. J. (1978) *British Journal of Anaesthesia* **501**, 1091.
8. Larrabee, M. G. and Posternak, J. M. (1952) *Journal of Neurophysiology* **15**, 91.
9. Goldstein, A. (1978) *Anesthesiology* **491**, 1.
10. Angel, A. (1984) In *The Neurobiology of Pain* (eds A. V. Holden and W. Winslow), p. 359. Manchester: Manchester University Press.
11. Wyke, B. D. (1965) In *General Anaesthesia*, 2nd edn (eds F. T. Evans and T. C. Gray), London: Butterworths.
12. Sebel, P. S., Heneghan, C. P. and Ingram, D. A. (1985) *British Journal of Anaesthesia* **57**, 841.
13. Janig, W. (1985) *European Journal of Anaesthesia* **2**, 319.
14. Schmidt, R. F. (ed.) (1985) *Fundamentals of Sensory Physiology*, 3rd edn. Berlin: Springer-Verlag.
15. Kehlet, H. (1982) *Regional Anesthesia* **7** (Suppl.), S38.
16. Prys-Roberts, C. (1987) *British Journal of Anaesthesia* **59**, 1341.
17. Merkel, G. and Eger, E. I. (1963) *Anesthesiology* **24**, 346.
18. de Jong, R. H. and Eger, E. I. (1975) *Anesthesiology* **42**, 384.
19. Evans, J. M., Bithell, J. F. and Vlachnikolis, I. G. (1987) *British Journal of Anaesthesia* **59**, 1346.
20. Eger, E. I. (1974) *Anesthetic Uptake and Action*. Baltimore: Williams and Wilkins.
21. Morgan, M. (1983) *Anaesthesia* **38** (Suppl.), 1.
22. Sear, J. W. and Prys-Roberts, C. (1979) *British Journal of Anaesthesia* **51**, 867.
23. Spelina, K. R., Coates, D. P., Monk, C. R., Prys-Roberts, C., Norley, I. and Turtle, M. J. (1986) *British Journal of Anaesthesia* **58**, 1080.
24. Humbert (1875) quoted by Marcenac and Lemetayer (1930) *Bulletin Veterinaire Français* **3**, 141.
25. Hall, L. W. and Weaver, B. M. Q. (1954) *Veterinary Record* **656**, 289.
26. Hall, L. W. (1957) *Veterinary Record* **69**, 615.
27. Nunn, J. F. (1977) *Applied Respiratory Physiology*, 2nd edn. London: Butterworths.
28. Tusiewicz, K., Bryan, A. C. and Froese, A. B. (1977) *Anesthesiology* **47**, 327.
29. Knill, R. L. and Gelb, A. W. (1978) *Anesthesiology* **49**, 244.
30. Nunn, J. F. (1985) *Lectures in Anaesthesiology 1985/2* (ed. J. S. M. Zorab). Oxford: Blackwell Scientific.
31. Hall, L. W. (1984) *Equine Veterinary Journal* **16**, 89.
32. Rugh, K. S., Garner, H. E., Hatfield, D. G. and Herrold, D. (1964) *Equine Veterinary Journal*, **16**, 185.
33. Hall, L. W. and Trim, C. M. (1975) *British Journal of Anaesthesia*, **47**, 819.
34. Bastron, R. D., Perkins, R. M. and Pyne, J. L. (1977) *Anesthesiology*, **29**, 142.
35. Burgher, B. M., Hopkins, T., Tullock, A. and Hollenberg, N. K. (1976) *Circulation Research*, **38**, 196.
36. Hughes, R. L. (1979) *Proceedings of the Association of Veterinary Anaesthetists of Great Britain and Ireland* **8**, 55.
37. Freeman, J. (1962) *British Journal of Anaesthesia* **34**, 832.
38. Sackner, M. A., Hirsch, J., Epstein, S. and Rynolin, A. M. (1976) *Chest* **69**, 164.
39. Ayers, L. N., Tierney, D. F. and Imagawa, D. (1973) *American Review of Respiratory Diseases* **107**, 955.
40. Nunn, J. F. (1977) *Applied Respiratory Physiology*, 2nd edn. London: Butterworths.

CHAPTER 4

PRINCIPLES OF SEDATION, ANALGESIA AND PREMEDICATION

There is considerable confusion concerning the terminology applied to sedative, tranquillizing and hypnotic drugs, and no single classification yet exists. Formerly, *a hypnotic* was defined as a depressant of the central nervous system which enabled the patient to go to sleep more easily, or a drug used to intensify the depth of sleep. *A sedative* was a drug which relieved anxiety and as a result tended to make it easier for the patient to sleep — in fact they were usually associated with drowsiness. *A tranquillizer* was a drug with a predominant action in relieving anxiety without producing undue sedation. With this classification many drugs fall into more than one category, the differentiation usually being related to dose [1]. This is particularly so for the sedatives and hypnotics and usually these are considered as one group, best exemplified by chloral hydrate or xylazine where low doses cause drowsiness and higher doses cause sleep. The term 'tranquillizer' was usually employed for drugs which affected mood or behaviour but in recent years this term has become unpopular [2] and indeed the classification of tranquillizers as 'major' and 'minor' as suggested by the World Health Authority is now rarely used. In current pharmacological texts [3–5] classification is now based on medical clinical uses of the drugs. Three categories are recognized, these being antianxiety drugs (anxiolytics), antipsychotic drugs and the classical sedative/ hypnotics. Benzodiazepines are considered both as antianxiety drugs and as sedative/hypnotics. Drugs now classified as 'antipsychotic' are those previously termed 'neuroleptics' which reduce psychomotor agitation, curiosity and apparent aggressiveness in animals, exerting their effects by blocking dopamine-mediated responses in the central nervous system. Overdose causes marked extrapyramidal symptoms and parkinsonian-type tremor [6, 7]. Drugs of the butyrophenone and phenothiazine groups are neuroleptic agents and are now categorized as antipsychotics.

The multiplicity of definitions is confusing and it is more important that the veterinarian understands the major actions of the drugs than is able to categorize them, for in this way it is possible to appreciate the limitations of the drugs in use. For example, if drugs such as the benzodiazepines are used for premedication they will not quieten the animal, but may make it more difficult to handle by removing its inhibitions, thus making vicious animals more likely to bite, and even friendly animals may become uncontrollable. Phenothiazine drugs, by reducing nervousness, may make an animal more liable to sleep, but will not have this effect in the vicious animal no matter what the dose used. Thus the term 'tranquillizer' is still loosely used in clinical anaesthesia [8] to cover both the antianxiety and antipsychotic drugs, and will continue to be used in places in this text.

SEDATION

Effective sedation depends on the careful selection of the drug appropriate for the procedure, the species of animal, its temperament and condition and must allow for possible side-effects. Where sedation is to control an animal so that it may undergo surgery under local analgesia, comparatively high doses of drugs may be used, but where sedation fails to be adequate, resort may have to be made to drug combinations (see p. 70) or to general anaesthesia. Where sedative and 'tranquillizing' drugs are used for premedication, lower doses are usually utilized and their effect on the subsequent anaesthetic (even where there is no apparent preanaesthetic sedation) must be taken into account (see p. 76). In all cases it is important that the animal is left undisturbed for an adequate period of time after administration of the sedative because stimulation during the onset of the drug's action may prevent the full effect from developing. To sedate an animal that is in pain a suitable analgesic must be used.

During the past decade there have been major pharmacological advances in the recognition of specific receptor sites and of the actions resulting from their stimulation or blockade. These advances have been followed by the synthesis of potent drugs which act as agonists or as antagonists at such sites. Where receptors are involved in sedation and anaesthesia, these advances have included a better understanding of the actions of existing drugs, availability of newer and more potent agonist drugs, and of antagonists to enable the reversal of some sedative agent effects.

Phenothiazine derivatives

Drugs of this group are classified as antipsychotics (or in older terminology as 'neuroleptics'). All drugs of this group have a wide range of central and peripheral effects, but the degree of activity in different pharmacological actions varies from one compound to another. These actions and side-effects have been well reviewed [2, 7]. As dopamine antagonists they have their calming and mood-altering (antipsychotic?) effects, and also a powerful antiemetic action, particularly against opioid-induced vomiting. The degree of sedation produced varies markedly between drugs. For many uses in medical practice, sedation is an unwanted side-effect but in veterinary medicine the phenothiazine derivatives are used primarily for this purpose. In general, the phenothiazines do not have analgesic activity, although methotrimeprazine is claimed to be a powerful analgesic in man. Their major cardiovascular side-effects are related to their action in blocking α_1 adrenoceptors, and thus having an antiadrenaline effect. This results in marked hypotension primarily due to peripheral vasodilation. They exert an antiarrhythmic effect on the heart [9, 10] which was originally thought to be due to a quinidine action on the cardiac membrane [7], but has more recently been suggested as being caused by a blocking action on cardiac α-arrhythmic receptors [11, 12]. They have a spasmolytic action on the gut although, at least in the horse gut, motility is not reduced (J. Davis, personal communication). However, as they cause relaxation of the cardiac sphincter, in ruminants they increase the chance of regurgitation should the animal become recumbent. They have varying degrees of antihistamine activity and also produce a partial cholinergic block. All phenothiazine derivatives cause a fall in body temperature partly due to increased heat loss through dilated cutaneous vessels and partly through resetting of the thermoregulatory mechanisms.

In spite of all their side-effects the phenothiazines are well tolerated by the majority of normovolaemic animals. The choice of any one of the group is governed by its specific potency in the desired field (e.g. promethazine as an antihistamine, acepromazine

as a sedative), its duration of action or suitability of presentation.

Acepromazine

Acepromazine is probably the most extensively used phenothiazine in veterinary practice. It is the 2-acetyl derivative of promazine and has the chemical name 2-acetyl-10-(3-dimethylaminopropyl)phenothiazine: it is prepared as the maleate, a yellow crystalline solid.

The drug has marked sedative properties, which are responsible for its popularity in veterinary medicine. Like all phenothiazine drugs, with low doses there are effects on behaviour, and as the dose is increased sedation occurs [13, 14], but the dose–response curve rapidly reaches a plateau after which higher doses do not increase but only lengthen sedation and increase side-effects [2, 15]. Further increase in doses may cause excitement and extrapyramidal signs. In many animals sedation may be achieved with doses as low as 0.03 mg/kg by intramuscular injection although the drug has been used safely at very much higher doses (0.3 mg/kg) when prolonged effects were required. A calming effect on the behaviour of excitable animals can be seen at doses even below 0.03 mg/kg, making acepromazine a drug liable to abuse, particularly in the equine sporting field. The length of action is prolonged. Clinically obvious sedation lasts 4–6 hours after doses of 0.2 mg/kg, but in horses Parry and coworkers [14] considered that there were detectable residual effects for 12 hours after doses of 0.1 mg/kg, and for 16–24 hours after 0.15 mg/kg intramuscularly. Owners of giant breeds of dog often complain that their animals are sedated for several days following acepromazine administration, but scientific substantiation of these reports is not available. In practice, the dose is chosen in relation to length of sedation and the purpose for which sedation is required. However, the drug cannot be relied upon to give sedation in all animals; some individuals fail to become sedated and, in these, other drugs or drug combinations must be employed.

A reason for the popularity of acepromazine in veterinary medicine is that, compared with many other drugs of the phenothiazine group [15–17], excitement reactions are rare. However, excitement reactions have been reported occasionally in horses after intravenous [2] or intramuscular [18] injection of the drug.

Other central effects of acepromazine include hypothermia and a moderate antiemetic effect. Acepromazine is said to reduce the threshold at which epileptiform seizures occur but Dundee [1] claimed that in man the phenothiazines have an anticonvulsant effect. It is difficult to reconcile these two statements but in veterinary medicine it seems to be generally agreed that acepromazine should be avoided in animals with a history of fits or which are in danger of convulsions for any reason (e.g. after myelography).

In all species of animals, acepromazine causes a marked fall in blood pressure and this property has been particularly well documented in the horse [14, 19–21]. This property is thought to be through vasodilatation brought about by peripheral α_2-adrenoceptor block. In most fit and healthy animals the cardiovascular effects are well tolerated but in shocked or hypovolaemic animals a precipitous and even fatal fall in arterial pressure can occur. The effects of clinical dose rates of acepromazine on heart rate are generally minimal, most investigators having found a slight rise [14, 18, 20, 22] or no change [23]. However, Popovic and coworkers in 1972 [24] reported that in dogs doses of 1 mg/kg acepromazine caused bradycardia and even sinoatrial arrest, and atrioventricular block has been noted in horses (L. W. Hall, unpublished observations). These differences in reports could be due to the route of administration, dose (1 mg/kg is high compared with most clinical dosage) or individual animal sensitivity. Changes in cardiac output appear to be minimal [10, 23]. Like other phenothiazines, acepromazine has antiarrhythmic effects on the heart and protects against adrenaline-induced fibrillation [9] and this property must be an advantage when acepromazine is used for preanaesthetic medication.

Fainting and cardiovascular collapse has been reported to occur occasionally in all species of animal following the use of even low doses of acepromazine. In some cases it may have been due to administration to a hypovolaemic animal but in others it has not been explained. The boxer dog is renowned for 'fainting' after very small doses of acepromazine given by any route, and it has been suggested that this may be due to orthostatic hypovolaemia or to vasovagal syncope.

Clinical doses have little effect on respiration and although sedated animals may breathe more slowly the minute volume of respiration is usually unchanged [2, 9, 14].

Acepromazine has little antihistamine activity but has a powerful spasmolytic effect on smooth muscle including that of the gut. It it metabolized by the liver and both conjugated and non-conjugated metabolites are excreted in the urine.

The drug causes protrusion of the flaccid penis from the prepuce and in bulls and stallions was often given to facilitate examination of this organ. In horses, however, physical damage to the dangling penis may result in swelling and failure of the organ to return within the prepuce when the drug action ceases. This event, which may eventually necessitate amputation of the penis, has been reported as occur-

ring in horses following the use of several phenothiazine drugs. More recently priapism has been reported as occurring in stallions following the use of acepromazine, usually but not always as part of the neuroleptanalgesic mixture 'Large Animal Immobilon' [25]. In most reports the stallion was being castrated but priapism has been encountered in other circumstances, for example immediately after induction of anaesthesia with an intravenous barbiturate in acepromazine-premedicated animals [26]. G. B. Edwards and K. W. Clarke (unpublished observations) have encountered three cases of priapism in horses which had not been given acepromazine undergoing surgery for relief of colic. Most reports involving the association of acepromazine alone fail to differentiate between priapism and flaccidity with physical injury but Sharrock [27] reported priapism in a gelding given acepromazine 0.07 mg/kg by intravenous injection and found that detumescence followed the administration of benztropine. As both priapism and flaccid paralysis with subsequent physical injury are equally calamitous in valuable breeding stallions the manufacturers now specifically contraindicate the use of the drug in these animals. Members of the Association of Anaesthetists of Great Britain and Ireland discussed the use of acepromazine and concluded that, despite possible side-effects involving the equine penis, the drug remains a useful sedative in male horses. It was, however, recommended that only minimal doses of acepromazine should be administered, preferably by intramuscular rather than intravenous injection, and in the event of priapism or prolonged prolapse of the flaccid penis the condition must be treated quickly and efficiently [28].

In the UK acepromazine is available as 2 and 10% solutions for injection and as tablets for oral use. The injectable forms are non-irritant and are effective by intravenous, intramuscular and subcutaneous routes. Following intravenous injection sedation is usually obvious within 5 minutes but in some cases the full effects may not be apparent for 20 minutes and when the drug is used for premedication by this route at least this period should be allowed to elapse before anaesthetic agents are given. Maximal effects are seen 30–45 minutes after intramuscular and subcutaneous injection. It has been claimed that absorption from subcutaneous sites is poor and the fact that, at least in small animals, it works very well when given by this route may indicate that even the minimum recommended doses are larger than necessary. Given by the oral route, absorption, and therefore its effects, is very variable and much higher doses need to be administered (e.g. 1–3 mg/kg in dogs and cats).

Acepromazine has been very widely used in all species of animals as a sedative and premedicant, as well as in combination with etorphine as 'Large

Animal Immobilon'. Very small doses have been used to treat behavioural problems in dogs and horses but the dose required in any individual case can only be found by trial and error. Its antiemetic properties make it a useful drug for the prevention of motion sickness in dogs and cats and its spasmolytic properties have led to its use in spasmodic colic in horses. Parenteral doses of acepromazine for sedative and premedicant purposes in most domestic animals are in the range 0.025–0.1 mg/kg, the lower doses being used by the intravenous route. Higher doses of up to 0.2 mg/kg may be used safely by intramuscular injection. Recommended doses for specific purposes will be discussed in the chapters relating to the individual species of animal.

Propionylpromazine

This compound, 10–(3–dimethylaminopropyl)–2–propionylphenothiazine, has been widely used on the Continent of Europe and in Scandinavia for sedation and premedication of both small and large animal patients. Its actions, the sedation it produces and its side-effects are very similar to those of acepromazine. In horses it is used in doses of 0.15 to 0.25 mg/kg and in dogs the dose ranges from 0.2 to 0.3 mg/kg. It has also been widely used in combination with methadone.

Chlorpromazine

This compound, 2–chloro–10–(3–dimethylaminopropyl)phenothiazine hydrochloride, was used extensively in veterinary practice [29] but has largely been replaced by acepromazine and propionylpromazine. Its actions and side-effects are similar to those of acepromazine, but it is less potent (doses of up to 1 mg/kg have been used), has a longer duration of action and produces relatively less sedation. It is particularly unreliable in horses, giving rise to what appears to be a state of panic due to the muscle weakness it supposedly causes. It is still widely used in human medicine for its antipsychotic actions, as in psychotic patients its weak sedative properties constitute a desirable feature.

Promazine

This is 10–(3–dimethylaminopropyl)phenothiazine hydrochloride and has actions similar to those of chlorpromazine but it gives better sedation with fewer side-effects. It was often preferred to chlorpromazine in horses since it seldom produced excitement or recumbency [17, 30–32]. For premedication it was administered at doses of up to 1 mg/kg.

Methotrimeprazine

This is a typical phenothiazine but it is also a potent analgesic having about 0.7 times the potency of morphine. In veterinary practice in the UK it is used in combination with etorphine as the neuroleptanalgesic mixture 'Small Animal Immobilon' (p. 72).

Promethazine

This drug, 10–(2–dimethylaminopropyl)phenothiazine hydrochloride, was probably the first phenothiazine derivative to be used in veterinary anaesthesia. Solutions of promethazine are irritant to the tissues and should be injected deeply in a large muscle mass 40–60 minutes before anaesthesia. In emergencies the drug can be given, after dilution with isotonic saline, by very slow intravenous injection. Rapid intravenous injection causes a profound fall in blood pressure which may be fatal in shocked animals.

Promethazine is used in veterinary medicine primarily for its potent antihistamine activity; it is employed for premedication prior to the administration of anaesthetic drugs which cause histamine release.

Butyrophenones

In man the butyrophenone group of compounds were classed as major tranquillizers (neuroleptics) but they can cause very unpleasant side-effects, including hallucinations, loss of body image, restlessness, mental agitation, and even feelings of aggression. These side-effects are often not obvious to an observer and only become known when the human patient recovers from the drug and complains, often bitterly, about the experience. The incidence of these side-effects is dose related and increases with increase of dose. Overdose results in dystonic reactions. We do not know whether the subjective effects produced in animals are similar to those known to occur in man, but the unpredictable aggressive behaviour shown by some animals when under the influence suggests they may be.

Cardiovascular and respiratory effects of the butyrophenones are minimal, although slight hypotension may result from α-adrenergic block. They are potent antiemetics, acting on the chemoemetic trigger zone to prevent drug-induced vomiting, such as may be caused by opioid analgesics. It is this latter property which makes the butyrophenones the drugs of choice for the neuroleptic component of neuroleptanalgesia (p. 71).

From experience of their use in man it seems doubtful whether butyrophenones should ever be used on their own as tranquillizing agents, but in veterinary medicine they have been used in this way as well as in neuroleptanalgesic combinations.

Azaperone

Azaperone, 4'–fluoro–4–(4–(2–pyridyl)–1–piperazinyl)butyrophenone, is a drug which is marketed to be used in pigs where its intramuscular administration produces a good, dose-related, sedative effect up to the maximum recommended dose for clinical use [33, 34]. Pigs may show excitement during the first 20 minutes following injection, particularly if disturbed during this period. Intravenous administration of the drug frequently results in a vigorous excitement phase.

In horses intramuscular administration at a dose of 0.4–0.8 mg/kg can sometimes give good sedation [35] but some horses develop muscle tremors and sweat profusely following its use [18, 36] and in practice azaperone often proves unsatisfactory in this species of animal. Intravenous injection of the drug frequently causes violent excitement in horses [37]. Although Dodman and Waterman [37] suggest that the cause of excitement may be the horse's reaction to the ataxia produced, the fact that pigs show a similar reaction, coupled with the known central nervous effect in man, suggests that the excitement is due to a direct effect of the drug.

Azaperone in clinical doses has minimal effects on respiration, such effect as there is being that of slight stimulation [38].

Clarke [38] reported a consistent small fall in arterial blood pressure in pigs following the intramuscular injection of 0.3–3.5 mg/kg of the drug. The effect is presumably due to the α-adrenergic block common to all butyrophenones. Reductions in cardiac output and heart rate in pigs were reported to be clinically insignificant [18, 33] but in horses an increase in heart rate has been reported.

When azaperone is used as a sedative or for premedication before caesarean section in pigs, the piglets may appear sleepy for some hours after delivery. However, provided they are kept warm they breathe well and there is usually no problem due to this sleepiness.

In pigs, azaperone is widely used both as a sedative and as a premedicant [39]. In particular, it is given to this species of animal prior to the use of metomidate (p. 278). It is also sold directly to farmers to be used to sedate pigs before transportation and to prevent fighting following the mixing of pigs or calves in one pen.

It should not be used in horses for, should an excitement reaction be encountered, an extremely dangerous situation might arise in which injury to the horse and/or its handlers might occur.

Droperidol

Droperidol is a potent neuroleptic agent with an action of 6–8 hours duration [40]. It is an extremely potent antiemetic and is said to antagonize the respiratory depressant effects of morphine-like compounds by increasing the sensitivity of the respiratory centre to carbon dioxide. Although it was claimed that extrapyramidal side-effects were rare, they are produced by overdosing — but are sometimes delayed for up to 24 hours after administration of the drug. Doses of 0.1–0.4 mg/kg give useful sedation in pigs for 2–5 hours [41]. However, in this species of animal, droperidol has been superseded by the less expensive azaperone. The main use of droperidol in veterinary medicine is in neuroleptanalgesia techniques when it is combined with fentanyl (p. 71).

Fluanisone

This drug 4'–fluoro–4–(4–(o–methoxy)phenyl)–1–piperazinyl butyrophenone, is used in combination with fentanyl for neuroleptanalgesic techniques (p. 71).

Benzodiazepines

Chlordiazepoxide was first introduced in 1955 [5] and since this time drugs of the benzodiazepine group have been widely used in human and veterinary medicine, although their veterinary applications appear to have been more limited. In man, drugs of this group are utilized for certain specific properties, these being (1) an antianxiety action, (2) sedation and hypnosis, (3) anticonvulsant effects, (4) muscle relaxation and (5) retrograde amnesia. A very wide range of different compounds now exist which are employed for one or more of these effects, these drugs differing primarily in bioavailability, permissible route of administration and length of action.

Benzodiazepine compounds exert their main sedative effects through depression of the limbic system, and their muscle-relaxing properties through inhibition of the internuncial neurones at spinal levels. Their action is thought to be through stimulation of specific benzodiazepine (BZ) receptors, which then potentiates the effect of the inhibitory transmitter γ-aminobutyric acid (GABA). GABA acts on the chloride channel, increasing the flow of chloride ions into the cell, causing hyperpolarization and therefore making the cell more refractory to other stimuli. These actions have been the subject of numerous reviews [5, 8, 42–45]. Current opinion [42] suggests that there is more than one type of BZ receptor and that different receptors may be responsible for some of the different actions, such as sedation and muscle relaxation [42]. The possibility of such heterogeneity of receptors has been taken as the rationale for the production of certain benzodiazepines, such as zolazepam, which are claimed to be more hypnotic with less anxiolytic properties. However, Dundee and Wyant [8] consider this difference in action from antianxiety to hypnosis is simply one of dose dependence.

As these drugs act at specific sites, specific antagonists have been developed and one, flumazenil, is now used clinically as a benzodiazepine antagonist. Other compounds act as 'inverse agonists' [5, 42] causing anxiety and convulsions as well as having analeptic properties (i.e. they have the opposite actions to the classical benzodiazepine drugs).

The primary use of benzodiazepines in anaesthetic practice in man is as anxiolytics, for premedication and for induction of anaesthesia. The advantages of their use is that at clinical doses they have minimal respiratory effects and although after intravenous use there may be some vasodilation and hypotension, in general cardiovascular effects are limited and the drugs are very safe. However, despite the common use of these compounds as induction agents there is a question as to whether it is possible to induce anaesthesia with benzodiazepines alone. Dundee and Wyant consider that they do usually cause anaesthesia but admit that whilst sedation is predictable, anaesthesia is not and that young, fit patients may be particularly resistant to their effects. In contrast, standard texts [5, 44] suggest that true anaesthesia does not result from their use, but that retrograde amnesia prevents human patients from complaining. Certainly it is very difficult, if not impossible, to induce anaesthesia with benzodiazepine drugs in fit healthy animals [46] although they do combine with almost any other central nervous depressant drug to give anaesthesia. Both in man and animals it is in combinations such as with opioid drugs, that they are generally employed. Certainly, when used for premedication at subsedative doses, they do markedly reduce the dose required of subsequent anaesthetic agents, but when they are used in such combinations their advantage of causing minimal cardiovascular and respiratory effects may be lost [8].

Most benzodiazepines have a high oral bioavailability, and many can also be given by the intramuscular and intravenous routes. Their action when given intravenously is not within one circulation time; there are marked differences between individuals in sensitivity and it may take several minutes for maximal effects to become apparent. Metabolism is in the liver and in many instances the metabolites are as active, or more active, than the parent compound; actions therefore tend to be prolonged.

In animals the compounds were first used for their action in taming wild animals, including ungulates and the larger Felidae [47]. They have also been used at low doses to treat behavioural problems and widely used as anticonvulsants. In fit animals they do not, on their own, cause sedation and indeed their anxiolytic properties may result in animals becoming uncontrollable (a phenomenon also noted in people [8]). They are used in combination with other drugs such as opioids to produce sedation and analgesia for intensive care and to counteract the convulsant and hallucinatory properties of ketamine. Benzodiazepines have the property of stimulating appetite [48, 49] in a variety of animals. Diazepam has been particularly widely used for this in cats showing anorexia following illness and doses of up to 1 mg/kg have claimed to be successful in restoring normal feeding habits in these animals. However, in debilitated cats intravenous doses of 0.05–0.1 mg/kg are usually adequate and doses of 0.4 mg/kg should not be exceeded if deep sedation is not to result.

Of the available benzodiazepine drugs, diazepam, midazolam, climazolam and zolazepam have been most utilized in veterinary anaesthesia.

Diazepam

Diazepam is probably the most widely used of the benzodiazepines. It is, like all other compounds of this group, insoluble in water and solutions for injection contain solvents such as propylene glycol, ethanol, and sodium benzoate in benzoic acid. Intravenous injection may give rise to thrombophlebitis and this is thought to be due to solvents rather than to diazepam itself. An emulsion specially prepared for intravenous injection is claimed not to be irritant to veins, but the bioavailability of this preparation is reduced compared with that of the other formulations. Because of the problems of solubility diazepam should not be diluted with water or mixed with solutions of other drugs.

The effects of diazepam in domestic animals have been poorly documented. A rise in plasma concentration, coupled with a return of clinical effects, occurs 6–8 hours after administration and is thought to be due to enterohepatic recycling of the drug and/or its metabolites [8]. Premedication with diazepam increase the length of action of other anaesthetic agents and the drug is particularly useful prior to ketamine anaesthesia to reduce the hallucinations which seem to occur with this dissociative anaesthetic agent.

The sedative and hypnotic effects of diazepam appear to be minimal or absent in fit, healthy dogs and attempts to use it for hypnosis or as an intravenous induction agent in this species of animal have been unsuccessful. Lees [46] recorded a personal communication from MacKenzie reporting that the administration of doses of 2 mg/kg given intravenously to greyhounds resulted in no obvious sedation, marked ataxia, and violent struggling when restrained. The authors' experiences are in agreement with her findings.

At clinical dose rates diazepam has no significant effect on the circulation or respiratory activity but does produce some muscular relaxation due to its action at the internuncial neurones. It has a very low toxicity and large doses given to dogs for prolonged periods do not produce any changes in kidney or liver function.

Diazepam has a major role in veterinary practice in the control of convulsions of any origin. Averill [50] recommends that dogs in status epilepticus should be given 5 mg by slow intravenous injection, followed if necessary by a further 5 mg, and Kay and Fenner [51] recommend doses of 10–35 mg for this purpose. In dogs and cats the drug has been used both for premedication as a preventive measure, and post-operatively to control convulsions caused by radiographic techniques involving the introduction of contrast media into the spinal canal. Convulsions of toxic origin in cats have also been treated successfully with the drug.

The use of diazepam as a premedicant, sedative and tranquillizer is less well documented. Oral doses of up to 5 mg/day have been used in dogs to control behavioural problems without producing unwanted sedation. It has been used for premedication prior to the use of ketamine in dogs and horses [52, 53], and during anaesthesia to abolish ketamine-induced convulsions in cats [54]. It has proved to be useful for postoperative sedation in dogs, especially when sedation has to be maintained for prolonged periods [55]. Provided postoperative pain has been relieved by the appropriate use of analgesic agents, diazepam may be given intravenously in doses of up to 1 mg/(kg h), for at least the first 6 hours, to control restlessness and facilitate the carrying out of necessary nursing.

Diazepam has not been widely used in large animals, and in horses its muscle-relaxing properties may be associated with induced panic [56, 57].

Midazolam

Midazolam (8–chloro–6–(2–flurophenyl)–1–methyl–4H–imidazo(1, 5–a)(1, 4)benzodiazepine, is a water-soluble compound which is not painful on intravenous injection and does not cause thrombophlebitis. It is metabolized in the liver and in man its half-life is considerably shorter than that of diazepam, and thus it is less cumulative and recovery is more rapid. These properties have led to its being used for intravenous sedation and 'induction of anaesthesia'. Like most benzodiazepines it has minimal respiratory and cardio-vascular effects and in combination with opioids has been widely used in man for cardiac surgery [8].

Although literature relating to its use is sparse, midazolam has been used fairly extensively in small animal patients, especially with ketamine in cats [58]. It has also been shown that the combination of midazolam (0.25 mg/kg) and metoclopramide (3.3 mg/kg) will produce good sedation in pigs even though neither drug on its own will produce sedation in these animals [59]. Again in pigs, midazolam (0.3 mg/kg) has been used by intramuscular injection with droperidol (0.5 mg/kg) to produce excellent sedation [60].

Climazolam

Climazolam is a potent benzodiazepine which following intravenous administration has a very rapid onset of effect. It has been used in a wide variety of animals including cattle, sheep, horses and dogs [61–63]. In cattle, 5 mg/kg orally cause sedation and ataxia but much lower doses by the intravenous or intramuscular route give useful sedation. Horses, however, panic (presumably from the feeling of muscle weakness) and the drug is contraindicated on its own for these animals, although it is useful in anaesthetic combinations, being particularly effective for use with ketamine [63]. Climazolam (1–1.5 mg/kg) has also been used in combination with fentanyl (5–15 µg/kg) for anaesthesia in the dog [62].

Zolazepam

This drug is claimed to have marked hypnotic effects in man. It is now being used in animals combined, in a fixed ratio, with the dissociative agent tiletamine [63, 64].

Flumazenil (benzodiazepine antagonist)

Originally developed for the treatment of benzodiazepine overdose in man, flumazenil is a potent and specific benzodiazepine antagonist and in medical practice is now being widely employed to reverse midazolam sedation in 'day case' patients.

Flumazenil has been reported to reverse diazepam or climazolam sedation in sheep and cattle [63] and has also been used in combination with naloxone to reverse climazolam/fentanyl combination anaesthesia [62]. Although to date the veterinary use of flumazenil has been limited there is no reason why it should not be employed in any situation where it may become necessary to reverse the effects of a benzodiazepine drug.

α_2–Adrenoceptor agonists

Xylazine has been used as a sedative in animals since 1968 [65] but at that time the mechanisms of its complex actions and side-effects were not understood. When it was described as 'both excitatory and inhibitory of adrenergic and cholinergic neurones' [66] this statement appeared more than a little confusing. A similar drug, clonidine, was originally used in man for its powers of peripheral vasoconstriction, but later became (and still is) used as an antihypertensive [67]. These actions and the correctness of the above description only became explicable in 1974 when Langer [68] suggested the existence of receptor sites situated presynaptically on the noradrenergic neurones which, when stimulated by noradrenaline, inhibited the further release of this transmitter, thus forming a negative-feedback mechanism. Langer suggested further that these presynaptic inhibitory receptors differed from the previously recognized α adrenoceptors and should therefore be termed α_2 adrenoceptors. There is now convincing evidence for the presence of postsynaptic and presynaptic α_2 adrenoceptors in both central and peripheral sites. The distinction between α_1 and α_2 adrenoceptors is made on sensitivity to specific agonists and antagonists. Adrenaline and noradrenaline stimulate both types. For α_1 adrenoceptors, phenylephrine and methoxamine are considered to be fairly specific agonists and prazosin to be a specific antagonist. Classically, for pharmacological tests clonidine is considered a specific α_2-adrenoreceptor agonist and yohimbine and idazoxan, antagonists. However, very few drugs are absolutely specific in their actions and the vast majority can only be described as showing selectivity, thus at higher doses the alternative α receptors may also be stimulated or blocked, a factor possibly explaining some of the side-effects and aberrant reactions occasionally seen with the clinically used drugs.

α_2 Adrenoceptors are currently the subject of extensive research, the majority of which is well beyond the scope of this book. Some excellent reviews of the basic pharmacology do explain the major actions and side-effects and the interested reader is referred to some of these [69, 70].

As the presynaptic α_2 adrenoceptors inhibit noradrenaline release, it might be expected that the action of agonists would be the opposite of the classical effects of sympathetic stimulation. However, where postsynaptic α_2 adrenoceptors exist they often exert a stimulating action similar to that exerted by α_1 adrenoceptors at the same site. The major central and peripheral actions most relevant to anaesthetic practice of stimulation of the α_2 adrenoceptors are summarized in Table 4.1 and the clinical effects seen with

Table 4.1 Results of α_2-adrenoreceptor stimulation

CNS	Sedation, analgesia, hypotension, bradycardia
CVS	Peripheral vasoconstriction $\rightarrow$ initial hypertension
	Central bradycardia and vasomotor depression $\rightarrow$ hypotension
Gut	Relaxation, decreased motility
Salivation	Decreased
Gastric secretion	Reduced
Uterus	Stimulation
Eyes	Mydriasis, decreased intraocular pressure
Hormones	Reduced release of insulin, renin and antidiuretic hormone (ADH)
Platelets	Aggregation

After Livingstone *et al.* [69]

drugs which are agonist at this site are the result of the balance of these actions.

Clinical actions of α_2-adrenoreceptor agonists

In recent years many new potent and highly selective α_2-adrenoreceptor agonists have been developed for both medical and veterinary use. In veterinary practice the major drugs used are xylazine, detomidine and medetomidine; clonidine, although primarily used in medical practice has also been studied in animals in some detail.

The major actions and side effects of all these drugs are similar, although there may be differences in length of action, and in the extent and significance of some of the side-effects seen. There are variations between the drugs in their specificity for α_2 and α_1 receptors and this explains some of the differences in observed clinical effects. There is also marked variation in species sensitivity to their actions. For example, cattle are approximately 10 times more sensitive to xylazine than are horses or dogs, but are equally sensitive to medetomidine as are dogs, and equally or less sensitive to detomidine than are horses. Pigs appear to be very resistant to all the drugs so far tested. There is as yet no convincing pharmacological explanation for these differences in species sensitivity, which makes generalized comparisons of their potency meaningless except in the context of a stated species of animal.

The α_2-adrenoreceptor agonists are used primarily for their central effect of profound sedation (even of hypnosis in some species of animals) but they also give analgesia through both spinal and central actions. In earlier editions of this book doubt was expressed as to the degree of clinical analgesia produced by xylazine as sedation is so profound that analgesia is most difficult to assess. However, the analgesic

Xylazine

Detomidine

Medetomidine

Clonidine

effects of α_2-adrenoreceptor agonists even in subsedative doses are now well documented [70–72].

The major side-effects of the α_2-adrenoreceptor agonists are on the cardiovascular system. Although the majority of investigations have been into the actions of xylazine, the evidence to date with the newer compounds suggests that their actions are, in the main, similar. In all species there is marked bradycardia due to central stimulation and mediated through the vagus nerves. The effects on arterial blood pressure depend on the relative effects of the central and peripheral stimulation. There is often an initial hypertensive phase, the extent and duration of which depends on the particular drug, its dose, route of administration and species of animal concerned, followed by a more prolonged period of arterial hypotension, again dependent on the drug and the species of animal. Cardiac output falls (but the drugs seem to have little direct action on the myocardium) and the circulation appears to be slowed. The exact state of the peripheral circulation is more complicated and dose dependent. During the early phase of arterial hypertension with bradycardia, peripheral resistance is increased, presumably through shutdown of blood vessels. How long this poor peripheral

perfusion lasts is difficult to ascertain and probably depends on the species of animal, the drug and the dose used, because in the hypotensive phase peripheral resistance is said to be reduced.

The bradycardia, which can be severe, has given rise to much discussion. Many authorities have recommended medication with anticholinergics prior to sedation with these drugs in order to prevent the fall in heart rate but recent evidence has thrown doubt on the soundness of this advice. To be effective the anticholinergic must be given an adequate time prior to the α_2-adrenoreceptor agonist; arrhythmias or tachycardia often result and the hypertensive phase of the agonist's action may be enhanced in the absence of bradycardia. In cats it has been shown that anticholinergics further decrease cardiac output, presumably due to the resulting tachycardia preventing adequate filling of the heart during diastole [73], but this does not necessarily apply in larger animals. Recent work involving continuous recording of the ECG (L. W. Hall, unpublished observations) has shown pulse rates of normal sleeping dogs and horses to drop to values similar to those seen in animals sedated by α_2-adrenoceptor agonists; the bradycardia in the sedated animal can be over-ridden by toxaemia or by the administration of some anaesthetics. Thus, the use of anticholinergics remains controversial and more study of the possible combinations is necessary before an informed judgement of their use can be made. The question of the possible direct effects of α_2-adrenoceptor agonists on the myocardium is also an open one. There have been reports of animals which were in a very excited state at the time of xylazine administration suffering sudden cardiac arrest and the suggestion has been made that this drug might sensitize the heart to adrenaline-induced arrhythmias. Indeed Muir and Piper [74] showed this to be the case in halothane-anaesthetized dogs but failed to show the same effect with xylazine in horses. It must be noted here that pharmacological studies have failed to demonstrate α_2-adrenoceptors in the heart but their presence in the coronary vessels has been established.

Respiratory effects appear to differ between species of animal. Although with doses which cause deep sedation in dogs, cats and horses, respiratory rates may be reduced, there is no serious fall in P_aO_2 [73, 75, 76]. In ruminants tachypnoea may occur, breathing appears to require a considerable effort and the P_aO_2 shows desaturation of the haemoglobin [77–79]. This hypoxaemia does not seem to be due to changes in blood pressure or in ventilation and, indeed, has been shown to occur following clonidine injection in anaesthetized artificially ventilated sheep [80]. Thus, intrapulmonary mechanisms have been postulated as the cause, hypoxaemia being accompanied by a marked increase intrapulmonary shunt. Xylazine causes a marked increase in airway resistance in sheep [81] but not in cattle [82].

All these drugs cause an increase in urination, thought to be through inhibition of antidiuretic hormone (ADH) release but, when high doses are used, diuresis is possibly assisted by hyperglycaemia. Gut motility ceases almost completely. These side-effects must be taken into account when these drugs are used to facilitate investigations such as barium meals and glucose tolerance tests. Another important side-effect of α_2-adrenoceptor agonists is that many (but not all) cause significant uterine stimulation and their administration is, therefore, contraindicated in very early or late pregnancy for they may induce abortion.

In doses which produce clinical sedation most of these drugs cause hypothermia but the mechanism by which this is produced appears to differ between drugs and species of animal. Xylazine-induced hypothermia has been shown to be antagonized by the antagonist idazoxan whilst clonidine-induced hypothermia is intensified by this antagonist [83]. In rats, low doses of detomidine cause hypothermia which can be reversed by the antagonist yohimbine [84], but higher doses cause hyperthermia probably due to an α_1-adrenoceptor-stimulating action.

When α_2-adrenoceptor agonists are used for premedication they greatly reduce the dose requirements of inhalation anaesthetics [84] or intravenous agents. They also combine with opioids to produce deep sedation or even anaesthesia (p. 71).

Xylazine

Xylazine, 2–(2,6–dimethylphenylamino)–4*H*–5,5–dihydro–1,3–thiazine, was enthusiastically received as a sedative and over the past 20 years it has maintained its popularity as a generally reliable sedative and premedicant in a wide range of animal species [85–89].

The drug is a typical α_2-adrenoceptor agonist and exerts its effects accordingly. However, there are marked variations in susceptibility to it between the various domestic species of animal. Horses, dogs and cats require 10 times the dose needed in cattle and even then the degree of sedation achieved in horses is considerably less. Pigs are even more resistant than horses [65]. It is possible that lesser variations in sensitivity may occur in breeds within a single species and that this might contribute to the occasional failure of the drug to produce sedation.

Xylazine can be given by intravenous, intramuscular or subcutaneous injection although the subcutaneous route is not very reliable. Injections are non-irritant although minor temporary swellings have been reported at the site of intramuscular injections of concentrated solutions in horses. Although never proved by laboratory testing most users of the drug are satisfied that the potency of available commercial solutions decreases with age, and that this deterioration is enhanced by increased environmental temperature (J. Van Dieten, personal communication).

In horses the drug is usually used in doses that enable the animal to remain standing (although with marked ataxia) but in ruminants and small animals sedation is dose dependent and higher doses are used which may cause recumbency, unconsciousness and a state close to general anaesthesia. After these high doses sedation is very prolonged and is accompanied by marked cardiovascular and respiratory depression — i.e. they constitute overdoses. The sedative effects of xylazine appear to be synergistic with a variety of sedative, analgesic and anaesthetic drugs and such combinations (p. 70) are much preferable to overdoses of xylazine for the production of these effects).

Although the drug can be a potent analgesic, claims as to the degree of analgesia achieved at clinical dose rates are conflicting. Sedative doses appear to produce a short period of intense analgesia in horses [10, 90] and there is considerable experimental and clinical evidence that the drug produces excellent analgesia in equine colic [91]. However, others [85, 86] have found that horses deeply sedated with xylazine may respond violently to manipulations or even attempts to inject local analgesics. It may be that such reactions are a response to touch rather than pain as non-painful procedures such as hair clipping or the placing of a radiographic plate may cause a horse to respond with a well-directed kick. Cattle and small animals do not show this marked response to touch. However, analgesia is not adequate for minor surgery and in cats Arbeiter *et al.* [88] found that even massive doses of xylazine sufficient to cause prolonged unconsciousness were inadequate to abolish all reaction to painful stimuli in the majority of animals. Thus, despite the undoubted analgesic properties of the drug, in the opinion of the authors where surgery is to be performed local analgesia must be used to supplement its effects.

The cardiovascular effects of xylazine are typical of this group of drugs and appear to be similar in all species of animal [85, 92–94]. An initial rise in arterial blood pressure following its intravenous injection is short lived and the pressure falls to 10–20% below initial resting levels. This hypertensive phase is not always evident after intramuscular injection. Cardiac output falls due to bradycardia and heart block is usually observed. The advisability of using anticholinergic drugs to counteract bradycardia is disputed [75, 95]. Xylazine appears to have little direct effect on the myocardium but causes a dose-related depression of respiration. Falls in P_aO_2 are species specific, being particularly severe in ruminants, while the muscle-relaxing properties make the drug contraindicated in animals suffering from upper airway obstruction.

Other side-effects of xylazine include: muscle twitching when sedation is deep; sweating in horses at the time sedation is diminishing; vomiting at the onset of sedation in dogs and cats; hyperglycaemia; decreased intraocular pressure and gut motility; and increased urine production. Xylazine also causes uterine contractions and should not be used in late pregnancy for it may induce premature labour. Increase in uterine tone may contraindicate it in cattle or horses receiving ovum transplants since this may reduce the chance of implantation.

Xylazine has proved to be a very safe sedative in a wide variety of animals but some serious reactions have been reported. There have been reports of violent excitement or collapse in horses associated with its intravenous injection. Some of these mishaps may have been due to inadvertent intra-arterial injection, but it is probable that a few have been genuine drug reactions. Fainting through extreme bradycardia has been suggested as a possible cause of collapse, but this is unlikely because the greatest bradycardia is coupled with arterial hypertension. Deaths have also been reported in cattle and the problems of recumbency in ruminants must be increased by the hypoxaemia caused by α_2-adrenoceptor agonists and the advent of the opportunity to limit the duration of recumbency by the reversal of sedation with drugs such as yohimbine or atipamezole should increase the safety of xylazine in these animals. In small animals, deaths have mainly resulted from the use of xylazine for premedication.

In most species of animal, xylazine is a useful drug for premedication prior to induction of anaesthesia with one of a wide variety of agents. Its use greatly reduces the dose of anaesthetic required, and although the reduction can often be predicted from the degree of sedation achieved, it may still be present in animals which have responded poorly to the drug. In heavily sedated animals circulation is slowed, the effects of subsequent anaesthetic agents is delayed and overdose of the anaesthetic may result. Thus, particular care is needed when this sedative is followed by intravenous agents such as the barbiturates, Saffan or propofol. Xylazine is particularly useful in combination with ketamine for its muscle-relaxing properties help to reduce the rigidity caused by the dissociative agent and xylazine/ketamine combinations have proved useful in a wide range of animal species [96–104].

Detomidine

Detomidine, 4–(2,3–dimethylphenyl)methyl–1*H*–imidazole hydrochloride, is an imidazole derivative which has been developed as a sedative/analgesic for animals. It is supplied in multidose bottles at a concentration of 10 mg/ml and may be given by the intravenous or intramuscular routes. It is not effective if given orally, but it is when administered sublingually because it is readily absorbed through mucous membranes.

In a variety of laboratory animals its sedative potency has been shown to be of a similar order to that of clonidine and approximately 10 times that of xylazine [105]. (These relative potencies are not necessarily the same in domestic animals, for in cattle, unlike xylazine, it is no more potent than it is in horses.)

The properties of detomidine are well recorded in *Acta Veterinaria Scandinavica*, Supplement 82/1986 (20 papers). Its analgesic powers have been shown in a number of pain models and it is particularly effective as an analgesic in equine colic [106–109]. Cardiovascular changes are typical of an α_2-adrenoreceptor agonist in that there is marked bradycardia and following doses of 20 µg/kg arterial blood pressure is elevated for about 15 minutes but falls significantly below control values within 45 minutes of injection of the drug [110, 111]. Higher doses of the drug are followed by more prolonged arterial hypertension but as yet there have been no investigations into whether this is followed by prolonged hypotension. Work to date in horses shows that arterial pressure during anaesthesia after detomidine premedication appears to be dependent on the anaesthetic agents used [107]. Like xylazine, detomidine causes a minimal fall in equine P_aO_2 [107] but marked hypoxaemia in sheep [112]. In horses, other side-effects include muscular twitching, sweating, piloerection, hyperglycaemia, a marked diuresis and reduced gut motility. Side-effects increase in frequency and duration with increased dose.

One difference between xylazine and detomidine appears to be in their effect on the uterus. Whereas xylazine appears to have marked ecbolic effects, detomidine, at doses of 20 µg/kg intravenously, slows electrical activity in the pregnant bovine uterus, although 40–60 µg/kg causes an increase in electrical activity [113]. Thus low doses of detomidine may prove to be safe for use in pregnant animals but further trials are needed to confirm this.

Detomidine is primarily used as a sedative for horses. In early work, doses between 10 and 300 µg/kg were employed, horses remaining standing after the highest doses, although sedation and side-effects (bradycardia, arterial hypertension, ataxia, sweating, piloerection, muscle tremor and diuresis) were unacceptably prolonged. This early work serves to demonstrate the very high therapeutic index of the drug as subsequent clinical experience has shown that intravenous doses of 10–20 µg/kg give adequate sedation for about an hour with much more limited side-effects [110]. The drug has also been widely used in horses for premedication prior to induction of anaesthesia with agents such as ketamine, thiopentone and propofol [114, 115]. A more detailed description of the effect and uses of detomidine in horses is given in Chapter 11.

The doses of detomidine required in cattle appear to be similar to those in horses. Again, early experimental work suggested that high doses were needed for adequate sedation but subsequent trials have shown that doses of up to 30 µg/kg are satisfactory. In the authors' limited experience, doses of 10 µg/kg intravenously produce sedation in cattle very similar to that seen in horses, i.e. cattle remain standing but show marked ataxia. The relative lack of a hypnotic effect with detomidine means that cattle are more likely to remain standing than after xylazine and this probably led to an initial misapprehension that cattle required higher doses. Low doses of detomidine may probably be used safely in early and late pregnancy in cattle (Chapter 12).

Medetomidine

This compound, 4–(1–(2,3–dimethylphenyl)ethyl)–1*H*–imadazole, is a very potent, efficacious and selective agonist of α_2 adrenoreceptors in the central and peripheral nervous system. Its actions and uses were the subject of a symposium (*Acta Veterinaria Scandinavica,* Supplement 85/1989 (30 communications)) and the reader is referred to this for detailed references. It is a mixture of two optical isomers, the dextrorotatory isomer being the active component, and is used in a wide variety of animals as a sedative, hypnotic, analgesic and premedicant. It is available for veterinary use as a 1 mg/ml solution of the racemic mixture. Dextromedetomidine is said to be a useful premedicant and anxiolytic in man [116, 117].

Apart from the required actions of sedation, hypnosis and analgesia [118] it has the usual marked cardiovascular effects of this group of drugs (bradycardia, arterial hypertension followed by hypotension and reduced cardiac output). All the other typical side-effects, such as vomiting in small animals, muscular twitching, hypothermia, decreased gut movement and hyperglycaemia have been noted [119, 120].

In most animals medetomidine slows respiration and, indeed, dogs may show a form of periodic breathing [120]. Nevertheless, at normal sedative doses in non-ruminant animals arterial oxygenation is adequately maintained, the P_aCO_2 does not rise to an excessive level and there is less depression of the ventilatory response to carbon dioxide than is commonly seen in anaesthetized animals. It has not yet been established whether medetomidine is safe for use in pregnant animals but in bitches the electrical activity of the uterine muscle is depressed at doses of 20 µg/kg, while at higher doses (40–60 µg/kg) there is an initial increase in this activity for some 5–7 minutes followed by depression; pregnant bitches do not abort [121]. Medetomidine markedly reduces the MAC of volatile agents given subsequently for anaesthesia and a similar synergism must be expected with intravenous agents whenever medetomidine premedication is used.

The solution is non-irritant and can be administered by intravenous, intramuscular or subcutaneous injection. Intravenous injection gives the fastest and most reliable results and vomiting is less common than with other routes of administration. Vomiting occurs in 10–20% of dogs and 50–65% of cats given intramuscular medetomidine and although some sedation may be evident within 5 minutes, maximal sedation is not achieved until 20 minutes have elapsed. The subcutaneous route seems to be unreliable [122]. Although medetomidine is ineffective when given by mouth, as it is inactivated by passage through the liver, it is absorbed through mucous membranes and can be administered effectively sublingually (L. W. Hall, unpublished observations).

Following its administration in the dog, the animal rapidly becomes ataxic, then stands quietly with its head down. Vomiting may occur at this time, but tends to be of short-lived duration compared with that induced by xylazine. Next, the dog becomes recumbent but even if apparently very deeply sedated it can be made to arise and walk around in a most ataxic manner before resuming recumbency. Muscle twitching may occur, being most marked in the most deeply sedated animals. In the medium-sized dog, maximal sedation is achieved with intramuscular doses of 40 µg/kg (or half this amount by intravenous injection), higher doses lengthening the duration of sedation but up to 80 µg/kg also contributing to futher analgesia. Smaller animals appear more resistant to the effects of the drug and require higher doses so that it has been suggested that doses should be calculated on the basis of milligrams/body surface area rather than on bodyweight. Sedation is less effective in noisy or disturbing surroundings but, once sedated, dogs are not usually responsive to sound.

In cats higher doses (80–150 µg/kg intramuscularly) are needed to produce sedation. Sedation is usually excellent but the animals are capable of being aroused. The intravenous use of medetomidine in cats has apparently not been explored.

The drug has been widely used in combination with other drugs to prolong recumbency. In the dog, combinations with opioids have proved to be successful [123] but the most popular combinations have been with ketamine, even 1–2 mg/kg of this drug being adequate to ensure prolongation of recumbency.

Medetomidine has been used in sheep and cattle; intravenous doses of 10–20 μg/kg causing sedation similar to that seen after 0.1–0.2 mg/kg of xylazine (K. W. Clarke and G. C. W. England, unpublished observations). In wild animals higher doses are required and the drug has usually been used in combination with ketamine when administered by dart gun for immobilization. Indeed, medetomidine/ketamine combinations have been found to provide excellent immobilization and relaxation in a wide range of species of animals, while the ability to reverse the sedation with α2-adrenoreceptor antagonists has proved to be particularly useful [124–126].

The drug has also been used in many rodents and other laboratory animals and there is marked species variation in susceptibility to its effects, the guinea pig being most resistant. Once again, combinations with ketamine are more effective than the sedative alone.

Romifidine

This drug, developed from clonidine, has typical α2-adrenoreceptor agonist effects. It has undergone clinical trials in Germany and Switzerland as a sedative and premedicant for horses. Maximal sedation is achieved with intravenous doses of 80 μg/kg. When compared with horses given intravenous xylazine (1 mg/kg) or detomidine (20 μg/kg) it produces less ataxia and the head is not lowered to the same extent, but response to imposed stimuli is reduced to the same degree by all three drugs. At these doses, the duration of effect is longest with romifidine, horses remaining quieter than normal for some considerable time after obvious sedation has waned.

α2-Adrenoceptor antagonists

The central and peripheral effects of the α2-adrenoceptor agonists can be reversed by the use of equally specific antagonists. Of these, the most extensively studied has been yohimbine, but new and more potent compounds have been developed recently.

The ability to awaken xylazine- or detomidine-sedated subjects has proved to be particularly useful in wild animals where prolonged sedation may be fatal [127], and in domestic ruminants [128] where prolonged recumbency is again unwelcome. However, in some clinical situations the α2-adrenoceptor antagonists may be useful in small animal practice.

The antagonists used include yohimbine [129], idazoxan [129, 130], RX821002A and atipamezole [123, 127], the most potent and specific being atipamezole, idazoxan and RX821002A [124, 127, 129].

Atipamezole

When using antagonists in the clinical situation it is necessary to consider the pharmacokinetics of the drugs involved, as if the antagonist is eliminated faster than the agonist, resedation will occur; this is most serious in wild animals which are not under observation and vulnerable to predators. The dose rates of antagonist drugs for reversing sedation will obviously vary with the dose of sedative used and the length of time since it was administered. With all antagonists investigated, higher doses are required to reverse cardiopulmonary effects than to reverse sedation [129, 131]. The situation is complicated by the fact that there may be species differences in antagonist effects and it is, therefore, very difficult to be certain of the exact dose of antagonist necessary in any particular case. For this reason it is important that no side-effects occur should the antagonist be overdosed. Convulsions have occasionally been reported after yohimbine, idazoxan and RX821002A but in most reports ketamine, which is not influenced by the α2-adrenoceptor antagonists, was part of the sedative combination used and may have been the cause of this side-effect.

Of the α2-adrenoceptor antagonists, yohimbine and atipamazole are the most easily available to the veterinary profession.

Yohimbine has been used in a wide variety of animals, doses of 0.1 mg/kg generally being employed to reverse xylazine sedation in small animals; high doses have caused excitement in dogs [132]. It has sometimes been used in combination with 4-aminopyridine but the combination appears to have no advantages over the use of the antagonist alone.

Atipamezole has mainly been used to reverse medetomidine sedation in dogs [123, 131], cats [133] and wild animals. Serious relapse into sedation has not been noted, although with low doses of the drug animals have been described as appearing 'tired'. Overdose of atipamezole does not appear to cause problems in most species of animal, injection into the unsedated dog [123] causing mild muscular tremors but little else and convulsions have never been noted in the absence of ketamine. However, although atipamezole appears to have little effect in unsedated cats when used to reverse medetomidine sedation a few cats have been described as being 'over-reversed' but overt excitement has not been seen. Atipamezole has also been shown to be effective in reversing detomidine sedation in horses, and xylazine sedation in wild animals, sheep and cattle.

Tameridone

This purine alkyl piperidine derivative has undergone extensive clinical and pharmacological investigations in cattle and in these animals intravenous doses of 0.05 mg/kg or intramuscular doses of 0.1–0.2 mg/kg produce good sedation for 90–120 minutes [134]. Sedation appears to be dose dependent in depth and takes longer to appear than sedation after xylazine administration. The drug appears to be equally effective in cattle of all breeds and temperaments but cows at full term undergoing caesarian section appear particularly sensitive to the drug, intravenous doses of 0.03 mg/kg readily causing recumbency. Pharmacological studies [135] showed that tameridone (0.05 mg/kg intravenously) caused a fall in arterial blood pressure and respiratory depression similar to that seen after equipotent doses of xylazine. However, in contrast to the effects of xylazine, tameridone causes a slight increase in pulse rate, no change in pulse-pressure product and any decrease in ruminal motility is very short lived.

Tameridone has been tried extensively in the USA for the capture and transport of wild ruminant animals. Results have been variable, doses and depth of sedation achieved differing between species of animal. When compared with xylazine in these circumstances, tameridone gives less sedation but appears to have a better and more prolonged calming effect. It is unlikely to be adequate for capture of animals but has proved to be useful when given to animals initially immobilized with opioid drugs (W. R. Lance, Wildlife Laboratories Inc., personal communication).

ANALGESIA

The anaesthetist is concerned in providing analgesia before, during and after surgery. Although the animal may be deemed to be unconscious during general anaesthesia and, therefore, incapable of appreciating pain, there is now evidence that the use of analgesic drugs during general anaesthesia assists in a smooth, pain-free recovery. The mechanisms of pain perception are detailed in most textbooks of physiology and have been well reviewed [136, 137].

All general anaesthetics undoubtedly have an analgesic action but apart from this analgesia can be provided by four main methods:

1. Use of local analgesics
2. Use of opioid drugs
3. Use of α_2-adrenoceptor agonists
4. Use of non-steroidal anti-inflammatory drugs (NSAIDs)

With all of these there is now convincing evidence that they are more effective if administered before pain becomes manifest [138].

Local analgesics used during surgery may also provide outstanding postoperative analgesia, particularly if of the long-acting group of drugs, e.g. bupivacaine. α_2-Adrenoceptor agonists, when used parenterally at analgesic doses will also cause deep sedation (which is not always a disadvantage in the postoperative period) and bradycardia. (In man, these α_2-adrenoreceptor agonists are now being administered by the epidural route to limit their side-effects). Non-steroidal anti-inflammatory drugs (NSAIDs) act primarily by inhibiting prostaglandin release at the site of trauma and by reducing inflammation and swelling — themselves a major source of postoperative pain. Details of the very large number of NSAIDs, their uses, limitations and toxicity are beyond the scope of this book; however, they are well reviewed in current standard pharmacological texts. The use of flunixine meglamate and phenylbutazone for postoperative analgesia after surgery of the limbs is widespread. To date, in small animal anaesthesia NSAIDs have been considered to provide insufficient analgesia in the immediate postoperative period, although they are considered to be useful later on. Possible reasons for their neglect in small animal practice is their high toxicity if overdoses are given, but if used correctly and with due care, they can make a most useful contribution to postoperative analgesia.

Opioid analgesics

In the form of opium, opioids have been used as painkillers in man for at least 2000 years and the refined and processed extracts, morphine and heroin, still have a major role as analgesics. There is now a wide range of both naturally occurring and synthetic opioids that differ in potency, pharmacokinetics and, in some cases, side-effects, so that the clinician has an enormous range of choice.

The principal reason for employing opioids is to provide analgesia but some are used as cough suppressants. Unfortunately, these drugs have a wide range of side-effects, the most serious of which is respiratory depression. Even more unfortunately, in man these drugs cause euphoria and addiction, rendering them liable to abuse and resulting in controls on their use in attempts to limit this abuse. Abuse is not a feature of their use in veterinary patients but they have other undesirable side-effects, including the production of nausea and vomiting (in dogs), constipation, pruritis and in some cases dysphoria. Whilst in dogs they invariably cause sedation, in cats and horses higher doses cause excitement, although clinical doses can be used quite safely in these species of animal, being particularly unlikely to produce excitement when pain is present.

The use of nalorphine as an antidote to morphine poisoning in man was first reported in 1951 [139] and since then other agents which antagonize the effects of morphine have been produced. Many of these have partial antagonist activity, sufficient for them to be used as analgesics, and often they are less liable to abuse and, therefore, subject to fewer controls over their use. Pure antagonists, such as naloxone, will reverse the effects of morphine at doses which have no intrinsic activity when given alone.

In recent years the discovery of specific receptor sites of action for the opioids (first suggested by Martin *et al.* in 1976 [140]) and the identification in the central nervous system of endogenous ligands such as encephalins, endorphins and dynorphin which act at these receptors, has led to a better understanding of the multiple actions of agonist and partial agonist opioid drugs, as well as providing the possibility of the development of more specific drugs with fewer side-effects. On the basis of response to specific drugs Martin *et al.* initially postulated the existence of three opioid receptors termed μ, κ and σ (Table 4.2). Other multiple receptors have since been postulated and of these it is now accepted that the one known as the δ receptor is of importance. Also, many authorities now do not consider the σ receptor to be a true opioid receptor. The actions which are suggested to occur on activation of these various receptors have been the subject of many reviews [136–146] and Table 4.3 summarizes, in a very simplified form, the suggested actions following stimulation of the receptors.

It is thought that analgesia results primarily from stimulation of the μ and κ receptors while stimulation of the δ receptors modulates the effects at the μ receptors.

Table 4.2 Receptor selectivity (agonist and antagonist) of some opioid drugs

Drug	μ Receptor	κ Receptor	σ Receptor
Morphine	+++	+/−	−
Fentanyl	+++	−	−
Pethidine	++	−	−
Methadone	+++	−	+
Buprenorphine	+++	?	?
Butorphanol	++	++	−
Nalbuphine	+++	+	−
Pentazocine	++	+	+
Diprenorphine	++	++	++
Nalaxone	+++	+	+

Table 4.3 Actions suggested to occur on stimulation of various receptors

Receptor	Suggested action
μ	Spinal and supraspinal analgesia
	Respiratory depression
	Euphoria
	Nausea and vomiting
	Changes in gut motility
	Miosis
	Addiction
	? Sedation
κ	Supraspinal analgesia
	Sedation
	Addiction (mild)
	Miosis
	Dysphoria? Psychomimetic effects
δ	?
σ	Dysphoria and psychomimetic effects
	Mydriasis

Drugs classified as pure agonists, e.g. morphine, cause analgesia by stimulation of the μ and κ receptors, although they may have actions elsewhere. Naloxone is antagonistic at all receptors where it is active. The partial agonists/antagonists show a range of activity. Some may act as agonists at one type of receptor whilst antagonizing at another; some have partial agonist actions at a single type of receptor, low doses stimulating the receptor but higher doses antagonizing this effect. Unfortunately, in intact animals, unlike in pharmacological preparations, responses may not be so clear cut. For example, butorphanol is said to have no μ activity but it induces a 'walking' response in horses, which is said to be a μ effect [147]. Nevertheless, despite discrepancies, a knowledge of the range of activity at different receptors is helpful in arriving at an understanding of the actions, side-effects and reversibility of the wide range of opioids available for clinical use.

Increasing the dose of pure agonists increases analgesia but, unfortunately, also increases respiratory depression. Moreover, all the drugs which have potent μ-agonist activity appear to have effects which give rise to abuse by humans. It has been suggested that μ receptors are of two types, μ_1 and μ_2: stimulation of μ_1 resulting in analgesia whilst μ_2 stimulation leads to respiratory depression and abuse [142]. The drug meptazinol was claimed to be a pure μ_1 agonist [148] but this drug does not appear to have lived up to early expectations and is now thought to act also by other mechanisms [142].

Partial agonists have a limit to the analgesia they can produce, increasing doses sometimes antagonizing the analgesia of lower doses (i.e. the dose–response curve is bell shaped). However, the respiratory depression produced by the partial agonists is also limited, maximal depression reaching a plateau at high doses. Unfortunately, the maximal respiratory depression may still be of some clinical significance. Partial agonists are less liable to human abuse, primarily because many produce unpleasant dysphoric and hallucinatory effects. Psychomimetic and hallucinatory effects have generally been considered signs of σ-receptor stimulation. Recently, pure κ agonists have become available and it was hoped that these drugs would have the analgesic advantages of an opioid agonist without causing respiratory depression or having a major potential for abuse. Regrettably, all the drugs available to date cause unacceptable dysphoria in man and as a result it is now postulated that some of their actions attributed to σ-receptor stimulation may in fact be a property of κ-receptor stimulation. As animals cannot complain of dysphoric or hallucinatory experiences it behoves veterinarians to exercise care when using drugs likely to cause such effects.

General actions of opioid agonists in animals

At least in man it seems that the euphoric effects of morphine-like drugs contribute to the analgesia they produce, patients being unconcerned by any residual pain. Whether this is also true in animals can only remain a speculation. The pure agonists produce dose-dependent respiratory depression but it must be emphasized that in the case of chest pain low doses may improve respiratory activity through their analgesic effect. In ambulatory humans, dogs and cats morphine and some other opioid agonists cause vomiting and as they also produce marked depression of the cough reflex care must be taken to ensure that inhalation of vomit does not occur. Opioid agonists increase the tone of the gut, particularly of the sphincters, and decrease transit time, causing constipation. Their use is generally contraindicated for biliary or ureteric pain as they cause spasm of the bile and ureteric ducts. Cerebrospinal fluid pressure is elevated, so their use is also contraindicated in head injuries. The pure agonists' effects of causing tolerance and addiction in man results in their use being subject to tight statutory controls.

In humans, dogs and rabbits opioid agonists tend to cause central nervous depression whilst in cats and horses excitement may predominate. This species difference reflects in many of the properties of the drugs. High doses of morphine will sedate dogs, but not horses and cats. Opioid agonists generally cause miosis, and do so in the dog, but generalized excitement in horses and cats may sometimes be accompanied by mydriasis. The effects on the cardiovascular system are very variable and depend on the drug, its dose and the species of animal concerned. In general, however, at high doses they cause bradycardia, thought to be mediated via vagal mechanisms, and this is regularly seen in dogs. They have minimal direct effect on the heart and their effects on arterial blood pressure may be very variable. Release of histamine by morphine and pethidine may cause arterial hypotension in dogs. Opioid agonists usually cause arterial hypertension and tachycardia in horses — presumably manifestations of the excitement reaction although under some circumstances bradycardia can occur [149, 150].

High doses of opioids produce muscle rigidity in all species of animals, including dogs.

It must be emphasized again that the presence or absence of pain can have a major influence on the response to opioids, and horses and cats in pain when these drugs are given may show no adverse reactions to doses which would cause excitement in normal animals.

Use and choice of opioid analgesics

Opioid drugs may be used to provide analgesia before, during and after surgery as well as in combination with sedative drugs for 'chemical control'. The choice of opioid will depend on the degree of analgesia needed, the speed of onset of the drug's action and the length of action required, as well as on the side-effects that can be tolerated in the circumstances. When analgesia is needed during surgery, an opioid with a fairly long action may be used for premedication (e.g. morphine or buprenorphine), or a short-acting drug such as fentanyl or alfentanil given during surgery. Where potent agonists such as fentanyl or etorphine are used to provide a major component of anaesthesia for surgery, respiratory depression may be severe but can be counteracted by providing supplemental oxygen and IPPV as necessary. A similar degree of respiratory depression during the recovery period is unacceptable if less support is available. As all opioids cross the placenta, care must be taken if they are used at parturition, although naloxone may be used to antagonize respiratory depression in the neonate.

Dysphoric or hallucinatory effects will not be a problem during general anaesthesia and are often prevented in conscious animals by the use of sedatives, but may cause distress if drugs causing these effects are given to unsedated, ambulatory animals. Because opioids often have a synergistic depressant action in combination with sedatives or anaesthetics, doses (particularly of the more potent agents) may need to be reduced when combinations of these drugs are used. The use of partial agonists is encouraged by their freedom from statutory controls.

Epidural opioids

In man, opioids are used by the epidural route in order to try to achieve analgesia without central and respiratory depression. Although useful, respiratory depression may occur and sometimes is seriously delayed, occurring at a time when the patient is not under close observation. Another common side-effect is pruritis in 67–100% of patients, although only serious in 1–10% [151]. Epidural opioids can be effective in animals and they may have a role to play in the provision of prolonged analgesia in experimental animals but in veterinary practice the problems of maintaining asepsis in the management of indwelling epidural catheters may limit their usefulness.

When they are used by epidural injection care must be taken to ensure that the solution used does not contain a preservative, for this may damage nerves.

Opioid agonists

Morphine

Morphine, the principal alkaloid found in opium (the partially dried latex from the unripe capsule of *Papaver somniferum*) is still the 'gold standard' against which other analgesics are assessed. As the alkaloid itself is insoluble in water it is supplied for use as a water-soluble salt, usually the sulphate or hydrochloride. It is strongly addictive because of its euphoric properties in man and its use is, therefore, subject to controls.

Its major properties are those of producing analgesia, respiratory depression and constipation. Small doses have but minimal effects on the cardiovascular system but higher doses may cause bradycardia and hypotension in dogs. In these animals histamine release may contribute to its hypotensive action. In horses, hypertension may occur with minimal changes in heart rate [150].

Doses of 0.1–0.3 mg/kg by intramuscular injection will usually provide good analgesia for about 4 hours in most species of animal if they are in pain when the drug is given, but in cats it may be safer to restrict the dose to 0.1 mg/kg. Excitement reactions, bradycardia and histamine release are more common when the drug is given by the intravenous route and even after intravenous injection analgesia may not become apparent for some 15 minutes [144].

Papaveretum ('Omnopon')

Papaveretum, a preparation containing all the alkaloids of opium, is said to cause less vomiting than morphine in ambulatory dogs. It is most commonly used with hyoscine in the preparation 'Omnopon–Scopolamine', a time-honoured premedication in medical anaesthesia, which contains 20 mg of the alkaloids with 0.4 mg of hyoscine ('Scopolamine') per millilitre. For many years it has been used with acepromazine to control vicious dogs (for large dogs, a 1 ml vial of the Omnopon–Scopolamine mixture with 3 mg of acepromazine) and this has proved to be as effective as any of the more recently available combinations of drugs.

Pethidine

Pethidine (meperidine in North America) is only one-tenth as potent as morphine and although its primary actions are typical of agonist opioids it also appears to have atropine-like properties. Unlike morphine, it appears to relax intestinal spasm and so is particularly useful in equine spasmodic colic. It rarely, if ever, causes vomiting in dogs or cats and has little effect on the cough reflex. Doses given by intramuscular injection have little effect on arterial blood pressure but pethidine is a potent histamine liberator and because of this its intravenous injection can result in severe hypotension in dogs.

In large animals, doses of 1 mg/kg by intramuscular injection and, in dogs, doses of 1–2 mg/kg produce satisfactory analgesia. In cats, intramuscular doses of 10–20 mg per cat may be given. Pethidine appears to have a short half-life in animals [152, 153] and these doses only give pain relief for 1.5–2 hours.

Methadone

Methadone is a synthetic agonist, approximately equipotent to morphine in terms of analgesia, although it produces less sedation in dogs and more ataxia in horses. It is less likely to cause anaphylactoid reactions than is pethidine. It has been widely used in horses at intravenous or intramuscular doses of 0.1 mg/kg, higher doses carrying an increased risk of ataxia and excitement. The dose for the dog is generally accepted to be 0.25 mg/kg.

Methadone has frequently been used in dogs and horses as part of sedative/opioid combinations. A preparation used on the Continent of Europe, 'Polamivet', contains 2.5 mg of the laevorotatory isomer together with 0.125 mg of an atropine-like compound, diphenylpiperidonoethylacetamide hydrochloride, per millilitre of solution and this mixture is widely used in combination with the phenothiazine derivative, propionyl promazine, 'Combelen', for sedation of horses and dogs.

Fentanyl

This drug is about 50 times as potent as morphine. It is a pure agonist capable of producing a high level of analgesia, sufficient to allow surgery [147]. Effective following intravenous, intramuscular and subcutaneous injection, it is also rapidly absorbed across mucous membranes. Following intravenous injection it is effective in 4–7 minutes and, although claimed to be short acting (15–20 minutes) this is largely due to redistribution in the body so that cumulative effects occur with prolonged or high dosages.

The pharmacology of fentanyl in animals has been well described [147, 148]. In dogs, rats and primates it produces sedation and myosis, whilst in mice, cats and horses it causes excitement with mydriasis. Horses show a very marked locomotor response, pacing increasing with dosage, yet they show very little ataxia [147]. As with all opioid agonists, analgesia is accompanied by respiratory depression and when the drug is used in dogs during general anaesthetic IPPV is usually necessary if the dose used exceeds 0.2 mg/kg. Fentanyl has little effect on the cardiovascular system but usually causes some slowing of the pulse. Occasionally severe bradycardia occurs, necessitating the administration of anticholinergics.

In veterinary practice, fentanyl has been primarily used as a part of neuroleptanalgesic mixtures for dogs [154] but it is now becoming popular in balanced anaesthesia techniques and for postoperative analgesia in intensive care. In man, the use of adequate opioid analgesia has been shown to reduce the stress and catabolic responses to anaesthesia and surgery, and to reduce morbidity. There is some evidence that a similar reduction in the stress response occurs in animal patients given opioid analgesics during surgery.

Alfentanil

This fentanyl derivative is only one-quarter as potent an analgesic as fentanyl itself but has the advantage of being rapidly effective (1–2 minutes following intravenous injection). It has been claimed to be shorter acting than fentanyl although pharmacological studies of its pharmacokinetics in dogs throw some doubt on this since it has been shown to be more cumulative following repeated doses [155]. Alfentanil plasma levels decay triphasically in dogs ($t_{1/2 B} = 104$ minutes), and less than 1% of the drug is excreted unchanged as alfentanil, metabolism into a large number of inactive metabolites being rapid [156]. Analgesia is accompanied by respiratory depression and very severe bradycardia may occur [157].

In dogs, alfentanil may be used to reduce the induction dose of an intravenous anaesthetic although this may entail production of several minutes of apnoea. For example, mixing 10 µg/kg of alfentanil with 0.3 or 0.6 mg of atropine and injecting this mixture some 30 seconds before injecting propofol can reduce the dose of propofol needed to induce anaesthesia to less than 2 mg/kg, but apnoea of up to 3 minutes of duration may occur [158]. Similar results follow when alfentanil at this dose is used prior to the injection of thiopentone. However, with these intravenous anaesthetics apnoea is not nearly so prolonged when the alfentanil dose is reduced to 5 µg/kg, while there is still a desirable reduction in the dose of anaesthetic needed to allow endotracheal intubation. Alfentanil is now often used in intermittent doses to provide an 'analgesic element' in anaesthetized dogs about to be subjected to intense surgical stimulation but in spontaneously breathing animals the individual doses should not exceed 5 µg/kg if there are no facilities for prolonged IPPV of the lungs.

In Munich, Erhardt [159] has used etomidate/alfentanil to produce short periods of anaesthesia followed by a rapid recovery in dogs, cats, rats, rabbits, sheep, goats and calves.

Other fentanyl derivatives

Sufentanil is approximately 10 times as potent as fentanyl, while *lofentanil* has a very potent and exceptionally long-lasting effect. Neither of these drugs has been used extensively in veterinary medicine. *Carfentanil* is one of the most potent opioids known. It is said to be 3–8 times as potent as etorphine and has proved to be useful in elephants [160] although at the concentrations used it is a dangerous drug to handle since it is rapidly absorbed across mucous membranes. An antagonist suitable for use in humans should be readily available whenever carfentanil is used.

Etorphine is a very potent derivative of morphine which is claimed to be effective in a dose of about 0.5 mg per 500 kg. It appears to have all the properties of morphine but equipotent doses cause more respiratory depression. Its very great potency constitutes its sole advantage in that an effective dose for a very large animal can be dissolved in a very small volume of solvent, enabling it to be used in dart-gun projectiles for immobilizing wild game animals. In anaesthetic practice this very same potency makes it a difficult drug to handle and constitutes a hazard to the anaesthetist.

Etorphine is an extremely long-acting compound and recovery from its effects is also delayed by enterohepatic recycling. Its action is usually terminated by the use of diprenorphine, a specific antagonist. The drug has the highly undesirable property of producing stimulation of the central nervous system before depressing it and this results in a period of excitement. In an attempt to overcome this, etorphine is marketed in fixed-ratio combinations with phenothiazine tranquillizers and these potent neuroleptanalgesic mixtures will be discussed later on p. 72.

Buprenorphine

Buprenorphine is a partial agonist that is popular as a premedicant and postoperative analgesic in cats, dogs and laboratory animals [161, 162] where it is used by the intravenous, intramuscular and subcutaneous routes. Although in man it is given in the form of a sublingual tablet, oral administration is ineffective in animals as the drug is broken down during the first pass through the liver.

This drug is unusual in that its association and dissociation with receptors is very slow. Thus, even after intravenous injection it has a prolonged outset of action (30 minutes or longer), a fact often forgotten in its use. Its long duration of action (known to be about 8 hours in man) is due to its slow dissociation from receptors and analgesia remains long after it can no longer be detected in the blood by most assay methods. This tight binding to receptors means that its actions are very difficult to reverse with naloxone, although pretreatment with naloxone will prevent its effects. Should respiratory depression result from the use of buprenorphine it should be treated with IPPV of the lungs, or with non-specific respiratory stimulants such as doxapram.

The analgesic dose–response curve is bell shaped, higher doses antagonizing analgesia already produced by lower doses; however, higher doses do not antagonize the respiratory depression once this has reached a plateau. In the authors' experience serious respiratory depression is rare with the usual clinical doses but as its onset may be delayed when it does occur, it is important that any animal given the drug remains under close observation for at least 2 hours after its administration. On its own, in clinical doses, it does not appear to cause sedation, or to cause excitement in susceptible species of animal, but its use towards the end of surgery slows recovery from

anaesthesia. Its effects on the cardiovascular system are minimal.

Doses used in dogs and cats vary from 6 to 10 µg/kg and in horses the authors have found it an effective analgesic at doses of 6 µg/kg for orthopaedic cases. However, the bell-shaped nature of the dose–response curve must be considered and if these doses are inadequate for pain relief, they may be followed by doses of a pure agonist drug. Buprenorphine has also been extensively used with α_2-adrenoceptor agonists in sedative combinations (p. 195).

The popularity of the drug in the UK has undoubtedly been due to its prolonged length of action, that it provides better analgesia that can be obtained with other partial agonists and, until recently, its freedom from control under the Misuse of Drugs Act 1971.

Butorphanol

In the UK this drug is currently not subject to controls under the Misuse of Drugs Act 1971. It is used in cats, dogs and horses for analgesia and in sedative combinations with α_2-adrenoceptor agonists. Butorphanol is also used in dogs for its antitussive effect. In dogs and horses it is said to have minimal effects on the cardiovascular system [163, 164] but caution may be in order here for in man it causes increased pulmonary vascular resistance and, at high doses, hypertension, so it is not recommended for patients with cardiovascular disease.

In experimental horses it has been used in doses of 0.1–0.4 mg/kg but the higher doses caused restlessness and apparent dysphoria [165] and the dose currently used clinically is 0.1 mg/kg by intravenous injection, which seems to be particularly effective for the relief of mild colic. However, in the authors' experience even this dose may induce walking behaviour in unrestrained animals.

Doses of 0.1–0.5 mg/kg by intramuscular or subcutaneous injection have been found to give effective analgesia for about 4 hours in both dogs and cats [132]. In experimental studies [166, 167] visceral analgesia was found to be superior to somatic analgesia, and lower doses superior to higher doses, possibly indicating that, like buprenorphine, the dose–response curve is bell shaped. Butorphanol may be given orally for analgesia although doses 5–10 times those by injection are required to produce an equivalent effect.

Pentazocine

In man this partial agonist has lost its earlier popularity due to producing a high incidence of dysphoria and hallucinatory responses, coupled with causing a marked increase in pulmonary vascular resistance. Like buprenorphine, in the UK its use is controlled under the Misuse of Drugs Act 1971. Although it is impossible to assess dysphoria in animals most veterinarians with extensive experience of pentazocine have seen signs they associate with such an effect, particularly following high doses.

Despite these problems pentazocine has been quite widely used in veterinary practice, doses of 1–3 mg/kg being said to give 1–3 hours of pain relief [132, 161, 166]. Pentazocine can be given orally but first-pass liver metabolism means that high doses are necessary. In the experimental horse colic model, doses of 0.5–4 mg/kg have been tested, the higher doses giving rise to ataxia and muscle tremors [161]. The currently recommended dose for the relief of colic pains in horses is 0.33 mg/kg intravenously, followed 15 minutes later by a similar intramuscular dose [142].

Nalbuphine

Although this drug has minimal cardiovascular effects and appears to cause few dysphoric reactions it has a low ceiling of analgesia and is not to be recommended for relief of severe pain. In experimental dogs it has been found that doses of 0.75 mg/kg give reasonable visceral analgesia; somatic analgesia is poor and analgesia is always inferior to that provided by butorphanol. Currently the drug is being evaluated as part of a sedative combination for use in horses and in the doses being used for this nalbuphine alone produces no discernible unwanted effects in pain-free horses.

Sequential analgesia

Sequential analgesia is a term introduced to describe the use of partial agonists subsequent to pure agonists (usually fentanyl) in an attempt to reverse residual respiratory depression whilst maintaining analgesia. First attempted with pentazocine, buprenorphine and nalbuphine have also been used for this purpose [138]. On theoretical grounds, buprenorphine should be the least efficient and nalbuphine the most because of their μ-agonist and -antagonist properties (Table 4.2) and nalbuphine has been widely recommended for use in man for this purpose [144]. In laboratory practice, buprenorphine has been used to reverse the effects of high doses of fentanyl [162].

The idea of agonist/antagonist analgesia is not new, for many years ago a combination of pethidine together with its antagonist levallorphan was marketed, but was found to produce no less respiratory depression than pethidine alone at equianalgesic doses. It is clear that the final outcome of sequential analgesia must be the result of a delicate balance of activities at the various receptors and the 'reversing' drugs must be given with great care according to the need of the individual patient [144].

Opioid antagonists

Pure antagonists

Naloxone is a pure antagonist at all opioid receptors and so will reverse the effect of all opioid agonists but it is less effective against partial agonists. In man, reversal of opioid actions with naloxone is sometimes accompanied by tachycardia but there are no reports of this in the veterinary literature. The drug is fairly short acting and its effects may wear off before those of the previously administered agonist so that repeated doses may be needed. This is particularly important in veterinary medicine where large and frequent doses of naloxone are needed to counter the effects of the very potent long-acting agent etorphine.

Naloxone given to an animal that has not received an opioid may temporarily alter behaviour and it has been claimed that the drug is effective in stopping horses crib biting [142]. Naloxone is thought by some to have a role in the treatment of shock [142].

Naltrexone is a long-acting derivative of naloxone and although not currently used in veterinary practice it could prove useful should a long-acting pure antagonist be required.

Partial agonists used as antagonists

Some partial agonists, which either give poor analgesia or produce dysphoria sufficient to preclude their use as analgesics are used *for* their antagonistic properties. *Nalorphine* was the first to be used as an opioid antagonist but has now been superseded by naloxone. *Diprenorphine* is marketed as a specific antagonist of etorphine and in animals it appears to be very efficient in this role. However, as it causes hallucinations in man it is only licensed for use in animals and in medical practice naloxone remains the drug of choice for countering the effects of etorphine.

Sedative/opioid combinations

When opioids are combined with sedative drugs, synergism seems to occur, sedation and analgesia being greater than that capable of being achieved by either drug alone. The use of the sedative will often also prevent any excitement effects that might occur with the opioid alone. There is nothing new about the

Table 4.4 Composition of some commercially available neuroleptanalgesic mixtures

Commercial name	Analgesic	Neuroleptic
Innovar Vet	Fentanyl 0.4 mg/ml	Droperidol 20 mg/ml
Thalamonal	Fentanyl 0.05 mg/ml	Droperidol 2.5 mg/ml
Hypnorm	Fentanyl 0.315 mg/kg	Fluanisone 10 mg/ml
Immobilon L.A.	Etorphine 2.45 mg/ml	Acepromazine 10 mg/ml
Immobilon S.A.	Etorphine 0.074 mg/ml	Methotrimeprazine 18 mg/ml

use of such combinations, veterinarians having used them for many years to make animals more manageable [168]. The range of sedative/opioid mixtures in use for sedation and control of animals is now enormous, α_2-adrenoceptor agonists, neuroleptic agents and benzodiazepines all having been combined with a wide variety of agonist and partial agonist opioids. Depth of sedation achieved depends primarily on the opioid employed, partial agonists or less potent agonist combinations giving sedation, whilst, where large doses of the potent opioids such as fentanyl or alfentanil are used, anaesthesia can be achieved, although severe respiratory depression may accompany the use of these high-dose opioid techniques. Suitable combinations for sedation, control and anaesthesia in each species of animal are given in later chapters of this book.

The term neuroleptanalgesia has been used to describe the combination of opioids with phenothiazines or butyrophenones (neuroleptics). The principles of their use are the same as outlined above for any sedative/opioid combination but the neuroleptic agents have the specific property of reducing opioid-induced vomiting in dogs. Neuroleptic techniques can be used in two ways. At comparatively low opioid dose rates they can be used for control, or as premedication before general anaesthesia; at higher dose rates they can be used to produce sufficient depression of the central nervous system to enable surgery to be performed. This latter use is sometimes termed 'neuroleptanaesthesia' and was the way in which the technique was first used in veterinary medicine [154], but is associated with profound respiratory depression and should not be used unless facilities for ventilatory support are available.

To obtain the best results the neuroleptic should be administered first and, when it is fully effective, the analgesic should be given to produce the desired result. In veterinary medicine, however, for convenience it is usual to employ commercially available fixed-ratio mixtures of the two drugs and it must be accepted that this ratio may not be optimal for any particular animal.

The compositions of three commercially available mixtures of fentanyl/butyrophenone tranquillizer are given in Table 4.4. All have similar properties and may be considered together. They are used in dogs, primates and small rodents, but they are contraindicated in cats because fentanyl may cause violent excitement in these animals. They are usually used to produce deep sedation with profound analgesia sufficient for procedures such as endoscopy, or the lancing of a superficial abscess; however, they are inadequate for major surgery. The rationale for using the short-acting fentanyl with long-acting butyrophenones is not obvious, but the combination appears effective in both man and animals.

Fentanyl has been used with fluanisone (see p. 294) for neuroleptanalgesia in dogs as a 1:50 mixture (Fluanisone Comp.). Given at a dosage level of 0.1 mg/kg of fentanyl with 5 mg/kg of fluanisone by slow intravenous injection it produced a period of surgical anaesthesia after short and mild excitement. Recovery was slow, the time varying from 2 to 10 hours before recovery of full consciousness.

In dogs it was found to be necessary to give atropine to prevent bradycardia caused by the intramuscular injection of a 1:50 fentanyl–droperidol mixture (Innovar-Vet). The analgesia, sedation and immobility produced by this mixture is sufficient for diagnostic procedures and minor surgery. Respiratory effects are variable, with both hyperpnoea and respiratory depression occurring. The advantages of the mixture are ease of administration, a wide safety margin, quiet postoperative state, reversibility with narcotic antagonists (such as naloxone), and tolerance by animals in poor physical condition. The disadvantages include variable response in certain breeds, the spontaneous movements which occur, the need, on occasion, to employ nitrous oxide or local analgesia when major surgery is to be performed, and the possibility of respiratory depression.

Fentanyl has also been used in the UK in combination with fluanisone, as the preparation Hypnorm. Diarrhoea has been reported to follow the administration of this mixture in over 24% of canine patients.

The effects of fentanyl with fluanisone and fentanyl with droperidol in pigs have been studied: neither mixture produced better sedation than droperidol given alone.

The results obtained by neuroleptanalgesic techniques are more impressive in monkeys. In these animals the technique may offer distinct advantages over the more conventional methods of anaesthesia, especially when skilled assistance is not available.

Etorphine/phenothiazine tranquillizer mixtures (Immobilon) are marketed for both small and large animal use, the concentrations of etorphine and the tranquillizer in each preparation being as shown in Table 4.4. At the doses recommended by the manufacturers the preparations cause intense central nervous depression with considerable analgesia, allowing major surgery to be carried out. When surgery is completed the effects of the etorphine (but not of the phenothiazine tranquillizer) are commonly reversed by the use of the specific antagonist, diprenorphine (Revivon). Revivon is also available in concentrations suitable for use in large and small animals, Large Animal Revivon containing 3.0 mg/ml and Small Animal Revivon, 0.272 mg/ml. These concentrations have been chosen so that, to reverse the effects of the appropriate Immobilon, a volume of Revivon equal to the volume of Immobilon used is needed.

The effects of Immobilon in horses are what might be expected to follow such high doses of an opiate drug in this species of animal, with excitatory effects predominating. Intramuscular injection regularly leads to excitement during induction; after intravenous injection the horse becomes recumbent within 1 minute and, although excitement may occur, it is much less marked. Once recumbent, intense muscular activity makes the animal very stiff and violent continuous tremors occur. The muscles relax somewhat after about 20 minutes. Blood pressure and heart rate increase to very high levels but respiration is severely depressed. Following the intravenous injection of Revivon most horses regain the standing position within a few minutes. Occasionally, horses become violently excited shortly after standing and a further excitement phase may occur several hours later. This later phase is thought to be due to enterohepatic recycling of etorphine and it is said that it can be prevented by the subcutaneous injection of a further dose of Revivon after the animal has recovered to the standing position.

In horses, this type of 'knockdown' with the advantage of the ability to produce almost immediate recovery by pharmacological reversal of the effects of the induction agent is obviously very attractive. However, the dangers inherent in the use of the very potent drugs required must be weighed very carefully against this advantage.

Although Immobilon has been recommended for clinical use in a wide variety of animals, little has been published concerning its pharmacology in them. In pigs and dogs, depressant effects predominate and etorphine rarely causes excitement. In pigs, the mortality rate following the use of Immobilon seems unacceptably high and work has shown that while in the majority of pigs arterial blood pressure is well maintained, in some it falls to such low levels that death is inevitable if the effect of the Immobilon cannot be rapidly reversed (Lees and Meredith, personal communication).

Immobilon, and other etorphine-containing mixtures, have been extensively used for the capture of wild game. Although generally used as 'knockdown' doses, as in horses, it is commonly used at lower dose rates whereby the animals (elephants and giraffes) become sedated but remain standing. Immobilon is not recommended for wild Felidea (nor domestic cats).

Once the effects of a long-acting neuroleptanalgesic combination of drugs, such as Immobilon, have been antagonized by the use of an opiate antagonist, problems arise if pain relief is needed or the animal has to be reanaesthetized (e.g. for the control of postoperative haemorrhage). Following the use of any opiate antagonist further doses of opiate analgesics are ineffective and pain must be relieved by other means.

In man, etorphine is extremely potent and the use of Immobilon constitutes a danger to the anaesthetist and assistants. Should an accident occur, naloxone is recommended as the drug of choice for treatment of human beings, but several doses may be needed to maintain respiration until medical help can be obtained.

ANTICHOLINERGIC AGENTS

Anticholinergic agents are widely used in anaesthesia to antagonize the muscarinic effects of acetylcholine and thus to block transmission at parasympathetic postganglionic nerve endings. The main purposes are:

1. To reduce salivation and bronchial secretions
2. To block the effects of impulses in the vagus nerves
3. To block certain of the effects produced by drugs which stimulate the parasympathetic system

The reduction of salivation and bronchial secretion is necessary if irritant volatile anaesthetics such as ether are used, but it is not essential with modern halogenated anaesthetics like halothane and methoxyflurane. However, in small dogs and in cats, even a little secretion may be enough to give rise to significant respiratory obstruction and in such patients it is probably advisable to administer anticholinergics before any anaesthetic. Ruminants produce large quantities of saliva but anticholinergic drugs merely make their saliva more thick and viscid and more likely to create respiratory obstruction, so such drugs should not be used in these animals.

Some drugs, in particular the α_2-adrenoceptor agonists and, in high doses, the opioids, can cause marked vagus-mediated bradycardia. Also, under light anaesthesia, surgery of the head and neck is prone to trigger vagal reflexes, and the horse and cat appear to be most at risk from these disturbances. In cats the oculocardiac reflex is well known to result in bradycardia and even cardiac arrest; stimulation of the nose or other similarly sensitive structures of the head region can have the same effect or cause laryngeal spasm. In horses, stimulation about the head and neck can produce sudden cardiac arrest without a prior warning of bradycardia.

Anticholinesterase drugs such as neostigmine are used to antagonize the block produced by competitive muscle relaxants and their use must be preceded or combined with one of the anticholinergic drugs to block the muscarinic effects of the released acetylcholine. Also, the depolarizing relaxant, suxamethonium, has effects similar to those of acetylcholine and an anticholinergic 'cover' should be employed when this relaxant is used.

In recent years the advisability of routine premedication with anticholinergic drugs has been questioned. These drugs certainly have side-effects and the tachycardia they induce may be undesirable. Disturbance of vision may cause a cat or horse to panic. Reduced gut motility may cause colic in horses. In man, considerable discomfort results from dry mouth in the postoperative period and, presumably, this may also be the case in animals. These disadvantages must be weighed against the advantages already mentioned.

Current medical practice, where ether is not used, suggests that it is preferable not to use anticholinergic drugs for routine premedication, but to reserve them for corrective measures should bradycardia occur during the course of the anaesthetic [169]. This, of course, assumes that monitoring is adequate to detect the bradycardia. However, it must be remembered that following intravenous injection, atropine may cause further bradycardia through a central effect before blocking at the vagal endings and increasing heart rate. The use of intravenous atropine or glycopyrrolate to correct some drug-induced bradycardias has been shown to be associated with further bradycardia and heart block [170]. Thus, in veterinary medicine the decision to include an anticholinergic agent in premedication may be based on the species of animal concerned, its size, the drugs to be used for and during anaesthesia, the likelihood of complications from bradycardia or vagal reflexes, the level of monitoring in use, and any specific contraindications. The main contraindications are in conditions associated with tachycardia and in certain forms of glaucoma which are aggravated by dilatation of the pupil.

Atropine

Atropine, the most important of the alkaloids obtained from *Atropa belladonna* (deadly-nightshade), is used in anaesthesia as the water-soluble sulphate. Its metabolism is not the same in all species of animal. When administered to dogs, atropine disappears very rapidly from the bloodstream. Part of the dose is excreted unchanged in the urine, part appears in the urine as tropine and the remainder is apparently broken down in the body to as yet unidentified products. In cats, atropine is hydrolysed by either of two esterases which are found in large quantities in the liver and kidneys. These esterases are also found in rabbits and rats.

Atropine inhibits transmission of postganglionic cholinergic nerve impulses to effector cells but inhibition is not equally effective all over the body, and atropine has less effect upon the urinary bladder and intestines than upon the heart and salivary glands.

The drug has unpredictable effects on the central nervous system. Certain cerebral and medullary functions are initially stimulated then later depressed by it, so that the final outcome depends on the dose used and on the route of administration. Clinical doses may produce an initial slowing of the heart due to stimulation of the vagal centres in the brain before its peripheral anticholinergic effects occur. Atropine overdose causes a 'central cholinergic syndrome' with fluctuations between hyperexcitability and depression.

Although atropine is, in general, a very safe drug with a wide therapeutic margin, occasional cases have been reported where an individual person or animal has appeared unduly sensitive to the central effects.

The main action of the drug is on the heart rate, which usually increases due to peripheral inhibition of the cardiac vagus; the initial slowing due to central action is only seen before the onset of the peripheral inhibition. Arterial blood pressure is usually unchanged, but if already depressed by vagal activity due to reflex or drug action (e.g. halothane) it will be raised by the administration of atropine. In man, an increase in the incidence of cardiac arrhythmias has been observed during anaesthesia following atropine premedication, but K. W. Clarke (unpublished observations) found that atropine reduced the incidence of ventricular extrasystoles in cats anaesthetized with a variety of halogenated volatile anaesthetics.

The minute volume of respiration is slightly increased due to central stimulation. Bronchial musculature is relaxed and bronchial secretions are reduced. Both anatomical and physiological dead-spaces are increased by atropine [171]. A report [172] that the administration of atropine was associated with hypoxaemia in the preoperative, operative and postoperative periods in man, was not confirmed by later studies [173, 174], and studies in dogs at the Cambridge Veterinary School and elsewhere have failed to show any hypoxaemia attributable to atropine administration.

Atropine has marked ocular effects. Mydriasis results from the local or systemic administration of atropine and thus it is probable that this drug should not be given to animals suffering from glaucoma. Except in dogs where the parenteral administration of the usual clinical doses does not alter pupillary size, the mydriasis may interfere with the so-called 'ocular signs' of anaesthesia (see p. 43). The ocular effects also result in visual disturbance and animals so effected must be approached with great caution as they may have problems in judging distances. This is particularly important in horses and cats as both these animals tend to panic in response to sudden movements which they do not see clearly.

Although atropine reduces muscle tone in the gastrointestinal tract, at the doses used for premedication this effect is minimal. The passage of barium meals along the gut of the dog is not appreciably slowed by atropine premedication but it is possible that the incidence of postanaesthetic colic in horses is increased by the use of this drug.

Because of the different ways in which they metabolize the drug, the effectiveness of a given dose varies according to the species of animal, but its therapeutic index is such that a wide range of doses can be recommended. In dogs, doses from 0.02 to 0.05 mg/kg are employed, while in cats doses of up to 0.3 mg (approximately 0.1 mg/kg for an adult cat for example) are perfectly safe. Pigs may be given from 0.3 to 1.8 mg according to size. The exact dose is largely determined by the fact that, at least in the UK, atropine sulphate for injection is still supplied in a solution containing 0.6 mg/ml — a legacy of earlier days when doses were measured in grains. A large animal preparation containing 10 mg/ml is now available, and this enables horses to be given doses between 10 and 60 mg much more conveniently than was previously possible.

To neutralize the muscarinic effects of the anticholinesterases such as neostigmine, in cats, dogs and pigs, 0.6–1.2 mg of atropine are given slowly intravenously 2–5 minutes before these agents are injected, or mixed in the syringe and injected with the anticholinesterase. In horses, doses of 10 mg appear to be adequate for this purpose.

Glycopyrrolate

Glycopyrrolate is a quaternary ammonium anticholinergic agent with powerful and prolonged antisialagogue activity. As an antisialagogue it is about five times as potent as atropine [175, 176]. In man, clinical doses have an almost selective effect on salivary and sweat gland secretion and cardiovascular stability is excellent, there being little change in heart rate, and a reduction in cardiac arrhythmias compared with their incidence after atropine. This cardiovascular stability was thought to make it particularly useful for combination with anticholinesterases for antagonizing competitive neuromuscular blocking agents and, indeed, as glycopyrrolate is claimed to have a more rapid onset of action than atropine, a preparation of neostigmine with glycopyrrolate is available for this purpose. However, later work [177] on anaesthetized human patients showed no difference in the cardiovascular effects of atropine and glycopyrrolate other than in the time of onset of action — glycopyrrolate taking 2–3 minutes to become effective following intravenous injection.

Glycopyrrolate has now been used widely in veterinary practice in doses of 0.01–0.02 mg/kg [176, 177]. However, although it has been satisfactory in preventing excessive salivation and bradycardia, it has proved disappointingly similar to atropine in its effects on the heart rate [170]. A comparison of atropine given intravenously at doses of 0.02–0.04 mg/kg with intravenous glycopyrrolate (0.02 and 0.01 mg/kg) in dogs with drug-induced bradycardia showed that both agents caused a high incidence of cardiac arrhythmia, including atrioventricular block, during the first 3 minutes after injection [176]. This is surprising since glycopyrrolate does not readily cross the blood–brain barrier and suggests that arrhythmias may be due to mechanisms other than central stimulation.

The fact that the drug does not readily cross the blood–brain barrier means that it has little central action, producing less effect on vision than other anticholinergic agents [178] and thus it could be the anticholinergic of choice in horses and cats.

Hyoscine

Hyoscine is an alkaloid resembling atropine, found in the same group of plants but usually obtained from the shrub henbane (*Hyoscyamus niger*). The peripheral actions of hyoscine resemble those of atropine. However, its relative potency at different sites differs from atropine. It is a more potent antisialagogue but less effective as a vagolytic so that its effect on heart rate is less than that of atropine when they are given in equipotent doses for their drying effects. The central effects of hyoscine are greater than those of atropine and in horses it may produce considerable excitement. In general, although hyoscine is used in man (in spite of its propensity to cause hallucinations) as a depressant of nervous activity, it is not suitable for this purpose in animals. It has been used as the hydrobromide for premedication in dogs in doses of 0.2–0.4 mg and it is often used with paraveretum (Omnopon–Scopolamine, Roche). This standard preparation contains 20 mg of paraveretum with a 0.4 mg of hyoscine per ml of solution.

PREMEDICATION

Preanaesthetic medication or 'premedication' helps both the anaesthetist and animal, for it makes the induction and maintenance of anaesthesia easier for the anaesthetist while at the same time rendering the experience safer and more comfortable for the patient. It implies the administration, usually before but sometimes at or immediately after the induction of anaesthesia, of sedatives, anxiolytics and analgesics, with or without anticholinergics.

The classical aims of premedication are:

1. To relieve anxiety, thus overcoming the apprehension, fear and resistance to anaesthesia.
2. To counteract unwanted side-effects of agents used in anaesthesia. Effects which may require modification depend on the species of animal and on the drugs used; they include vomiting (mainly in dogs and cats), poor quality of recovery, bradycardia, salivation and excessive muscle tone.
3. To reduce the dose of anaesthetic. In many, but not all cases, drug combinations may have a lower incidence of side-effects than a high dose of the anaesthetic would have on its own. However, occasionally (especially in the case of respiratory depression) side-effects may be additive.
4. To provide extra analgesia.

The use of anticholinergic agents for premedication has already been discussed (p. 72). Analgesic agents are essential if the patient is in pain in the preoperative period, but even when pain is absent, analgesics may increase preoperative sedation, reduce the subsequent dose of anaesthetic needed, contribute to analgesia during surgery and even, if sufficiently long acting, contribute to analgesia postoperatively. The use of long-acting analgesics such as buprenorphine is particularly popular for the contribution they make to all stages of the anaesthetic process. Very potent but short-acting opioids such as fentanyl and alfentanil will reduce the dose of anaesthetic required, but their short action means that further analgesia must be provided during recovery.

The sedative and anxiolytic drugs play the major role in premedication, improving the quality of anaesthetic induction and recovery, contributing to anaesthesia and in some cases counteracting unwanted side-effects such as the muscle rigidity produced by ketamine. By calming the animal in the preoperative period, the necessary clipping and cleaning is made more pleasant for the animal and nursing staff. Moreover, by controlling the emotional disturbance the release of catecholamines is reduced, thus decreasing the chance of adrenaline-induced cardiac arrhythmias, smoothing the course of anaesthesia and (usually) ensuring a quiet recovery.

The degree of activity of the central nervous system at the time when anaesthesia is induced determines the amount of anaesthetic which has to be administered to produce surgical anaesthesia. This activity is lowered by wasting disease, senility and surgical shock and increased by fear, pain, fever and conditions such as thyrotoxicosis. Sedatives and analgesics decrease the irritability of the central nervous system and thereby enhance the effects of the anaesthetic agents. In general, the depressant effects of the drugs used in premedication summate with those of the anaesthetic and unless this is clearly understood overdosage may occur. Most sedative drugs depress respiration, and if given in large doses before the administration of an anaesthetic which also produces respiratory depression (e.g. thiopentone sodium or halothane), respiratory failure may occur before surgical anaesthesia is attained. Premedication must, therefore, be regarded as an integral part of the whole anaesthetic technique, and never as an isolated event.

The type of sedative drug chosen for premedication will depend on a variety of factors. Phenothiazine derivatives such as acepromazine are good anxiolytics and reduce the incidence of vomiting. Their use usually results in a calm, but delayed, recovery and delayed recovery is to be avoided in horses and ruminants for in these animals prolonged recumbency gives rise to problems. To prevent recovery from being unacceptably delayed, doses of the phenothiazine derivatives used for premedication should be below those recommended for simply sedating animals when anaesthesia is not contemplated. Phenothiazine drugs undoubtedly increase the chance of regurgitation at induction of anaesthesia in ruminants.

The α_2-adrenoceptor agonists have a major effect in reducing the dose of subsequent anaesthetic required; doses at the lower end of the dosage range provide profound sedation and are useful in the animal which is particularly difficult to handle. They also provide some degree of muscle relaxation and are especially effective in counteracting the muscle tension associated with the use of drugs such as ketamine.

Benzodiazepines provide little obvious preoperative sedation but their muscle-relaxing properties are useful when drugs such as ketamine are to be used and they reduce the dose of subsequent anaesthetic needed.

Often more than one sedative drug is used in premedication. For example, α_2-adrenoceptor agonists and benzodiazepines may be combined prior to the use of ketamine. However, such polypharmacy must be used with care, as many such combinations may have synergistic activity and it is easy to administer an overdose of any anaesthetic agents given subsequently.

For premedication, drugs can be given by any one or more of the usual routes of drug administration. The choice is governed both by the nature of the drug to be used and the time which is available before anaesthesia is to be induced. If there is plenty of time the drugs may be given sublingually, by mouth or into the rectum. (The rectal route is not very satisfactory and is only used when for some reason the others are impracticable, but the sublingual route is surprisingly effective for the α_2-adrenoceptor agonists making it possible to subdue vicious animals by using a syringe to squirt the drugs into the animal's open mouth). If only 5–10 minutes will elapse before anaesthesia is induced then the intravenous route must be employed. It is always as well to ensure that the preliminary medication exerts its full effects before the administration of a general anaesthetic is begun; otherwise respiratory depression and respiratory failure may occur even during light anaesthesia.

In the past it was fairly simple to define the limits of premedication and to recognize when anaesthesia began. Today, with the wide range of different types of drugs available, such distinctions are no longer clear. Neuroleptanalgesic techniques may be considered as constituting premedication — but the more potent mixtures (e.g. Immobilon, p. 72) may enable surgery to be carried out without further resort to general anaesthetic agents. Dissociative agents such as ketamine may be regarded either as drugs for premedication or for the induction of general anaesthesia. Hypnotics (e.g. chloral hydrate or pentobarbitone) may be used at low doses for sedation, or at higher doses to produce hypnosis or even anaesthesia. In clinical practice, exact definitions of terminology are unimportant as long as the anaesthetist clearly understands the role played by each drug used, be it 'premedicant', 'dissociative agent' or 'anaesthetic', in the total process involved in bringing the animal to a state suitable for the performance of surgery, examination or whatever else is required.

Anxiolytics, sedatives, hypnotics and analgesics all have their place in this process. In any particular case, the choice of drugs, their dose and route of administration, gives the anaesthetist the opportunity to demonstrate artistry as well as scientific knowledge.

REFERENCES

1. Dundee, J. W. (1980) *General Anaesthesia*, 4th edn (eds Gray, Nunn and Utting), chapt. 13. London: Butterworths.
2. Tobin, T. and Ballard, S. (1979) *Journal of Equine Medicine and Surgery* **3**, 460.
3. Booth, N. H. (1982) *Veterinary Pharmacology and Therapeutics*, 5th edn (eds Booth and McDonald), chapt. 17. Ames: Iowa University Press.
4. Balderssarini, R. J. (1985) *The Pharmacological Basis of Therapeutics*, 7th edn (eds Gilman, Goodman, Rall and Murad), chapt. 19. New York: Macmillan.
5. Attia, R. R., Grogono, A. W. and Domer, F. R. (1987) *Practical Anesthetic Pharmacology*. Connecticut: Appleton-Century-Crofts.
6. Vickers, M. D., Schnieder, H. and Wood-Smith, F. G. (1984) *Drugs in Anaesthetic Practice*, 6th edn. London: Butterworths.
7. Lees, P. (1979) *Pharmacological Basis of Small Animal Medicine* (eds Yoxall and Hird), p. 825. London: Blackwell Scientific.
8. Dundee, J. W. and Wyant, G. M. (1989) *Intravenous Anaesthesia*. Edinburgh: Churchill Livingstone.
9. Muir, W. W., Werner, L. L. and Hamlin, R. L. (1975) *American Journal of Veterinary Research* **36**, 1299.
10. Muir, W. W. (1981) *Veterinary Clinics of North America: Large Animal Practice*, vol. 3, p. 17. Philadelphia: W. B. Saunders.
11. Maze, M., Hayward, E. and Gaba, D. M. (1985) *Anesthesiology* **63**, 611.
12. Dressel, P. E. (1985) *Anesthesiology* **63**, 582.
13. Carey, F. McL. and Sanford, J. (1985/6) *Proceedings of the British Equine Veterinary Association*, p. 52.
14. Parry, B. W., Anderson, G. A. and Gay, C. C. (1982) *Australian Veterinary Journal* **59**, 148.
15. Hall, L. W. (1971) *Wright's Veterinary Anaesthesia*, 7th edn. London: Baillière Tindall.
16. Martin, J. F. and Beck, J. D. (1956) *American Journal of Veterinary Research* **17**, 678.
17. Owen, L. N. and Neal, P. A. (1957) *Veterinary Record* **69**, 413.

18. MacKenzie, G. and Snow, D. H. (1977) *Veterinary Record* **101**, 30.
19. Glen, J. B. (1973) *Proceedings of the Association of Veterinary Anaesthetists of Great Britain and Ireland* **4**, 71.
20. Kerr, D. P., Jones, E. W., Holbert, M. S. and Huggins, K. (1979) *American Journal of Veterinary Research* **33**, 777.
21. Muir, W. W. and Hamlin, R. L. (1975) *American Journal of Veterinary Research* **36**, 1439.
22. Muir, W. W., Skarda, R. T. and Sheehan, W. C. (1979) *American Journal of Veterinary Research* **40**, 1518.
23. Lees, P. and Meradith, M. J. (1983) *Pharmacological Basis of Large Animal Medicine*. London: Blackwell Scientific.
24. Popovic, N. A., Mullane, J. E. and Thap, M. D. (1972) *American Journal of Veterinary Research* **33**, 1819.
25. Pearson, H. and Weaver, B. M. Q. (1978) *Equine Veterinary Journal* **10**, 85.
26. Lucke, J. N. and Sansom, J. (1972) *Veterinary Record* **104**, 21.
27. Sharrock, A. G. (1982) *Australian Veterinary Journal* **58**, 39.
28. Jones, R. S. (1979) *Veterinary Record* **90**, 613.
29. Scheidy, S. F. and McNally, I. C. S. (1958) *Cornell Veterinarian* **48**, 331.
30. Raker, C. W. and English, B. (1989) *Journal of the American Veterinary Medical Association* **134**, 19.
31. Cunningham, J. A. (1959) *Veterinary Record* **71**, 395.
32. Limont, A. G. (1961) *Veterinary Record* **73**, 691.
33. Marsboom, R. and Symoens, J. (1968) *Tijdsch. Diergenkde.* **93**, 3.
34. Marsboom, R. and Van den Brande, M. (1969) *Veterinary Record* **85**, 64.
35. Aitken, M. M. and Sanford, J. (1972) *Proceedings of the Association of Veterinary Anaesthetists of Great Britain and Ireland* **3**, 20.
36. Harris, C. (1977) Personal communication to KWC.
37. Dodman, N. H. and Waterman, A. E. (1979) *Equine Veterinary Journal* **11**, 33.
38. Clarke, W. W. (1969) *Veterinary Record* **85**, 649.
39. Marsboom, R. and Mortelmans, J. (1964) *Small Animal Anaesthesia*. Oxford: Pergamon Press.
40. Vickers, M. D., Wood-Smith, F. G. and Stewart, H. C. (1978) *Drugs in Anaesthetic Practice*. London: Butterworths.
41. Mitchell, B. (1966) *Veterinary Record* **78**, 651.
42. Petersen, E. N. (1987) *Drugs of the Future* **112**, 1043.
43. Stone, T. W. (1987) *Drugs in Anaesthesia* (eds Feldman, Scurr and Paton), p. 238.
44. Harvey, S. C. (1985) *Pharmacological Basis of Therapeutics* (eds Goodman, Gilman, Rall and Murad), chapt. 17. New York: Macmillan.
45. Baldessarini, R. J. (1985) *Pharmacological Basis of Therapeutics* (eds Goodman, Gilman, Rall and Murad), chapt. 19. New York: Macmillan.
46. Lees, P. (1979) *Pharmacological Basis of Small Animal Medicine* (eds Yoxall and Hird). London: Blackwell Scientific.
47. Smits, G. M. (1964) *Roy. Net. Ass. Tij. Dierg.* **89**, 195.
48. Macey, D. W. and Gasper, P. W. (1984) *Journal of the American Hospitals Association* **21**, 17.
49. Van Miet, A., Koot, M. and Van Duin, C. (1989) *Journal of Veterinary Pharmacology and Therapeutics* **12**, 147.
50. Averill, D. R. (1970) *Journal of the American Veterinary Medical Association* **156**, 432.
51. Kay, W. J. and Fenner, W. R. (1977) *Current Veterinary Therapy* (ed. Kirk), vol. VI. Philadephia: W. B. Saunders.
52. Muller, R. (1976) Inaugural Dissertation, Fachbereich Tiermedizin, Munchen.
53. Short, C. E. (1981) *Veterinary Clinics of North America: Equine Anaesthesia*. (ed. E. P. Steffey), p. 205. Philadelphia: W. B. Saunders.
54. Reid, J. S. and Frank, R. J. (1972) *Journal of the American Hospitals Association* **8**, 115.
55. Hall, L. W. (1976) *Journal of Small Animal Practice* **17**, 661.
56. Muir, W. W., Sams, R. A., Hoffman, R. H. and Woonan, J. S. (1982) *American Journal of Veterinary Research* **43**, 1756.
57. Rehm, W. F. and Schatzmann, U. (1984) *Proceedings of the Association of Veterinary Anaesthetists of Great Britain and Ireland* **12**, 93.
58. Chambers, J. P. and Dobson, J. M. (1989) *Journal of the Association of Veterinary Anaesthetists of Great Britain and Ireland* **16**, 53.
59. Watson, P. (1986) 5th Year Project Examination, Royal Veterinary College, University of London.
60. Jackson, P. G. G. (1990) Personal communication.
61. Komar, E. and Mouallem, H. (1988) *Journal of the Association of Veterinary Anaesthetists of Great Britain and Ireland* **15**, 127.
62. Erhardt, W., Stephen, M., Schatzmann, U., Westermayr, R., Schindele, M., Murisier, N. and Blumel, G. (1986/7) *Journal of the Association of Veterinary Anaesthetists of Great Britain and Ireland* **14**, 90.
63. Rehm, W. F. and Schatzmann, U. (1984) *Journal of the Association of Veterinary Anaesthetists of Great Britain and Ireland* **12**, 93.
64. Short, C. E. (1987) *Principles and Practice of Veterinary Anesthesia*. Baltimore: Williams and Wilkins.
65. Sagner, Von G., Hoffmeister, F. and Kronberg, G. (1968) *Deutsche Tierarztliche Wochenschrift* **22**, 565.
66. Kronberg, G., Oberdorf, A., Hoffmeister, F. and Wirth, W. (1966) *Naturwissenschaften* **53**, 502.
67. Schmitt, H. (1977) *Antihypertensive Agents* (ed. Gross), chapt. 7.
68. Langer, S. Z. (1974) *Biochemical Pharmacology* **23**, 1793.
69. Livingston, A., Nolan, A. M. and Waterman, A. E. (1986/7) *Journal of the Association of Veterinary Anaesthetists of Great Britain and Ireland* **14**, 3.
70. Scheinin, N. and Macdonald, E. (1989) *Acta Veterinaria Scandinavica*, Suppl. 85, p. 11.
71. Nolan, A. M., Waterman, A. E. and Livingstone, A. (1986/7) *Journal of the Association of Veterinary Anaesthetists of Great Britain and Ireland* **14**, 14.
72. Vainio, O., Palmu, L., Virtanen, R. and Wecksell, J. (1986/7) *Journal of the Association of Veterinary Anaesthetists of Great Britain and Ireland* **14**, 53.
73. Dunkle, N., Moise, N. J., Scarlettg-Kranz, J. and Short, C. E. (1986) *American Journal of Veterinary Research* **47**, 2212.
74. Muir, W. W. and Piper, F. S. (1977) *American Journal of Veterinary Research* **38**, 932.
75. Hsu, W. H. (1985) *American Journal of Veterinary Research* **46**, 856.
76. Symonds, H. W. and Mallinson, C. B. (1978) *Veterinary Record* **102**, 27.
77. DeMoor, A. and Desmet, P. (1971) *Veterinary Medicine Reviews (Leverkusen)*, p. 163.
78. Nolan, A. M., Waterman, A. E. and Livingstone, A. (1986/7) *Journal of the Association of Veterinary Anaesthetists of Great Britain and Ireland* **14**, 11.

79. Raptopoulos, D., Koutinas, A., Moustardas, N. and Papasteriadis, A. (1985) *Proceedings of the 2nd International Congress of Veterinary Anaesthesia*, Sacramento, p. 201.
80. Eisenach, J. C. (1988) *Journal of Pharmacology and Experimental Therapeutics* **244**, 247.
81. Nolan, A. M. and Waterman, A. E. (1985) *Journal of the Association of Veterinary Anaesthetists of Great Britain and Ireland* **13**, 122.
82. Watney, G. C. G. (1986/7) *Journal of the Association of Veterinary Anaesthetists of Great Britain and Ireland* **14**, 16.
83. Livingstone, A., Low, J. and Morris, B. (1984) *British Journal of Pharmacology* **81**, 189.
84. Virtanen, R. (1986) *Acta Veterinaria Scandinavia*, Suppl. 82, p. 35.
85. Clarke, K. W. and Hall, L. W. (1969) *Veterinary Record* **85**, 512.
86. Tronicke, R. and Vocke, G. (1970) *Veterinary Medical Reviews (Leverkusen)*, p. 247.
87. Rosenberger, G., Hemapel, E. and Baumeister, M. (1969) *Veterinary Medical Reviews (Leverkusen)*, p. 137.
88. Arbeiter, K., Szekely, H. and Lorin, D. (1972) *Veterinary Medical Reviews (Leverkusen)* **3**, 248.
89. Bauditz, R. (1972) *Veterinary Medical Reviews (Leverkusen)*, p. 204.
90. Pippi, N. L. and Lumb, W. V. (1979) *American Journal of Veterinary Research* **40**, 1082.
91. Lowe, J. E. (1978) *Journal of Equine Medicine and Surgery* **2**, 286.
92. Haskins, S. C., Patz, J. D. and Farver, T. B. (1986) *American Journal of Veterinary Research* **47**, 636.
93. Garner, H. H., Amend, J. F. and Rosborough, J. P. (1971) *Veterinary Medicine/Small Animal Clinician* **66**, 921.
94. Klide, A. M., Calderwood, H. W. and Soma, L. R. (1975) *American Journal of Veterinary Research* **36**, 931.
95. Kerr, D. D., Jones, E. W., Huggins, K. and Edwards, W. C. (1972) *American Journal of Veterinary Research* **33**, 525.
96. Amend, J. F., Klavano, P. A. and Stone, E. (1972) *Veterinary Medicine/Small Animal Clinician* **67**, 1305.
97. Haufmann, P. (1976) *Animal de Compagnie* **11**, 361.
98. Cullen, L. K. and Jones, R. S. (1977) *Veterinary Record* **101**, 115.
99. Muir, W. W., Skarda, R. T. and Milne, D. W. (1977) *American Journal of Veterinary Research* **38**, 195.
100. Muir, W. W., Skarda, R. T. and Sheehan, W. C. (1978) *American Journal of Veterinary Research* **39**, 1632.
101. Butera, T. S., Moore, J. N. and Garner, H. E. (1978) *Veterinary Medicine/Small Animal Clinician* **72**, 490.
102. Brouwer, G. J., Hall, L. W. and Kuchel, T. R. (1980) *Veterinary Record* **107**, 241.
103. Hall, L. W. and Taylor, P. M. (1981) *Veterinary Record* **108**, 489.
104. Waterman, A. E. (1981) *Veterinary Record* **109**, 464.
105. Virtanen, G. (1985) *European Journal of Pharmacology* **108**, 163.
106. Virtanen, G. (1986) *Acta Veterinaria Scandinavica*, Suppl. 82, p. 85.
107. Clarke, K. W. (1988) Clinical pharmacology of detomidine in the horse. Academic Dissertation, University of London.
108. Jochle, W. (1989) *Equine Veterinary Journal*, Suppl. 7, p. 117.
109. Jochle, W., Moore, J. M., Brown, J., Baker, G. J., Lowe, J. E., Fubini, S., Reeves, M. T., Watkins, J. P. and White, N. A. (1989) *Equine Veterinary Journal*, Suppl. 7, p. 111.
110. Clarke, K. W. and Taylor, P. M. (1987) *Equine Veterinary Journal* **18**, 366.
111. Sarazan, R. D., Starke, W. A., Krause, G. F. and Garner, H. E. (1989) *Journal of Veterinary Pharmacology and Therapeutics* **12**, 378.
112. Waterman, A. E., Nolan, A. M., and Livingstone, A. (1986/7) *Journal of the Association of Veterinary Anaesthetists of Great Britain and Ireland,* **14**, 11.
113. Jedruch, J. and Gajewski, Z. (1986) *Acta Veterinaria Scandinavica*, Suppl. **82**, p. 189.
114. Taylor, P. M. and Clarke, K. W. (1985) *Journal of the Association of Veterinary Anaesthetists of Great Britain and Ireland* **14**, 29.
115. Clarke, K. W., Taylor, P. M. and Watkins, S. B. (1986) *Acta Veterinaria Scandinavica*, Suppl. **82**, p. 167.
116. Scheinin, M., Kallid, A., Koulu, M., Viikari, J. and Scheinin, H. (1987) *British Journal of Clinical Pharmacology* **24**, 443.
117. MacDonald, E., Ruskoaho, H., Scheinin, M. and Virtanen, R. (1988) *Annals of Clinical Research* **20**, 298.
118. Stenberg, D., Salven, P. and Mettinen, M. V. J. (1987) *Journal of Veterinary Pharmacology and Therapeutics* **10**, 319.
119. Vainio, O., Palmu, L., Virtanen, R. and Wecksell, J. (1986/7) *Journal of the Association of Veterinary Anaesthetists of Great Britain and Ireland* **14**, 53.
120. Clarke, K. W. and England, G. C. W. (1989) *Journal of Small Animal Practice* **130**, 343.
121. Jedruch, J., Gajewski, Z. and Ratajska-Michalczak, K. (1989) *Acta Veterinaria Scandinavica*, Suppl. 85, p. 129.
122. England, G. C. W. and Clarke, K. W. (1989) *Journal of the Association of Veterinary Anaesthetists of Great Britain and Ireland* **16**, 32.
123. Clarke, K. W. and England, G. C. W. (1988) *Advances in Anaesthesia, Proceedings of the 3rd International Congress of Veterinary Anaesthesia*, Brisbane, p. 104.
124. Jalenka, H. H. (1988) *Journal of Zoo Animal Medicine* **19**, 95.
125. Jalenka, H. H. (1989) *Journal of Zoo and Wildlife Medicine* **20**, 163.
126. Jalenka, H. H. (1990) *Journal of the Association of Veterinary Anaesthetists of Great Britain and Ireland* **17** (in press).
127. Kock, R. A., Jago, M., Gulland, F. M. D. and Lewis, J. (1989) *Journal of the Association of Veterinary Anaesthetists of Great Britain and Ireland* **16**, 4.
128. Thompson, J. R., Hsu, W. H. and Kersting, K. W. (1989) *American Journal of Veterinary Research* **50**, 734.
129. Hsu, W. H., Hanson, C. E., Hembrough, F. B. and Schaffer, D. D. (1989) *American Journal of Veterinary Research* **50**, 1570.
130. Docherty, T. J., Ballinger, J. A., McDonell, W. N., Pascoe, P. J. and Valliant, A. E. (1987) *Canadian Journal of Veterinary Research* **51**, 244.
131. Vainio, O. and Vaha-Vaha, T. (1989) *Journal of Veterinary Pharmacology and Therapeutics* **13**, 15.
132. Paddleford, R. R. (1988) *Manual of Small Animal Anaesthesia*. Edinburgh: Churchill-Livingstone.
133. Virtanen, R. (1989) *Acta Veterinaria Scandinavica*, Suppl. 85, p. 29.
134. Degryse, A. D. and Ooms, L. A. A. (1986) *Journal of Veterinary Pharmacology and Therapeutics* **9**, 376.

135. Degryse, A. D. and Ooms, L. A. A. (1986) *Drug Development Research* **8**, 433.
136. Rang, H. P. and Dale, M. M. (1987) *Pharmacology*, chapt. 25. Edinburgh: Churchill Livingstone.
137. Smith, T. W. and Chapple, D. J. (1987) *Drugs in Anaesthetic Practice* (eds S. A. Feldman, C. F. Scurr and W. Paton), p. 292. London: Edward Arnold.
138. Mitchell, R. W. D. and Smith, G. (1989) *British Journal of Anaesthesia* **63**, 147.
139. Echenhoff, J. E., Elder, J. D. and King, B. D. (1951) *American Journal of Medical Science* **222**, 115.
140. Martin, W. R., Eades, C. C., Thompson, J. A., Huppler, R. E. and Gilbert, P. E. (1976) *Journal of Pharmacology and Experimental Therapeutics* **197**, 517.
141. Livingstone, A. (1985) *Journal of the Association of Veterinary Anaesthetists of Great Britain and Ireland* **131**, 89.
142. Booth, N. H. (1988) *Veterinary Pharmacology and Therapeutics*, 6th edn (eds Booth and McDonald), chapt. 15. Ames: Iowa University Press.
143. Stanley, T. H. (1985) *Proceedings of the 2nd International Congress of Veterinary Anaesthesia*, Sacramento, p. 18.
144. Hug, C. C. (1989) *General Anaesthesia*, 5th edn (eds J. F. Nunn, J. E. Utting and B. R. Brown), chapt. 11. London: Butterworth.
145. Dundee, J. W. and Wyant, G. M. (1988) *Intravenous Anaesthesia*, chapt. 13. London: Churchill Livingstone.
146. Jaffe, J. H. and Martin, W. R. (1985) *The Pharmacological Basis of Therapeutics*, chapt. 22. New York: Macmillan.
147. Tobin, T., Combie, J., Schults, T. and Dougherty, J. (1979) *Journal of Equine Medicine and Surgery* **3**, 284.
148. Sanford, J. (1984) *Journal of the Association of Veterinary Anaesthetists of Great Britain and Ireland* **12**, 48.
149. Clarke, K. W. and Paton, B. S. (1988) *Equine Veterinary Journal* **20**, 331.
150. Muir, W. W., Skarda, R. T. and Sheehan, W. C. (1978) *American Journal of Veterinary Research* **39**, 1632.
151. Morgan, M. (1989) *British Journal of Anaesthesia* **63**, 165.
152. Alexander, F. and Collett, R. A. (1974) *Research in Veterinary Science* **17**, 136.
153. Kalthum, W. and Waterman, A. E. (1988) *Journal of the Association of Veterinary Anaesthetists of Great Britain and Ireland* **15**, 39.
154. Marsboom, R. and Mortelmans, J. (1964) *Small Animal Anaesthesia*. Pergamon Press: Oxford.
155. Borel, J. D., Bentley, J. B., Gillespie, J., Gandolfi, A. J. and Brown, B. R. (1981) *Anesthesiology* **55**, A256.
156. Heykants, J., Meuldermans, W. and Michiels, M. (1982) *Proceedings of the VIth European Congress of Anaesthesiology*, London.
157. Arndt, J. O., Bednarski, B. and Parasher, C. (1986) *Anesthesiology* **64**, 345.
158. Chambers, J. P. (1989) *Journal of the Association of Veterinary Anaesthetists of Great Britain and Ireland* **16**, 14.
159. Erhardt, W. (1984) *15th Congress of the European Society of Veterinary Surgery*, Berne, Abstract, p. 11.
160. Bengis, R. G., de Vos, V. and van Niekerk, J. (1985) *Proceedings of the 2nd International Congress of Veterinary Anaesthesia*, p. 142.
161. Taylor, P. M. and Houlton, J. E. F. (1984) *Journal of Small Animal Practice* **25**, 437.
162. Flecknell, P. (1988) *Veterinary Annual* **28**, 43.
163. Trim, C. M. (1983) *American Journal of Veterinary Research* **44**, 329.
164. Robertson, J. T., Muir, W. W. and Sams, R. (1981) *American Journal of Veterinary Research* **42**, 41.
165. Kalpravidh, M., Lumb, W. V., Wright, M. and Heath, R. B. (1984) *American Journal of Veterinary Research* **45**, 211.
166. Sawyer, D. C. and Rech, R. H. (1987) *Journal of the American Hospitals Association* **23**, 438.
167. Lowe, J. E. (1978) *Journal of Equine Medicine and Surgery* **2**, 286.
168. Amadon, R. S. and Craige, A. H. (1936) *Journal of the American Veterinary Medical Association* **41**, 737.
169. Nunn, J. F., Utting, J. E. and Brown, B. R. (1989) *General Anaesthesia*, 5th edn. London: Butterworths.
170. Richards, D. L. S., Clutton, R. E. and Boyd, C. (1989) *Journal of the Association of Veterinary Anaesthetists of Great Britain and Ireland* **16**, 46.
171. Nunn, J. F. and Bergman, N. A. (1964) *British Journal of Anaesthesia* **36**, 68.
172. Tomlin, P. J., Conway, C. M. and Payne, J. P. (1964) *Lancet* **i**, 14.
173. Scott, D. B. and Taylor, S. H. (1964) *Lancet* **i**, 165.
174. Taylor, S. H., Scott, D. B. and Donald, K. W. (1964) *Lancet* **i**, 841.
175. Mirakhur, R. K., Jones, C. T. and Dundee, J. W. (1981) *Anaesthesia* **36**, 277.
176. Short, C. E., Paddleford, R. R. and Cloy, D. (1974) *Modern Veterinary Practice* **3**, 194.
177. Short, C. E. and Miller, R. L. (1978) *Small Animal Clinician*, p. 1269.
178. Sengupta, A., Gupta, P. K. and Pandy, K. (1980) *British Journal of Anaesthesia* **52**, 513.

CHAPTER 5

GENERAL PHARMACOLOGY OF INTRAVENOUS ANAESTHETIC AGENTS

The intravenous anaesthetics are particularly useful for the induction of anaesthesia which is to be continued by an inhalation technique, or where anaesthesia of only short duration is required. If serious overdosage of intravenous agents is to be avoided it is imperative that the anaesthetist shall not only be skilled in the technique of intravenous injection but also be familiar with the type of anaesthesia produced. With intravenous agents (particularly barbiturates), the clinical level of anaesthesia is more related to the intensity of stimulation than it is with most of the inhalation agents. An undisturbed animal may be breathing quietly and have marked relaxation of the jaw and abdominal muscles, giving a picture of deep unconsciousness. On application of a stimulus, however, the breathing may accelerate or deepen, muscle relaxation may be lost and reflex movement of a limb occur. Herein lies one of the major hazards of intravenous anaesthesia because if this animal is now given sufficient of the intravenous agent to abolish these reactions to stimulation, a dangerous degree of respiratory depression will occur when the stimulation ceases and prolonged unconsciousness can be expected. Although similar considerations apply to anaesthesia with some inhalation agents (e.g. halothane) it must always be borne in mind that a significant difference between the intravenous anaesthetics and those given by inhalation is that the action of intravenous agents is not as quickly reversible because unlike the inhalation agents they cannot be recovered from the patient.

Induction agents should, when given in adequate doses, produce loss of consciousness in one injection site/brain circulation time so that the dose can be titrated against the animals' requirements. Drugs with a slower onset of action such as chloral hydrate, which has to be metabolized to trichlorethanol before its effects become apparent, and ketamine are much more difficult to use as induction agents.

The terms 'ultrashort acting' and 'short acting' were used in the classification of the effects of barbiturates but they have come to be employed for a wider range of anaesthetic agents. They are both confusing and misleading and should be reserved for drugs which are indeed broken down rapidly in the body (propofol, for example). In contrast to these, return of consciousness following an intravenous barbiturate such as thiopentone (which was originally classified as an 'ultrashort-acting' compound) occurs with a large amount of active drug still in the body so that, if left undisturbed, animals tend to lapse back into a deep sleep from which they can only be aroused with difficulty.

BARBITURATES

It is more correct to regard barbituric acid as a pyrimidine derivative but it is usually depicted in either the keto or enol form (Fig. 5.1) Dundee and Clark [1] point out that the many variations are all derived by substitutions in the 1,2 and 5,5' positions and that four distinct groups of compounds can be recognized:

1. Barbiturates (or oxybarbiturates); $1 = H, 2 = O$
2. Methylated oxybarbiturates; $1 = CH_3, 2 = O$
3. Thiobarbiturates; $1 = H, 2 = S$
4. Methylated thiobarbiturates; $1 = CH_3, 2 = S$

Unconsciousness cannot be produced in one injection site/brain circulation time by the intravenous injection of an adequate dose of any of the group-1 compounds. They have a very limited use in veterinary practice as hypnotics or sedatives.

Group-2 compounds frequently, but not invariably, will produce unconsciousness in one injection site/brain circulation time. According to Dundee and Clark the methyl group confers convulsive activity, of

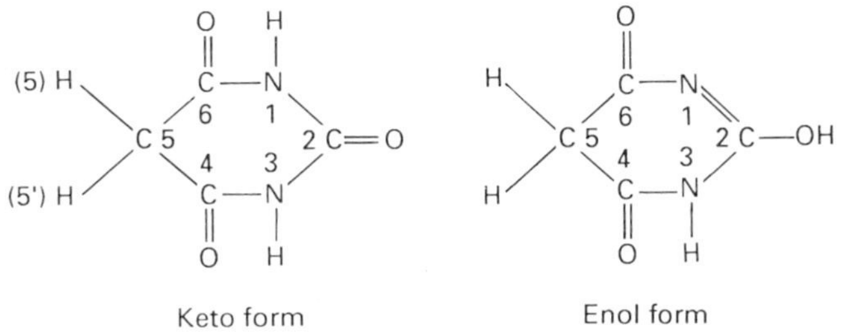

Keto form   Enol form

Fig. 5.1 Barbituric acid.

which tremor, involuntary muscle movement and hypertonicity are manifestations.

Intravenous injection of an adequate dose of one of the group-3 thiobarbiturates produces unconsciousness in one injection site/brain circulation time and return to consciousness is more rapid than after the same dose of the comparable oxybarbiturate.

Methylated thiobarbiturates of group 4 produce such severe convulsive manifestations as to preclude their use in clinical anaesthesia.

All barbiturates used as anaesthetics are prepared for clinical use as sodium salts and are usually available as powders to be dissolved in water or saline before use. Commercial preparations of most barbiturate anaesthetics contain a mixture of six parts anhydrous sodium carbonate and 100 parts (w/w) of the barbiturate to prevent precipitation of the insoluble free acid by atmospheric carbon dioxide. Aqueous solutions are strongly alkaline and are incompatible with acids such as most solutions of analgesics, phenothiazine derivatives, adrenaline and some preparations of relaxant drugs. Methohexitone is a colourless compound and its solution is readily distinguishable from the yellow solution of thiopentone and thiamylal.

The terminology applied to the barbiturates varies between North America and Britain, the former using the suffix '-al' and the latter '-one'.

Thiopentone sodium

In the UK thiopentone sodium was introduced into veterinary practice in 1937 [2, 3] and has come to be the most widely used induction agent, especially for dogs and cats. Studies of its pharmacology did not keep pace with progress in the clinical field and it was not until the 1950s that any notable contribution to an understanding of its clinical pharmacology was made when Brodie and his coworkers [4–7] followed the concentration of the drug in the urine and various body tissues both in dogs and in man. It was found that the liver and plasma concentrations of thiopentone, which were high almost immediately after a single injection, soon fell rapidly. The muscle con-

centration, although high almost immediately after injection, continued to rise for some 20 minutes, then fell — the fall being fairly rapid during the first hour but becoming progressively slower in the next 2 or 3 hours. In contrast to this, the concentration in the body fat, which was negligible at first, increased rapidly during the first hour and then more slowly until a maximum was reached in 3–6 hours. It was obvious that the concentration in the fat rose at the expense of that in the plasma and all other tissues. Although the brain concentration of thiopentone was below that of the blood plasma, both showed similar changes and therefore the depth of narcosis can be regarded as being related to the plasma concentration of the drug.

From these findings it is clear that the factors which govern the duration and depth of narcosis due to an injection of thiopentone are:

1. The amount of the drug injected
2. The speed of injection
3. The rate of distribution of the drug in the non-fatty tissues of the body
4. The rate of uptake of thiopentone by the body fat

The speed of injection and the quantity injected are related. For example, a small amount injected rapidly will produce a high plasma concentration and a parallel high brain level so that deep narcosis is induced rapidly. However, the drug soon becomes distributed throughout the non-fatty tissues of the body so that the plasma concentration and the brain concentration are reduced and there is a rapid decrease in the depth of narcosis. In contrast, a slow rate of injection of a larger quantity of the drug has the effect of maintaining the plasma level as the drug is distributed through the body tissues. This means that a larger amount of thiopentone will be necessary to obtain any given depth of narcosis and recovery will depend more on the uptake of the drug by the body fat and detoxication, since the concentration of thiopentone in the non-fatty tissues will already be high at the end of injection.

Thiopentone appears to cross the blood–brain barrier with very great speed. The factor which limits the time of response following an injection is the circulation time from the site of injection to the brain. The absence of any appreciable blood–brain barrier makes the rapid injection of the drug very useful for the production of short periods of narcosis with rapid recovery as redistribution occurs. Induction doses of thiopentone are usually between 5 and 10 mg/kg for most species of animal, but the anaesthetist always aims to combine the effects of injection speed and total dose in such a manner as to minimize the quantity needed by any individual animal for any given procedure, and takes full advantage of the reduction in dose offered by suitable premedication.

Carbon dioxide retention or the administration of this gas has the effect of reducing the plasma pH. Alteration of the plasma pH has a complex effect on the distribution of thiopentone in the body. Thiopentone is partially ionized and acts as a weak organic acid; the dissociation constant is such that a small change in pH will markedly affect the degree of ionization. If the plasma pH is lowered by carbon dioxide, the undissociated fraction of thiopentone is increased and since only this fraction is fat soluble, the decrease in pH results in an increase in the uptake of the drug by the fatty tissues. This lowers the plasma concentration and narcosis might be expected to lighten. However, this does not occur and Brodie has suggested that it is the undissociated fraction of the drug which is responsible for its pharmacological activity, for although the total plasma thiopentone is reduced, the concentration of the dissociated fraction remains roughly the same. A further mechanism may be implicated since thiopentone becomes bound to the plasma protein and the degree of binding depends on the protein concentration and the pH of the plasma. Protein binding is reduced by a reduction in pH and since the pharmacological activity resides in the unbound fraction narcosis might be expected to deepen when the plasma pH is reduced by carbon dioxide. To complicate the matter further, hyperventilation, which should have effects opposite to those of hypercapnia, has been shown to reduce the amount of thiopentone necessary for the maintenance of anaesthesia. This, of course, is not necessarily contradictory since all three factors, the uptake of thiopentone by the body fat, the degree of dissociation and the degree of binding by the plasma proteins, affect the concentration of active drug. It is unlikely that all three factors will be affected to the same degree and in the same way by changes in the pH of the plasma.

Comparatively little attention has been given to the reduction of plasma thiopentone concentration by detoxication. Animal experiments show prolongation of the action of large doses following liver damage caused by other agents, revealing the impor-

tance of the liver for recovery from thiopentone. Mark and coworkers [8] showed that up to 50% of thiopentone in the hepatic blood is removed in its passage through the human liver and although there are known to be marked species variations, the importance of hepatic metabolism in animals is now generally agreed. In dogs, Saidman and Eger [9] concluded that although the uptake in muscle still plays the dominant role in the early fall of arterial thiopentone levels, this is rivalled by the additive effect of metabolism and uptake in fat.

After intravenous injection, thiopentone rapidly reaches the central nervous system and its effects become apparent within 15–30 seconds of injection. Since the concentrations of the drug in the plasma and cerebrospinal fluid run parallel, the depth of narcosis can be assumed to be dependent on, and vary with, the blood level. However, this relationship is not a simple linear one, as acute tolerance to the drug develops. The plasma concentration of the drug at which the animal wakens increases as the duration of narcosis proceeds. Moreover, the depth and duration of narcosis bear some relation to the initial dose. When a large dose has been injected for the induction of narcosis, the animal will waken at a higher plasma level than after a small dose. This acute tolerance is probably the explanation for the clinical observation that recovery from the rapid injection of a given dose of thiopentone is quicker than if the same amount is given slowly. The initial concentration of the drug reaching the brain is greater when the drug is injected quickly so that consciousness returns at a higher plasma level than after a slower administration.

In clinical practice the intravenous injection of the drug is usually carried out at such a rate that surgical anaesthesia is reached within, at the most, 1–2 minutes. Apnoea sometimes occurs at a depth of anaesthesia which is sufficient to permit surgical intervention but excitement is very rarely seen during the induction of anaesthesia. The drug, like all barbiturates, has little, if any, analgesic action and reflex response to stimuli is not abolished until an appreciably greater depth of unconsciousness is reached than is required with many other agents. Because of the lack of analgesic properties thiopentone anaesthesia is more affected by premedication with analgesic drugs than is the case with other anaesthetic agents. This applies also to supplementation during anaesthesia with analgesics whether these be of the opioid type (alfentanil) or analgesic mixtures of nitrous oxide and oxygen. They reduce or abolish reflex response to stimuli and enable operative procedures to be performed at plasma levels of thiopentone which would be insufficient if the drug were given alone.

All barbiturate drugs cause respiratory depression

and a period of apnoea usually follows the intravenous injection of thiopentone. This is probably due to the central nervous depression caused by the initial high plasma concentration. The sensitivity of the respiratory centre to carbon dioxide is reduced progressively as narcosis deepens. As a result of the central depression the alveolar ventilation is diminished, raising the carbon dioxide tension of the arterial blood.

As with many other agents, anaesthesia in horses is often associated with a peculiar respiratory effect — a complete arrest of respiration for 20–30 seconds followed by four to eight respiratory movements. These bursts of activity followed by inactivity may persist throughout anaesthesia [10–14].

There is an apparent increase in the sensitivity of the laryngeal and bronchial reflexes under light thiopentone anaesthesia. This is generally attributed vaguely to parasympathetic preponderance under thiopentone narcosis. It would be wrong, however, to assume that thiopentone itself produces laryngeal and bronchial spasm for these are reflex phenomena, usually evoked by stimulation of the sensory afferent nerves by small amounts of mucus, regurgitated gastric contents or by foreign bodies such as endotracheal tubes. They may also be initiated by stimuli from other parts of the body. During anaesthesia these reflexes are depressed centrally and it is probable that thiopentone does not affect the afferent side of the reflex pathway as much as other agents do, so that deeper levels of unconsciousness are necessary for the suppression of these effects. Certainly, spasm is no more common in deep thiopentone anaesthesia than with other anaesthetic agents.

There is considerable disagreement among research workers concerning the effects of thiopentone on the cardiovascular system. This may well be due to the varying methods used for determinations of such things as cardiac output, differences of premedication, depth of narcosis and the degree of carbon dioxide retention, as well as on the speed of injection. It appears to be generally agreed, however, that the rapid intravenous injection of the drug causes a fall in blood pressure even in normovolaemic animals and that this can be serious in hypovolaemic states. After the initial fall the blood pressure returns to about the normal level but often with a persistent tachycardia.

The drug appears to have a direct depressant effect on the myocardium and in certain circumstances may produce cardiac arrhythmias such as ventricular extrasystoles. It is doubtful whether these have any clinical significance since they do not seem to progress to fibrillation and usually pass off quite spontaneously. In most instances only the electrocardiograph provides any indication of their presence. Where myocardial damage is present, it is unwise to use a very rapid rate of injection because this will submit the heart to a very high initial concentration of the drug.

In many types of anaemia the amount of thiopentone necessary for any given level of narcosis is reduced, for the plasma protein concentration as well as the haemoglobin level are low and decreased protein binding is then responsible for increased sensitivity to the drug.

Thiopentone modifies the vasomotor response to increase in intrathoracic pressure (Valsalva manoeuvre). In the absence of thiopentone, too vigorous controlled respiration will produce a fall in arterial blood pressure by increasing the mean intrathoracic pressure, although a degree of recovery ensues as the result of compensatory venoconstriction. This compensatory mechanism is impaired by thiopentone anaesthesia and persistent hypotension may result from injudicious positive pressure ventilation of the lungs.

Thiopentone does not effectively block motor nerve impulses and muscular relaxation can be provided only by excessive central nervous depression. Shivering is common in all species of animal in the recovery period and may be due to persistent cutaneous vasodilatation in a cold environment. It is probably a reflection of the lack of analgesic action because it is readily controllable by the use of small doses of analgesic drugs.

The incidence of hepatic damage after thiopentone anaesthesia is related to the dose administered and hepatic dysfunction always follows the use of large doses. However, the presence of liver damage does not make the use of the drug unsafe so long as only minimal doses are employed. The drug causes a small but sometimes persistent fall in plasma potassium concentration.

Uraemia increases the duration of thiopentone narcosis and the drug should be used with care, and in only minimal doses, in uraemic animals. Renal blood flow varies with the arterial blood pressure and prolonged hypotension caused by thiopentone can be followed by temporary oliguria.

Fetal respiration seems particularly sensitive to the depressant effects of thiopentone. It has never been clearly established whether, in animals, a long or short induction–delivery interval is beneficial to the offspring. At the Cambridge Veterinary School it has been used as an induction agent for obstetrical cases for over 35 years without evidence of serious harm to the offspring. Only minimal doses are administered and a relatively long induction–delivery interval is allowed. Other induction agents, with the possible exception of propofol, and in horses ketamine, appear to have no remarkable advantages.

Presentation

For many years thiopentone sodium was administered as a 5% solution in all but the larger farm animals but today it is generally agreed that it is always safer to employ a 2.5% solution (0.5 g in 20 ml) whenever possible in small animals, and even more dilute solutions for very small dogs and cats. The intravenous injection of a 5% or stronger solution causes spasm of the vein and its subcutaneous injection causes sloughing of the overlying skin. The use of a 2.5% solution does not cause venous thrombosis and ensures that accidental perivascular injection is much less likely to be followed by tissue necrosis. In small animals in which the total dose required is likely to be between 50 and 100 mg, further dilution of the solution up to 1.25% is advisable to give the injection bulk and ensure that the dose is not given too quickly. When it seems likely that more than 20 ml of a 2.5% solution will be required, thought should be given to the use of suitable premedication to reduce the thiopentone dose. It may be essential to use concentrated solutions (e.g. 10%) in horses and the larger farm animals but necrosis, sloughing and even aneurysms may follow their accidental perivascular injection [15]. It is a remarkable and as yet unexplained fact that the use of a 2.5% rather than a 5% solution halves the total dose of the drug which has to be administered to small animal patients. There is no completely acceptable explanation for this but it seems likely that acute tolerance may be involved.

The drug is usually supplied together with the appropriate quantities of sterile, pyrogen-free water to make a 2.5 or 5% solution. When prepared as a 2.5% solution and stored in multidose vials at room temperature the solution will generally remain fit for use for up to 4 or 5 days but freshly prepared 10% solutions may precipitate out at lower environmental temperatures.

Contraindications

In man, the harmful effects of barbiturates in porphyria are well known and an excellent review of the subject is that by Dundee and Wyant [16]. In the latent stage of the disease any barbiturate may provoke an acute exacerbation, the general course of which is of progressive acute demyelination of nerves, with clinical signs depending on those most affected. Progressive paralysis may end in the death of the patient. During these acute exacerbations, porphobilinogen is usually present in the urine and can be detected by a simple test in the absence of laboratory facilities. When first voided, urine containing porphobilinogen is usually normal in colour but it darkens when left standing in daylight for a few hours. The classical case presents with colicky abdominal pain and many are subjected to unnecessary laparotomy. Porphyria has been diagnosed in cattle and pigs [17] and while it is probably of little importance in these species, the anaesthetist must note that it has also been diagnosed in cats [18] although the exact type of porphyria was uncertain. In the light of our present knowledge, it seems that porphyria must be considered an absolute contraindication to the use of thiopentone in veterinary practice.

Thiamylal sodium

Thiamylal is a yellow crystalline substance which dissolves in water to give a clear yellow solution with a pH of 10.3. It closely resembles thiopentone in chemical structure except that while the latter is the ethyl derivative of the series, the former is the allyl compound. It is slightly more potent as an anaesthetic than thiopentone and has less of a cumulative effect.

Although it is usually prepared for clinical use in small animals as a 2.5% solution, a 2.0% solution is almost indistinguishable in use from 2.5% solutions of thiopentone. For horses and the larger farm animals 5–10% solutions are employed and these will cause tissue necrosis if accidently injected outside the vein.

It is claimed that in cats laryngeal spasm and apnoea are less troublesome than with thiopentone, while in dogs it is said to give rise to less excitement during induction and recovery but these supposed advantages are not readily apparent. Certainly this drug seems to cause more profuse salivation in small animals than does thiopentone and when using it the administration of atropine is almost essential.

Since it was first used in dogs [19] there have been many favourable reports of the use of thiamylal in the USA. In 1955 it was introduced into the UK [20] where it has since been used to only a very limited extent, probably because in dogs and cats it gives rise to more cardiac arrhythmias than thiopentone and, moreover, in the UK it has always been much more expensive.

Inactin

Although it has been in widespread use in Germany for a number of years, this agent, sodium 5-ethyl-5'-(1-methylpropyl)-2-thiobarbiturate, is apparently not used in English-speaking countries. It is a very satisfactory induction agent and, apart from being only about three-quarters as potent as thiopentone, the two drugs seem indistinguishable.

Methohexitone sodium

Methohexitone sodium is a racemic mixture of the α-*d* and α-*l* isomers of sodium 5-allyl-1-methyl-5-(1-methyl-2-ynyl)barbiturate, and differs from thiopentone in having no sulphur in the molecule. It is stable for at least 6 weeks in aqueous solutions kept at room temperature.

There are important differences between this and other barbiturates. The significant features characteristic of methohexitone sodium compared to thiopentone are:

1. Potency is two or three times greater
2. Shorter duration of effect
3. More rapid recovery to full alertness, even after prolonged anaesthesia

It is the only barbiturate drug for which there is convincing evidence of a more rapid recovery than from the 'standard' barbiturate, thiopentone.

In mice, rats, dogs, cats and monkeys, methohexitone sodium has been shown to be an ultrashort-acting intravenous anaesthetic that is about twice as potent (on a weight basis) as thiopentone. Its action is characterized by a rapid induction, satisfactory surgical anaesthesia and quick recovery. The total duration of the mean anaesthetic dose rarely exceeds 30 minutes. Unfortunately, in animals the recovery period is often complicated by muscle tremors or even frank convulsions. These undesirable features are not seen if the animal is allowed to recover quite undisturbed, or if recovery is prolonged by an opioid or a phenothiazine derivative given for premedication. Muscle tremors may also be seen in the induction period unless a rapid induction technique is practised.

The short duration of action depends both on marked fat solubility and also on a rapid rate of breakdown in the liver.

Methohexitone sodium is best administered to small animals as a 1% solution (10 mg/ml) in doses of 3–5 mg/kg but when large volumes of this solution would be required, a 2.5% (25 mg/ml) solution may be used. In large animals more concentrated solutions of up to 6% are more convenient to handle. Owing to differences in pH, solutions of methohexitone sodium should not be mixed with acid solutions such as atropine sulphate.

Rapid induction techniques, especially with the more concentrated solutions, usually produce temporary respiratory arrest. This is treated by maintaining the pulmonary ventilation until spontaneous respiration is resumed 30–60 seconds later. It is said that laryngospasm occurs less frequently with this than with the other intravenous anaesthetics. Rapid injection may produce transient hypotension but the blood pressure soon returns to normal levels.

Fowler and Stevenson [21, 22] and Fabry [23] have reported the use of methohexitone in small animal practice and there are some reports of its use in large animal patients. Tavernor [24] has used this agent in horses, and Robertshaw [5] demonstrated its value both as an induction agent and as a short-term anaesthetic for calves. Monahan [26] recorded the experiences of the Cambridge Veterinary School with methohexitone sodium as an induction agent in horses and cattle. Since then methohexitone has been used as an induction agent for more than 3000 horses at the Cambridge Veterinary School without one death attributable to its use.

Undoubtedly, there is a place in veterinary anaesthesia for an agent which can safely produce rapid anaesthesia with recovery which is fast and complete. Methohexitone sodium fulfills most of these requirements, although the occurrence of muscle tremors in animals recovering from its effects indicates that it is not the perfect agent. It seems to have an advantage over the thiobarbiturates in that recovery may be completed earlier as the animal is more alert and coordinated on regaining consciousness. It seems probable, however, that at least for small animal patients it will be superseded by propofol.

RAPIDLY ACTING NON-BARBITURATES

Saffan

Research into the anaesthetic activity of steroids produced a number of compounds which have hypnotic properties. Of these alphaxalone was the most promising.

Alphaxalone is virtually insoluble in water but it can be dissolved in Cremophor EL; the addition of another steroid, alphadolone, which itself has weak hypnotic properties, increases the solubility of alphaxalone in Cremophor EL more than three-fold. 'Saffan' is a mixture of the two steroids in Cremophor EL and this mixture has never been given an 'official' name. The name 'Saffan' is used in veterinary medicine; in human medicine the identical formulation was known as 'Althesin'. Each millilitre of Saffan contains 9 mg of alphaxalone and 3 mg of alphadolone. The ready-to-use solution is rather viscid, has a pH of about 7 and is isotonic with blood. Like all solutions made up in Cremophor EL it froths when drawn up into the syringe but is miscible with water. The dose of Saffan may be expressed in several ways but in veterinary anaesthesia it has been usual to record it as mg (total steroid)/kg body weight. Low water solubility of the steroids is undoubtedly a disadvantage and their solution in Cremophor EL led to the withdrawal of Althesin from medical anaesthetic practice, although many medical anaesthetists considered its withdrawal on this ground unwarranted.

Pharmacological studies in Glaxo Laboratories [27] led to the introduction of Saffan as an anaesthetic for cats, but it can be used in all domesticated animals, except dogs, without any major problems [28, 29].

The electroencephalographic pattern of cerebral depression is similar to that produced by other anaesthetics. Some evidence has been produced which suggests that Saffan selectively decreases cerebral oxygen consumption to an extent greater than can be attributed to a reduction in cerebral blood flow. Thus, it may be a useful agent for anaesthetizing animals other than dogs suffering from head injuries.

When given to cats by intravenous injection induction is not as smooth as with thiopentone and, in the authors' experience, retching and even vomiting may occur unless the induction dose is given rapidly. Twitching of limb and facial muscles is also seen but appears to have no clinical significance.

Saffan produces similar falls in arterial blood pressure, central venous pressure and stroke volume to thiopentone, but the hypotension is not dose related and is accompanied by tachycardia. It causes no significant changes in cardiac index or systemic vascular resistance [30]. With moderate doses the arterial hypotension is transient but large doses have a more prolonged effect. Foex and Prys-Roberts [31] observed a dose-related increase in pulmonary vascular resistance in goats and concluded that Saffan appeared to depress myocardial contractility to a comparable degree with anaesthetically equipotent doses of other induction agents. Sheep appear to be unduly sensitive to Saffan [32] for in these animals it produces a marked fall in cardiac output, pulse rate and arterial blood pressure, as well as respiratory depression. In dogs, Cremophor EL produces histamine release, thus causing a further fall in arterial blood pressure and making Saffan unsuitable for use without prior antihistamine medication; even then it cannot be recommended.

It is claimed that Saffan produces good muscle relaxation in cats without at the same time causing severe respiratory depression. Malignant hyperpyrexia-susceptible pigs have been safely anaesthetized with Saffan [33].

The only endocrine effect of Saffan is a weak anti-oestrogenic action. The major route of excretion of the two steroids is via the bile and in rats 60–70% of the steroids are excreted by this route within 3 hours of administration. There is some evidence that, like progesterone, the anaesthetic steroids are involved in enterohepatic circulation.

Information relating to the transfer of Saffan across the placental barrier is scanty but clinical results show very minor adverse effects on kittens when induction doses of up to 6 mg/kg are given to the mother. It has been claimed that kittens breathe almost immediately after delivery when the dose of Saffan given to the mother is restricted to less than 4 mg/kg.

Cats recovering from Saffan anaesthesia often show tremor of muscles, paddle and, if stimulated, may become extremely excited or convulse. This excitement and the convulsions disappear as soon as the stimulation ceases.

Oedema and/or hyperaemia of cats' ear pinnae and paws is common under Saffan anaesthesia. Measurement of paw and ear thickness suggests that this occurs more frequently than can be recognized by simple visual inspection. Currently, it has to be accepted that these side-effects result from some idiosyncrasy in some cats to some unidentified ingredient in the product. Informed opinion seems to be that this type of reaction, probably related to histamine release, is usually without clinical significance — although there have been occasional reports of ear pinna and paw necrosis.

Other reports of possible histamine release in cats cannot be dismissed so easily. These are clinical reports, only seldom supported by autopsy findings, associating the administration of Saffan with pulmonary oedema. However, in about 30 instances, lung oedema has been confirmed histologically at autopsy. Because these reports stem from a very few practitioners and it has been estimated that about 30 000 cats are anaesthetized with Saffan each month, Evans [34] has attributed this to an administration or administrator-associated problem. There seems to be no way of preventing its occurrence and because it is a potentially lethal complication others take the view that Saffan is not an acceptable alternative to thiopentone. In any discussion of this complication it is, perhaps, worthy of note that at least one region of the UK from which it is reported is one in which pulmonary oedema has been seen after thiopentone administration (J. B. Glen, personal communication), and this may indicate the operation of some factor peculiar to a geographical region. In such a region an endemic chronic infection may prime the complement systems, making them susceptible to activation by an intravenously administered compound [34]. This would lead to histamine release in affected animals by the so-called 'alternative pathway' [35] without involvement of immune recognition so no previous exposure to Saffan or to any other intravenous agent would be necessary for such a reaction as histamine-induced pulmonary oedema to occur. There are also reliable reports of laryngeal oedema following induction of anaesthesia with Saffan with no history of previous exposure to the steroids.

Although all the genus *Canis* show a dose-related anaphylactoid type of reaction to surface-active agents such as Cremophor EL, a constituent of Saffan, Corbett [36] has used this preparation in dogs after premedication with acepromazine and chlorpheniramine with apparent success, and claims that induction is pleasant, anaesthesia is of good quality and recovery is rapid and quiet. It is difficult to accept that the prior administration of an antihistamine merely to enable Saffan to be used is good practice, especially now that other and better agents are available for use in dogs, but the technique appears to have gained considerable popularity in Australia for caesarian section in bitches. It is claimed, without any scientific evidence, that pups delivered from a bitch under this combination of drugs are less depressed than with any other anaesthetic regimen. Attempts to follow the regimen in dogs in the UK have revealed a high incidence of skin erythema and vomiting.

The safety of Saffan as an anaesthetic for cats revealed in a recent survey carried out by the Association of Anaesthetists of Great Britain and Ireland probably stems from five important characteristics:

1. The high therapeutic index
2. Lack of cumulation in the body
3. Rapid, complete recovery of consciousness and appetite
4. Little respiratory depression with adequate muscle relaxation
5. Lack of local irritant properties and activity when given, accidentally, outside a vein

Unlike many induction agents Saffan may be given by intramuscular injection but, despite this possible use, there is no doubt that the prime role for the formulation is as an intravenous induction agent, or as a total anaesthetic (using incremental dosage or a continuous infusion technique), for the cat. Recovery from Saffan is due to both redistribution and breakdown and accumulation in the body is minimal. Metabolism is so fast that subcutaneous injections fail to produce any evidence of effect on the central nervous system, making it possible to disregard inadvertent perivascular injection as far as subsequent doses are concerned.

Metomidate

Metomidate (Hypnodil) is a non-barbiturate intravenous hypnotic synthesized in the laboratories of Janssen Pharmaceutica in Belgium. It was the first representative of a completely new group of anaesthetics, the imidazole derivatives, its formula being *dl*-1-(1-phenylethyl)-5-(methoxycarbonyl)imidazole hydrochloride. It is a white crystalline powder, freely soluble in water, but aqueous solutions are unstable and should be used within 24 hours of preparation unless stored in a refrigerator.

Introduced as a hypnotic for pigs [37–44] it has also been used experimentally in horses [45, 46] and for restraint for a variety of species of birds [47, 48].

Metomidate has strong central muscle relaxant properties but no analgesic activity so it has usually been used with other agents, such as fentanyl or azaperone, and it is difficult to establish the effects of the agent alone.

When given by intravenous injection it produces unconsciousness in one injection site/brain circulation time. In pigs, after azaperone premedication, induction of anaesthesia is smooth and side-effects are rarely seen. Occasionally muscle tremors occur and although they may persist for a few hours they appear to be of no clinical significance. Metomidate has also been given by intraperitoneal injection at the same time as an intramuscular injection of azaperone but the results are less predictable.

It is claimed that metomidate will, after azaperone premedication, produce analgesia of the skin, muscles and peritoneum of pigs but analgesia of the nose and the feet is said to be less complete. Experience at the Cambridge Veterinary School is that analgesia is always less than complete and violent reaction to surgical stimulation to any part of the body may occur unless an analgesic such as nitrous oxide is given.

Injection of metomidate is followed by slight hypotension, with a decreased pulse rate and a mild decrease of cardiac output. During anaesthesia there is remarkable stability of the cardiovascular system.

In pigs under azaperone-metomidate medication the minute volume of respiration is equal to that of the rested, conscious animal. The rate is decreased while the depth is slightly increased.

Muscle relaxation is produced by large doses of metomidate, presumably due to a central effect for no curare-like activity has been reported.

Piglets delivered by caesarean section from sows under metomidate hypnosis are sleepy but usually recover from this depressed state if they are kept warm. When high doses of metomidate are given to the sow the piglets may show tremors for several hours after birth.

Metomidate has a short duration of action, the peak effect being over by about 25 minutes after administration but animals may sleep for several hours. It is not clear whether sleep is due to metomidate or the drugs used for premedication. Recovery may be extremely violent, especially in horses.

Role

At present it seems that metomidate will never become widely used in veterinary anaesthesia. Although possibly indicated for pigs, there is currently little call for its use in the field because of present farm economics and although pigs are becoming widely used as experimental animals other agents are usually more satisfactory for laboratory purposes. It is possibly of some use in birds and some small laboratory animals.

Etomidate

Janssen Laboratories selected metomidate as an anaesthetic for birds and pigs but continued to work on the dextro- and laevorotatory isomers of other imidazole derivatives. The dextrorotatory isomer of etomidate, found to be the most potent of all substances tested, was chosen for development as an anaesthetic for man [49].

Etomidate is a whitish crystalline powder freely soluble in water. The commercial preparation Hypnomidate contains 20 mg dissolved in 10 ml of a mixture of 35% propylene glycol and 65% water (v/v), because injection of plain aqueous solutions causes pain. It is much more expensive than metomidate.

The pharmacokinetics of etomidate in animals other than rats have not been reported in detail. In dogs it is 76% bound to albumin and like thiopentone it quickly enters the brain and leaves rapidly as it becomes redistributed in the body. Of the total dose given, in rats 83% is excreted in the urine 20 hours (2% as unchanged etomidate) and 13% is excreted in the bile. It is quickly hydrolysed by esterases in the liver and plasma to pharmacologically inert metabolites.

In effective doses etomidate causes loss of consciousness in one injection site/brain circulation time. On a weight-for-weight basis it appears to be about 12 times more potent than thiopentone. Intravenous injection is associated with a high incidence of spontaneous involuntary muscle movement, tremor and hypertonus. Premedication with diazepam, fentanyl or pethidine reduces the incidence of these side-effects. The duration of anaesthesia is dose dependent and increasing the dose does not sig-

nificantly increase the occurrence of side-effects. The electroencephalographic changes produced by etomidate at induction are similar to those seen with barbiturates and no specific epileptogenic or convulsant action is observed on the tracing, so that the muscle movements cannot be attributed to these effects.

Lack of cardiovascular depression is claimed to be one of the outstanding features of etomidate [49, 50]. The drug does not release significant amounts of histamine and there is a very low incidence of thrombophlebitis after injection.

In unpremedicated human patients injection of etomidate is followed by coughing and hiccups in about 20% of cases but these effects are short lasting and do not interfere with the course of anaesthesia. Morgan *et al.* [51] report that injection is usually followed by a brief period of hyperventilation, then a period of respiratory depression, sometimes with apnoea, but it would appear that the effects of etomidate on respiration are less than those of other intravenous induction agents.

Pain on injection is frequent but its reported incidence varies widely and injection into a large vein is said to decrease the likelihood of pain being experienced by the patient.

A slight rise in serum potassium occurs when marked, persistent myoclonic movements occur but the main effect of importance, at least in man, is that etomidate inhibits increases in plasma cortisol and aldosterone concentrations during surgical stress, even when adrenocorticotropic hormone levels are normal or increased [52–54]. Similar effects probably occur in animals because adrenocortical function is suppressed 2 and 3 hours after the administration of etomidate to canine surgical patients [55]. Suppression of the endocrine response to surgical stress has been deemed by some to be beneficial, although this suppression has resulted in etomidate no longer being used for sedation of human patients in intensive care units.

Role

At present it is impossible to assess whether etomidate will have a place in veterinary anaesthesia. Erhardt [56] has reported acceptable results with a mixture of etomidate and alfentanil mixed in a ratio of 1 mg to 0.015 mg in dogs, cats, rats, rabbits, sheep, goats and calves but etomidate has so far failed to make any impact in veterinary practice in the UK.

Eugenols

The eugenols are related to oil of cloves and three derivatives have been subjected to clinical trials in man. The first, known as G29505 or Estil, was abandoned because of its deleterious effects on veins. Another derivative, Propinal, was abandoned very quickly because of its effects on respiration and the circulation. The third eugenol, propanidid (Epontol), became available in the UK in 1967. Doses of 5 mg/kg given to very small ponies by extremely rapid intravenous injection produced anaesthesia sufficient for castration followed by complete recovery in less than 10 minutes. Because of the extremely short duration of action it was found to be physically impossible to give the drug fast enough to produce anaesthesia in larger horses, and violent excitement followed the administration of subanaesthetic doses. In dogs, Epontol was found to produce severe respiratory depression and profound hypotension, probably because it contained Cremophor EL.

Propofol

Propofol is an intravenous anaesthetic agent unrelated to barbiturates, eugenols, or steroid anaesthetic agents. The active ingredient is 2,6-diisopropylphenol which exists as an oil at room temperatures. It was initially introduced in a preparation containing the surface-active agent Cremophor EL but it is now presented in an emulsion form. This preparation is a free-flowing oil-in-water emulsion containing 1% w/v 2,6-diisopropylphenol, 10% w/v soya bean oil, 1.2% w/v purified egg phosphatide and 2.25% w/v glycerol.

Details of pharmacological studies performed in rabbits, cats, pigs and monkeys have been published [57–59] and it is clear that like thiopentone it is a rapidly acting agent which produces anaesthesia of short duration without excitatory side-effects. Both agents produce equivalent cardiovascular and respiratory effects but unlike thiopentone, propofol does not produce tissue damage when injected perivascularly or intra-arterially. Pain on injection into small veins has been reported in man and occasionally dogs seem to resent its injection into the cephalic vein. Greater reflex depression and more pronounced electroencephalographic changes are associated with propofol than with thiopentone.

Propofol has been shown to be compatible with a wide range of drugs used for premedication, inhalation anaesthesia and neuromuscular block [58]. It lacks any central anticholinergic effect, is not potentiated by other non-anaesthetic drugs, does not affect bronchomotor tone or gastrointestinal motility and increases the threshold at which adrenaline causes cardiac arrhythmias.

The propofol blood-concentration profile following a single bolus dose can be described by the sum of three exponential functions representing: (i)

distribution from blood into tissues; (ii) metabolic clearance from the blood; (iii) metabolic clearance constrained by the slow return of propofol into blood from a poorly perfused tissue compartment. It is highly lipophilic and rapidly metabolized primarily to inactive glucuronide conjugates, the metabolites being excreted in the urine. In man, liver disease and renal failure have little effect on pharmacokinetic parameters and it seems likely that extrahepatic mechanisms contribute to the metabolism of propofol, but this has not been investigated in any detail in other animals.

The mean 'utilization rate' of propofol varies from species to species of animal (Table 5.1) and is probably related to differences in the rate of biotransformation and conjugation as the cat, with the smallest 'utilization rate' of the animals studied, has a deficiency in its ability to conjugate phenols [56].

Table 5.1 The main 'utilization rate' of propofol for various species of animal

Species	Mean utilization rate (mg/(kg min))
Mouse	2.22
Rabbit	1.55
Rat	0.61
Pig	0.28
Cat	0.19

Data supplied by J. B. Glen.

Propofol, subjected to preliminary clinical trials in ponies [60, 61], was found to be an effective agent for the smooth induction of anaesthesia. The original preparation of propofol in Cremophor EL used in these trials is slightly less potent than the current preparation but has very similar properties [62–64] and, since it is believed that Cremophor EL does not cause significant histamine release in horses, means that the emulsion preparation should not be very different. Following premedication with 0.5 mg/kg of xylazine the intravenous injection of 2.0 mg/kg produced anaesthesia which could be maintained with an infusion of propofol given at a rate of 0.2 mg/(kg min). Cardiovascular changes included a decrease in arterial pressure and cardiac output while respiratory depression was manifested by a decrease in rate and an increase in arterial carbon dioxide tension. Recovery after 1 hour of anaesthesia was rapid and smooth. No surgery was performed on the animals included in these trials but subsequent experience showed 0.2 mg/kg/min to produce satisfactory surgical conditions after the same xylazine premedication and propofol induction. The cost of propofol currently constitutes a marked deterrent but propofol is clearly worthy of further trials in horses.

Following initial trials [65–68] propofol is now accepted as a most useful agent in dogs and cats. The principal advantage of propofol over thiopentone is the more rapid recovery of consciousness. The drug is distributed and metabolized very quickly although, at least in man, concurrent administration of fentanyl reduces clearance and increases plasma concentrations [69].

The dose for induction of anaesthesia in unpremedicated dogs and cats is between 6 and 7 mg/kg. Premedication with between 0.02 and 0.04 mg/kg of acepromazine reduces this induction dose by about 30% in dogs but this effect is not so marked in cats premedicated with 0.04 mg/kg of acepromazine [68]. In dogs, anaesthesia maintained by continuous infusion appears to be less satisfactory than that maintained by halothane/nitrous oxide [67] although it is perhaps better when maintained by intermittent injections of the agent [66].

Following a single intravenous dose of 6 mg/kg, recovery in dogs is complete (awake, no ataxia) after about 20 minutes and acepromazine premedication does not appear to increase the recovery time. Recovery in greyhounds and other sight-hounds takes no longer than in other breeds. There is a suggestion that some families of boxers may be more susceptible to the drug since recovery was prolonged in some related animals of this breed [67]. In cats, recovery after a single dose is less rapid — about 30 minutes — presumably because of the cats' relative inability to conjugate phenols. In cats the incidence of postanaesthetic side-effects such as vomiting/retching and sneezing or pawing at the mouth is about 15% but this can be slightly reduced by acepromazine premedication [68]. Vomiting and retching may also be seen during recovery in dogs, the incidence being about 2% following a single injection or maintenance by intermittent injections and as high as 16% in dogs receiving a continuous infusion of propofol [67].

The great attraction for using propofol in dogs and cats is the rapid and complete, excitement-free awakening, irrespective of the duration of anaesthesia. Owners often comment on the bright, alert appearance of their animals within minutes of completion of the procedure necessitating the anaesthetic. A price must be paid for this, however. Animals require careful observation during the recovery period to ensure that they come to no harm from vomiting.

LESS RAPIDLY ACTING INTRAVENOUS AGENTS

The less rapidly acting intravenous agents include chloral hydrate, the dissociative agents and pentobarbitone sodium. In the past both have been used as anaesthetics but appropriate doses do not produce unconsciousness in one injection site/brain circulation time.

Chloral hydrate

Chloral hydrate is a white, translucent, crystalline substance which has a pungent smell and volatilizes slowly at room temperature. It is not deliquescent, but it is readily soluble in water and aqueous solutions are generally stable although the drug decomposes in the presence of alkali. Solutions may be sterilized by boiling for a short period. In the blood, chloral hydrate is reduced to 2,2,2-trichloroethanol (CCl_3CH_2OH) and its narcotic effect is generally attributed to this substance. When given by intravenous injection its effects are slow in appearing and this means that it is difficult to assess the degree of depression produced by a given dose as injection proceeds. Even following slow intravenous infusion of a dilute solution, narcosis continues to deepen for several minutes after the injection is terminated. Perivascular injection causes severe tissue reaction, often followed by sloughing of the overlying tissues.

Vladutiu [70] recorded the use of a mixture of equal parts of chloral hydrate and magnesium sulphate administered by intravenous injection as a general anaesthetic for a horse. Coffee [71] preferred three parts of chloral hydrate to one of magnesium sulphate. Millenbruck and Wallinga [72] recommended a mixture of chloral hydrate, magnesium sulphate and pentobarbitone.

Although chloral hydrate and these mixtures were widely used in large animals they are less used today because other agents are safer and more convenient to administer. Their properties as described in earlier editions of this book make this obvious.

Chloralose

Chloralose is prepared by heating equal quantities of glucose and chloral hydrate under controlled conditions so that two isomers are produced. Only α-chloralose has narcotic properties: β-chloralose can produce muscular pain. α-Chloralose is available commercially as a white, crystalline powder and it is used as a 1% solution in water or saline. The solution is prepared fresh immediately before use by heating to 60°C. Heating to above this temperature results in decomposition and precipitation occurs on standing.

Chloralose is still extensively used in physiological and pharmacological non-survival experiments. Because large volumes of solution have to be given before consciousness is lost anaesthesia is often induced with some other agent such as methohexitone. An intravenous dose of 80–100 mg/kg of chloralose causes loss of consciousness but spontaneous muscular activity is common. The peak narcotic action of chloralose is seen some 15–20 minutes after injection. The blood pressure is elevated and the activity of the autonomic nervous system is believed to be unaffected. The heart rate is often greatly increased and respiratory depression does not occur until very large doses are given. In the body chloralose is broken down to chloral and glucose and the safety margin is relatively wide.

Disadvantages are its relative insolubility, the long and comparatively shallow depth of anaesthesia and the slow recovery which is accompanied by struggling. It has no place in veterinary practice.

Urethane

Urethane, the ethyl ester of carbaminic acid, produces long-lasting light anaesthesia and is, therefore, like chloralose, used mainly for physiological and pharmacological experiments. It is believed to be carcinogenic and laboratory workers having contact with this compound are advised to handle it with care. Urethane is often given with chloralose to suppress the muscular activity which may occur when chloralose alone is used. It is claimed that urethane has little effect on respiration and arterial blood pressure.

Urethane has no place in veterinary anaesthesia but veterinarians may be called upon to advise on its use for experimental purposes. In dogs, cats and rabbits, light anaesthesia follows the intravenous injection of 500–1000 mg/kg.

Pentobarbitone sodium

Pentobarbitone sodium is the name given to sodium 5-ethyl-5-(1-methylbutyl)barbiturate. It is marketed as a sterile 6.5% solution containing propylene glycol, as a powder in gelatine capsules and, for euthanasia, in non-sterile solutions of about 20%.

The main action of pentobarbitone sodium is to depress the central nervous system, and effects upon other systems of the body only become important as the toxic limitations to the use of the drug are approached. It depresses the cerebral cortex and, probably, the hypothalamus. Because it depresses the motor areas of the brain it is used to control convulsive seizures. It has only a weak analgesic action and relatively large doses must be administered before pain reception is affected, thus, like all barbiturates, it is in fact primarily a hypnotic drug.

Pentobarbitone sodium takes an appreciable time to cross the blood-barrier and when given by intravenous injection the rate of injection must be slow if the full effects are to be assessed as injection proceeds.

The drug markedly depresses the respiratory centre and in pregnant animals it diffuses readily across the placenta into the fetal circulation, inhibiting fetal respiratory movements.

In sheep, pentobarbitone causes a marked decrease in stroke volume and in the acceleration of blood in the pulmonary artery. Pulse rate increases but this does not compensate for the fall in stroke volume so that cardiac output falls to an average of 64% of the resting volume in the conscious animal [32]. The blood pressure may subsequently rise due to hypercapnia consequent upon the respiratory depression produced by the drug.

Pentobarbitone sodium has no appreciable effect on the gastrointestinal system or on liver function but large doses may cause further injury to an already damaged liver. The drug is destroyed primarily in the liver although other tissues may have the power of breaking it down and some of the dose administered to an animal is excreted in the urine so that, if a diuresis can be produced by intravenous infusion of fluid, awakening may be accelerated. The drug has no direct action on the kidney but may inhibit water diuresis, probably by causing a release of antidiuretic hormone from the pituitary gland.

Recovery from pentobarbitone is always slow but the duration varies from species to species of animal. The drug is metabolized more rapidly in horses, sheep and goats than in pigs, dogs and cats. Convulsive movements, paddling of the limbs and vocalization may occur in the recovery period but such excitatory phenomena can usually be suppressed with analgesics or tranquillizers although these will further delay complete recovery.

Role

In horses, pentobarbitone is still often used to prolong the duration of chloral hydrate narcosis. In the field it is also used in cattle for anaesthesia of short duration. In dogs and cats it may be used on its own as a hypnotic or anaesthetic. Particularly in dogs, it is a valuable agent provided its potential dangers are understood and appropriate measures taken to avoid them. It is probably still the most widely used injectable anaesthetic for experimental work in dogs and cats despite its disadvantages and it is useful in canine practice where facilities for the administration of inhalation anaesthetics are unavailable.

DISSOCIATIVE AGENTS

Three cyclohexylamine derivatives have been used in several species of animal to produce a state which enables a surgical operation to be carried out. These substances, phencyclidine, tiletamine and ketamine, differ markedly both in chemical and physical properties as well as in their clinical effects from the non-inhalation agents already described. In man, they have been described as having a 'cataleptic, analgesic and anaesthetic action, but without hypnotic properties' [73]. Catalepsy is defined as a 'characteristic akinetic state with loss of orthostatic reflexes but without impairment of consciousness in which the extremities appear to be paralysed by motor and sensory failure'.

Another definition of the state produced by these agents is 'dissociative anaesthesia' which is characterized by complete analgesia combined with only superficial sleep [74]. Also in man, hallucinations and emergence delirium are known to occur. It cannot be known whether similar phenomena are experienced by animals but the state produced by these substances is clinically very different from anaesthesia produced by other agents. Spontaneous involuntary muscle movement and hypertonus are not uncommon during induction and purposeless tonic–clonic movements of the extremities may occur during anaesthesia. These movements of the extremities may be mistaken to indicate an inadequate level of anaesthesia and the need for additional doses; unless this possibility is recognized, overdoses may be given.

Electroencephalographic studies show a functional dissociation between the thalamoneocortical and limbic systems, the former being depressed before there is a significant effect on the reticular activating and limbic systems [75]. This differs from the effects of other non-inhalation anaesthetics and is manifested by the state of the animal. Hypertonus and muscle movement have already been mentioned; in addition, animals may remain with their eyes open and have a good tone in the jaw muscles with active laryngeal and pharyngeal reflexes, whilst analgesia appears to be extremely good.

Phencyclidine

Phencyclidine is phenylcyclohexylpiperidine, a compound which acts primarily on the central nervous system either by stimulation or depression, the overall effect produced varying considerably according to the species of animal concerned, and the dose rate used. Its pharmacology has been reported by Chen *et al.* [76]. Several workers have reported its use in monkeys [76–78]. In the veterinary field it has been used in pigs, goats [79, 80], chickens [81] and wild game animals [82]. However, because its effects in animals other than primates and lower monkeys have given cause for concern, it is today not recommended for general use in veterinary practice and, indeed, is no longer generally available.

Tiletamine

Tiletamine hydrochloride, known chemically as 2-(ethylamino)-2-(2-thienyl)cyclohexanone hydrochloride, is a cataleptic agent similar to phencyclidine hydrochloride.

The pharmacology of tiletamine has been reported by Chen and Ensor [83] and the compound has been subjected to numerous clinical trials in cats. Given by intramuscular injection in doses of 0.5–1.0 mg/kg it produces salivation (which is easily controlled with atropine), lacrimation, mydriasis and ataxia. Recovery, as indicated by the ability to walk without ataxia, occurs within 1–1.5 hours. At this dosage level the threshold to external stimuli is increased but there is no loss of consciousness or analgesia of the skin. Doses of 5–10 mg/kg produce observable sedation after 3 minutes. Loss of consciousness is not apparent at the lower end of the dosage scale but unconsciousness seems to be produced by doses of 10 mg/kg. Response to stimulation is generally absent and recovery occurs in 2–8 hours. High doses of 20–30 mg/kg given by intramuscular injection produce deep depression bordering on general anaesthesia which lasts 1–2 hours. The swallowing, pedal and palpebral reflexes are not abolished and muscle relaxation is absent. Recovery after these high doses takes 8–12 hours or even longer. Even very high doses of the drug have little effect on the cardiovascular system.

Although introduced for clinical trial as an anaesthetic agent for cats, it was not initially accepted in veterinary practice. At the high doses required to abolish response to stimulation, the respiratory depression together with the lack of muscle relaxation and long recovery period are serious disadvantages [84]. Another disadvantage of the preparation made available for trials was that its intramuscular injection caused pain.

Tiletamine has been used in combination with the diazepam analogue zolazepam in dogs and cats [85, 86]. This combination causes tachycardia with slight rises in blood pressure and cardiac output coupled with initial respiratory stimulation which is followed by mild depression of breathing. More recently, the combination has been used with xylazine to produce anaesthesia in horses [87]. Tiletamine–zolazepam may be useful in veterinary anaesthesia but the mixture has yet to be made available for clinical trials in the UK.

Ketamine

Ketamine is *dl*-2-(*o*-chlorophenyl)-2-(methylamino)-cyclohexanone hydrochloride. The molecule exists as two optical isomers and the racemic mixture is currently used clinically. It is available in 10, 50 and 100 mg/ml strengths and is suitable for intramuscular or intravenous injection. The 10 mg/ml solution is made isotonic with sodium chloride. In all species of animal, ketamine appears to have a much shorter duration of action than phencyclidine.

The effects of ketamine on the central nervous system are similar to those of phencyclidine. They become apparent rapidly, for the brain/plasma concentration ratio becomes constant in less than 1 minute [88]. Ketamine also rapidly crosses the placental barrier. Liver metabolism produces at least four metabolites which are excreted in the urine; they may have some slight additive effect to the action of the parent drug. Ketamine produces profound analgesia without muscle relaxation and tonic–clonic spasms of limb muscles may occur even in the absence of surgical or other stimulation. In horses and dogs convulsions are frequently seen during recovery and they sometimes occur in cats. Salivation is increased and saliva can obstruct the airway even though laryngeal and pharyngeal reflexes are retained. To eliminate these side-effects a variety of other compounds such as atropine, diazepam, acepromazine, xylazine and even the thiobarbiturates or an inhalation agent are commonly given concurrently with ketamine.

Mild respiratory depression has been reported and in clinical practice this is usually manifested by an increased rate which does not compensate for a decreased tidal volume. Although laryngeal reflexes may be present it is still necessary for the airway to be kept under close observation because the degree of protection of the upper airway is less than was once thought.

In contrast with the action of other intravenous induction agents, but like tiletamine and phencyclidine, ketamine causes a rise in arterial blood pressure and, on occasions, this rise can be alarming.

The rate of injection is not an important factor in the production of hypertension and intramusclar injection results in no less a rise in blood pressure than the intravenous route. The picture is one of stimulation by an agent which has a direct depressant action on the isolated heart preparation. This is probably due to an increase in circulating catecholamines caused by ketamine blocking the re-uptake of noradrenaline by adrenergic nerve terminals.

Cardiac arrhythmias are uncommon in animals under ketamine anaesthesia and the minimal arterial blood pressure value recorded during anaesthesia is always similar to and rarely less than the preoperative level.

Ketamine produces little, if any, muscle relaxation. There is generally an increase in skeletal muscle tonus and tendon reflexes are brisk. Athetoid limb movements occur without external stimuli and are not dose related.

There is no vidence of tolerance developing after repeated injections of ketamine and no significant cumulative effects have been reported. Daily injections of ketamine in rats, dogs and monkeys caused no alterations in haematological, urine or bone marrow values or in blood chemistry.

According to the manufacturers there were no adverse effects on the dam or the pups when pregnant bitches were given 25 mg/kg of ketamine twice a week over a 3 week period during each third of pregnancy and pregnant rabbits given ketamine daily during the period of organogenesis produced normal litters. There appears to be no published information regarding the use of ketamine for caesarian section in any species of animal but in the authors' experience lambs delivered from ewes that have had anaesthesia induced with ketamine behave as though they are unaware of their surroundings for up to 12 hours after delivery. Extreme difficulty has been experienced in getting them to suckle in the first 6 hours of life. For caesarian section in mares, induction of anaesthesia with ketamine after xylazine premedication seems to have little effect on the foal.

When ketamine was first introduced into veterinary practice in the UK it was not received with any great enthusiasm. This was probably because unnecessarily high dose rates were recommended and because it soon became apparent that the results claimed in experimental laboratories were not always reproduced in clinical situations. Over the years increasing familiarity with its effects and limitations, together with recognition that high doses merely prolong its effects without significantly improving operating conditions, have led to ketamine finding a place for certain purposes.

The difficulty in assessing the degree of unconsciousness coupled with the poor muscle relaxation produced by the drug make it doubtful whether ketamine should ever be used alone for surgical operations [89], although its ease of administration makes its use superficially attractive in animals such as sheep and cats. Ketamine alone in sheep, in the authors' experience and that of others [90, 91], fails to produce satisfactory anaesthesia, contrasting sharply with that reported from other centres [92, 93]. In cats it is doubtful if ketamine alone should be used except, possibly, to subdue a particularly wild individual.

However, there is general agreement that ketamine is the agent of choice for the sedation of reptiles [94–96], especially before halothane anaesthesia. Similarly, ketamine has proved to be of value in many species of birds [97–102].

Emphasis has now changed from the use of ketamine alone to its use in combination with other drugs to produce anaesthesia while avoiding the appearance of undesirable, or potentially dangerous, phenomena. Depending on the species of animal, α_2-adrenoceptor agonists (xylazine, detomidine, medetomidine) or benzodiazepines (diazepam, midazolam, zolazepam) are apparently the most satisfactory agents for combination with ketamine. The question whether atropine should also be used remains a matter for debate.

VOLUMES OF DISTRIBUTION OF INTRAVENOUS AGENTS

To be effective, an intravenous agent must attain and maintain an adequate therapeutic concentration at its site of action. A knowledge of its volume of distribution (V_d) makes it possible to calculate the doses to be administered initially and subsequently to achieve these concentrations. In theory, the volume of distribution is measured by injecting a known quantity of the drug and, after a period of time adequate for it to dilute in the total body water, determining its total concentration in the plasma (both free and combined). In practice, the equilibrium necessary is not attained because before it is complete the opposing processes of metabolism or excretion come into operation. To simplify calculations it is usually assumed that intravenous drugs are immediately distributed throughout the V_d and this is termed a 'single-compartment model'.

Secondary dispersion of highly lipid-soluble drugs such as the intravenous anaesthetic agents occurs as they cross cell membranes and the limiting factor to this process is the rate at which they are delivered to the cells — the blood flow to the tissues. Thus, organs with a rapid blood flow (e.g. brain, heart, liver, kidney) initially receive a high concentration of the drug but, with time, this is depleted as the agent redistributes into moderately and slowly perfused tissues (the muscles and fat, respectively). The greater the lipid solubility of the drug the more rapid its redistribution but even charged drugs can be redistributed. Redistribution also means that repeated doses of the drug can exert prolonged effects due to gradual passage over an extended period from the saturated sites where it is inactive back into the plasma. Plasma and the organs where blood flow is rapid can be taken to represent one 'compartment'; moderately and poorly perfused tissues represent second and third compartments.

PHARMACOKINETICS AND INTRAVENOUS AGENTS

Pharmacokinetics, the processes whereby drug concentrations at effector sites are achieved, maintained and diminished is of increasing importance today because of the use of computer models to study drug uptake and elimination, and of attempts to use microprocessors to control anaesthetic administration. For a detailed consideration of pharmacokinetics reference should be made to standard textbooks on pharmacology. The following simplified account draws mainly on *Lecture Notes in Pharmacology* by H. F. Grundy (Blackwell Scientific, Oxford).

Most drugs can be regarded as obeying what are known as *zero-order* or *first-order* kinetics. A zero-order process is one which occurs at a constant rate and is, therefore, independent of the quantity of drug present at the particular sites of absorption or removal. A zero-order process requires a large excess of drug available on the entry side (e.g. intravenous infusion) or, on the removal side a system which has a limited capacity. However, a first-order process is most common for both drug absorption and elimination. In a first-order process the rate of the reaction is exponentially related to the amount of drug available. In other words, a constant *fraction* of the drug is absorbed or eliminated in constant time. The rate constants (k_{ab} and k_{el}) are quantitative measurements of these fractions since they represent the fraction of the drug present which is absorbed or eliminated in unit time (usually in 1 minute or 1 hour).

A very simplified example of a first-order elimination is shown in Fig. 5.2 where the plasma concentration of an intravenous drug given by a single intravenous injection is plotted against time. Under these conditions a plot of log plasma concentration against time is linear. The time taken for the plasma concentration to halve ($t_{1/2}$) is known as the plasma half-life. The V_d can be calculated for the initial concentration (i.e. that at zero time) and from this, by assuming V_d to be constant over the whole time period (which, in practice, it seldom is), the clearance from the plasma can be calculated. A more accurate method assumes

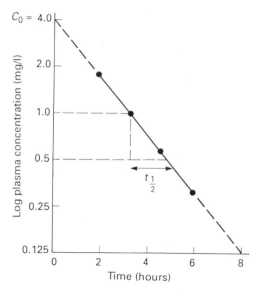

Fig. 5.2 Simplified diagram of first-order elimination from the plasma of an intravenous drug. Dots indicate measured plasma concentrations at given time intervals after injection. The plot of log plasma concentration versus time is linear.

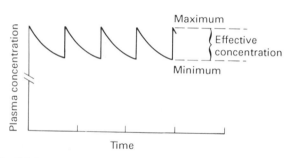

Fig. 5.3 Intermittent intravenous dosage to maintain an effective anaesthetic concentration. Single-compartment model.

(usually incorrectly) that the clearance from the plasma is a constant fraction of the instantaneous level, thus:

$$\text{Plasma clearance} = \frac{\text{Original dose}}{\text{Area under curve to complete elimination}}$$

The area under the curve is obtained from a graph of actual concentration (not log concentration) against time.

What is known as 'the plateau principle' applies when a drug undergoes zero-order absorption and first-order elimination. Under these conditions it can be shown that when the concentration of the drug being administered is changed, the time taken to reach a steady-state (plateau) level is determined solely by the reciprocal of the rate constant of elimination (k_{el}). The height of the plateau reached depends on the concentration of the drug administered and when this height is attained the amount of drug given is reduced to maintain it. Similar principles apply when loading doses are followed by subsequent doses to maintain this level (Fig. 5.3). It should be noted that about 97% of the drug administered will be eliminated from the plasma in about $5 \times t_{1/2}(50 + 25 + 12.5 + 6.25 + 3.125\%)$.

Ideally, the anaesthetist would like to know the concentration of the anaesthetic agent attained and maintained at the site of its effect (i.e. the brain) but as may be guessed from the above considerations this is rarely possible. All that can be said is that the plasma drug concentration is *often* related to, and is a valid measure of, the required quantity so that the $t_{1/2}$ is, usually, the paramount determinant of dose frequency when intermittent administration is the method employed.

Although the actual plasma concentration-effect approach of the pharmacologist is undoubtedly rational, the question arises as to whether the anaesthetist may not work better with a dose–effect relationship [103]. This is a somewhat regressive pharmacological approach to the system but offers a simpler model for everyday use.

REFERENCES

1. Dundee, J. W. and Clarke, R. S. J. (1979) *General Anaesthesia*, 4th edn (eds T. C. Gray, J. F. Nunn and J. E. Utting). London: Butterworths.
2. Sheppard, M. and Sheppard, D. H. (1937) *Veterinary Record* **49**, 424.
3. Wright, J. G. (1937) *Veterinary Record* **49**, 27.
4. Brodie, D. D. (1952) *Federation Proceedings. Federation of American Society of Experimental Biology* **11**, 632.
5. Brodie, D. D., Burn, J. H., Epstein, H. G., Feigan, G. A. and Paton, W. D. M. (1957) *British Medical Journal* **ii**, 479.
6. Brodie, D. D., Burnstein, E. and Mark, L. C. (1952) *Journal of Clinical Investigation* **105**, 421.
7. Brodie, D. D., Mark, L. C., Papper, E. M., Lief, P. A., Bernstein, E. and Rovenstine, E. A. (1950) *Journal of Pharmacology and Experimental Therapeutics* **98**, 85.
8. Mark, L. C., Brand, L., Kanvyssi, S., Britton, R. C., Perel, J. M., Landrau, M. A. and Dayton, P. G. (1965) *Nature, London* **206**, 1117.
9. Saidman, L. J. and Eger E. I. (1966) *Anesthesiology* **27**, 118.
10. Longley, E. O. (1950) *Veterinary Record* **62**, 17.
11. Waddington, F. G. (1950) *Veterinary Record* **62**, 100.
12. Ford, E. J. H. (1951) *Veterinary Record* **63**, 636.
13. Jones, E. W., Johnson, L. and Heinze, C. D. (1960) *Journal of the American Veterinary Medical Association* **137**, 119.

14. Tyagi, R. P. S., Arnold, J. P., Usenik, E. A. and Fletcher, T. F. (1964) *Cornell Veterinarian* **54**, 584.
15. Neal, P. A. (1963) *Veterinary Record* **75**, 289.
16. Dundee, J. W. and Wyant, G. M. (1988) *Intravenous Anaesthesia*, 2nd edn. Edinburgh: Churchill Livingstone.
17. Blood, D. C. and Henderson, J. A. (1961) *Veterinary Medicine*. London: Baillière, Tindall and Cox.
18. Tobias, G. (1964) *Journal of the American Veterinary Medical Association* **145**, 462.
19. Reutner, T. F. and Grulzit, O. M. (1948) *Journal of the American Veterinary Medical Association* **113**, 357.
20. Crawshaw, H. A. (1955) *Veterinary Record* **67**, 266.
21. Fowler, N. G. and Stevenson, D. E. (1961) *Veterinary Record* **73**, 917.
22. Fowler, N. G. and Stevenson, D. E. (1964) *Small Animal Anaesthesia*. Oxford: Pergamon Press.
23. Fabry, A. (1963) *Veterinary Record* **75**, 1049.
24. Tavernor, W. D. (1962) *Veterinary Record* **74**, 595.
25. Robertshaw, D. (1964) *Veterinary Record* **76**, 357.
26. Monahan, C. M. (1964) *Veterinary Record* **76**, 1333.
27. Child, K. J., Currie, J. P., Davis, B., Dodds, M. G., Pearce, D. R. and Twissell, D. J. (1971) *British Journal of Anaesthesia* **43**, 2.
28. Hall, L. W. (1972) *Postgraduate Medical Journal* **48**(Suppl. 2), 55.
29. Eales, F. A., Hall, L. W. and Massey, G. M. (1974) *Proceedings of the Association of Veterinary Anaesthetists of Great Britain and Ireland* **5**, 1.
30. Dyson, D. H., Allen, D. A. Ingwersen, W., Pascoe, P. J. and O'Grady, M. (1987) *Canadian Journal of Veterinary Research* **51**, 236.
31. Foex, P. and Prys-Roberts, C. (1972) *Postgraduate Medical Journal* **48**(Suppl. 2), 24.
32. Clarke, K. W. and Hall, L. W. (1975) *Proceedings of the 20th World Veterinary Congress*, Thessaloniki.
33. Hall, L. W., Trim, C. M. and Woolf, N. (1972) *British Medical Journal* **ii**, 145.
34. Evans, J. M. (1979) *Proceedings of the Association of Veterinary Anaesthetists of Great Britain and Ireland* **8**, 73.
35. Watkins, J., Padfield, A. and Alderson, J. D. (1978) *British Medical Journal* **i**, 1180.
36. Corbett, H. (1977) *Australian Veterinary Practitioner* **7**, 184.
37. Marsboom, R. and Symoens, J. (1968) *Netherlands Journal of Veterinary Science* **1**, 124.
38. Clarke, K. W. (1969) *Veterinary Record* **85**, 649.
39. Symoens, J. and van den Brande, M. (1969) *Veterinary Record* **85**, 64.
40. Diminger, J. and Reetz, I. (1970) *Deutsche Tierarztliche Wochenschrift* **77**, 445.
41. Prasse, R. (1970) Prakt. *Tierarzteblatt* **51**, 278.
42. Callear, J. F. F. and Van Gestel, J. F. E. (1971) *Veterinary Record* **89**, 453.
43. Roztocil, V., Nemecek, I. and Pavlica, J. (1971) *Veterinary Medicine (Praha)* **16**, 591.
44. Jones, R. S. (1972) *Veterinary Record* **90**, 613.
45. Cox, J. E. (1973) *Veterinary Record* **92**, 143.
46. Hillidge, C. J., Lees, P. and Serrano, L. (1973) *Veterinary Record* **93**, 307.
47. Houston, D. C. and Cooper, J. E. (1973) *International Zoo Yearbook* **13**, 269.
48. Cooper, J. E. (1974) *Veterinary Record* **94**, 437.
49. Janssen, P. A. J., Niemegeers, C. J. E. and Marsboom, R. P. H. (1975) *Archives of International Pharmacodynamics and Therapeutics* **214**, 96.
50. Nagel, M. L., Muir, W. W. and Nguyen, K. (1979) *American Journal of Veterinary Research* **40**, 193.
51. Morgan, M., Lumley, J. and Whitwam, J. G. (1977) *British Journal of Anaesthesia* **49**, 233.
52. Wagner, R. L. and White, P. F. (1984) *Anesthesiology* **61**, 647.
53. Fellows, I. W., Yeoman, P. M., Selby, C. and Byrne, A. J. (1985) *European Journal of Anaesthesiology* **2**, 285.
54. Moore, R. A., Allen, M. C., Wood, P. J., Rees, L. L. H. and Sear, J. W. (1985) *Anaesthesia* **40**, 124.
55. Kruse-Elliott, K. T., Swanson, C. R. and Aucoin, D. P. (1987) *American Journal of Veterinary Research* **148**, 1098.
56. Erhardt, W. (1984) *Journal of the Association of Veterinary Anaesthetists of Great Britain and Ireland* **12**, 196.
57. Glen, J. B. (1980) *British Journal of Anaesthesia* **52**, 731.
58. James, R. and Glen, J. B. (1980) *Journal of Medicinal Chemistry* **123**, 1350.
59. Glen, J. B. and Hunter, S. C. (1984) *British Journal of Anaesthesia* **5**, 617.
60. Nolan, A. (1982) *Proceedings of the 1st International Congress of Veterinary Anaesthesia*, Cambridge, p. 204.
61. Nolan, A. and Hall, L. W. (1985) *Equine Veterinary Journal* **171**, 394.
62. Glen, J. B., Hunter, S. C., Blackburn, T. P. and Wood, P. (1985) *Postgraduate Medical Journal* **61**(Suppl. 3), 7.
63. Cummings, G. C., Dixon, J., Kay, N. H., Windsor, J. P. W., Major, E. D., Morgan, M., Sear, J. W., Spence, A. A. and Stephenson, D. K. (1984) *Anaesthesia* **39**, 1168.
64. Jessop, E., Grounds, R. M., Morgan, M. and Lumley, J. (1985) *British Journal of Anaesthesia* **57**, 1173.
65. Hall, L. W., (1984) *Journal of the Association of Anaesthetists of Great Britain and Ireland* **11**, 115.
66. Watkins, S. B., Hall, L. W. and Clarke, K. W. (1987) *Veterinary Record* **120**, 326.
67. Hall, L. W. and Chambers, J. P. (1987) *Journal of Small Animal Practice* **281**, 623.
68. Brearley, J. C., Kellagher, R. E. B. and Hall, L. W. (1988) *Journal of Small Animal Practice* **29**, 315.
69. Cockshott, I. D. (1985) *Postgraduate Medical Journal* **61** (Suppl. 3), 45.
70. Vladutiu, O. (1938) *Revista Veterinara Militara*, Nos 2, 3. (1939) *Abstract Record Medicin Veterinaire* **115**, 236.
71. Coffee, W. F. (1949) *Journal of the American Veterinary Association* **114**, 291.
72. Millenbruck, E. W. and Wallinga, M. H. (1966) *Journal of the American Veterinary Medical Association* **108**, 148.
73. Chen, G. M. (1965) *Archives of International Pharmacodynamics and Therapeutics* **157**, 193.
74. Corsenn, G. (1969) *Anaesthetist* **18**, 25.
75. Corssen, G., Miyasaka, M. and Domino, E. G. (1968) *Current Researches in Anesthesia and Analgesia* **47**, 746.
76. Chen, G. M., Ensor, C. R., Russell, D. and Bohner, B. (1959) *Journal of Pharmacology and Experimental Therapeutics* **128**, 241.
77. Chen, G. M. and Watson, J. K. (1960) *Anesthesia and Analgesia* **39**, 132.
78. Rutty, D. A. and Thurley, D. C. (1962) *Veterinary Record* **74**, 883.
79. Spalding, V. T. and Heymann, C. S. (1962) *Veterinary Record* **74**, 158.
80. Wilkins, H. H. (1961) *Veterinary Record* **73**, 767.

81. Wright, A. and Jordan, F. T. W. (1963) *Veterinary Record* **75**, 471.
82. Harthoorn, A. M. (1962) *Veterinary Record* **74**, 410.
83. Chen, G. M. and Ensor, C. R. (1968) *American Journal of Veterinary Research* **29**, 863.
84. Garmer, L. N. (1969) *Research in Veterinary Science* **10**, 382.
85. Bree, M. M., Cohen, B. J. and Rowe, S. E. (1972) *Laboratory Animal Science* **22**, 878.
86. Wars, G. S., Johnsen, D. O. and Roberts, C. R. (1974) *Laboratory Animal Science* **24**, 737.
87. Hubbell, J. A. E., Bednarski, R. M. and Muir, W. W. (1989) *American Journal of Veterinary Research* **50**, 737.
88. Green, C. J., Knight, J., Precious, S. and Simpkin, S. (1981) *Laboratory Animals* **15**, 163.
89. Nowrouzian, I., Schels, H. G., Ghodsian, I. and Karimi, H. (1981) *Veterinary Record* **108**, 354.
90. Taylor, P., Hopkins, L., Young, M. and McFadyen, I. R. (1972) *Veterinary Record* **90**, 35.
91. Thurman, J. C., Kumar, A. and Link, R. P. (1973) *Journal of the American Veterinary Association* **162**, 293.
92. Glenn, J. L., Straight, R. and Snyder, C. C. (1972) *American Journal of Veterinary Research* **33**, 1901.
93. Cooper, J. E. (1974) *Veterinary Record* **95**, 37.
94. Harding, K. A. (1977) *Veterinary Record* **100**, 289.
95. Bree, M. M. and Gross, N. B. (1969) *Laboratory Animal Care* **19**, 500.
96. Borzio, F. (1973) *Veterinary Medicine — Small Animal Clinician* **68**, 1364.
97. Gerlach, H. (1969) *Veterinary Record* **84**, 342.
98. Kittle, E. L. (1971) *Modern Veterinary Practice* **52**, 40.
99. Mattingly, B. E. (1972) *Raptor Research* **61**, 51.
100. Mandelker, L. (1973) *Veterinary Medicine — Small Animal Clinician* **68**, 487.
101. Klide, A. M. (1973) *Veterinary Clinics of North America*, vol. 3, p. 175. Philadelphia: W. B. Saunders.
102. Boever, W. J. and Wright, W. (1975). *Veterinary Medicine — Small Animal Clinician* **70**, 86.
103. Waud, B. E. and Waud, D. R. (1986) *Anesthesiology* **65**, 355.

CHAPTER 6

GENERAL PHARMACOLOGY OF THE INHALATION ANAESTHETICS

An inhalation anaesthetic cannot be introduced into the brain without at the same time being distributed through the entire body, and this distribution exerts a controlling influence over the rate of the uptake or elimination of the anaesthetic by brain tissue. All the gaseous and volatile substances used as anaesthetics may be regarded as inert gases as far as uptake and elimination are concerned so to regulate anaesthesia in a rational manner the anaesthetist should have a clear understanding of the processes involved in the exchange of inert gases in the body.

TERMINOLOGY

In the account which follows, frequent reference is made to tensions, solubilities and concentrations of gases in solution. These terms may perhaps be best explained by considering certain specific examples.

The tensions of agents dissolved in a liquid. This is the pressure of the agent in the gas with which the liquid should be in equilibrium. (A liquid and a gas, or two liquids, are in equilibrium if, when separated by a permeable membrane, there is no exchange between them.) The statement that 'the tension of nitrous oxide in the blood is 380 mmHg (50.5 kPa)' means that if a sample of blood were placed in an ambient atmosphere containing nitrous oxide at a concentration of 50% v/v (and, therefore, according to Dalton's law, exerting a partial pressure of 380 mmHg (50.5 kPa)) there would be no movement of nitrous oxide into or out of the blood. 'Tension' is a term used by physiologists and anaesthetists, while physicists speak of 'partial pressure'.

Solubility coefficients of gases. At any given temperature the mass of a gas dissolved in a solution, i.e. its concentration in the solution, varies directly with its tension (Henry's law) and is governed by the solubility of the gas in the particular solvent. The solubility of anaesthetics varies widely and, therefore, at any one tension, the quantities of the different anaesthetics in the solvent are not equal.

The solubility of anaesthetics in the blood and tissues are best expressed in terms of their partition, or distribution, coefficients. For example, the blood–gas partition coefficient of nitrous oxide is 0.47. This means that when blood and alveolar air containing nitrous oxide at a given tension are in equilibrium, there will be 47 parts of nitrous oxide per unit volume (say per litre) of blood for every 100 parts of nitrous oxide per unit volume (litre) of alveolar air. In general, the partition coefficient of a gas at a stated temperature is the ratio, at equilibrium, of the gas's concentration on the two sides of a diffusing membrane or interface. In the brain and all other tissues (except fat) gases have very nearly the same solubility as they have in blood; their tissue–blood partition coefficients are close in unity. Exceptions are substances like halothane which are exceptionally soluble in fat. Halothane is about 60 times as soluble in fat as it is in blood (i.e. fat–blood coefficient is 60) and because of the lipoid nature of brain tissue, the brain–blood partition coefficient for halothane is 2.6.

Concentration of a gas in solution. The concentration of a gas in solution may be expressed in a variety of ways including:

1. The volume of gas which can be extracted from a unit of volume of solution under standard conditions (v/v)

2. The weight of dissolved gas per unit volume of solvent (w/v)
3. The molar concentration i.e. the number of gram-molecules of gas per litre of solvent

The molar concentration is the most useful — equimolar solutions of gases of different molecular weights contain equal concentrations of molecules. This would not be so if their concentrations in terms of w/v were equal.

SIMPLIFICATIONS

If some factors are reduced to their simplest possible terms, and certain assumptions are made, it is possible to give approximate predictions relating to inert gas exchange in the body. These predictions are sufficiently realistic for practical purposes and will serve to illustrate the main principles involved. Once these are understood, more elaborate expositions found elsewhere [1–5] should become reasonably easy to follow. It is possible, once these certain assumptions have been made, to give a mathematical description of uptake under certain conditions and this line of approach has been admirably reviewed by Kety [6] in an account which includes his own, very large, contributions to this field of knowledge. It is mainly on this review and one

other paper [7] that the following outline is based.

For simplicity, the physiological variables such as cardiac output and tidal volume must be assumed to be unaffected by the presence of the gas, and to remain uniform throughout the administration. Allowance cannot be made for alterations in the tidal volume as uptake or elimination proceeds. The blood supply to the grey matter of the brain must be assumed to be uniform and the gas to be evenly distributed throughout the grey matter. Finally, although in practice anaesthetics are seldom administered in this way, the anaesthetic must be assumed to be given at a fixed inspired concentration, and, what is more, it must be assumed that no rebreathing of gases occurs.

UPTAKE OF ANAESTHETICS

Kety has pointed out that when an inert gas is suddenly introduced at a fixed partial pressure into the inspired air in a non-breathing system, the tissues of the body do not immediately acquire the gas at this tension. The tensions of the gas in the alveolar blood and tissues all tend to move towards inspired tension but a number of processes, each of which proceeds at its own rate, intervene to delay the eventual saturation of the tissues. In other words, the tension of the gas in the brain follows, with a slight delay, its tension in the alveolar air. Since both the rate of induction and recovery from inhalation anaesthesia are governed by the rate of change of the tension of the anaesthetic in the brain, and this in turn is governed by the rate of change of its tension in the alveoli, the factors which determine the tension of the anaesthetic in the alveoli are obviously of very great importance to the anaesthetist.

The rate at which the tension of an anaesthetic in the alveoli air approaches its tension in the inspired air depends on the pulmonary ventilation, the uptake of the anaesthetic by the blood and tissues and the inspired concentration. First, by means of pulmonary ventilation the gas is inhaled, diluted with functional residual air, and distributed to the alveolar membrane. This is where diffusion occurs and normally the alveolar gas equilibrates almost immediately with the pulmonary blood which is then distributed throughout the body. A second diffusion process occurs across the capillary membranes of the tissues into the

interstitial fluid and from there through the cell membranes into the cells themselves. Venous blood leaving the tissues is in equilibrium with the tissues. The blood from the tissues returns to the lungs, still carrying some of its original content of anaesthetic, and is again equilibrated with alveolar gas which now contains a slightly higher tension of the anaesthetic. It is in this manner that the alveolar (or arterial) and venous (or tissue) tensions of the anaesthetic in question gradually, and in that order, rise towards eventual equilibrium with the inspired tension.

As this complex process proceeds, the tension of the anaesthetic in the alveolar air increases continuously, but not at a uniform rate. Plotted against time, alveolar tension rises in a curve that, in general, is the same for every inert gas (Fig. 6.1). In Kety's terminology this curve has an initial rise (which is steep), a knee and a tail, which slopes gradually upwards until, after several hours or even days, depending on the anaesthetic in question, complete equilibrium is reached. The steep initial rise represents the phase in which ventilation is moving anaesthetic into the lungs, i.e. the so-called 'pulmonary washout' phases. The slowly rising tail represents the more gradual process of tissue saturation. The knee marks the point at which lung washout gives place to tissue saturation as the most important influence. The tail can be very long if the anaesthetic in question has a very high fat–blood partition coefficient.

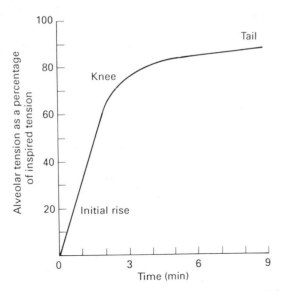

Fig. 6.1 Typical alveolar tension curve for an inert gas inhaled at a constant tension from a non-rebreathing system.

Effect of blood solubility on alveolar tension

The shape of curve obtained with any given anaesthetic depends on a number of factors. These include such things as: the minute volume of respiration; the functional residual capacity of the lungs; the cardiac output; the blood flow to the main anaesthetic absorbing bulk of the body — the muscles and the fat. However, one single physical property of the anaesthetic itself is considerably more important than all of these factors — the solubility of the anaesthetic in the blood. This is the factor which determines the height of the knee in the alveolar uptake curve. With anaesthetics of low blood solubility the knee is high; with those of high blood solubility the knee is low. This may be illustrated by consideration of the hypothetical extremes of solubility.

A totally insoluble gas would not diffuse into the pulmonary blood and would not be carried in it away from the lungs. If such a gas were inhaled at a constant inspired tension in a non-breathing system, its alveolar tension would increase exponentially as lung washout proceeded until, after a very short time, alveolar tension equalled inspired tension. The curve obtained would be all initial rise, and there would be no tail (Fig. 6.2, curve A). Such a gas could not, of course, ever be an anaesthetic, since none would ever reach the brain. A gas of extremely low blood solubility (Fig. 6.2, curve B) would give an almost identical curve. The loss into the pulmonary blood stream of only a minute amount of the gas contained in the lungs at any moment would bring the tension of the gas in the blood into equilibrium with the tension

in the alveolar air. The capacity of the blood for such a gas would be extremely small. Likewise, the capacity of the entire body tissue (with the possible exception of fat) would be small since, as already pointed out, the tissue–blood partition coefficients of most anaesthetics are close to unity. If such an agent, even when given at the highest permissible inspired concentration of 80% with 20% of oxygen, only produced a faint depression of the central nervous system, it could nevertheless be looked upon as a very active agent because it would be deriving its effect through the presence in the brain of only a minute trace.

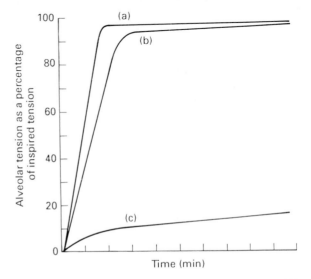

Fig. 6.2 Alveolar tension curves for a totally insoluble gas (A), a gas of low solubility (e.g. nitrous oxide) (B), and a gas of extremely high solubility (C), all breathed at a constant inspired tension from a non-rebreathing circuit.

At the other hypothetical extreme would be a gas of very nearly infinite solubility in blood.

All but a very small fraction of the gas in the lungs at any one moment would dissolve in the pulmonary blood as soon as the blood arrived at the alveoli. The capacity of the blood and body tissues for such a gas would be vast. The alveoli tension curve (Fig. 6.2, curve C) would be very flat, with virtually no initial rise, a knee virtually on the baseline and a very slowly rising tail. Given time enough for full equilibrium, it might be possible to achieve very deep anaesthesia by using a minute inspired tension but, of course, in one sense the gas would be a very weak anaesthetic, since its concentration in the brain would be enormous.

Ranging between these hypothetical extremes of solubility are the gaseous and volatile anaesthetics. Their solubilities in blood and tissues as far as they have been determined are shown in Table 6.1.

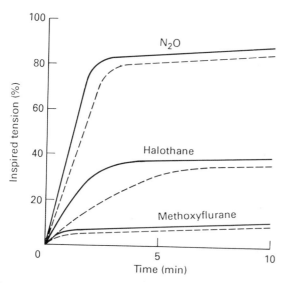

Fig. 6.3 Effect of blood solubility on alveolar (——) and grey matter (– – –) tension curves of anaesthetics administered at a constant inspired tension from a non-rebreathing system.

The effect of the different solubilities on the alveolar tension when the agents are administered at a constant inspired tension are shown in Fig. 6.3. (It must be appreciated that the curves have not been drawn accurately and are only intended to represent approximate, relative curves. Similar curves, drawn from data computed on an electrical analogue, a device for predicting actual values in man, have been constructed by Mapleson [1]).

The tension of anaesthetic agents in brain tissue

In addition to the alveolar tensions, the anaesthetist is also concerned with the tissue tension, and particularly with the tension of anaesthetic agents in the grey matter of the brain. In the lungs (unless pathological changes are present) diffusion from the alveolar air to the blood is almost instantaneous, as has already been pointed out. This means that the tension of the agent in the blood leaving the lungs, that is to say in the arterial blood, may for all practical purposes be regarded as equal to the tension in the alveolar air. Only when the body has become absolutely saturated does the arterial tension equal the tissue tension. During the saturation process, and after the administration is stopped, the tissue tension is accurately represented by the tension of the agent in the venous blood leaving that tissue. This lags behind the arterial tension by an amount which depends mainly upon the blood supply of the tissue. Fatty tissues are exceptions to this rule, for in them the relative solubilities play an important part. In organs with a

rich blood supply, such as the brain and the heart, the venous tension rises quite quickly to the arterial tension. After about 20 minutes (in man) with anaesthetics whose solubility in grey matter is about equal to that in blood, or perhaps 40 minutes in the case of agents like halothane which are a little more soluble in grey matter, arterial and grey matter tensions, during uptake and during elimination, are almost equal (Fig. 6.3).

It follows from these considerations that if a gas has a low blood solubility, any change in its tension in the alveolar air is quickly reflected in the grey matter in the brain, whereas if the blood solubility is high there will be a considerable delay because the whole body will act as a very large buffer. Thus, with an inhalation anaesthetic, the speed with which induction of anaesthesia can be carried out (when the inspired tension is kept constant) is governed by the solubility of the anaesthetic in the blood. Low solubility (nitrous oxide or cyclopropane) favours rapid induction, whereas high blood solubility (ether) leads to slow induction. The important point to note here is, of course, that so far all the arguments have been based on the assumption that the inspired concentration is maintained constant. In fact, alteration of the inspired tension can do much to overcome the slow induction with agents of high blood solubility. For example, if, in man, ether were given at the concentration which would give satisfactory anaesthesia after full equilibration, induction might take as long as 24 hours. It would be a very long time before the patient even lost consciousness. The difficulty is, of course, in practice, overcome by starting the administration not with this concentration, but with one which is much higher and which would if administered indefinitely kill the patient. As the desired level of anaesthesia is approached the inspired concentration is gradually reduced. Even so, induction with this very soluble agent is slow. In dogs, light anaesthesia is produced by tensions of ether in the brain of the order of 23 mmHg (3.1 kPa), while tensions of about 30 mmHg (4.0 kPa) produce deep anaesthesia, yet Haggard [10] had to administer this anaesthetic for about 20 minutes at more than five times these concentrations before these brain tensions were obtained.

It is in fact standard practice to hasten induction of inhalation anaesthesia in this way. However, the maximum concentration which can be administered is limited by the volatility of the anaesthetic, and its pungency. Many anaesthetics are so pungent or irritant that they cannot be inhaled in high concentrations.

Recovery from an inhalation anaesthetic cannot be subjected to the same treatment. When the administration of the anaesthetic is terminated its concentration in the inspired air cannot be reduced to below zero. Although the full buffering effect of the body tissues will not be seen after accelerated inductions and brief administration (those tissues with a poor blood supply or high tissue–blood partition coefficient will then be only very incompletely saturated), elimination of the more soluble anaesthetics must take time and will be slow. Low blood solubility leads to rapid elimination of nitrous oxide and rapid recovery from anaesthesia. Fink [11] studied the elimination of this gas from the lungs at the end of anaesthesia and found that the volume eliminated was such that the minute volume of expiration exceeded the inspired volume by as much as 10% in the first 10 minutes. This outpouring of nitrous oxide diluted the alveolar oxygen and if the patient was breathing room air, the alveolar oxygen tension fell to levels as low as 85 mmHg (11.3 kPa), resulting in arterial oxygen saturation of only 92%. This phenomenon, which has been named 'diffusion hypoxia', can also happen if nitrous oxide is cut off during anaesthesia. Theoretically, it can happen with any agent, but it is unlikely to have any ill effects with ether, because of the small volumes involved and the slow excretion of ether. The danger will be greatest if two insoluble agents such as nitrous oxide and isoflurane are administered together.

SAFETY OF INHALATION ANAESTHETICS

Blood solubility is not only important as a factor influencing the speed of induction and recovery. It has wider implications; it determines (in an inverse manner) the extent to which tissue tension keeps pace with alterations in inspired tension and thus it controls the rate at which anaesthesia can be deepened or lightened. With a very soluble agent such as ether no sudden change in tissue tension is possible; if gross overdosage is given the anaesthetist has plenty of time in which to observe the signs of deepening unconsciousness and to reduce the strength of the inhaled mixture. With an anaesthetic of low blood solubility such as desflurane, however, increase in tissue tension follows very quickly on the heels of an increase in the inspired tension; anaesthesia may deepen rapidly and a gross overdose may be almost instantly fatal. It is, therefore, very important with the less soluble anaesthetics to consider carefully the factors that favour the giving of an overdose, the chief of which must be volatility and potency.

Volatility governs the potential strength of the inspired mixture for obviously the more volatile the anaesthetic the greater the risk of its being administered at a high concentration. Gaseous anaesthetics and liquid anaesthetics which have low boiling points are, therefore, potentially dangerous. Because gases are passed through flowmeters the danger is, in their case, rather less, since the anaesthetist has an accuracy of control only possible with volatile liquids by the use of special, often expensive, vaporizers.

Potency determines the magnitude of a possible overdose. With a weak anaesthetic such as nitrous oxide overdose is impossible; if it were not for lack of oxygen, nitrous oxide could be given at 100% concentration without danger. However, a concentration of 80% of an agent which was fully effective when given at a concentration of say 5% would constitute a gross overdose. This is, of course, self-evident, but as has been pointed out by Bourne [2], anaesthetists have in the past paid insufficient attention to the precise meaning and measurement of potency, so that there is much confusion. An acceptable definition of potency would do much to clarify thought relating to safety of inhalation anaesthetics.

UPTAKE AND ELIMINATION OF INHALATION ANAESTHETICS IN CLINICAL PRACTICE

The various assumptions made for the purpose of theoretical or mathematical predictions of anaesthetic uptake and elimination cannot, of course, be made in everyday anaesthetic practice. Many of the factors which have to be regarded as constant if any mathematical prediction is to be made, do, in fact, vary considerably during the course of anaesthesia. Such factors include the tidal volume; the physiological dead-space; the functional residual capacity (i.e. that volume of gas in the lungs which dilutes each single breath of anaesthetic); the thickness and permeability of the alveolar–capillary membrane; the cardiac output and pulmonary blood flow (which may be different, especially in pathological conditions of the lungs); regional variations in ventilation/perfusion relationships in the lungs; the blood flow through the tissues of the body, the partition coefficients of the anaesthetic between the gaseous (or vapour) state, and lung tissue or blood, and between blood and the body tissue; and the blood flow, diffusion coefficient and diffusion distance for each of the tissues of the body.

In addition, it must be remembered that the anaesthetics themselves may modify many of the variables as administration proceeds. For example, most anaesthetics depress breathing and decrease the cardiac output.

Considerations such as these indicate only too clearly why it is not yet possible to give a complete account of the uptake and elimination of inhalation anaesthetics as encountered in clinical practice.

Gas pockets in the body

The study of the pulmonary exchange of gases has led to an explanation of certain complications of nitrous oxide anaesthesia. Severe abdominal distension may occur in animals suffering from intestinal obstruction when they are anaesthetized with nitrous oxide, and the subarachnoid injection of air for pneumo-encephalography may, during nitrous oxide anaesthesia, cause a marked rise in cerebrospinal fluid pressure [12, 13]. Intrathoracic pressure in cases of pneumothorax is increased by the administration of nitrous oxide and so is middle ear pressure [14, 15]. The volume of air which must be injected intravenously into rabbits to cause death during nitrous oxide anaesthesia is much less than the lethal volume in rabbits anaesthetized with halothane [16]. These hazards of nitrous oxide are explained by the fact that nitrous oxide is 35 times more soluble in blood than is nitrogen. If an air pocket exists anywhere in the body, nitrous oxide will diffuse into the pocket as nitrogen is reabsorbed during the denitrogenation of the body. While, because of its low solubility, the amount of nitrogen reabsorbed is negligible, the amount of nitrous oxide diffusing into the pocket will be far from negligible. It can be demonstrated that at equilibrium, which is virtually complete in 10–20 minutes, the volume of any gas pocket which existed is doubled if 50% and quadrupled if 75% nitrous oxide is administered. Thus, when nitrous oxide is used, air embolism and the presence of air pockets in the body (e.g. in pneumothorax and paralytic ileus) may constitute major hazards.

GENERAL APPRAISAL OF INHALATION ANAESTHETIC AGENTS

Detailed consideration of the pharmacology of the inhalational anaesthetic agents may be found in standard textbooks on pharmacology and this section simply outlines the virtues of the agents and the criteria for their appraisal. The anaesthetist needs to know at least the properties especially relevant to the clinical use of the agents in current use and the possibility of improving on their characteristics.

Non-flammability

Modern anaesthetics must be non-flammable in the range of concentrations and gas mixtures (usually of oxygen and nitrous oxide) used in clinical practice. In the past, quenching gases such as helium were used to make otherwise explosive mixtures of agents such as cyclopropane safe for clinical purposes [17] but today non-flammability is usually achieved by halogenation — in particular, fluorination — of the agent. In most cases this does not greatly change flammability limits but it does greatly increase the energy necessary to ignite the agents and it is this which renders these agents non-flammable in clinical use [18]. They require a spark having an energy of 10–30 J to ignite them and a static spark released within an anaesthetic system has an energy of only a few hundred millijoules. Thus, the halothane/oxygen mixture within the vaporizing chamber of a plenum-type vaporizer (see p. 156) may contain about 33% of halothane at 20°C which is well within the flammable range for halothane but it could only be ignited by a powerful energy source which cannot be present during normal use [18].

Nitrous oxide increases the flammability of organic vapours because it is an endothermic compound whose decomposition results in the evolution of heat together with the production of an oxygen-rich mixture (33% oxygen). Thus, although the lowest concentration of halothane in oxygen which can be ignited is around 14% it has been found that in pure nitrous oxide 2% of halothane vapour is ignitable by an ignition energy as low as 0.3 J [19].

Promising anaesthetic agents have often been rejected on the grounds of flammability. For example, hexafluorobenzene [20] has been abandoned because it burns at a concentration of 4% in nitrous oxide. This must be contrasted with trichloroethylene which in the UK has been used extensively and successfully as a 'non-flammable agent' although it burns in nitrous oxide at 5%.

Chemical stability

The use of completely closed breathing circuits (see p. 163) for prolonged periods imposes a severe test of the chemical stability of an agent because of the continuing passage over hot, moist, very alkaline soda lime. A compound which is toxic to mice in the concentration range 100–5000 ppm has been detected at a concentration of 5 ppm after 1 hour of closed-circuit halothane anaesthesia [21, 22] but halothane has now been used extensively with soda lime without any reports of harmful effects. Halothane is, however, broken down by ultraviolet light and samples removed from an anaesthetic circuit for analysis by an ultraviolet absorption meter should not be returned to the circuit.

Biotransformation of anaesthetic gases and vapours

It was formerly believed that, with the exception of trichloroethylene, anaesthetic gases and vapours were chemically inert and were mainly excreted unchanged through the lungs. However, the studies of Van Dyke, Chenoweth and their colleagues in 1965 [23] showed this to be untrue for cyclopropane and ethylene and since that time considerable work has been done on the metabolism of anaesthetic vapours, particularly the halogenated hydrocarbons and ethers. Diethyl ether is broken down first into ethanol and acetylaldehyde, which are subsequently metabolized to form carbon dioxide [24]. Metabolism of halothane has been demonstrated in man and animals and *in vitro* studies show that hepatic enzyme systems can metabolize it by dechlorination. Repeated exposures to halothane increases the hepatic-drug-metabolizing enzyme activity. Schimassek *et al.* [25] showed that for halothane the induced enzyme activity involves mitochondrial enzymes rather than the microsomal enzyme system. Methoxyflurane is also metabolized by hepatic enzyme systems [23].

A distinction must be made between direct toxicity produced by an unchanged administered substance and toxicity produced indirectly by its biotransformation to toxic metabolites. Except in sensitivity reactions the toxicity of an unchanged compound is normally directly related to the concentration present and decreasing the concentration will decrease its toxicity. Metabolite formation is more complicated and may be faster when the concentration of the parent compound is low. The mechanism of this concentration dependence is unknown but it seems that biotransformation reaches a maximum at relatively low concentrations of anaesthetic [26] and later as its concentration in the liver increases the efficiency of the enzyme system decreases. The plateau in biotransformation rate could be because the amount of enzyme available becomes the rate-limiting factor or its activity is depressed either by inhibition due to the anaesthetic substrate or the metabolites produced. The important implication for toxicity caused by metabolism of anaesthetics is that greater quantities of metabolites may be produced by subanaesthetic concentrations than by exposure to an anaesthetizing concentration when each is administered for the same

number of MAC hours (see p. 44). Furthermore, increasing the duration of anaesthesia does not proportionally increase the quantity of metabolites produced in the body. Finally, while a large reduction in the concentration of an administered anaesthetic might reduce direct toxicity to below threshold for harm, this might not be the case for indirect toxicity due to metabolites.

Depression of vital body functions

In experiments on isolated organs all anaesthetics have a depressant effect but in an intact animal these depressant effects may be modified or even controlled by various mechanisms. With the exception of nitrous oxide all the inhalational anaesthetic agents produce a concentration-dependent depression of respiration and there is some difference between the agents currently used and their tendency to produce this effect. In clinical practice this effect is offset by surgical stimulation so that all the standard agents can be used in spontaneously breathing animals without undue accumulation of carbon dioxide provided excessively deep levels of central nervous depression are avoided. As far as the cardiovascular system is concerned, all the inhalational agents have a directly depressant action and the differences in their overall effects can be attributed to differences in their action on baroreceptor activity and on the activity of the sympathoadrenal system as reflected in plasma adrenaline and noradrenaline. The direct effects on the cardiovascular system are opposed by sympathetic activity resulting from surgical stimulation and the changes in cardiovascular function seen will depend on the balance between inhibitory and excitatory influences.

Table 6.1 Physical characteristics and approximate MAC values for some anaesthetic agents

Name	Partition coefficient			Boiling point (°C)	MAC (vol. %)
	Water–gas	Blood–gas	Oil–gas		
Chloroform	4.00	8.00	400.0	61.2	0.77
Cyclopropane	0.21	0.55	11.5	−34	9.2
Enflurane	0.78	1.90	98.00	56.5	1.68
Ether	13.00	12.00	65.00	34.6	1.92
Halothane	0.80	2.40	220.00	50.2	0.75
Desflurane	0.23	0.42	18.7	?	5.72
Isoflurane	0.62	1.40	97.00	48.5	1.15
Methoxyflurane	4.50	11.00	950.00	104.7	0.20
Nitrous oxide	0.47	0.47	1.4	−89	>100
Sevoflurane	0.36	0.60	53.00	58.5	2.5
Trichloroethylene	1.70	9.00	714.00	86.7	0.23

Values taken from various sources in the literature but mainly from: Halsey, M. J. (1981) *British Journal of Anaesthesia* **53**, 43S; Steward, A. *et al.* (1973) *British Journal of Anaesthesia* **45**, 282; Eger, E. I. (1987) *Anesthesia and Analgesia* **66**, 971; Data Sheets, May and Baker/Ohio Medical Products.
[a] MAC values vary slightly with species of animal.

Volatility

Volatility may be expressed by the boiling point or the saturated vapour pressure at 20°C. In general, the more potent the agent, the higher the boiling point. As can be seen from Table 6.1 the boiling points of halothane, enflurane and isoflurane lie within the range 48–58°C.

With highly volatile agents, oxygen enrichment of the inspired gas becomes more important until in the extreme case of nitrous oxide, which has a boiling point of −89°C at normal atmospheric pressure, less than about 75% of 1×MAC (depending on the species of animal) can be administered in the presence of 21% of oxygen. It seems to be generally agreed that for various reasons a minimum inspired oxygen concentration of about 33% is desirable during general anaesthesia and on that assumption an anaesthetic concentration of 1.3×MAC should be attainable without risk of any degree of hypoxia [27].

Interaction with other drugs

All muscle relaxants are potentiated by inhalational anaesthetics in a dose-dependent manner and since muscle relaxation quite adequate for most operations can be produced by inhalation agents alone it is reasonable to assume that at least part of this potentiation is due to the central nervous depression produced by the anaesthetic agent. In addition it has been shown that inhalational agents decrease the sensitivity of the postjunctional membrane of the neuromuscular junction and possibly act at a more distal site such as the muscle membrane itself [28]. The different anaesthetic agents differ in the extent to which they potentiate relaxants. For example, enflurane and isoflurane are considerably more potent in potentiating *d*-tubocurarine in man than are halo-

thane or nitrous oxide [29]. The reason for this is quite unknown but, clearly, it may be considered advantageous for an inhalational agent to contribute to a neuromuscular block since its component can be removed by ventilation of the lungs with a non-rebreathing circuit, so increasing the flexibility of control because there are then at least two methods of reducing or abolishing the block — use of an anti-cholinesterase and ventilation.

The sensitization of the myocardium to adrenaline, both endogenous and exogenous, by the inhalational agents has been the subject of much investigation and it can be concluded that while straight-chain hydrocarbons tend to sensitize the heart to these catecholamines, the ethers, especially if fluorinated, do not have this effect. Indeed, the fluorinated ethers in current use, enflurane and isoflurane, have the most desirable attribute of conferring good stability to adrenaline.

Analgesia

For as yet unknown reasons subanaesthetic concentrations of agents such as ether, methoxyflurane and nitrous oxide produce marked analgesia, whereas others such as halothane do not [30]. It may be speculated that this effect depends on the release of endorphins (enkephalins) but except for nitrous oxide evidence for this is lacking. If an agent having a good analgesic action has a high solubility (e.g. methoxyflurane) then elimination of it will be slow and analgesia will be present during recovery. Unfortunately, less desirable effects such as respiratory depression and hypotension are also prolonged so that it is usually better to rely on specific analgesic drugs in the postoperative period rather than the retention of the anaesthetic agent.

INDIVIDUAL INHALATION ANAESTHETICS

Diethyl ether

Diethyl ether, commonly known simply as 'ether', was one of the earliest inhalational anaesthetics introduced into clinical practice but its use is currently declining. The chief reason for this is its flammability and also its great water and blood solubility which, together with its irritant smell, make for a slow induction and recovery. Nevertheless, ether has always had the justified reputation of being a very safe anaesthetic agent.

It is a transparent, colourless liquid with a vapour which is highly flammable and twice as heavy as air.

Ether is decomposed by air, light and heat; the liquid is therefore stored in amber-coloured bottles kept in a cool, dark place. Its heavy vapour tends to pool on the floor and unless ventilation is good the possibility of fires is very great. Sparks of static electricity or sparks from faulty connections in electrical switches and apparatus can easily ignite ether–air mixtures, and ether–oxygen mixtures are explosive. Fires have resulted from the vapour rolling along the floor into an adjoining room and being ignited there. Ether should not be administered in any place in which electrical equipment such as radiographic apparatus or diathermy is to be used, and in these places the ether vaporizer should be removed from the anaesthetic machine; it is not sufficient to merely turn the control to the 'off' position.

Ether is safe in the presence of adrenaline. Indeed, its administration is associated with sympathoadrenal stimulation which opposes its negative inotropic effect and the concurrent administration of β-adrenergic blocking drugs allows this effect to become dangerous. Normally, cardiac output is well maintained even at deep levels of unconsciousness.

During light levels of unconsciousness, ether does not depress respiration. The spleen contracts while the intestines become dilated and atonic. The blood sugar level rises due to the mobilization of liver glycogen under the influence of the increased secretion of adrenaline. Liver and kidney function is depressed but these organs usually recover their normal function within 24 hours. The inhalation of ether causes metabolic acidosis and ketone bodies may appear in the urine. Although ether does undergo some metabolism it contains no halogens so that its intermediate metabolites are such relatively non-toxic substance as ethyl alcohol, acetic acid and acetaldehyde.

Ether possesses many disadvantages. Its inhalation provokes the secretion of saliva and of mucus within the respiratory tract. Postanaesthetic nausea appears to be pronounced and animals will not eat for several hours afterwards. On the other hand, ether has been in continuous use for well over 100 years and millions of operations must have been performed on animals under ether anaesthesia. The number of deaths directly attributable to ether, apart from accidents (e.g. explosions and fires) and errors of technique, is very small indeed. It must be considered a safe agent for the inexperienced anaesthetist because, in addition to being slow in action, it produces the graded series of signs which were formerly used to indicate depth of anaesthesia. Ether anaesthesia is usually associated with reasonably good skeletal muscle relaxation and postoperative analgesia.

Chloroform

Chloroform is a most powerful anaesthetic which has largely fallen into disuse although it is still used to some small extent in equine anaesthesia for operations of very short duration

The record of chloroform undoubtedly accounts of many disasters and it is probable that if it had been subjected at the time of its introduction into anaesthesia to the full battery of tests which are applied to potential anaesthetics today, it would never have been accepted for clinical use. Chloroform has a toxic effect on the liver and kidneys, causing cloudy swelling and even acute fatty change in the cells.

When severe these changes give rise to delayed poisoning, the symptoms of which develop some 24–48 hours after administration. It is characterized by acute acidosis, severe vomiting (in dogs and cats), acetonuria, albuminuria, mild pyrexia and icterus, and frequently terminates fatally with severe hyperpyrexia. In addition, chloroform sensitizes the myocardium to the effects of catecholamines and sudden death has occurred from ventricular fibrillation during induction or recovery from chloroform anaesthesia.

Most anaesthetists agree that chloroform is much more dangerous than any other of the anaesthetics available today.

Halothane

Halothane was introduced into veterinary anaesthesia in 1956 [31] and was so greatly superior to existing agents that it soon became universally used in the western world. It is probable that halothane has been subjected to more investigational studies than any other anaesthetic agent. In the veterinary field there are now many such papers including those of Fisher and Jennings, Vasko, Auer, and Steffey and his colleagues [32–38].

Vapour concentrations of 2–4% in the inspired air produce smooth and rapid induction of anaesthesia in all species of domestic animal. Anaesthesia can then be maintained with inspired concentrations of 0.8–2%, the MAC (see p. 44) being about 0.8%. Recovery from short-duration halothane anaesthesia is also reasonably rapid and free from excitement although unrelieved pain can give rise to restlessness during the recovery period. When no other agents are administered most animals are able to walk without ataxia in 15–30 minutes depending on the duration of anaesthesia and the degree of obesity of the animal. Blood concentrations are around 14 mg/dl during the maintenance of anaesthesia and fall rapidly during recovery so that levels of 4–6 mg/dl have been recorded 15 minutes after discontinuance of anaesthesia.

The mucosa of the respiratory tract is not irritated by halothane and the agent has been shown to produce bronchodilatation and an increase in expiratory reserve volume in ponies [39]. The arterial carbon dioxide tension is directly related to the alveolar concentration of halothane when this is above 0.7% [40].

Halothane causes a dose-dependent depression of cardiac output and arterial blood pressure due mainly to a negative inotropic effect [41, 42] although it does cause some block of transmission at sympathetic ganglia [43]. Evidence for the mode of action of halothane on the peripheral vasculature is still both controversial and more than a little confusing. In dogs, Perry and coworkers [44] showed that halothane decreases plasma catecholamine levels and this may explain the reduction of arterial pressure and decreased myocardial contractility and cardiac output.

Dose-dependent respiratory depression occurs, both the depth and rate being decreased so that the minute volume of respiration is greatly reduced, leading to a progressive rise in arterial carbon dioxide tension until equilibrium between production and elimination of this gas is reached. Except in horses, respiratory failure from overdose precedes cardiac failure by a considerable margin.

Adaptation of both cardiovascular and respiratory function occurs with time [38]. After about 4 hours cardiac output in horses increases by about 40% from that at 30 minutes and the values for arterial carbon dioxide tension and the ratio of inspired-to-expired gas flow become significantly higher than those after 30 minutes of anaesthesia.

Bradycardia is common during halothane anaesthesia due, apparently, to activity in the vagus nerves. Usually a perfectly normal ECG persists throughout anaesthesia although ventricular extrasystoles and bigeminal rhythm have been reported as occurring in dogs; these can largely be prevented by premedication with acepromazine [45]. In cats atrioventricular dissociation with interference and extrasystoles may occur [46]. Arrhythmias are usually associated with carbon dioxide accumulation from respiratory depression, hypoxia, catecholamine release and overdosage. Changes in heart rate and rhythm should not be treated with atropine as a routine since the abolition of vagal tone may accentuate their severity and even induce ventricular fibrillation. Catecholamine-induced arrhythmias may be treated with propranolol [47].

Halothane has minimal neuromuscular blocking effect and the muscle relaxation seen during halothane anaesthesia (which is only moderate at deep levels of central nervous depression) appears to be central in origin. It does, however, potentiate the effects of non-depolarizing muscle relaxants and antagonize those of depolarizing agents [48]. Shivering is often seen in all species of domestic animals during recovery from halothane anaesthesia but the reason for it is unknown. It does not seem to be related to body or environmental temperature and its only importance is that it may be harmful by increasing oxygen demands in animals suffering from respiratory and/or cardiovascular diseases which limit oxygen uptake when they are breathing air.

Because of its lack of analgesic properties halothane anaesthesia is more affected by premedication with analgesic drugs than is the case for many other agents. This also applies to supplementation during anaesthesia with analgesics, whether these be of the opioid type or analgesic mixtures of nitrous oxide and oxygen. Postoperative analgesia during recovery is not a feature of unsupplemented halothane anaesthesia.

Minimal pathological changes have been found in the liver and kidneys of dogs, horses and sheep anaesthetized for long periods with halothane [49, 50]. The question of hepatotoxicity in man has been much discussed but its actual incidence remains unknown. Cascorbi *et al.* [51] considered that anaesthetists may metabolize halothane to a greater extent than other persons because they excrete more breakdown products in the urine. If so, it is likely that this may result from hepatic enzyme induction, but it is uncertain whether it is beneficial or harmful to an individual to have increased ability to metabolize halothane. Recurrent hepatitis apparently due to halothane sensitization has, however, been reported in an anaesthetist [52].

Halothane and ether form an azeotropic mixture (31.7% diethyl ether and 68.3% halothane, v/v) with a boiling point of 51.5°C. This mixture was once employed in veterinary anaesthesia [53] but it is an illogical one and is no longer used.

Enflurane

Enflurane was introduced into clinical practice in 1958 and is now quite widely used in human medicine. Fears about its possible epileptogenic properties [36, 54–58] have not been realized although some anaesthetists have reported muscle twitching in enflurane anaesthetized dogs. Like halothane, it depresses cardiovascular function in a dose-dependent manner, and the effects of the two drugs are comparable. Both agents produce a negative inotropic effect on the heart of the intact dog, which is accompanied by decrease in myocardial oxygen demand. In equipotent concentrations enflurane causes slightly greater impairment of left ventricular function than does halothane [59]. There is inhibition of adrenal medullary catecholamine secretion during enflurane anaesthesia and this may account for the hypotension which is often a conspicuous feature [34, 50]. Under light anaesthesia surgical stimulation produces an immediate rise in arterial blood pressure, possibly due to sympathetic activity.

Subcutaneous injection of adrenaline by the surgeon for haemostasis is unlikely to cause serious cardiac irregularities under enflurane anaesthesia because enflurane is a halogenated ether and ethers do not markedly sensitize the heart to the effects of catecholamines. In addition, when adrenaline is given as a continuous infusion for its positive inotropic action arrhythmias are seen much less commonly than under halothane anaesthesia.

Although there is muscular relaxation during clinical anaesthesia with enflurane, muscle relaxants should be used rather than higher concentrations of enflurane to provide good muscle relaxation. All the commonly used muscle relaxants are compatible with this agent but the actions of the non-depolarizing relaxants may be markedly enhanced so that smaller doses become adequate.

The degree of metabolic biotransformation is much less than with many other inhalation agents. The production of inorganic fluoride is probably not great enough to constitute a threat to the health of normal kidneys. Any potential hazard from fluoride toxicity is most unlikely to occur if high vapour strengths are avoided, but 'enflurane hepatitis' has been reported [60].

The ability to produce rapid changes in the depth of anaesthesia coupled with rapid recovery and the apparent absence of adverse side-effects suggested that this agent might be useful in veterinary practice, particularly for horses and small animals undergoing surgery on a day patient basis [61, 62]. However, in horses recovery is unpleasant [63], and in small animals its advantages over halothane appear to be marginal, so it seems likely to fall into disuse.

Isoflurane

Isoflurane is similar to enflurane in general, physical and chemical properties. A great deal of experimental work has been carried out in evaluating isoflurane and comprehensive reviews of its pharmacological properties are those of Eger [64], Wade and Stevens [65] and Forrest [66].

It may be administered with oxygen or nitrous oxide/oxygen mixtures and because it is a potent anaesthetic an accurately calibrated vaporizer should be used. Isoflurane has a pungent odour but animals breathe it without breath holding or coughing. Clinical signs of anaesthesia resemble those seen with halothane.

Like most inhalation agents it undergoes some biotransformation, the main metabolites being trifluoroacetic acid and inorganic fluoride, but this appears to be minimal, rendering the possibility of fluoride nephrotoxicity very remote [67].

Respiratory and cardiovascular depression are dose dependent. Respiratory depression in the unstimulated subject is greater than with halothane but, clinically, surgical stimulation counteracts this and tends to equalize respiratory rates under anaesthesia with the two agents. Arterial blood pressure is as well maintained as it is under halothane anaesthesia. However, heart rate is increased and cardiac output and stroke volume are reduced less than they are with halothane; a greater fall in peripheral resistance must be responsible for the similarity of the blood pressure response, for at clinical concentrations halothane has

little effect on total peripheral resistance. There is evidence that at 1.5% and 2.0 × MAC isoflurane lowers peripheral resistance and maintains or increases blood flow to organs and muscle. Arrhythmias have not been reported and because it is an ether irregularities following the injection of adrenaline are less likely to occur than under halothane anaesthesia.

In horses a limited number of tests have shown minimal or no toxicity [68] and recovery is usually quiet [37] although problems have been reported, particularly after the use of ketamine as an induction agent before maintenance with isoflurane. The quick elimination of isoflurane allows foals to nurse shortly after completion of surgery.

The high volatility of isoflurane, coupled with its low blood solubility, provide for relatively rapid induction and recovery and easy control of the depth of anaesthesia. Its low solubility in fatty tissues avoids accumulation in obese subjects. It increases splanchnic blood flow and thus enhances hepatic oxygenation. Renal blood flow is well maintained during isoflurane anaesthesia and because there is very little production of fluoride ions, coupled with less than 1% elimination via the kidneys, it can generally be administered quite safely to patients with renal dysfunction.

It seems probable that isoflurane will completely replace enflurane in veterinary practice because, in addition to having greater muscle-relaxing effects, its lower partition coefficients result in more rapid recovery for small animal day patients and horses. Whether, when it becomes less expensive, it will replace halothane is more uncertain for in dogs recovery from isoflurane is no more rapid than from halothane [69].

Sevoflurane

Sevoflurane is another halogenated ether which has lower distribution coefficients than isoflurane and a MAC between 1.7 and 2.3%. It is metabolized and unstable in the presence of soda lime [70], and there are indications that emergence excitement can easily be provoked in the recovery period. It seems possible that a more satisfactory agent can be found with even lower solubilities.

Desflurane (I-653)

A new agent, desflurane has the same structure as isoflurane except for the substitution of fluorine for chlorine on the α carbon of the ethyl moiety. It has an exceptionally low solubility (blood–gas partition coefficient 0.42), is flammable at a concentration of 17% and has a relatively high vapour pressure of around 700 mmHg (93.3 kPa) at 22–23°C [71]. Its properties indicate that it should have a MAC of about 5.8%. There is currently no information concerning its use in veterinary anaesthesia.

Methoxyflurane

Methoxyflurane is a halogenated ethyl methyl ether. It is a clear, colourless liquid which boils at 104.65°C at 760 mmHg (101 kPa) and freezes at −35°C. Although the boiling point is slightly higher than that of water it volatilizes more readily as a result of a low latent heat of vaporization (205 J/g). It is non-explosive and non-flammable in air or oxygen at the temperatures and conditions encountered in anaesthesia.

It is chemically stable and is not decomposed by air, light, moisture or alkali such as soda lime. It may, however, slowly form a brownish discoloration due to the antioxidant used in its formulation but this does not affect the anaesthetic properties. Contact with copper, brass or bronze may also cause discoloration but without apparent effect on safety or toxicity. The odour of methoxyflurane has been described as 'fruity' and is well accepted and tolerated by animals.

The saturated vapour pressure of methoxyflurane is only 25 mmHg (3.3 kPa) at 20°C. and because of this it is not satisfactory as an induction agent.

Blood concentrations and tissue levels during and after surgical anaesthesia in dogs have been studied [71] and its MAC (see p. 44) is about 0.16% It persists in the blood even after apparent complete recovery 24 hours after anaesthesia and since it has good analgesic properties this can provide worthwhile postoperative analgesia.

The maximum vapour concentration obtainable is only mildly irritating to inhale so that stimulation of secretions in the respiratory tract is minimal. Like halothane, it produces dose-dependent respiratory depression. As a result of the low vapour pressure, respiratory depression and rate of uptake by the tissues, it is extremely difficult to produce respiratory arrest in dogs and cats allowed to breathe spontaneously.

Heart rate and rhythm are not altered until anaesthesia becomes very deep, when the rate becomes very slow. Bagwell and Woods [72] reported cardiovascular depression in dogs, but the sympathetic nervous system was not blocked by methoxyflurane.

Chenworth *et al.* [71] have shown that the urine contains only minute traces of methoxyflurane, but polyuric renal dysfunction (high-output renal failure) has been reported in humans and certain laboratory animals. It follows the prolonged administration of high concentrations of the compound and is due to the release of free fluoride by its metabolism in the body. It has not been reported in veterinary anaesthesia but has resulted in the withdrawal of methoxyflurane from medical practice.

Trichloroethylene

In its effects trichloroethylene resembles chloroform but it is much less potent and less toxic. The ratio between the anaesthetic and the minimal lethal dose is high. In the presence of soda lime its use is contraindicated for in an absorber it may be broken down to such toxic products as hydrochloric acid, dichloracetylene, phosgene and carbon monoxide.

It produces a very high degree of analgesia and the main use of trichloroethylene in veterinary anaesthesia was to reinforce the analgesic properties of nitrous oxide. It seems likely that trichloroethylene will be withdrawn by the manufacturers when anaesthetists can be persuaded to accept its departure from the anaesthetic scene.

Nitrous oxide

Nitrous oxide is a colourless gas with a faint, rather pleasant smell. It is not flammable or explosive but it will support combustion, even in the absence of free oxygen. Compressed into cylinders at 40 atm pressure it liquifies so that the amount in a cylinder can only be determined by weighing since the pressure of the gaseous nitrous oxide above the liquid level remains constant as long as any liquid remains. Thus, a pressure gauge screwed into the cylinder outlet will register a constant pressure until all the nitrous oxide has vaporized and after this the reading drops rapidly to zero as gas leaves the cylinder. Some type of 'regulator' or pressure-reducing valve must be attached to the cylinder before the rate of flow of the gas can be accurately adjusted or measured.

It is not irritant to the respiratory mucosa and because it is non-toxic it has been administered for very long periods although it has been known since 1956 that exposure to it for several days causes bone marrow depression. It is now recognized that this is due to oxidation of vitamin B_{12} [74].

The results of several studies suggest that nitrous oxide does not depress and may even increase pulmonary ventilation [75–77]. The tachypnoea produced by the gas may result from direct central stimulation similar to that postulated for potent inhalation agents but the impact of nitrous oxide appears to be greater than that of other inhaled anaesthetics. In man, the greater increase in respiratory rate and minute ventilation associated with its use is also found when it is combined with some of the inhaled anaesthetics but not with the newer narcotics. Respiratory rate and minute ventilation are greater at a given MAC level when nitrous oxide and isoflurane are combined than when isoflurane is given alone [78]. This tendency is also encountered when the gas is given with halothane [79] but not enflurane [80].

Adding nitrous oxide to a stable level of alfentanil anaesthesia seems to produce no effect [81].

As already discussed (p. 103) the gas tends to enter gas-filled spaces in the body at a greater rate than nitrogen can diffuse out. This is of considerable importance in herbivores and in the presence of a closed pneumothorax.

During the induction of anaesthesia a large gradient exists between the tension of nitrous oxide in the inspired gas and the arterial blood so that in the early moments of induction the blood takes up large volumes of the gas. Its rapid removal from the alveoli by the blood elevates the tension of any remaining (second) gas or vapour such as oxygen or halothane, and augments alveolar ventilation. Thus, during the first few minutes of nitrous oxide administration anaesthetic uptake is facilitated because the enhanced tension of the second gas ensures a steeper tension gradient for its passage into the blood. This is known as 'the second-gas effect'.

The phenomenon known as 'diffusion hypoxia' occurs immediately following anaesthesia when the gas is being rapidly eliminated from the lungs. Nitrous oxide may form 10% or more of the volume of the expired gas, and the outward diffusion of nitrous oxide into the alveoli lowers the partial pressure of oxygen in the lungs. This effect appears to have little clinical significance in healthy animals but the hypoxia may be dangerous in elderly animals or in those suffering from pulmonary or cardiovascular disease and such animals should have an oxygen-enriched mixture administered for some 10 minutes after the termination of a long nitrous oxide/oxygen anaesthetic.

According to Steffey and Howland [82] the anaesthetic potency in horses is only about half that in human beings in that 80% nitrous oxide produces the anaesthetic equivalent in a young healthy horse of only about 40% of nitrous oxide in a healthy, young human subject. In dogs it is claimed [83] that nitrous oxide has a less useful role as an anaesthetic supplement than in man but there can be no doubt that most veterinary anaesthetists agree that its analgesic properties enable excessive dosage of the more potent agents to be avoided and concurrent cardiopulmonary depression minimized.

Cyclopropane

Cyclopropane is as inflammable as ether and mixtures with both air and oxygen are explosive. It has solubility characteristics closer to the ideal than any other inhalation agent in use today but it produces marked respiratory depression.

The administration of cyclopropane to dogs and other domestic animals for physiological experiments was developed by Professor R. A. Gregory of Liverpool and in the 1950s it was extensively employed in veterinary hospitals in the UK. However, the explosion risk associated with its use is a very real one and its use has declined. It seems probable that it will soon be withdrawn by the manufacturers since with the advent of agents such as isoflurane there is much less indication for its use.

FUTURE DEVELOPMENTS

There is a tendency to assume that the development of inhalational anaesthetics has peaked with isoflurane and that the rapidly mounting costs of research and development together with the costly and extensive tests demanded by governmental drug-licensing authorities make it no longer worthwhile for the pharmaceutical industry to persist in trying to develop new agents. Although it is probably true that there is not much room for improvement in agents having the characteristics of halothane or isoflurane it is likely that for several reasons search for agents with lower solubility characteristics will continue. The lowest possible solubility in blood carries the greatest benefit both in speed of induction and recovery with minimization of after-effects. Furthermore, the lowest possible solubility minimizes the total quantity of agent which has to be introduced into the body to produce anaesthesia and this reduces the possibility of damage by harmful metabolites in two ways. First, it minimizes their quantity and, secondly, it minimizes the time available for their production since an agent of low solubility is only present in the body for a short time.

The most likely candidate would seem to be a substance which is a gas at ambient temperature. Compressed and delivered from a cylinder, precise control of its inspired concentration could be provided by accurate flowmeters and expensive vaporizers would no longer be necessary. Any such gas must, of couse, be non-explosive and non-flammable and its MAC value must be such as to allow it to be administered with at least 30% oxygen.

REFERENCES

1. Mapleson, W. W. (1963) *Uptake and Distribution of Anesthetic Agents*. New York: McGraw-Hill.
2. Bourne, J. G. (1964) *Anaesthesia* **19**, 12.
3. Butler, R. A. (1964) *British Journal of Anaesthesia* **36**, 193.
4. Eger, E. I. (1964) *British Journal of Anaesthesia* **36**, 140.
5. Epstein, R. H. (1964) *British Journal of Anaesthesia* **36**, 172.
6. Kety, S. S. (1950) *Anesthesiology* **11**, 517.
7. Kety, S. S. (1951) *Pharmacological Reviews* **3**, 1.
8. Bourne, J. G. (1960) *Nitrous Oxide in Dentistry*. London: Lloyd-Luke.
9. Larson, C. P., Eger, E. I. and Severinghaus, J. W. (1962) *Anesthesiology*, **23**, 349.
10. Haggard, H. W. (1924) *Journal of Biological Chemistry* **59**, 737.
11. Fink, B. R. (1955) *Anesthesiology* **16**, 511.
12. Eger, E. I. and Saidman, L. J. (1965) *Anesthesiology* **26**, 61.
13. Saidman, L. J. and Eger, E. I. (1965) *Anesthesiology* **26**, 67.
14. Hunter, A. R. (1955) *Proceedings of the Royal Society of Medicine* **48**, 765.
15. Thomsen, K. A., Terhildsen, K. and Arnfred, I. (1965) *Archives of Otolaryngology* **82**, 609.
16. Munsen, E. S. and Merrick, H. C. (1966) *Anesthesiology* **27**, 78.
17. Warren, A. G. (1960) Thesis, Zurich.
18. Larsen, E. R. (1972) *Modern Inhalation Anaesthetics. Handbook of Experimental Pharmacology*, vol. 30 (ed. M. B. Chenoweth). Berlin: Springer-Verlag.
19. Brown, T. A. and Morris, G. (1966) *British Journal of Anaesthesia* **38**, 164.
20. Hall, L. W. and Jackson, S. R. K. (1973) *Anaesthesia* **28**, 155.
21. Raventos, S. and Lemon, R. G. (1965) *British Journal of Anaesthesia* **37**, 716.
22. Sharp, J. H., Trudell, J. R. and Cohen, E. N. (1979) *Anesthesiology* **50**, 2.
23. Van Dyke, R. A. and Chenoweth, M. B. (1965) *Anesthesiology* **26**, 384.
24. Greene, N. M. (1968) *Anesthesiology* **29**, 123, 327.
25. Schimassek, H., Kunz., W. and Gallowitz, D. (1966) *Biochemical Pharmacology* **15**, 1957.
26. Halsey, M. J. (1979) *General Anaesthesia*, 4th edn (eds T. C. Gray, J. F. Nunn and J. E. Utting). London: Butterworths.
27. White, D. C. (1986) *Anaesthesia Review*, vol. 3, p. 110 (ed. L. Kaufman). London: Churchill Livingstone.
28. Ngai, S. H. (1975) *Muscle Relaxants* (ed. R. Katz). Amsterdam: Excerpta Medica.
29. Ali, H. H. and Savarese, J. J. (1976) *Anesthesiology* **45**, 216.
30. Dundee, J. W. and Moore, J. (1960) *British Journal of Anaesthesia* **32**, 453.
31. Hall, L. W. (1957) *Veterinary Record* **69**, 615.
32. Fisher, E. W. and Jennings, S. (1961) *American Journal of Veterinary Research* **22**, 279.
33. Vasko, K. A. (1962) *American Journal of Veterinary Research* **123**, 248.
34. Steffey, E. P., Gillespie, J. R., Berry, J. D., Eger, E. I. and Rhode, E. A. (1975) *American Journal of Veterinary Research* **36**, 197.
35. Steffey, E. P., Gillespie, J. R., Berry, J. D., Eger, E. I. and Schalm, O. W. (1976) *Americal Journal of Veterinary Research* **37**, 959.
36. Steffey, E. P., Howland, D., Giri, S. and Eger, E. I. (1977) *American Journal of Veterinary Research* **38**, 1037.
37. Auer, J. A., Garner, H. E., Amend, J. F., Hutcheson, D. P. and Salem, C. A. (1978) *Equine Veterinary Journal* **10**, 18.
38. Steffey, E. P., Kelly, A. B. and Woliner, M. J. (1987) *American Journal of Veterinary Research* **48**, 952.
39. Watney, G. C. G., Jordan, C. and Hall, L. W. (1987) *British Journal of Anaesthesia* **59**, 1022.
40. Merkel, G. and Eger, E. I. (1963) *Anesthesiology* **24**, 346.
41. Sugai, N., Shimosato, S. and Etsten, B. E. (1968) *Anesthesiology* **29**, 267.
42. Prys-Roberts, C., Gersh, B. J., Baker, A. B. and Rueben, S. R. (1972) *British Journal of Anaesthesia* **44**, 634.
43. Burn, J. H., Epstein, H. H., Feigan, G. A. and Paton, W. D. M. (1957) *British Medical Journal* **ii**, 479.
44. Perry, L. B., Van Dyke, R. A. and Theye, R. A. (1974) *Anesthesiology* **40**, 465.
45. Wiersig, D. O., Davis, R. H. and Szabiniewicz, M. (1974) *Journal of the American Veterinary Medical Association* **165**, 341.
46. Muir, B. J., Hall, L. W. and Littlewort, M. C. G. (1959) *British Journal of Anaesthesia* **31**, 488.
47. Tavernor, W. D. and Lees, P. (1969) *Archives of International Pharmacodynamics* **180**, 89.
48. Graham, J. D. P. (1958) *British Medical Bulletin* **14**, 15.
49. Stephen, C. R., Margolisd, G., Fabian, L. W. and Bourgeois-Gavardin, M. (1958) *Anesthesiology* **19**, 770.
50. Wolff, W. A., Lumb, W. V. and Ramsaya, K. (1967) *American Journal of Veterinary Research* **28**, 1366.
51. Cascorbi, H. F., Blake, D. A. and Helrich, M. (1970) *Anesthesiology* **32**, 119.
52. Klatskin, G. and Kimberg, D. V. (1969) *New England Journal of Medicine* **280**, 515.
53. Hime, J. M. (1963) *Veterinary Record* **75**, 426.
54. Vitue, R. W., Lund, L. O., Phelps, M. K., Vogel, J. H. K., Beckwich, H. and Heron, M. (1966) *Canadian Anaesthetists Society Journal* **13**, 233.
55. Joas, T. A., Stevens, W. C. and Eger, E. I. (1971) *British Journal of Anaesthesia* **43**, 739.
56. Michenfelder, J. D. and Cucchiara, R. F. (1974) *Anesthesiology* **40**, 575.
57. Schettini, A. and Wilder, B. J. (1974) *Anesthesia and Analgesia* **53**, 951.
58. de Jong, R. H. and Heavner, J. E. (1971) *Anesthesiology* **35**, 474.
59. Horan, B. F., Prys-Roberts, C., Bennett, M. J. and Foex, P. (1977) *British Journal of Anaesthesia* **49**, 1179.
60. Lewis, J. H., Hyman, J. *et al.* (1983) *Annals of Internal Medicine* **98**, 984.
61. Cribb, P. H., Hird, J. F. R. and Hall, L. W. (1970) *Veterinary Record* **101**, 50.
62. Hunter, J. M., Jones, R. S. and Utting, J. E. (1981) *Research in Veterinary Science* **31**, 177.
63. Taylor, P. M. and Hall, L. W. (1985) *Equine Veterinary Journal* **17**, 51.
64. Eger, E. I. (1981) *Anesthesiology* **55**, 559.
65. Wade, J. G. and Stevens, W. C. (1981) *Anesthesia and Analgesia* **60**, 666.
66. Forrest, J. B. (1983) *Clinics in Anesthesiology* **1/2**, 251.

67. Davidkova, T., Kikucchi, H., Fujii, K., Mukaida, K., Sato, N., Kawachi, S. and Motio, M. (1988) *Anesthesiology* **69**, 218.
68. Steffey, E. P., Zinkl, J. and Howland, D. (1979) *American Journal of Veterinary Research* **30**, 1646.
69. Zbinden, A. M., Thomson, D. A., Westenskow, D. R., Frei, F. and Maertens, J. (1988) *British Journal of Anaesthesia* **60**, 395.
70. Eger, E. I. (1987) *Anesthesia and Analgesia* **66**, 971.
71. Chenworth, M. B., Robertson, D. N., Erley, D. S. and Golhke, M. S. (1962) *Anesthesiology* **23**, 101.
72. Bagwell, E. E. and Woods, E. F. (1962) *Federation Proceedings: Federation of the American Society for Experimental Biology* **20**, 313.
73. Mazze, R. I. and Cousins, M. J. (1973) *Canadian Anaesthetists Society Journal* **20**, 64.
74. Brodsky, J. B. (1923) *Clinics in Anesthesiology* **1/2**, 455.
75. Eckenhoff, J. E. and Helrich, M. (1958) *Anesthesiology* **19**, 240.
76. Hornbein, T. F., Eger, E. I., Winter, P. M., Smith, G., Wetstone, D. and Smith, K. H. (1982) *Anesthesia and Analgesia* **61**, 553.
77. Hall, L. W. (1988) *British Journal of Anaesthesia* **60**, 207.
78. Dolan, W. M., Stevens, W. C., Eger, E. I., Cromwell, T. H., Halsey, M. J., Shakespeare, T. F. and Miller, R. D. (1974) *Canadian Anaesthetists Society Journal* **21**, 557.
79. Hornbein, T. F., Martin, W. E., Bonica, J. J., Freund, F. G. and Parmentier, P. (1969) *Anesthesiology* **3**, 250.
80. Lam, A. and Knill, R. L. (1981) *Anesthesia and Analgesia* **60**, 261,
81. Andrews, C. J. H., Sinclair, M., Dye, A., Dye, J., Harvey, J. and Prys-Roberts, C. (1982) *British Journal of Anaesthesia* **54**, 1129.
82. Steffey, E. P. and Howland, D. (1978) *American Journal of Veterinary Research* **39**, 1141.
83. Steffey, E. P., Gillespie, J. R., Berry, J., Eger, E. I. and Munson, E. S. (1974) *Journal of Applied Physiology* **36**, 530.

CHAPTER 7

RELAXATION OF THE SKELETAL MUSCLES DURING ANAESTHESIA

To relax skeletal muscles it is necessary to abolish voluntary muscle contractions and modify the slight tension which is the normal state (the 'tone' or 'tonus' of the muscle). Tone is maintained by many complex mechanisms but, briefly, it can be said that all result in the slow asynchronous discharge of impulses from cells in the ventral horn region of the spinal cord. This discharge gives rise to impulses in the α motor neurones which cause the muscle fibres to contract. The activity of these ventral horn cells is controlled by impulses from the higher centres (cerebrum, cerebellum or medulla oblongata) exciting the α motor neurone direct, or by impulses through the small motor nerve fibre system (the γ efferents) which activate them directly via the stretch reflex arc. Movements controlled by the γ-fibre system are essentially directed towards governing the length of

the muscle. Voluntary movement, on the other hand, involving direct activity in the α fibres, results in muscle tension of a given magnitude.

The relevance to anaesthesia lies in the fact that the small motor nerve fibre system is, like the motor fibres to the skeletal muscles themselves, a cholinergic one. Any drug which can affect the neuromuscular junction may, therefore, also interfere with the effect of the γ fibres on the muscle spindles. A paralysis of the γ-fibre/muscle spindle junction will have, as a major consequence, a reduction in the afferent inflow from the muscle spindles and the mere reduction of such a flow to the brain stem may have subtle effects. For example, there seems to be a possibility that a drug which paralyses the γ fibres and so reduces muscle spindle proprioceptive inflow to the higher centres actually contributes to a sleep-like state.

METHODS OF ABOLISHING MUSCLE TONE AND ABILITY TO CONTRACT

During anaesthesia abolition of muscle tone and ability to contract can be brought about in three ways. The first of these is by the use of anaesthetic agents which act centrally, the second and third utilize drugs which have a peripheral rather than a central action:

1. The anaesthetic agents, by producing depression of the central nervous system, cause decreased activity of the ventral horn cells in the spinal cord and, thus, muscle relaxation. A profound degree of muscle relaxation can be obtained when a potent narcotic drug is adminstered in doses which produce a deep generalized depression of the whole central nervous system. However, consequences of such a generalized depression are widespread. For example, depression of the medullary vasomotor centre contributes to the advent of circulatory failure during an operation, for in deeply narcotized animals severe hypotension is caused by the loss of relatively small quantities of blood. Furthermore, the deeply narcotized animal lacks the ability to

compensate for circulatory disturbances caused by sudden changes of posture. Deep narcosis impairs or even abolishes the activity of the medullary respiratory centre and although this may be of little significance during an operation when respiration can be maintained by artificial means, should it persist postoperatively it can have serious consequences. Finally, after deep narcosis there is likely to be a period of depression and immobility which can predispose to complications such as pneumonia in horses and the aspiration of regurgitated ingesta in ruminants or of stomach acid in other animals.

Other centrally acting drugs such as guaiphenesin produce muscle relaxation by selectively depressing the transmission of nerve impulses at the internuncial neurones of the spinal cord, brain stem and subcortical regions of the brain.

2. The second method of producing muscle relaxation utilizes drugs which have a peripheral action. Local analgesics injected directly into a muscle

mass, or around nerve fibres or nerve endings, block the transmission of impulses and the muscle fibres are effectively isolated from nervous influences. This is strikingly demonstrated by paravertebral nerve block in cattle. At the same time this method also has its disadvantages. The temperament of some animals is such as to render them unsuitable subjects for the use of local analgesics alone, especially when limb muscles are involved, and even in docile animals immobility of the whole body can only be assured when local analgesia is combined with general anaesthesia or very deep sedation. The injection of local analgesics is a time-consuming procedure and even after the simplest of techniques there is a delay before the full degree of relaxation is obtained. In addition to these disadvantages, techniques such as anterior epidural and subarachnoid blocks cause a loss of control of much of the circulatory system as a result of paralysis of sympathetic nerves.

3. The third way of producing muscle relaxation is by the use of drugs having an effect at the neuro-muscular junction itself. These drugs are known as 'neuromuscular blockers' or, more simply, as 'relaxants'. In general it may be said that they have no significant action in the body other than at the neuromuscular junction, and by their use it is possible to produce quickly, and with certainty, any degree of muscle relaxation without influencing the excitability and functioning of the central nervous and cardiovascular systems. In order that their mode of action be understood it is essential that the phenomena which occur at the neuro-muscular junction upon the arrival of an impulse in the motor nerve should be appreciated. The following brief review of neuromuscular transmission is concerned with such details of the process as are of importance in anaesthesia. For a detailed study of these phenomena reference should be made to standard texts on physiology.

THEORY OF NEUROMUSCULAR TRANSMISSION

It is now well established that acetylcholine is synthe-sized and stored in the motor nerve and is released as a result of a propagated impulse in the nerve fibre. Acetylcholine depolarizes the end-plate region, giving rise to an end-plate potential which in turn produces a propagated action potential and muscle contraction. Curare, long known to block neuro-muscular transmission, antagonizes acetylcholine at the end-plate. The anticholinsterases reverse curare

block, and this was satisfactorily interpreted as causing an increase in the effective local concentration of acetylcholine at the end-plate, thus shifting the competitive balance between curare and acetylcholine in favour of the latter. This description is, however, a simplification and indeed it is not established with any certainty whether the receptor sites for curare-like drugs are different from those for acetylcholine or whether they are the same receptors in an altered

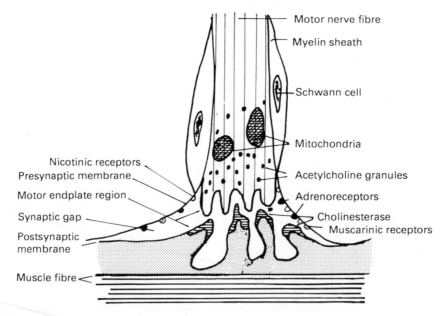

Fig. 7.1 Diagramatic representation of the modern view of the neuromuscular junction.

mode or special position. It is becoming increasingly important for the anaesthetist to have a more detailed understanding of drug action and interaction at the neuromuscular junction. Unfortunately, the whole subject is still bedevilled by speculation and hypothesis in regard to finer details but, nevertheless, sufficient is known to have considerable bearing on the clinical use and application of especially the newer neuromuscular blocking drugs. In particular, the anaesthetist needs to know more about transmitter release and synaptic function, especially the role of calcium ions and their binding protein, calmodulin, in the mobilization and release of acetylcholine.

Calcium ions are capable of generating action potentials, but only at the presynaptic terminal, and these action potentials are accompanied by the release of transmitter [1]. In the absence of extracellular calcium ions the injection of calcium salts into the presynaptic terminal causes postsynaptic depolarization [2]. Thus calcium is an essential intermediary, linking depolarization of the presynaptic membrane to transmitter release. Secretion is triggered by an increase in the concentration of intracellular calcium ions. Depolarization opens channels in the membrane that allow calcium ions to pass into the cell, possibly through cyclic adenosine monophosphate (cAMP) mechanism. Thus, it is generally believed that depolarization activates membrane-bound adenyl cyclase which converts ATP to cAMP and that the latter acts on a protein kinase which causes opening of the calcium channel. Calcium itself does not cause transmitter mobilization and release — an essential intermediary is calmodulin, a calcium-binding protein which regulates its action. The binding of four calcium ions to calmodulin changes its shape and activates it. Activated calmodulin combines with an inactive receptor protein, activating it by changing its shape and this activated form is known to be associated with the aggregation of acetylcholine vesicles and their subsequent interaction with the presynaptic membrane. It seems probable that the release of transmitter (exocytosis) is also depended on calcium ions and calmodulin.

Drugs may interact with this complex system in many ways. For example, calcium antagonists such as verapamil may act by inhibiting calmodulin combination with calcium. One molecule of this drug may be enough to block the uptake of several thousand calcium ions. There is evidence that the change in quantal content of acetylcholine released is proportional to the fourth power of the change in calcium ion concentration [3]. In dogs a dose of 0.1 mg/kg of verapamil produces a significant interaction with the non-depolarizing agent, pancuronium, which persists long beyond the period of the calcium antagonist's cardiac effects [4]. Volatile anaesthetics

may be considered to be non-specific calcium antagonists [5, 6] and so it is not surprising that these agents produce and potentiate neuromuscular blockade [7, 8].

In recent years there has been an increasing awareness that there are prejunctional receptors which have an influence on normal neuromuscular transmission. One theory holds that prejunctional nicotinic receptors are involved in the mobilization of transmitter from the reserve stores to the readily releasable store [9]. To complicate the picture further there are muscarinic and adrenoreceptors on the motor nerve ending and these may be involved in modulating synaptic function [10, 11]. Thus, drugs such as noradrenaline may be expected to have some effect on neuromusclar transmission and, indeed, noradrenaline is known to increase transmitter output in skeletal muscle. The catecholamine effect on the motor nerve endings is thought to be an α effect

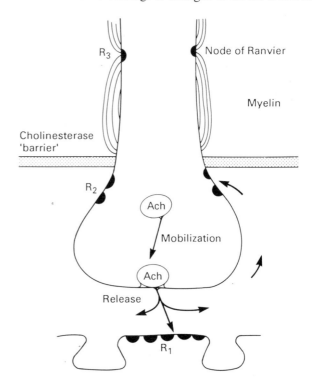

Fig. 7.2 Diagramatic representation of prejunctional (R_2) and postjunctional (R_1) cholinoceptors. R_2 receptors are hypothetical — it is suggested that their stimulation by released acetylcholine hastens mobilization of acetylcholine stored in the nerve terminal and maintains transmitter output during high frequencies of nerve stimulation. R_3 receptors, postulated to occur at the node of Ranvier, would be normally protected by a cholinesterase barrier but might be stimulated after anticholinesterase administration, thus producing local depolarization to generate an action potential propagating in both directions from this site. (From suggestions by W. C. Bowman (1980) *Pharmacology of Neuromuscular Function*, Chapt. 3. Bristol: Wright.

[12] in the presynaptic region contributing to an anticurare action; it contrasts with the β effect on the postsynaptic membrane which leads to hyperpolarization and a deepening of non-depolarizing neuromuscular block.

A remarkable property known as 'desensitization' is displayed by the acetylcholine receptor of striated muscle and its associated systems. This appears as the waning of a stimulant effect or the development of repolarization (usually partial but under some circumstances complete) despite the continued presence of acetylcholine or some other depolarizing substance at the end-plate. The rate of this repolarization increases with the concentration of the drug [13, 14]. It has been proposed that receptors can exist either in their normal state or in some conformationally different desensitized state. Katz and Thesleff [14] concluded from a kinetic analysis that a model such as

$$D + R \; \leftrightharpoons \; DR$$
$$\Updownarrow \qquad\qquad \Updownarrow$$
$$D + R^1 \; \leftrightharpoons \; DR^1$$

was applicable where D is the drug, R the normal receptor, R^1 the desensitized receptor, and DR and DR^1 the drug–receptor complexes of each kind. The extent of desensitization appears to vary both between species and between individuals of any one species. Repolarization occurs faster when the extracellular concentration of calcium is high and acetylcholine has been shown to change the affinity of the receptor for certain blocking agents in a way which may be connected with the desensitization process.

NEUROMUSCULAR BLOCK

Consideration of the mechanisms of neuromuscular transmission outlined above suggests many ways in which the process may be modified to produce failure or block of transmission.

Non-depolarizing, antagonist, curare-like or competitive block results when the drug reduces the degree of depolarization of the postsynaptic membrane caused by acetylcholine following motor nerve stimulation. When the reduction in the degree of depolarization is such that a threshold depolarization is not achieved, a neuromuscular block is present. As the effect is 'all or none' for each motor end-plate, what is seen in any particular muscle during this type of block represents a spectrum of these thresholds. For completed suppression of the motor response to occur even the most resistant synapses must be blocked.

In normal neuromuscular transmission an excess of acetylcholine is produced by motor nerve stimulation. There also exist many more receptors than necessary for the production of a total increase in cation conductance required to trigger an action potential. This results in a substantial 'safety factor' [5]. It has been shown that under certain conditions in cat tibialis muscle four or five times as much acetylcholine is released as is needed for threshold action. Expressed in terms of receptors this means that 75–80% of the receptors must be occluded before the threshold is reached [16].

The existence of a safety factor has obvious practical significance. It means, for example, that the action of the drug is far from terminated at the time when transmission is apparently normal. There is likely to be considerable 'subthreshold action' which is only detectable when a tetanic stimulus is applied to the motor nerve or when some other drug is potentiated.

It also explains the properties of muscles partially blocked by competitive drugs, such as the fall of tension during a tetanus (see p. 124), the sensitivity of the depth of block to anticholinesterases, catecholamines, previous tetanization, anaesthesia and a wide range of drugs.

Depolarizing drugs will increase the variation of safety factor. Slightly depolarized fibres become more excitable, i.e. their safety factor becomes greater than normal. Conversely, deeply polarized fibres become less excitable; if the depolarization is sufficient, the propagation threshold may rise above the maximum depolarization which can be achieved by acetylcholine and the safety factor becomes zero. It is likely that this underlies the general insensitivity of partial depolarization block.

Some drugs will produce depolarization and then prevent the passage of excitation from motor nerve to muscle fibre. Such drugs have been termed 'depolarizing agents' and the analysis of their actions brought to light a variety of stimulant effects analogous to those of acetylcholine itself, and attributable to end-plate depolarization. In themselves, however, these effects do not explain how synaptic block is produced, nor even why the overt signs of stimulation (such as fasciculations and limb movements) are quite transient, although the depolarization persists. During the block produced by a depolarizing agent there is a decrease of electrical excitability of the membrane of the end-plate region as a result of the persisting depolarization [17].

Depolarization block may be followed by an alteration of the threshold of the end-plate region to depolarization by acetylcholine. This 'raised-threshold block' was originally described by Zaimis [18] as 'dual block'. Foldes *et al.* [19] suggested the term 'phase-II block' to indicate that it follows 'phase I' which is the depolarizing activity of the drug. Phase-II block following prolonged suxamethonium depolarization may be due to 'channel block', the molecule of the drug being small enough to actually penetrate the open ion channels.

In the past, neuromuscular block has been classified as 'depolarizing' or 'competitive' solely on characteristics such as the response to an anticholinesterase, the behaviour during and after the application of a tetanic stimulus, and interaction with other drugs. This now seems a dangerous outlook. Erosion of the safety factor from some causes makes it possible for a block to develop from quite a small rise in propagation threshold produced by a depolarizing drug without greatly increasing the variation in safety

factor; such a block would show many of the characteristics of a competitive block. When it is realized that some neuromuscular blocking agents may be 'partial agonists' (i.e. possessing limited ability themselves to depolarize as well as an ability to compete) and that drugs may act presynaptically as well as postsynaptically, it becomes clear that under clinical conditions many situations will rise where the underlying mechanisms can only, at the moment, be guessed. To interpret the effect of neuromuscular blocking drugs clinically it is necessary to assess contributions due to depolarization, competitive antagonism and presynaptic action produced by the various drugs used and to be aware of the safety factors of transmission in the absence of such drugs [16].

PATTERN OF NEUROMUSCULAR BLOCK

One feature of neuromuscular block which appears to be reasonably constant and common to all species of animal and all types of relaxant drugs is the sequence of events as each muscle group becomes involved (Fig. 7.3). Usually, the muscles of facial expression, the jaw and the tail become paralysed within 30–60 seconds of the intravenous injection of the drug. Paralysis of the limb and neck muscles follows next and then the swallowing and phonatory muscles are affected. Soon after this the abdominal muscles become involved, then the intercostals fail and finally the diaphragm becomes paralysed. The reasons for this pattern of response to neuromuscular blocking

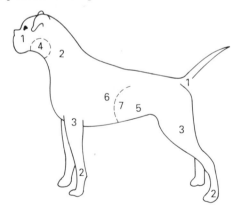

Fig. 7.3 Usual sequence of muscle paralysis: 1, the muscles of expression, the jaw muscles and tail muscles; 2, the neck and distal limb muscles; 3, the proximal limb muscles; 4, the swallowing and phonatory muscles; 5, the muscles of the abdominal wall; 6, the intercostal muscles; 7, the diaphragm. This pattern is not invariable and the sequence of recovery is not always the reverse of that of onset — for example, it is most important to note that in horses the block may wear off in the facial muscles before power has returned to the muscles of the limbs.

drugs are largely unknown and although this is the commonly accepted sequence of the paralysis, individual lightly unconscious animals have been observed to be able to make chewing movements or to move a limb although 'curarized' to the point of respiratory arrest. Moreover, the sequence of events on recovery is not always the exact reverse of paralysis. Function may return to the facial muscles of horses before it returns to the limb muscles.

In the past attempts were made to take advantage of the response pattern by giving doses of relaxants which were just enough to paralyse the abdominal muscles without paralysis of the intercostal muscles and diaphragm. However, useful relaxation of the abdominal muscles is invariably associated with a marked diminution in the tidal volume of respiration. The animal may compensate for this respiratory impairment, when it is of a minor degree, by an increase in respiratory rate. The breathing which results is characterized by a pause between inspiration and expiration, producing a rectangular pattern when recorded spirometrically. The increased respiratory rate is accompanied by over-activity of the diaphragm resulting in very turbulent conditions for intra-abdominal surgery. Larger doses of the relaxant will result in respiratory depression which cannot be compensated for by an increase in rate. Because of the oxygen-rich mixtures commonly used in breathing circuits hypoxia may not occur but, nevertheless, the decreased minute volume of respiration will lead to an inefficient elimination of carbon dioxide. The results are likely to be a rising blood pressure, an increased oozing from cut cutaneous vessels and distressed respiratory efforts. Thus, it is now generally agreed that if the abdominal muscles are to be relaxed by the use of a neuromuscular blocking drug some form of artificial respiration will be required. Consequently, for abdominal surgery there is little point in attempting to assess the exact dose of drug in any individual animal, for any spontaneous respiratory movements may interfere with efficient intermittent positive pressure ventilation of the lungs, and all that is required is to ensure that the dose given is sufficiently large to produce complete respiratory arrest.

AGENTS WHICH PRODUCE NON-DEPOLARIZING (COMPETITIVE) BLOCK

d-Tubocurarine chloride

A purified, biologically standardized preparation of curare (Intocostrin) was used in human patients by Bennett [20] to soften the convulsions of psychiatric convulsive therapy, and later during cyclopropane anaesthesia by Griffith and Johnson [21]. It was, however, a relatively crude substance, and only in 1944 was the pure quaternary alkaloid *d*-tubocurarine used in anaesthesia [22]. After intravenous injection the maximum activity is apparent within 2–3 minutes and lasts for 35–40 minutes in most species of animal. Some 30–40% of the dose is excreted unchanged in the urine within 3–4 hours. Plasma proteins have the power of binding *d*-tubocurarine chloride [22] and Utting [23] demonstrated in dogs that the blood concentration of tubocurarine is low in alkalaemia and high in acidaemia. The change in the reaction of the blood from acid to alkaline will apparently drive tubocurarine out of the blood, presumably to specific and non-specific receptors. A full discussion of the fate of tubocurarine in the body has been given by Kalow [24].

In 1951, Pickett [25] reported the use of 0.12 mg/kg body weight in 250 dogs, but it soon became apparent that this dose is inadequate for the production of really useful relaxation. Use of an effective dose, ED_{90}, i.e. the dose that corresponds to 90% depression of twitch response (see p. 125) under light general anaesthesia, showed that in dogs *d*-tubocurarine chloride has actions other than at the neuromuscular junction for although even large doses of the drug do not affect the canine myocardium [26] it causes a severe fall in blood pressure and an increase in heart rate. The fall in arterial blood pressure appears to be due to block of impulse transmission across autonomic ganglia — hence the tachycardia from vagal block — and/or the release of histamine.

A similar fall in arterial blood pressure occurs when the drug is adminstered intravenously to cats. In pigs, doses of the order of 0.3 mg/kg cause complete relaxation with respiratory paralysis without at the same time causing any marked fall in arterial blood pressure. Although unlikely to be of any use in clinical porcine anaesthesia, *d*-tubocurarine chloride has proved to be a useful agent for the production of relaxation required for experimental surgery.

Little is known about the action of *d*-tubocurarine chloride in ruminant animals. Young lambs and calves appear very sensitive to the paralysing action of the drug but doses of up to 0.06 mg/kg have been given to these animals without harmful effects being noted.

Booth and Rankin [27] studied the action of a crude curare preparation in horses during chloral hydrate narcosis and came to the conclusion that this combination of drugs had no value in equine anaesthesia. However, once again if the dose of curare used (about 0.12 mg/kg when expressed in terms of the pure alkaloid *d*-tubocurarine) was much less than what is today regarded as the minimal effective dose. Doses of the order of 0.22–0.25 mg/kg produce good relaxation with respiratory arrest in anaesthetized horses breathing 0.8–1% halothane or 0.4–0.6% methoxyflurane, and no significant hypotension is encountered.

Certain antibiotics, notably the aminoglycosides, may produce neuromuscular block and increase sensitivity to *d*-tubocurarine chloride (and to other non-depolarizing agents) [28–31].

In veterinary anaesthesia it seems to be a 'dirty' drug with many actions, such as an ability to produce ganglionic blockage and histamine release in addition to its main activity, so that with the advent of newer drugs it has largely fallen into disuse.

Gallamine triethiodide

In 1947, Bovet and his coworkers [32] described the neuromuscular blocking properties of the first satisfactory synthetic neuromuscular blocking drug — gallamine triethiodide. It blocks cardiac muscarinic activity which can be useful during halothane anaesthesia since halothane tends to stimulate the vagus nerve. Tachycardia occurs within 1–1.5 minutes after the intravenous injection of gallamine and in dogs and pigs the heart rate increases by 10–20%. The rise in heart rate is sometimes accompanied by a rise in the arterial blood pressure. It is not detoxicated in the body and is excreted unchanged in the urine. In cats 30–100% of the total dose injected can be recovered from the urine within 2 hours [33]. Gallamine does not give rise to histamine release so that it is a useful non-depolarizing relaxant in dogs.

In dogs doses of 1.0 mg/kg by intravenous injection usually cause complete relaxation for 15–20 minutes. Apart from a slight tachycardia, the drug appears to produce few side-effects, but occasionally hypertension follows its administration. In cats 1.0 mg/kg provokes apnoea of 10–20 minutes duration. Pigs are very resistant to the effects of gallamine and doses of 4 mg/kg are needed to produce complete relaxation with apnoea. In horses, doses of 0.5–1.0 mg/kg produce complete paralysis with apnoea of 10–20 minutes duration. Young lambs and calves have been given doses of 0.4 mg/kg without harmful effect but in these animals apnoea may be prolonged.

Alcuronium chloride

This compound is diallylnortoxiferine, a derivative of the alkaloid toxiferine obtained from calabash curare. It has a relatively long duration of action.

Alcuronium has been used quite extensively in dogs and horses and seems to have no significant histamine-liberating or ganglionic blocking effects. During light halothane anaesthesia the dose required to produce complete relaxation with respiratory arrest is 0.1 mg/kg. Intravenous injection produces no change in heart rate, arterial blood pressure or central venous pressure. The return of spontaneous breathing is apparently followed by a prolonged period of partial paresis; because of this, reversal of the myoneural block with a anticholinesterase is obligatory. If only one dose of alcuronium chloride has been given during the course of an operation, the block is very readily reversed by drugs such as neostigmine, but when more than one dose of alcuronium has been administered some difficulty may be experienced in antagonizing its effects. It is, therefore, probably advisable to limit the use of alcuronium chloride to anaesthesia for operations which can be completed in the 70 ± 18 minute period of relaxation which follows one injection of the drug [34].

Pancuronium bromide

Pancuronium bromide, an amino steroid free from any hormonal action, fulfills the need for a rapidly acting, non-depolarizing neuromuscular blocker with a relatively rapid onset and medium duration of activity. It has no major undesirable side-effects.

A study in 1970 of the effects of pancuronium bromide in dogs, cats and horses (G. M. Thompson, personal communication) showed that the intravenous injection of the drug causes minimal change in heart rate or central venous pressure and no alteration of the ECG. During light anaesthesia doses of 0.06 mg/kg have been found to produce complete relaxation with apnoea in dogs [35] and horses of about 40 minutes' duration together with a short-lived rise in arterial blood pressure. A similar period of apnoea follows a second dose of 0.03 mg/kg. The delay in achieving maximum effect after intravenous administration is much less than is found with *d*-tubocurarine or alcuronium. Complete antagonism with neostigmine (always given with an anticholinergic) is readily obtained and no cases of relapse into neuromuscular block have been encountered. Care should be taken in dogs suffering from chronic nephritis and other conditions which impair kidney function, because pancuronium is, in part, excreted unchanged in the urine. Its action is also prolonged in cases of biliary obstruction [36].

Vecuronium

Vecuronium is a monoquarternary analogue of pancuronium, the only difference in structure between the two being that in this compound the nitrogen in the piperidine group (Fig. 7.4) attached to the steroid nucleus is not quarternary and positively charged whereas in pancuronium it is. Due to the instability of the 3-acetyl group in high concentrations in solution the drug is marketed as a freeze-dried buffered powder with water in a separate ampoule. The powder can be kept on the shelf at room temperature without deterioration. Vecuronium is currently the most specific neuromuscular blocking drug in clinical use and is more potent and shorter acting than pancuronium [35, 37]. It shows a low propensity to liberate histamine and possesses a negligible ganglionic blocking action, hence cardiovascular side-effects are unlikely to be observed during clinical use of the drug.

Although the mechanism and exact pathway of inactivation in the body is not fully understood, by

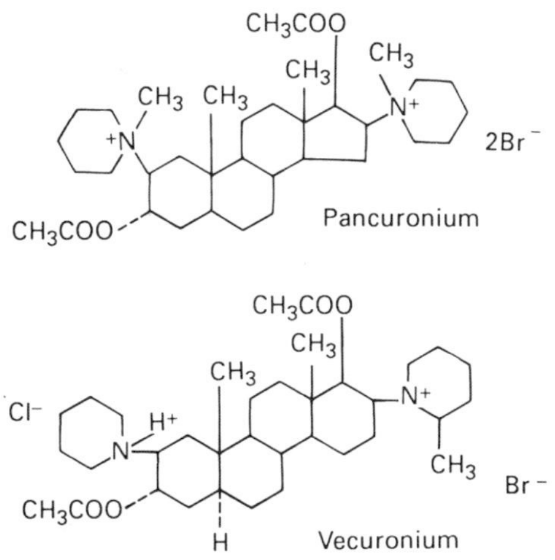

Fig. 7.4 Formulae of pancuronium and vecuronium.

analogy with pancuronium there are likely to be three main metabolites that could arise by deacetylation to the corresponding alcohol. The principal metabolite appears to be the 3-hydroxyl derivative for up to 10% of an injected dose may appear in this form in the urine.

In dogs doses of 0.06 mg/kg produce an initial block of about 20 minutes [38] and in horses this dose appears to produce apnoea of 20–30 minutes duration. Although the ED_{90} of vecuronium is about 0.04 mg/kg compared with 0.05 mg/kg for pancuronium, at this dose the recovery from neuromuscular block to 50% twitch depression (see p. 124) is less than 10 minutes and the relaxation produced is less than adequate for most surgical procedures, whereas that produced by pancuronium is much longer lasting. As a result it is necessary to use a bolus dose of vecuronium to produce a rather greater initial block than with pancuronium if useful relaxation is to be obtained.

According to Duveldestin *et al.* [39], in spite of the greater lipophilicity of vecuronium the placental transfer rate is lower than that of pancuronium. In man, the ratio of umbilical vein to maternal plasma contraction is about 1:10 (i.e. well below that needed to produce a clinical effect in the fetus) when doses of up to 0.1 mg/kg are given to the mother.

Vecuronium has both hepatic and renal pathways for excretion but renal failure has little effect on its clearance. Biliary excretion accounts for about 50% of the injected dose so clearance is much reduced in severe hepatic disease [40]. In the absence of renal and hepatic disease it is not markedly cumulative upon repetitive doses and, indeed, in healthy dogs up to six incremental doses of 0.04 mg/kg have been shown to be non-cumulative [41].

Atracurium

Atracurium is available as a solution in an acidic medium. It deteriorates slowly at room temperature and so should be kept at 4°C. As it is inactivated at alkaline pH it should not be mixed with thiopentone in the same syringe and, when using sequential injections through a butterfly needle or indwelling cannula, the thiopentone should be cleared with saline before the atracurium is injected. Because of its propensity to release histamine, atracurium cannot be administered in multiples of its ED_{50} to give the same sort of flexibility of duration of action associated with vecuronium where a large single bolus dose can be used to provide relaxation for a moderately prolonged operation. It is in short procedures that its relatively rapid onset, short duration of action and rapid recovery are most useful. The paralysing dose for the dog is from 0.3 to 0.5 mg/kg and recovery from these doses occurs in about 40 minutes, although there is a very wide range in the duration of effect. The reason for this wide variability in duration is unknown. Atracurium appears to be more potent in horses, doses of 0.04 mg/kg producing paralysis of about 90 minutes' duration.

Atracurium is unique in that its degradation depends on neither renal nor hepatic activity. At body pH and temperature, the drug is unstable; it breaks down by rapid Hofmann degradation to produce a monotertiary and a monoquaternary derivative, both of which are inactive at the neuromuscular junction. The half-life of this process in cats is about 19 minutes [42]. Coupled with uptake by the liver, kidney and other tissues, this produces a rapid plasma clearance and an apparent large rapid distribution volume. Because of this, the Hofmann degradation process does not need an enzyme system and attains a linear relationship between the dose of drug and the rate of metabolism irrespective of the substrate load. Obviously, the reason why the duration of block is unaffected by hepatic disease or anuria is because neither process involves liver metabolism or renal excretion. Some anxiety has been expressed about a possible central nervous system effect of the tertiary metabolite of atracurium. This compound, laudanosine, does penetrate the blood–brain barrier and, in higher concentrations than are likely to be produced with clinical doses in normal animals, it can cause analeptic or convulsant effects. To date, no reports of side-effects attributable to laudanosine have been described in the veterinary literature.

Pipecuronium

Pipecuronium bromide, a non-depolarizing neuromuscular blocking agent, is an analogue of pancuronium. Its properties in dogs when administered in doses of 0.05 and 0.025 mg/kg and its interactions with suxamethonium have been investigated by Jones [43, 44]. It is not widely available outside Eastern Europe and, therefore, is of less interest than vecuronium and atracurium.

Dimethyl ether of *d*-tubocurarine

The dimethyl ether of *d*-tubocurarine [45] has been used as a relaxant during anaesthesia in dogs, cats, pigs and horses. It appeared to be two to three times as potent as *d*-tubocurarine chloride but the duration of neuromuscular blockade was slightly shorter. It never gained a wide popularity and has not been available in the UK since about 1965 but it is still available in the USA under the name of 'Metocurine'.

Fazadinium bromide

Fazadinium bromide, a non-depolarizing neuro-muscular blocking agent, was introduced for clinical trials in man in 1972 [46, 47]. It was claimed to have a rapid onset of action coupled, at low dosage, with short duration of action. The results of trials in dogs and cats [48] were disappointing. It is no longer available.

Mivacurium

For a number of years, Savarese and colleagues in Massachusetts have been investigating a series of bulcy diester compounds which are non-depolarizing and metabolized by plasma cholinesterase. One of these, mivacurium, has a significantly shorter duration of action than atracurium or vecuronium and is undergoing clinical trials in man. It will be interesting to see whether it is free from the problems of histamine release associated with other members of the benzylisoquinoline group (which includes atracurium).

PHARMACOKINETICS OF NON-DEPOLARIZING AGENTS

Studies of the pharmacokinetics of the non-depolarizing relaxants are still at an early stage and more research is needed to account for the large variation seen in their pharmacokinetics and effects. It is now possible to measure the small concentrations of non-depolarizing agents present in the plasma following intravenous injection and the information gained from studying the plasma decay curves should give some help in understanding the variability of the responses to drugs and in the effects of diseases.

The elimination half-lives of some agents in common use (gallamine, pancuronium, alcuronium) apparently do not differ significantly. Their initial volumes of distribution are similar and seem to equate to that of the extracellular fluid volume, while their clearances (with the exception of vecuronium which has a much higher clearance) are similar. Thus, it would seem that from the pharmacokinetic viewpoint, the non-depolarizing relaxants in clinical use do not differ greatly. Biexponential curves have been fitted to the decay curves for most of the non-depolarizing relaxants but as with any biological investigations there is variation in the pharmacokinetic parameters and, unfortunately, much of the published information relates to only a few subjects [49]. Predictions can be made using the two-compartment model as to the effect of either increasing the dose of the drug or of using more than one dose. Increasing dose besides producing more effect will also progressively increase the duration of effect. Repeated doses will also lead to progressively increasing duration of effect [50].

AGENTS WHICH PRODUCE DEPOLARIZING BLOCK

Muscle paralysis due to depolarization differs from that caused by non-depolarizing drugs in the following respects:

1. The paralysis is preceded by the transient stimulation of muscle fibres, probably caused by the initial depolarization. The muscle twitching which results from this is visible in animal subjects.
2. Substances which antagonize the non-depolarizing agents tend to potentiate the depolarizing ones and thus in clinical practice it is important to note that drugs such as neostigmine may actually prolong the action of depolarizing relaxants.
3. In a nerve–muscle preparation it can be demonstrated that after partial paralysis with a non-depolarizing drug there is a rapid decay of an induced tetanus, whereas after a corresponding degree of paralysis caused by a depolarizing agent an induced tetanus is sustained.
4. It is unlikely that the depolarizing agents ever produce a pure type of neuromuscular block. For example in dogs they cause both depolarization and desensitization.
5. In the cat, rat and mouse, the depolarizing agents affect the red muscles more than the white, whereas non-depolarizers have the opposite effect.

From a study of the pharmacological properties of a series of polymethylene-bis-trimethyl ammonium compounds, Paton and Zaimis [51] considered that the decane compound decamethonium iodide might be a useful substitute for *d*-tubocurarine but it never made any impact in anaesthesia. Bovet and his colleagues [52, 53] and, independently, in the UK, Buttle and Zaimis [54] found that the esters of choline, notably the succinyl derivatives, caused neuromuscular block of short duration by depolarization in certain animal species. The two compounds concerned were dimethylsuccinylcholine and diethylsuccinylchloline. Edridge [55] suggested that the former substance should be known as suxamethonium and the latter as suxethonium. The two compounds resemble each other pharmacologically, with the sole difference that the paralysis caused by the suxethonium compound is rather more rapid in onset and of slightly shorter duration. The first two of the compounds to be used in veterinary anaesthesia was suxethonium bromide [56] but the suxamethonium compound is the one more generally employed today.

Suxamethonium

There is some slight variation in the response of the various muscle groups but the diaphragmatic muscle is usually the last to be affected. Suxamethonium causes marked muscle fasciculation and in man these contractions frequently lead to muscle pains which are obvious to the patient on the day after operation. Conscious volunteers given suxamethonium for experimental purposes have reported that the muscle fasciculations are extremely painful. There is evidence to suggest that suxamethonium produces actual muscle injury. Airaksinen and Tammisto [57] reported myoglobinuria after intermittent administration of the drug and muscle damage is also indicated by the finding that serum creatine kinase levels are raised by the use of suxamethonium during halothane anaesthesia [58].

There are wide species differences between the various domestic animals in their sensitivity to the neuromuscular blocking action of suxamethonium. The horse, pig and cat are relatively resistant, but dogs, sheep and cattle are paralysed by small doses of the drug. Like acetylcholine, suxamethonium is hydrolysed by cholinesterases and this hydrolysis is believed to be responsible for recovery from its effects. It has been shown in dogs that the injection of a purified pseudocholinesterase preparation produces a marked increase in resistance to the effect of the drug [59]. Because of this, attempts have been made to correlate the sensitivity of an animal to suxamethonium with the levels of cholinesterase present in its blood.

The ability of plasma cholinesterase to hydrolyse butyrylthiocholine can be used to predict sensitivity to suxamethonium in man but it has not been of value in animals [60]. Faye [61] has made an extensive study of the role of cholinesterase in the explanation of differing species sensitivity to suxamethonium. In her opinion the affinities of cholinesterase for different substrates are different between species (Tables 7.1 and 7.2) and, furthermore, although the hydrolysis of various assay substrates parallels that of suxamethonium in man, they do not in other species of animal. Therefore, the substrates used to study cholinesterase activity in man cannot be used to draw conclusions regarding suxamethonium sensitivity in other animals and for this to be done Faye considers it most important that the substrate used for assay is suxamethonium itself.

Table 7.1 Mean values for plasma cholinesterase as determined by the use of different substrates

Species	Propionyl thiocholine	Benzoyl choline	Butyryl thiocholine	Succinyl choline
Sacred baboon	4.20	0.85	7.01	89.70
Chimpanzee	5.65	0.93	6.15	76.50
Bottle-nosed dolphin	0.04	None	0.02	47.90
Pig	0.34	0.03	0.32	43.13
Horse	4.18	0.27	4.46	33.10
Dog	2.13	0.36	2.33	8.01
Cat	1.36	–	–	7.24
Indian elephant	0.01	None	0.05	7.00
Goat	0.14	0.04	0.02	6.70
Sheep	0.05	None	None	1.47
Cow	0.06	–	–	0.95

By courtesy of Dr Sherry Faye, Senior Biochemist, Bristol Royal Infirmary.

Table 7.2 Plasma cholinesterase activities determined using different substrates expressed as per cent of appropriate mean human reference range. Mean cholinesterase activity for human Elu homozygotes taken as: propionylthiocholine activity 4.58 units/ml, benzoylcholine activity 0.88 units/ml, butyrylthiocholine activity 5.04 units/ml and succinylcholine activity 58.6 units/ml

Species	Propionyl thiocholine activity	Benzoyl choline activity	Butyryl thiocholine activity	Succinyl choline activity
Red deer	1.3	4.5	0.5	6.8
Goat	2.9	4.5	0.5	6.7
Fallow deer	1.0	–	1.3	12.4
Bottle-nosed dolphin	0.9	–	0.4	81.7
Indian elephant	0.2	–	0.9	11.9
Sacred baboon	91.7	96.6	139.1	153.1
Patas monkey	9.2	5.7	13.5	45.9
White rhino	29.7	12.5	34.3	26.4
Donkey	99.3	62.5	124.4	61.6
Muscovy duck	8.5	7.9	6.9	18.9

By courtesy of Dr Sherry Faye, Senior Biochemist, Bristol Royal Infirmary.

Because cholinesterase is formed in the liver, the existence of severe liver damage, cachexia or malnutrition may prolong the duration of action of suxamethonium. In man, atypical forms of pseudocholinesterase are recognized. Although they have been found in animals their significance and mode of inheritance have not been determined.

Suxamethonium is so closely related to acetylcholine that it might be expected to have actions in the body in addition to its effects at the neuromuscular junction and this is indeed the case. Injection of suxamethonium causes a rise in blood pressure in all animals, although in some species the rise may be preceded by a fall. In cats there is an immediate marked fall in arterial blood pressure, followed by a slower rise to above the resting level. The fall in blood pressure can be prevented by the prior administration of atropine, and the rise by hexamethonium so that the prior administration of both these drugs prevents any blood pressure change. Blood pressure changes are seen after each successive dose of suxamethonium but with progressively diminishing severity. Pulse rate changes are variable, both bradycardia and tachycardia being observed, sometimes in the same animal, and often the heart rate does not change. In horses and dogs the nicotinic response predominates [62, 63] — very occasionally a fall in blood pressure with bradycardia is seen, but an increase in both blood pressure and heart rate is the usual response.

Cardiac arrhythmias are frequently seen after the intravenous injection of suxamethonium and usually take the form of atrioventricular nodal rhythm. Stevenson [64] demonstrated that one injection of suxamethonium causes a rise in the level of serum potassium and since this was not abolished by adrenalectomy, ganglionic blockade, adrenolytic drugs or high epidural block it is likely to be due to the release of potassium ions from muscle. This rise in serum potassium may also be associated with cardiac irregularities. Prolonged adminstration of suxamethonium, on the other hand, causes a large decrease in serum potassium in dogs, but the reason for this is unknown [64].

In horses intravenous doses of 0.12–0.15 mg/kg usually cause paralysis of the limb, head and neck muscles without producing diaphragmatic paralysis.

In most horses double this dose will cause total paralysis but the exact effect produced in any individual animal will depend on the depth of anaesthesia at the time when the relaxant is administered. After a single dose paralysis generally lasts for about 4–5 minutes although limb weakness may persist for several more minutes. In cattle doses of about one-sixth of this quantity (0.02 mg/kg) produce paralysis of the body muscles without diaphragmatic paralysis and this relaxation lasts 6–8 minutes. Once again, double this dose will cause complete paralysis in most animals. In sheep, doses similar to those used in cattle are employed. Pigs require much larger doses; to facilitate endotracheal intubation the dose required is about 2 mg/kg which produces complete paralysis of 2–3 minutes' duration. In cats, 3–5 mg quantities of suxamethonium chloride (total dose) produces 5–6 minutes of complete paralysis. The dog is comparatively sensitive to suxamethonium and doses of 0.3 mg/kg produce total paralysis of 15–20 minutes' duration. A single dose may produce phase-II block in dogs and phase-II block may also be produced when more than one dose of the drug is given to other animals. It is believed that the response of the motor end-plate gradually alters with each successive dose but the precise time and dose relationship is not yet known.

Apart from its use to produce good conditions for endotracheal intubation in pigs and cats, it seems that there are, today, no good indications for suxamethonium in veterinary anaesthesia.

MONITORING OF NEUROMUSCULAR BLOCKADE

In view of the enormous variation in the response to a given dose of neuromuscular blocking agent and the rate of spontaneous recovery from neuromuscular block, it is not surprising that many attempts have been made to determine the nature, degree and duration of the block produced during clinical anaesthesia. Techniques developed for use in pharmacological laboratories are generally not suitable for clinical use and others such as electromyographic recording are usually beyond the capabilities of the clinician in the operating theatre. As a result, there is rather little information relating to the accurate evaluation of neuromuscular block during clinical anaesthesia.

A technique of mechanical measurement of response evoked by peripheral nerve stimulation in horses, cattle and dogs was described by Bowen [65] and Jones and Prentice [66] used a similar technique in horses. A comparison of the evoked electrical and mechanical responses in peripheral nerve stimulation was used [67] to investigate neuromuscular function in hypocalcaemic cows and parathyroidectomized

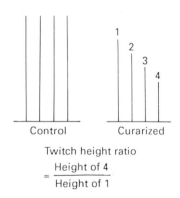

Fig. 7.5 'Train-of-four' stimulation of the motor nerve.

dogs and a very similar technique has been used to study the action of muscle relaxants in dogs [68, 69].

A method known as 'train-of-four' stimulation was developed (Fig. 7.5) and applied to the study of neuromuscular blockade during anaesthesia of human subjects by Ali *et al.* [70]. The method as developed by these workers involves recording four twitch responses evoked in a muscle by supramaximal stimulation of its motor nerve at the rate of 2 Hz. This particular stimulation frequency enables observation of depletion of acetylcholine in the absence of the rapid mobilization which occurs at higher stimulation rates. The fourth twitch in the 'train-of-four' is said to be as strong as the first when 25–30% of the receptors are free of neuromuscular blocking drug. By contrast, stimulation of the nerve at, say 30–50 Hz for 5 seconds results in sustained tension when only 20–25% of the receptors are free. Thus, it is claimed that 'train-of-four' responses are more useful than recordings of sustained contractions produced by higher-frequency stimulation in the evaluation of neuromuscular blockade. The 'train-of-four' technique has been used by Cullen and Jones [71–73] to study the nature of suxamethonium neuromuscular block in dogs but its value in other animals has been questioned. According to Klein [74], in halothane anaesthetized horses there may be very obvious 'fade' during 50 Hz stimulation when no fade exists at 2 Hz. She claims that stimulation at the higher rate is a much more sensitive method to indicate a slight blockade, but it must be recognized that tetanic stimulation induces recovery in the muscles stimulated so that all subsequent events are shifted towards normality [75]. A tetanic stimulation of 50 Hz for 5 seconds stresses neuromuscular function to much the same extent as does maximal voluntary effort and it may be possible to decide, by visual or tactile means, whether there is any fade in response to tetanic stimulation. A sustained tetanus is known to correlate with a train-of-four (T_4) ratio (ratio of the fourth twitch in the train to the first) of 0.7 or greater [76]. It seems certain that fade represents the interaction of neuromuscular blockers with different sites within the neuromuscular junction [77]. A site of action at presynaptic nicotinic receptors or ion channels could impede the mobilization and/or release of the transmitter in response to repeated stimulation of the motor nerve; ion channel blockade at the postsynaptic membrane might also be involved.

The importance of routine monitoring of neuromuscular block is now widely recognized. There can be little doubt that the reliance on simple clinical evaluations of the degree of neuromuscular blockade (using such criteria as the respiratory efforts in the anaesthetized animal) is inadequate. There is a remarkably wide variation in the sensitivity of individuals to relaxant drugs and after spontaneous or evoked recovery from neuromuscular blockade routine monitoring allows the prediction of which individuals are likely to be able to maintain and clear their airways. For example, a T_4 ratio of 0.5 is generally accepted as being compatible with clinically safe recovery.

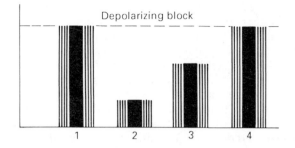

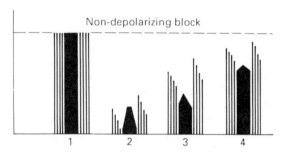

Fig. 7.6 Top: depolarizing blockade muscle response pattern. A sequence of train-of-four, tetanic stimulation at 50 Hz and train-of-four is repeated at intervals 1, 2, 3 and 4. The intensity of the responses is represented by the height of the lines in the diagram. The intensity and not the character of the response is changed by depolarizing agents. Bottom: non-depolarizing blockade muscle response pattern. Applying the sequence of stimulation as above. At 2 the initial response to a single train-of-four rapidly diminishes and may disappear completely while the tetanus response is poorly sustained but the response to a train-of-four stimulus after the tetanic stimulation is increased (post-tetanic facilitation). Post-tetanic facilitation can be detected at 3 and 4.

During the onset of neuromuscular blockade, routine monitoring also allows more accurate judgement of the achievement of proper muscle relaxation. This is important, for ordinary reflex responses depend not only on the degree of neuromuscular blockade but also on the depth of central nervous depression. Using the standard anaesthetic sequence of premedication followed by barbiturate induction and maintenance with nitrous oxide/oxygen plus volatile supplement complete abolition of the twitch response is necessary to provide relaxation of the abdominal muscles.

When the newer, relatively short-acting agents are administered by infusion or frequent incremental doses, routine monitoring of the degree of neuromuscular blockade becomes almost essential.

Clinical monitoring

Using a nerve stimulator

Several inexpensive peripheral nerve stimulators are commercially available, and a typical one is shown in

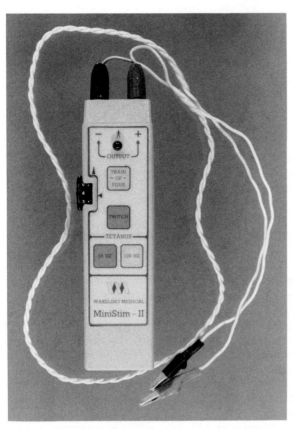

Fig. 7.7 MiniStim nerve stimulator. This is typical of the small, inexpensive nerve stimulators used for monitoring neuromuscular block.

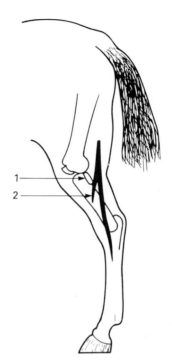

Fig. 7.8 Site for stimulation of the peroneal nerve in the horse. The nerve crosses the shaft of the tibia just distal to the head of the fibula and is often palpable at this site.

Fig. 7.7. They have the ability to deliver single twitch, train-of-four and tetanic stimuli so that selection of the mode of stimulation presents no problem. In horses the peroneal nerve may be stimulated where it crosses the shaft of the fibula just distal to the head of that bone (where it is palpable) (Fig. 7.8), and the facial nerve ventral to the eye (Fig. 7.9). In dogs probably the best nerve to stimulate is the ulnar nerve at its most superficial location on the medial aspect of the elbow (Fig. 7.10).

Determination of the muscle response is more difficult. Under experimental conditions frames and transducers may be used to record the response in loaded muscles. The accurate calculation of the ratio of the first to the fourth twitch height requires that a permanent copy of the twitch response is made or a twitch response analyser is used. The transducers and circuitry involved are unlikely to be available in veterinary practice so it is usually necessary to rely upon visual assessment and/or palpation of the muscle activity in unloaded muscles.

With both visual assessment and palpation when

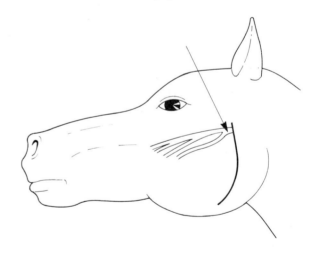

Fig. 7.9 Site for stimulation of the facial nerve in the horse.

train-of-four stimulation is used marked degrees of fade (up to 60%, i.e. a T_4 ratio of 0.4) may not be detectable even by experienced observers and it is important to note that fade of this degree indicates that there is a significant degree of block present. Some attempt has been made to quantify the extent of neuromuscular blockade by counting the twitches in response to train-of-four stimulation but this approach suffers from some obvious drawbacks. One of these is that individual relaxants may be associated with

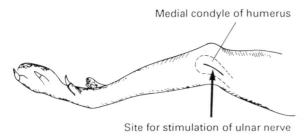

Medial condyle of humerus

Site for stimulation of ulnar nerve

Fig. 7.10 Site for stimulation of the ulna nerve in the dog and cat.

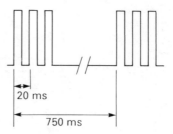

20 ms

750 ms

Fig. 7.11 Preferred pattern of double-burst stimulation [79]. In each burst three impulses are given at a frequency of 50 Hz and the two bursts are separated by 750 ms.

different degrees of T_4 ratio fade and hence the presence or absence of the fourth twitch of the train may be associated with different absolute degrees of block, depending on the relaxant used [78]. Also, although it may be easier to decide by touch, rather than visually, how many responses are present to train-of-four stimulation it is almost impossible to estimate the T_4 ratio in this manner. Many anaesthetists are, therefore, of the opinion that the most convenient and safest way of assessing the degree of neuromuscular block present during clinical anaesthesia is by the application of tetanic stimulation to the nerve (50 Hz for 5 seconds), when it is usually quite simple to decide by visual or tactile means whether there is any fade in response to the tetanic stimulation. Other anaesthetists have adopted a different approach to this problem and have developed a technique known as 'double-burst stimulation' or 'DBS' [79]. The DBS consists of two short-lasting, 50 Hz tetanic stimuli or bursts separated by a 750 ms interval. The response to this pattern of stimulation is two single separated muscle contractions of which the second is less than the first during non-depolarizing neuromuscular blockade. The DBS with three impulses in each burst is most suitable for clinical use and it is claimed that it is easier to detect fade manually than is the case with train-of-four stimulation (Fig. 7.11).

When any nerve stimulator is used supramaximal stimulation must be employed (e.g. 200 to 300 V for 0.3 ms) and the results of stimulation should be observed before neuromuscular block is induced to ascertain that the placing of the electrodes is correct and that twitches can be obtained.

Without the use of a nerve stimulator

In clinical practice depression of diaphragmatic activity is frequently used in the assessment of the degree of blockade because this muscle is generally regarded as being the most resistant to paralysis by neuromuscular blocking drugs. Abolition of diaphragmatic activity can thus be taken to indicate complete muscle paralysis. If an animal can move its limbs in such a way as to indicate that the muscles are capable of producing a sustained contraction (e.g. maintain itself in sternal recumbency) it usually means that, at the most, only partial neuromuscular block is present but short, jerky movements are often seen in animals where diaphragmatic activity is not in evidence and marked block exists. To assess the ability of a partially paralysed animal to breathe, the airway may be occluded and the subatmospheric pressure generated in the trachea during an attempt at inspiration measured with an anaeroid manometer. Depending on the depth of anaesthesia and the prevailing arterial carbon dioxide tension, a pressure of -10 to -20 cmH$_2$O can usually be taken to indicate that block is insufficient to produce respiratory insufficiency. However, although gas exchange may be adequate in an animal whose airway is safeguarded by an endotracheal tube, the degree of neuromuscular block may not leave enough margin of safety after extubation if the animal subsequently develops an obstructed airway.

FACTORS AFFECTING THE ACTION OF NEUROMUSCULAR BLOCKING DRUGS

Factors such as age, concurrent administration of other drugs, body temperature, extracellular pH, neuromuscular disease and genetic abnormalities may influence the response to muscle relaxant drugs. These have been well reviewed by Ali and Savarese [75].

Body temperature

The effect of muscle and body temperature on the potency and duration of action of muscle relaxants is difficult to assess because any effect of change in body temperature on neuromuscular block may be complicated by changes in regional blood flow. Reduction in body temperature decreases the renal, hepatic and biliary elimination of non-depolarizing relaxants and during hypothermia reduced doses may be needed to produce a given degree of neuromuscular block. In clinical practice it certainly seems that the requirements of non-depolarizing agents are decreased during moderate hypothermia. Reduction of muscle blood flow in hypothermic animals may lead to delay in onset time of the block and, unless allowance is made for this, gives rise to the risk of serious overdosing if the drug is being given in incremental doses to assess its effects as administration proceeds.

Administration of other drugs

Any drug which has anticholinesterase properties will prolong the action of suxamethonium and tend to antagonize non-depolarizing neuromuscular blockade. Several antibiotics, especially neomycin and the aminoglycosides (p. 118) may produce or enhance non-depolarizing block, possibly by binding calcium to produce hypocalcaemia, or by influencing the binding of calcium at presynaptic sites. However, antibiotic-induced or -enhanced competitive block is not invariably antagonized by anticholinesterase drugs or by the administration of calcium.

General anaesthetics may have a marked effect on neuromuscular block. Halothane, methoxyflurane and isoflurane potentiate non-depolarizing relaxants such as pancuronium.

Extracellular pH

Hypercapnia augments tubocurarine block and opposes its reversal by neostigmine. Alcuronium and pancuronium block is apparently unaffected by changes in arterial blood carbon dioxide tension, but block due to suxamethonium may be potentiated by acidosis.

A number of explanations have been advanced to account for these findings and it seems likely that factors such as protein binding, ionization of the relaxant and ionization of receptor sites may be important.

Neuromuscular disease

Animals suffering from myasthenia gravis are resistant to depolarizing blockers and are more than normally sensitive to competitive blocking agents. A myopathy has been described in a horse [80] where a generalized muscle spasm was produced by the administration of extremely small doses of suxamethonium.

Genetic factors

Genetic factors in relation to the response to suxamethonium have been described in humans.

Blood pressure and flow

Recovery from the effects of neuromuscular blocking drugs is likely to be more rapid if blood flow through the muscle is high and thus maintains a steep concentration gradient between the tissues and the blood by removing molecules of the agent as soon as they are freed from the receptor sites.

Electrolyte imbalance

A deficiency of calcium, potassium or sodium retards the depolarization of the motor end-plate and by thus inhibiting neuromuscular transmission will increase the blocking effects of the non-depolarizing muscle relaxants. On the other hand, hyperkalaemia and hypernatraemia render muscles more resistant to them.

EVOKED RECOVERY FROM NEUROMUSCULAR BLOCKADE

Many anaesthetists administer an anticholinesterase at the end of anaesthesia to counteract the effects of non-depolarizing neuromuscular blocking drugs as otherwise the relaxant might still occupy a variable but possibly significant number of receptor sites in the immediate postoperative period. In the absence of monitoring of the neuromuscular block, the anaesthetist often assesses neuromuscular function by using respiratory measurements such as tidal volume, respiratory rate or inspiratory and expiratory airway pressures with a temporarily occluded airway. Unfortunately tidal volume and respiratory rate are influenced by many factors unrelated to neuromuscular

function, and the presence of what appears to be adequate spontaneous breathing is in itself no guarantee of adequate recovery from neuromuscular blockade. Non-depolarizing agents have a sparing effect on the diaphragm so that spontaneous breathing can occur in the presence of marked peripheral neuromuscular blockade. This is a particular problem in horses for these animals appear to have a psychological need to stand immediately on recovery from anaesthesia and the presence of even a small degree of peripheral neuromuscular blockade can result in violent excitement and floundering about as the animal tries, unsuccessfully because of muscle weakness, to get to its feet.

There are no effective antidotes to those agents which act by depolarization, but certain anticholinesterases are effective antidotes to the non-depolarizing relaxants and possibly to the 2nd phase block following the use of suxamethonium. The administration of anticholinesterases when dual block is suspected but not proven is not to be recommended since prolonged paralysis requiring several hours of ventilatory support may result.

The three anticholinesterase drugs used today to antagonize the effects of non-depolarizing neuromuscular blockers are neostigmine, edrophonium and pyridostigmine. They may be used to:

1. Restore full respiratory activity at the end of an operation when non-depolarizing agents have been used
2. Antagonize the effects of non-depolarizing agents in an unexpectedly short operation — e.g. when a prolonged operation is contemplated but is found, on surgical exploration, to be impracticable or unnecessary
3. Abolish the occasional long-lasting effects of curarization

The classical view is that their inhibitory action on acetylcholinesterase in the region of the motor endplate results in accumulation of acetylcholine, allowing it to win the competition with the neuromuscular blocking drug for the receptor sites [81]. However, they also induce repetitive firing of the motor nerve terminal, enhancing acetylcholine mobilization and release. There is still some uncertainty as to whether the effect on neuromuscular transmission is due to acetylcholinesterase inhibition or to the blocking of ion channels so as to increase the prejunctional output of acetylcholine. The reversal of neuromuscular blockade by these agents has been well reviewed by Jones [82].

Neostigmine

Neostigmine is probably the most widely used anticholinesterase antagonist of non-depolarizing neuromuscular block. The time course of the antagonizing effect of neostigmine is roughly half-way between that of edrophonium and pyridostigmine, being about 7–10 minutes [83].

Unless neuromuscular block is being monitored by a motor nerve stimulation technique, neostigmine should never be given until there is some sign of spontaneous respiratory activity, otherwise there is no way of assessing its effects and the possibility of passing from a non-depolarization to a depolarization block exists.

An anticholinergic should always be given to counteract the muscarinic effects of neostigmine (bradycardia, salivation, defaecation and urination). Atropine sulphate may be mixed in the syringe with neostigmine and the mixture given in small repeated doses until full respiratory activity is established or monitoring reveals a satisfactory T_4 ratio. It is customary to mix atropine and neostigmine in the ratio of approximately 1:2 (e.g. 1.2 mg of atropine with 2.5 mg of neostigmine, or glycopyrollate with neostigmine). This practice is safe because the anticholinergics exert their effects before the onset of neostigmine activity.

Neostigmine, even if given with full doses of atropine, may cause serious cardiac arrhythmias if there has been gross underventilation during anaesthesia or if carbon dioxide has been allowed to accumulate at the end of the operation with a view to ensuring the return of spontaneous respiration. Hypercapnia also increases the neuromuscular block of non-depolarizing agents and so antagonism is likely to be less effective under these conditions. It has been shown that after anaesthesia in which pulmonary ventilation has been used to lower the carbon dioxide tension of the arterial blood, spontaneous breathing returns at low carbon dioxide tensions, provided that no depressant drugs have been used. This is probably due to the effect of stimuli arising in the trachea and bronchi, skin and, perhaps, to the effect of a sudden increase of afferent nerve impulses resulting from the return of proprioceptive activity in the muscle, as the muscle tone is restored following the administration of neostigmine.

To ensure satisfactory antagonism there must be some return of muscle tone before neostigmine is given: indeed it should not be injected after full doses of the commonly used competitive blocking drugs unless there are obvious signs of return of muscle tone. If necessary, 'reversal' of the block should be delayed and pulmonary ventilation continued until such a time as all four twitches in the train-of-four are visible, or decreasing total chest compliance, attempts at spontaneous breathing or response to stimuli such as movement of the endotracheal tube in the trachea are observed.

In the absence of facilities for the monitoring of neuromuscular block reliance must be placed on clinical signs to assess when reversal is adequate. The signs of residual neuromuscular block include tracheal tug, paradoxical indrawing of the intercostal muscles during inspiration similar to that seen in cases of airway obstruction, and a 'rectangular' breathing pattern in which the inspiratory position is held for some time before expiration begins. The atropine–neostigmine mixture should be given in small doses, with a pause between each, until these signs disappear.

Glycopyrrolate in doses of 0.01 mg/kg may be used

as an alternative to atropine for counteracting the muscarinic effects of neostigmine.

Edrophonium

Recent studies with edrophonium indicate that it is an effective and reliable antagonist to the non-depolarizing agents. Earlier impressions that its effects were too short lasting were probably due to the use of inadequate doses. Doses of edrophonium in excess of 0.5 mg/kg appear to be similar in effect to that of neostigmine but the onset of action is considerably shorter (about 1–3 minutes) making it easier to titrate more accurately its administration to full reversal of the blockade. It is usual to administer it in conjunction with atropine or glycopyrrolate although it may have fewer and more transient muscarinic effects than neostigmine [84].

Pyridostigmine

In the USA pyridostigmine has found favour in some centres. It has a longer duration of action but its long onset time of around 10–15 minutes means that assessment of reversal is difficult if it is administered by a titration method. Katz [85] believed it to have fewer muscarinic effects on the bowel and myocardium than neostigmine, but Fogdall and Miller [86] found no difference. In veterinary practice, it appears to have no significant advantages over neostigmine.

'Recurarization'

'Recurarization' is a term often used to describe relapse into a partially or completely paralysed state following apparently successful reversal of a neuromuscular block. The term is probably not strictly correct for it is possible under certain circumstances to reintroduce neuromuscular block with anticholinesterases. The neuromuscular blocking properties of neostigmine have been known for many years [87] and it is possible to reintroduce neuromuscular block with both neostigmine and edrophonium. The block so introduced following neostigmine may last for up to 30 minutes which is long enough to be clinically significant and may be the explanation for some reports of 'neostigmine-resistant' curarization. In contrast, neuromuscular block reintroduced under similar conditions following edrophonium is not as constant and is much shorter in duration [88].

USE OF NEUROMUSCULAR BLOCKING DRUGS IN VETERINARY ANAESTHESIA

Indications

The general indications for the use of muscle relaxants during anaesthesia in veterinary clinical practice are as follows:

1. To relax the skeletal muscles for easier surgical access.
2. To facilitate control of respiration during intrathoracic surgery.
3. To assist the reduction of dislocated joints. Clinical experience shows that not only are dislocations more easily reduced if the muscles are paralysed but also that reluxation is facilitated by the absence of muscle tone. The reduction of fractures, on the other hand, is seldom eased by the administration of relaxants.
4. To limit the amount of general anaesthetic used when muscular relaxation itself is not the prime requisite. For example, in dogs no muscle relaxation is required during the operation of aural resection but the surgical stimulation is intense and results in head shaking unless the animal is very deeply anaesthetized. The judicious use of muscle relaxant prevents head shaking by weakening the muscles of the neck so very much smaller quantities of anaesthetic or analgesic can be employed. In these circumstances all that is required of the anaesthetic is to produce unconsciousness, and thus the detrimental effects of deep depression of the central nervous system are avoided.
5. To ease the induction of full inhalation anaesthesia in animals already unconscious from intravenous narcotic drugs. For example, when thiopentone is used to induce loss of consciousness in horses before the administration of an inhalant such as halothane, there is a period when the effect of the thiopentone is waning and the uptake of the inhalation agent is not yet sufficient to prevent movement of the limbs. The careful use of small doses of relaxant can do much to 'smooth out' this transitional period by paralysing the limb muscles.
6. To facilitate the performance of endotracheal intubation and endoscopy. Although animals can be intubated without the use of relaxants, the use of these drugs may make endotracheal intubation very much easier, especially in cats and pigs.

Contraindications

It must be very clearly understood that a relaxant should never be administered unless facilities which enable immediate and sustained artificial respiration to be applied to the animal are available. The administration of even small doses of these drugs may, on occasion, be followed by respiratory paralysis. An animal cannot be ventilated efficiently for very long by the application of pressure to the chest wall and artificial respiration must be carried out by the application of intermittent positive pressure to the lungs through an endotracheal tube — the use of a face-mask is not really satisfactory because it is all too easy to inflate the stomach as well as the lungs.

In addition, it must be clearly recognized that neuromuscular blocking drugs have no narcotic or analgesic properties. It is impossible to overemphasize the importance of ensuring beyond all reasonable doubt that during *any surgical operation* an animal is unconscious and incapable of appreciating pain or fear throughout the whole period of action of any neuromuscular blocking drug which may be employed. Fortunately, provided due care is taken, it is a relatively simple matter to ensure this, but any doubt about the maintenance of the unconscious state must constitute an absolute contraindication to the use of neuromuscular blockers.

Experience has shown that caution should be exercised in the use of these drugs in animals suffering from electrolyte imbalance (e.g. cases of intestinal obstruction) or respiratory obstruction.

Technique of use

Several points in the use of relaxant need emphasis and detailed consideration.

Premedication

The induction of anaesthesia by intravenous medication is simple and pleasant for the animal so that heavy sedation with large doses of narcotic or ataractic drugs is neither necessary nor desirable. When, however, the use of an intravenous agent is deemed undesirable and anaesthesia is to be induced with an inhalation agent, somewhat heavier premedication is indicated. In these cases, too, the neuromuscular blocker may be given as soon as consciousness is lost to avoid the occurrence of narcotic excitement with its associated struggling. Atropine or glycopyrollate should always be given to avoid the troublesome salivation and increased bronchial secretion which may otherwise follow the administration of depolarizing agents.

Induction and maintenance of anaesthesia

Induction of anaesthesia with a drug given by intravenous injection has very few contraindications pro-

vided that only minimal doses are employed. The dose used should be only just sufficient to produce loss of consciousness and relaxation of the jaw muscles. Dogs, horses and ruminants may then be intubated. In cats and pigs, the injection of the barbiturate is immediately followed by that of the neuromuscular blocking agent and the animal allowed to breathe oxygen through a close-fitting face-mask until respiration ceases and atraumatic intubation can be performed. These animals are perhaps best intubated under suxamethonium-induced relaxation and full respiration should be allowed to return before a further dose, or another relaxant, is administered.

Endotracheal intubation is most desirable when relaxant drugs are to be used because:

1. A perfectly clear airway is required at all times.
2. Owing to relaxation of oesophageal muscle, the stomach contents are apt to be regurgitated and their passage to the lungs is facilitated by the absence of the protective reflexes of the pharynx and larynx.
3. If the endotracheal tube is not used the stomach and even the intestines may be inflated by gases forced down the oesophagus when positive pressure is applied to the airway at the mouth and nostrils. This may be dangerous and is always a nuisance in abdominal surgery.

Maintenance of anaesthesia involves the administration of further doses of the neuromuscular blocking agent whenever these are indicated, and ensuring that the animal remains lightly anaesthetized throughout the operation.

The indications for supplementary doses of relaxant are relatively easy to state. The drugs are always best given by the intravenous injection of repeated small doses until the desired degree of relaxation is obtained. One exception to this rule is that a dose given prior to endotracheal intubation must be large enough to abolish respiratory movements so that the tube may be introduced between completely relaxed vocal cords. During the operation more neuromuscular blocker is given if muscle relaxation becomes inadequate, or if forceful spontaneous respiratory movements return. When an animal is being maintained in complete apnoea, the dose of relaxant drug used should be such that if given the opportunity (by temporarily suspending IPPV), the animal is just capable of making feeble respiratory efforts. Resistance to inflation of the lungs, in the absence of other obvious causes (e.g. obstruction of the airway), indicates that forceful respiratory efforts are imminent and that a further small dose of relaxant should be given. This sign is readily observable in horses, and in these animals when pressure-cycled ventilators are in use waning relaxation manifests itself by hypoxia and hypercapnia which are easily noted if the blood gases are being monitored. Supplementary doses of neuro-muscular blocking agents given during the course of an operation should, in general, not exceed half the initial dose.

The maintenance of a light plane of anaesthesia throughout the operation is of very great importance. Allowing the animal to awaken to consciousness during the course of an operation clearly cannot be tolerated, yet deep central nervous depression must be avoided if full benefit is to be derived from the use of any relaxant drug. Probably the best agent with which to maintain a light level of unconsciousness is nitrous oxide since this agent can never, in the absence of hypoxia, produce profound depression of the central nervous system. However, nitrous oxide/oxygen mixtures alone may fail to maintain uncon-sciousness, and on these occasions some supplemen-tation will be required. The indications for the supplementation of nitrous oxide/oxygen mixtures when relaxants are being used include:

1. The appearance of signs of vasovagal syncope (pallor, hypotension).
2. A rise in pulse rate which cannot be accounted for by such factors as haemorrhage or tachycardia due to gallamine.
3. The occurrence of reflex movements. Contractions of limb or facial muscles either spontaneously, or in response to stimulation, must be regarded as indicating that the animal is awakening. It is most important to note that these movements can always be seen, even when clinically paralysing doses of neuromuscular blocking drugs have been given, if the depth of unconsciousness becomes too shallow. The reason for this is unknown, but it is tempting to speculate that the γ-fibre endings (see p. 113) are more sensitive to the action of relaxant drugs than are the α-fibre endings, for if this is so the neuromuscular blockers might abolish muscle tonus and produce relaxation without entirely preventing contraction of the muscles due to impulses in the α motor neurones.

The effect of nitrous oxide/oxygen mixtures may be reinforced in three ways:

1. *By overventilation of the animal.* The majority of anaesthetists now believe that overventilation should involve simply hyperinflation of the lungs while the arterial dioxide tension is kept as near normal as possible. Separation of lung inflation from the production of hypocapnia is achieved by ventilating at about twice the spontaneous tidal and minute volumes with increased apparatus dead-space, partial bypass of the soda lime or, in non-rebreathing circuits, with the addition of 4–5% of carbon dioxide to the inspired gases. Use of this technique has shown that the clinically beneficial effects of hyperventilation do not depend on hypocapnia.

2. *By intravenous injections of barbiturates and anal-gesics.* Small intravenous injections of thiopen-tone or an analgesic such as pethidine or fentanyl may be administered as required, and the anaesthetist is then completely aware of the total amounts of all central nervous depressants which have been given. When vigorous overinflation of the lungs without the induction of hypocapnia is practised only very small quantities of intravenous supplements will be required.

3. *By adding other inhalation agents.* Anaesthesia can always be deepened by adding other inhala-tion agents to the nitrous oxide/oxygen mixture. However, unless accurately calibrated vaporizers are used with non-rebreathing circuits, the anaes-thetist is unaware of how much of the agent is being administered to the animal. When halothane or isoflurane is added to nitrous oxide in a circle absorber system with low gas flow rates, a meter such as the EMMA Analyser must be used to monitor the end-tidal concentration, but such meters are not generally available to the veterinary anaesthetist. As a general rule it may be said the use of supplementary inhalation agents with nitrous oxide/oxygen, and the use of more potent agents instead of nitrous oxide to maintain anaes-thesia, are both unwise. Much more needs to be known about the rate of uptake of inhalation agents in domestic animals before their forced administration to any animal can be undertaken with safety. Although under certain circumstances the experienced anaesthetist may safely add low concentrations of the volatile inhalational agents to the inspired nitrous oxide/oxygen mixture in a rebreathing system, this cannot be recommended to the less experienced unless the actual inspired concentration of the agent can be measured.

It must be emphasized that the danger of an animal becoming fully awake during an operation when neuromuscular blocking agents are being used, although always present, should never be allowed to deter the anaesthetist from making full use of them. There should never be any doubt that the animal is unconscious during the whole opera-tion period.

Mixing of muscle relaxants

Theoretically, it is unwise to use drugs of differing actions at the myoneural junction in the same animal at any one time. There is some clinical evidence to support this view yet with a proper appreciation of the risks involved and the avoidance of certain sequences, drugs such as suxamethonium and pancuronium can be given with safety to the animal during one operation. For example, in pigs it is often desirable to produce total paralysis rapidly with suxamethonium so as to obtain the best possible conditions for intubation of the trachea and yet to obtain relaxation throughout the subsequent operation with a non-depolarizing drug. Provided the effects of suxamethonium have worn off (as judged by the respiratory activity) few, if any, harmful effects are seen when the non-depolarizing (competitive) relaxant is given. On the other hand, the use of suxamethonium at the end of a long operation when a non-depolarizing drug has provided the relaxation up to the last few minutes, seems to involve considerable risk of the production of persistent apnoea. The presence of clinically unrecognizable concentrations of non-depolarizing agents at the neuromuscular junction will markedly increase the resistance towards the blocking effects of subsequently administered depolarizing compounds.

Under these circumstances, excessive doses of depolarizing relaxants have to be administered before the desired degree of relaxation can be obtained.

During any operation cumulative effects should not be forgotten — if it is necessary to administer a second dose, the quantity given should not exceed half the total dose used initially to secure the desired degree of relaxation. Various antibiotics (e.g. neomycin, streptomycin) may also have an additive effect at the neuromuscular junction with those of the neuromuscular blocking agent used.

The response of young animals to neuromuscular blocking drugs is different from that of adults. The muscles of a 7 day old kitten are about 10 times less sensitive to depolarizing drugs than those of a normal adult cat but very sensitive to tubocurarine [89]. Lim *et al.* [90] found that the anaesthetic drugs themselves have an age-dependent effect upon neuromuscular transmission so that the complementary relaxation provided by some anaesthetics is variable and important.

POSTOPERATIVE COMPLICATIONS ASSOCIATED WITH THE USE OF NEUROMUSCULAR BLOCKING AGENTS

The most important complication is prolonged apnoea. The best prevention of this complication is the avoidance of excessive doses. The potentially troublesome desensitization of the postjunctional membrane can be avoided if the anaesthetist does not persist with the administration of increasingly larger doses of depolarizing agents in the face of obvious tachyphylaxis to their blocking effect. In the presence of postoperative apnoea, the animal should be ventilated until the cause of the apnoea can be ascertained and treated. If non-depolarizing agents were used during the operation and the cause of apnoea seems to be due to paralysis of the respiratory muscles, it may be treated by the intravenous injection of atropine and an anticholinesterase. There is no antidote to the phase-I block of the depolarizing drugs and the only treatment is ventilation until the return of adequate spontaneous breathing.

When an anticholinergic agent is ineffective but the apnoea appears to be due to neuromuscular block caused by non-depolarizing agents, or is due to a phase-II block, the effects of the intravenous administration of potassium and/or calcium may be tried. In the absence of a urinary output potassium should be given cautiously and if possible myocardial activity should be continuously monitored for incipient electrocardiographic evidence of hyperkalaemia (e.g. high, spiking T waves, shortening of the S-T segment). If the administration of potassium is not effective and there is reason to believe that the plasma level of ionized calcium has been diminished (e.g. after the transfusion of large quantities of citrated blood), calcium gluconate or calcium chloride solutions may be given.

The commonest cause of prolonged apnoea following the use of non-depolarizing agents appears to be hypothermia. Unless precautions are taken to maintain the body temperature it falls in just those operations for which the use of relaxant drugs is indicated — laparotomy and thoracotomy. This fall is particularly great in small animal patients and there is often difficulty in antagonizing the effects of non-depolarizing drugs in these animals until they are rewarmed. Animals should not be left in the postoperative period with any residual neuromuscular block. Harroun *et al.* [91] found that if dogs were returned to their cages with any residual curarization, pulmonary atelectasis invariably developed. Estimation of the tone of the masseter muscle, by gentle traction on the mandible, has proved to be a useful test for detecting slight degrees of muscular weakness. If the masseter tone is good there is unlikely to be trouble with respiration.

CENTRALLY ACTING MUSCLE RELAXANTS

Mephenesin

Mephenesin is a colourless, odourless, crystalline solid soluble in alcohol and propylene glycol. The intravenous injection of a 10% solution leads to a high incidence of venous thrombosis and also to haemolysis which may cause haemoglobinuria, oliguria, uraemia and death. The drug is partly detoxicated in the liver and partly excreted unchanged in the urine. Mephenesin mixed with pentobarbitone was introduced for canine and feline anaesthesia but the mixture did not prove to have any significant advantage over pentobarbitone alone. Mephenesin has many side-effects and it is no longer used in anaesthesia.

Guaiphenesin BP

Guaiphenesin is a mephenesin-like compound which has been used in Germany for many years [92–95] and is now used widely throughout the world. Its effects in horses have been extensively studied [96–99]. Concentrated solutions (over 10%) in water or 5% in glucose have been associated with haemolysis, haemoglobinuria and venous thrombosis [98, 99] and although the recently introduced 15% stabilized solutions are said to be free from these effects there is evidence that they cause thrombosis. Solutions of 10% in water have minimal haemolytic effect — they have an osmolality of 242 mOsm/kg which is closer to the osmolality of equine plasma than the formerly recommended 5% solution or those in dextrose [100]. Injection into the tissues causes swelling, pain, abscesses and necrosis so that accurate intravenous injection is essential. Venous thrombosis is potentially very serious; it is a delayed complication and may be related to the speed of injection since it has been reported as occurring with all formulations of guaiphenesin, particularly when they were infused under pressure [99].

Cardiovascular depression has been shown to be dose dependent. In healthy horses, heart rate is increased and arterial blood pressure decreased when guaiphenesin is administered with minimal doses of thiobarbiturate [101–103]. Respiration is also depressed by guaiphenesin, an increase in frequency being insufficient to compensate for a reduction in tidal volume so that the arterial carbon dioxide tension rises [104, 105]. The duration of action in male horses is 1.5 times that in mares but there is apparently no sex difference in the doses required to produce relaxation [106]. In contrast to the neuro-muscular blocking agents, significant amounts of the drug cross the placental barrier.

Following premedication with acepromazine (0.04 mg/kg intravenously) or xylazine (0.6 mg/kg intravenously) a mixture of guaiphenesin and thiobarbiturate given 'to effect' will produce about 20 minutes of immobilization in horses. The usual dose requirement is about 4 mg/kg of the thiobarbiturate and 100 mg/kg of guaiphenesin. Completing the induction of anaesthesia with halothane often produces marked arterial hypotension but the pressure recovers slowly over the next 20–30 minutes. The abdominal relaxation obtained with doses of guaiphenesin which do not interfere with respiratory activity is never as good as can be produced with the proper use of neuromuscular blocking drugs, but it may be useful in situations where inhalation anaesthesia cannot be used or the services of a specialist anaesthetist are not available. For short operations, doses in excess of 50 mg/kg of guaiphenesin may be associated with marked ataxia in the recovery period and this can give rise to excitement unless a small dose of a sedative such as xylazine is given at the end of operation.

In horses under chloral hydrate narcosis, intravenous doses of 3–4 g/50 kg of guaiphenesin are claimed to produce surgically useful degrees of abdominal relaxation lasting 10–15 minutes, without at the same time causing significant respiratory depression [107]. Relaxation of the pharyngeal and laryngeal muscles is sufficient to facilitate endotracheal intubation.

The drug may be used to cast cattle. If these animals are premedicated with tranquillizers and analgesics the necessary dose for casting purposes is 4–5 g/50 kg, i.e. about 1 litre of the 5% solution in any animal weighing 500 kg. Towards the end or after the completion of this intravenous injection the animal starts to sway and then falls relaxed. Barbiturates may be mixed with the solution (e.g. 0.25 g of thiobarbiturate per 50 kg body weight) but as the two drugs potentiate each other most animals then fall during the infusion, which is completed in the cast position.

Guaiphenesin has been used in other species of animal but its administration is rendered difficult by the large volumes of solution which must be infused. Even in horses and cattle this is a considerable disadvantage associated with its use, for ataxia develops as the solution is run into the vein and care has to be exercised to avoid the type of injury to the animal resulting from stumbling when the hind legs are crossed.

REFERENCES

1. Katz, B. and Miledi, R. (1965) *Proceedings of the Royal Society (London)* **183**, 421.
2. Miledi, R. (1973) *Proceedings of the Royal Society (London)* **183**, 421.
3. Dodge, F. A. J. and Rahamimoff, R. (1967) *Journal of Physiology* **193**, 419.
4. Lawson, N. W., Kraynack, B. J. and Gintautas, J. (1983) *Anesthesia and Analgesia* **62**, 504.
5. Jones, R. M. (1984) *Anaesthesia* **39**, 747.
6. Lynch, C., Vogel, S. and Sperelakis, N. (1980) *Anesthesiology* **53**, S420.
7. Auer, J. and Meltzer, S. J. (1914) *Journal of Pharmacology and Experimental Therapeutics* **5**, 521.
8. Pollard, B. J. and Millar, R. A. (1973) *British Journal of Anaesthesia* **45**, 404.
9. Koelle, G. B. (1962) *Journal of Pharmacy and Pharmacology* **14**, 65.
10. Das, M., Ganguly, D. K. and Vedasiromoni, J. R. (1978) *British Journal of Pharmacology* **62**, 195.
11. Standaert, F. G. and Dretchen, K. L. (1979) *Federation Proceedings* **38**, 2183.
12. Bowman, W. C. and Nott, M. W. (1969) *Pharmacological Reviews* **21**, 27.
13. Fatt, P. (1950) *Journal of Physiology* **111**, 408.
14. Katz, B. and Thesleff, S. (1967) *Journal of Physiology* **138**, 63.
15. Paton, W. D. M. and Waud, D. R. (1967) *Journal of Physiology* **191**, 59.
16. Cookson, J. C. and Paton, W. D. M. (1969) *Anaesthesia* **24**, 395.
17. Burns, B. D. and Paton, W. D. M. (1951) *Journal of Physiology* **115**, 41.
18. Zamis, E. J. (1952) *Nature, London* **170**, 617.
19. Foldes, F. F., Wnuck, A. L., Hamer-Hodges, R. J., Thesleff, S. and de Beer, E. J. (1957) *Anesthesia and Analgesia* **36**, 23.
20. Bennett, A. E. (1940) *Journal of the American Medical Association* **114**, 322.
21. Griffith, H. R. and Johnson, G. E. (1942) *Anesthesiology* **3**, 418.
22. Gray, T. C. and Halton, J. (1946) *Proceedings of the Royal Society of Medicine* **39**, 400.
23. Utting, J. E. (1963) *British Journal of Anaesthesia* **135**, 706.
24. Kalow, W. (1959) *Anesthesiology* **20**, 505.
25. Pickett, D. (1951) *Journal of the American Veterinary Medical Association* **119**, 346.
26. Gray, T. C. and Gregory, R. A. (1948) *Anaesthesia* **3**, 17.
27. Booth, N. H. and Rankin, A. D. (1953) *American Journal of Veterinary Research* **14**, 51, 59.
28. Lee, C., Chen, D., Barnes, A. and Katz, R. L. (1976) *Canadian Anaesthesia Society Journal* **23**, 527.
29. Pittinger, C. and Adamson, R. (1972) *Annual Review of Pharmacology* **12**, 169.
30. Singh, Y. N., Marshall, I. G. and Harvey, A. L. (1978) *British Journal of Anaesthesia* **501**, 109.
31. Singh, Y. N., Marshall, I. G. and Harvey, A. L. (1979) *British Journal of Anaesthesia* **51**, 1027.
32. Bovet, D., Depierre, F. and De Lestrange, Y. (1947) *Academy of Science, Paris* **225**, 74.
33. Mushin, W. W., Wien, R., Mason, D. F. J. and Langston, G. T. (1949) *Lancet* **i**, 72.36.
34. Jones, R. S., Heckmann, R. and Wuersch, W. (1978) *Research in Veterinary Science* **25**, 101.
35. Booiji, L. H. D. J., Edwards, R. P., Yung, J. S., Sohn, M. D. and Miller, R. D. (1980) *Anesthesia and Analgesia* **30**, 26.
36. McLeod, K., Watson, J. J. and Rawlins, M. D. (1976) *British Journal of Anaesthesia* **48**, 341.
37. Westra, P., Houwertjes, M. C., DeLang, A. R., Scaf, A. H. J., Hindriks, F. R. and Agoston, S. (1980) *British Journal of Anaesthesia* **52**, 747.
38. Jones, R. S. (1985) *Research in Veterinary Science* **38**, 193.
39. Duveldestin, P., Demetrion, M. and Depoix, J. P. (1983) *Clinical Experiences with Norcuron* (ed. S. Agoston), p. 92. Exerpta Medica.
40. Westra, P., Houwertjes, M. C., Wessling, H. and Meyer, D. F. K. (1981) *British Journal of Anaesthesia* **53**, 407.
41. Jones, R. S. and Seymour, C. J. (1985) *Journal of Small Animal Practice* **26**, 213.
42. Payne, J. P. and Hughes, R. (1981) *British Journal of Anaesthesia* **53**, 45.
43. Jones, R. S. (1987) *Research in Veterinary Science* **43**, 101.
44. Jones, R. S. (1987) *Research in Veterinary Science* **43**, 308.
45. Collier, H. O. J. (1950) *British Medical Journal* **i**, 1293.
46. Savege, T. M., Blogg, C. E., Ross, L. A., Lang, M. and Simpson, B. R. (1973) *Anaesthesia* **28**, 253.
47. Simpson, B. R., Savege, T. M., Foley, E. I., Ross, L. A., Strunin, L., Wallon, B., Maxwell, M. P. and Harris, D. M. (1973) *Lancet* **i**, 516.
48. Clarke, K. W. (1977) *Proceedings of the Association of Veterinary Anaesthetists of GB and Ireland* **7**, 1.
49. Norman, J. (1982) *Anaesthesia Review* (ed. L. Kaufman), vol. 1, p. 84. Edinburgh: Churchill Livingstone.
50. Norman, J., Katz, R. L. and Seed, R. F. (1970) *British Journal of Anaesthesia* **42**, 702.
51. Paton, W. D. M. and Zaimis, E. J. (1948) *Nature, London* **162**, 810.
52. Bovet, D., Bovet-Nitti, F., Guarino, S., Longo, V. G. and Fuaco, R. (1951) *Archives of International Pharmacodynamics* **88**, 1.
53. Bovet, D., Courvoisier, S. and De Lestrange, Y. (1949) *Archives of International Pharmacodynamics* **80**, 172.
54. Buttle, G. A. H. and Zaimis, E. J. (1949) *Journal of Pharmacology* **1**, 991.
55. Edridge, A. (1952) *Proceedings of the Royal Society of Medicine* **45**, 869.
56. Hall, L. W. (1952) *Veterinary Record* **64**, 491.
57. Airaksinen, M. M. and Tammisto, T. (1966) *Clinical Pharmacology* **7**, 583.
58. Tammisto, T., Leikkonen, P. and Airaksinen, M. (1967) *Acta Anaesthesiologies Scandinavica* **11**, 333.
59. Hall, L. W., Lehmann, H. and Silk, E. (1953) *British Medical Journal* **i**, 134.
60. Hansson, C. H. (1957) *Nordisk Veterinarmedicin* **9**, 753.
61. Faye, S. (1988) Ph.D. Thesis, University of Leeds.
62. Adams, A. K. and Hall, L. W. (1962) *British Journal of Anaesthesia* **34**, 445.
63. Adams, A. K. and Hall, L. W. (1962) *Proceedings of the 1st European Congress of Anaesthesia*, Vienna.
64. Stevenson, D. E. (1960) *British Journal of Anaesthesia* **32**, 364.

65. Bowen, J. M. (1969) *American Journal of Veterinary Research* **30**, 857.
66. Jones, R. S. and Prentice, D. E. (1976) *British Veterinary Journal* **132**, 226.
67. Bowen, J. M., Blackman, D. M. and Heaver, J. E. (1970) *American Journal of Veterinary Research* **31**, 831.
68. Hechmann, R., Jones, R. S. and Wuersch, W. (1977) *Research in Veterinary Science* **23**, 1.
69. Jones, R. S., Hechmann, R. and Wuersch, W. (1978) *Research in Veterinary Science* **25**, 101.
70. Ali, H. H., Utting, J. E. and Grey, T. C. (1971) *British Journal of Anaesthesia* **43**, 473.
71. Cullen, L. K. and Jones, R. S. (1980) *Research in Veterinary Science* **29**, 266.
72. Cullen, L. K. and Jones, R. S. (1980) *Research in Veterinary Science* **29**, 277.
73. Cullen, L. K. and Jones, R. S. (1980) *Research in Veterinary Science* **29**, 281.
74. Klein, L. V. (1981) *Veterinary Clinics of North America*, vol. 3, No. 1, p. 152. Philadelphia: W. B. Saunders.
75. Ali, H. H. and Savarese, J. J. (1976) *Anesthesiology* **45**, 216.
76. Ali, H. H., Savarese, J. J., Lebowitz, P. W. and Ramsey, F. M. (1981) *Anesthesiology* **54**, 294.
77. Jones, R. M. (1985) *Anesthesiology* **40**, 964.
78. Williams, N. E., Webb, S. N. and Calvey, T. N. (1980) *British Journal of Anaesthesia* **52**, 1111.
79. Engbaek, L., Ostergaard, D. and Vibay-Mogensen, J. (1989) *British Journal of Anaesthesia* **62**, 274.
80. Jones, R. S. and Ritchie, H. E. (1965) *British Journal of Anaesthesia* **37**, 142.
81. Randall, L. O. and Lehman, G. (1950) *Journal of Pharmacology and Experimental Therapeutics* **99**, 16.
82. Jones, R. S. (1988) *Journal of the Association of Veterinary Anaesthetists* **15**, 80.
83. Baird, W. L. M. and Kerr, W. J. (1983) *British Journal of Anaesthesia* **55**, 63S.
84. Cronelly, R., Morris, R. B. and Miller, R. D. (1982) *Anesthesiology* **57**, 261.
85. Katz, R. I. (1967) *Anesthesiology* **28**, 528.
86. Fogdall, R. P. and Miller, R. D. (1973) *Anesthesiology* **39**, 504.
87. Briscoe, G. (1936) *Journal of Physiology* **86**, 48P.
88. Astley, B. (1987) *Anaesthesia Review* (ed. L. Kaufman), vol. 4, p. 188. Edinburgh: Churchill Livingstone.
89. Maclagan, J. and Vrbova, G. (1966) *Journal of Physiology* **182**, 131.
90. Lim, H. S., Davenport, H. T. and Robson, J. G. (1964) *Anesthesiology* **25**, 161.
91. Harroun, P., Berkert, G. E. and Hathaway, H. R. (1946) *Anesthesiology* **7**, 24.
92. Frey, R., Gopfert, R. and Raule, P. (1952) *Anaesthetist* **1**, 33.
93. Marcus, G. H. and Lobermeyer, G. (1955) *Anaesthetist* **4**, 167.
94. Dietz, O., Krause, W. and Sattler, H. G. (1959) *Monatshefte fur Veterinarmedicin* **14**, 363.
95. Krause, H. and Illing, K. (1960) *Monatshefte fur Veterinarmedicin* **15**, 22.
96. Westhues, M. (1960) *Tieraerztl Wochenschrift* **73**, 463.
97. Fritsch, R. (1961) *Deutsche Tierarztliche Wochenschrift* **68**, 123.
98. Funk, K. A. (1973) *Equine Veterinary Journal* **5**, 1.
99. Schatzman, U. (1974) *Equine Veterinary Journal* **6**, 164.
100. Grandy, J. L. and McDonell, W. N. (1980) *Journal of the American Veterinary Medical Association* **176**, 619.
101. Heath, R. B. and Gabel, A. A. (1970) *Journal of the American Veterinary Medical Association* **157**, 1486.
102. Wright, M., McGrath, C. J. and Raffe, M. (1979) *Veterinary Anaesthesia* **VI**, 41.
103. Schatzman, U. (1980/1) *Proceedings of the Association of Veterinary Anaesthetists of Great Britain and Ireland* **9**, 153.
104. Muir, W. W., Skarda, R. T. and Milne, D. W. (1977) *American Journal of Veterinary Research* **38**, 195.
105. Muir, W. W., Skarda, R. T. and Sheehan, W. (1978) *American Journal of Veterinary Research* **39**, 1274.
106. Davis, L. E. and Wolff, W. A. (1970) *American Journal of Veterinary Research* **31**, 469.
107. Westhues, M. and Fritsch, R. (1961) *Die Narkose der Tiere: Allgemeinnarkose*. Berlin: Paul Parey.

CHAPTER 8

ARTIFICIAL VENTILATION OF THE LUNGS

Special techniques to ventilate the lungs when the respiratory muscles are paralysed by neuromuscular blocking drugs or rendered inactive by central nervous depression have evolved gradually over a number of years. Today, they usually involve endotracheal intubation together with periodic inflation of the lungs and the commonest method used is known as 'intermittent positive-pressure ventilation of the lungs' or 'IPPV'. It was first employed during intrathoracic surgery but it is now much more widely used in anaesthesia. It is also a routine technique used in intensive care whenever respiratory failure occurs. There are certain differences between IPPV when the thoracic cage is opened widely at thoracotomy from when it is intact, and the anaesthetist must appreciate what these differences are if IPPV is to be correctly managed under all circumstances.

OPENING OF THE PLEURAL CAVITY

When a normal-size unilateral thoracotomy incision is made the ipsilateral lung collapses, spontaneous respiratory movements become more vigorous and the mediastinum moves from side to side with each respiratory effort. Unless proper measures are applied without delay death from hypoxaemia is inevitable.

Collapse of the lung

Distension of the lungs to fill the thoracic cavity is due to the existence of a pressure gradient between the airway and the pleural cavity. The airway pressure is usually atmospheric and the intrapleural pressure subatmospheric due to the outward recoil forces of the chest wall and the limited expansibility of the lungs. This distending force is opposed by what has been termed the 'elasticity' of the lung tissue, although the term 'elasticity' is not strictly applicable because surface tension in the alveoli contributes in a most important manner to the lung retractive force. When the chest is opened and atmospheric pressure allowed to act directly in the pleural cavity, the normal pressure gradient is abolished and the retractive forces cause the lung to collapse (Fig. 8.1). Blood flowing through the collapsed lung returns unoxygenated to the arterial side of the circulation.

Mediastinal movement

In any normal animal the mediastinum is not a rigid partition between the two halves of the chest. Veterinary anatomists have made much of the presence or

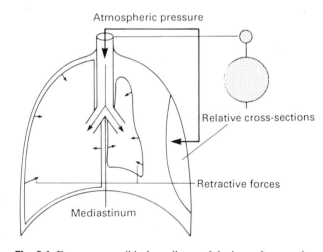

Fig. 8.1 Forces responsible for collapse of the lung after opening of the chest wall.

absence of fenestration in the mediastinum but in practice this seems unimportant and the behaviour of each half of the chest during respiration is always dependent on the conditions prevailing in the other half. Unilateral pneumothorax can occur in all domestic animals and its presence causes the mediastinum to move towards the intact side during inspiration and the opposite way during expiration. This movement of the mediastinum results in obstruction of the thin-walled great veins and thus impedes the venous return to the heart. However, this impediment poses little problem and death is usually due to the effects of hypoxia rather than circulatory failure.

Paradoxical respiration

Paradoxical respiration is seen at thoracotomy or after disruption of the chest wall by trauma. The paradox is that during spontaneous breathing the lung on the damaged side of the chest becomes smaller on inspiration and larger on expiration.

When the thorax enlarges at inspiration its increased volume comes to be occupied by:

1. Air which enters the lungs
2. Blood which enters the right atrium and great veins

In the presence of an open pneumothorax air enters not only into the lungs via the trachea but also through the chest wall defect into the pleural cavity. The proportion of air entering by each route is largely governed by the relative sizes of the trachea and chest wall defect. When the opening in the chest wall is large, or when there is any degree of airway obstruction, the greater volume of air will enter through the defect into the pleural cavity and the mediastinum will be pushed towards the intact side of the chest.

During inspiration, pressure in the collapsed lung is greater than in the trachea because the pressure created by the retractive forces of that lung is added to that of the atmosphere. Thus, on inspiration the increased volume on the intact side of the chest is occupied by air from the collapsed lung as well as from the atmosphere (Fig. 8.2). The exposed lung, therefore, becomes smaller. On expiration the reverse

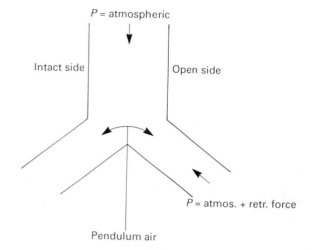

Fig. 8.2 Unilateral pneumothorax: effect on intrabronchial pressures.

occurs and air from the lung on the intact side is discharged partly into the collapsed lung which becomes larger. In this way an animal with an open pneumothorax breathing spontaneously shuttles air from one lung to the other at each breath. This 'pendulum air' produces, in effect, an increase in respiratory dead-space, and the animal's respiratory efforts are less effective in producing proper pulmonary ventilation.

ARTIFICIAL LUNG VENTILATION

Prior to the introduction of IPPV, the gross mediastinal movement, hypoxia and circulatory disturbance resulting from the events described above were nearly insurmountable obstacles in intrathoracic surgery. This surgery only really became practicable when it was shown that raising the pressure in the trachea to above atmospheric during inspiration and lowering it to atmospheric or subatmospheric during expiration causes air to flow into both lungs at inspiration and from both during expiration; 'pendulum air' is no longer a problem and surgically embarrassing mediastinal movement is abolished. The introduction of muscle relaxants necessitated the use of IPPV during other types of surgery.

IPPV is easily applied during anaesthesia by rhythmical compression of the reservoir bag of a breathing circuit. This is most simply achieved by manual squeezing, but machines have been designed and built to relieve the anaesthetist of the bag-squeezing duty. If the bag is squeezed as the animal breathes in, the tidal volume may be augmented ('assisted

respiration'). The increased ventilation produced results in 'washout' of carbon dioxide and the arterial carbon dioxide tension falls below the threshold for stimulating the respiratory centre so that spontaneous breathing movements cease and the anaesthetist can impose whatever respiratory rhythm is required — 'controlled respiration'.

A properly used machine undoubtedly provides the most efficient means of ventilating the lungs for prolonged periods, but to use a machine properly, or even to squeeze a bag correctly, it is essential to understand the principles underlying IPPV and to know under what circumstances any possible harmful effects may arise.

Compliance has been defined in many ways but the simplest definition is that of Comroe *et al.* [1] — 'volume change produced by unit pressure change'. Ideally the measurements necessary for the calculation of this value should be made when no air is flowing into or out of the lungs (i.e. at the end of inspiration). As Comroe *et al.* point out very clearly, compliance measurements cannot be compared unless related to a lung volume such as the functional residual capacity (FRC). Unfortunately, measurement of FRC is not a simple procedure and such measurements as have been made in large animals [2, 3] have omitted this refinement. As normally measured, compliance has two components and compliance values can be found for both the lungs themselves and the thoracic cage but, of course, during thoracotomy the total compliance measured approaches that of the lungs alone. During anaesthesia the compliance may be altered by assistants resting their weight on the chest, by the use of retractors and by the degree of muscle relaxation. Airway resistance has to be overcome to deliver air to the alveoli at inspiration and to expel it during expiration. Unlike compliance, airway resistance must be measured during air flow. It becomes less as lung volume increases [1] and is less during inspiration than expiration.

Airway resistance during anaesthesia is increased by the resistance of apparatus, such as endotracheal tubes, which may be used. Animals with pulmonary disease may also have increased resistance and, for example, Gillespie *et al.* [4] have shown that 'broken-winded' horses have a rapid increase in airway resistance at the end of expiration. The effects of a sudden increase in airway resistance at the end of expiration must be clearly understood by the anaesthetist if trouble is to be avoided during IPPV. If the expiratory period of the IPPV is too short the lungs may not have time to empty completely because the increase in resistance will delay the expulsion of air from the lungs. This will mean that the lung volume will be greater at the start of the next inspiration. Thus, there will be a steady increase in FRC until the retractive force of the lungs, which increases with increase in lung volume [5], becomes sufficient to empty the lungs to a new FRC in the time available and the inspiratory and expiratory tidal volumes become equal. While conscious, the 'broken-winded' horse empties the lungs by active expiratory movements but when anaesthetized and under the influence of a muscle relaxant expiration may become passive and, consequently, longer in duration. The pattern of IPPV used must make allowance for this, and large tidal volumes should be delivered with long expiratory pauses between each inspiration.

Airway resistance is frictional in nature due to the movement of gas molecules through the air passages, but the tissues of the lungs and chest wall must also offer a resistance to movement due to their displacement during the breathing cycle. However, Comroe *et al.* consider that the magnitude of this resistance is seldom likely to interfere with pulmonary function. These workers found that in healthy young men the pulmonary tissue resistance afforded only about 20% of the total pulmonary resistance; the airway resistance was responsible for the remainder.

To overcome pulmonary resistance a driving force has to be applied to the upper airway (conveniently referred to as 'the mouth') to produce an airflow through the respiratory passages. An analogy can be drawn with Ohm's Law, where, $R = E/I$, and the formula written: Resistance = Driving pressure/Flow. During spontaneous breathing the driving pressure must be atmospheric less the alveolar pressure during inspiration and, during expiration, the alveolar pressure less atmospheric pressure. During IPPV the driving pressure or force during inspiration will be atmospheric pressure plus the pressure exerted on the reservoir bag less the alveolar pressure, but during expiration the driving pressure will be alveolar less atmospheric pressure unless a subatmospheric pressure is applied at the mouth.

Consideration of the 'flow formula' where Resistance = Driving pressure/Flow shows that if the resistance is low and a small volume has to be delivered only a small driving pressure is required. If, however, the resistance is increased and/or a greater flow is required, the driving pressure must be greater. This is important, for registration of the pressure in the upper airway is often used to monitor the tidal volume delivered by a ventilator — increasing the pressure is assumed to increase the tidal volume delivered. While this may be so if the pulmonary resistance is low, considerable caution must be exercised in translating a pressure reading taken somewhere in the upper airway into a volume of gas actually reaching the alveoli. Mushin *et al.* [6] have clearly explained how a high gas flow into the lungs, or a high airway resistance, can lead to the peak pressures recorded in the upper airways being much higher than the final peak alveolar pressure so that lung compliance cannot be easily calculated from upper airway pressures and consequently, related changes in lung volume cannot be assumed.

Airway resistance also depends on the nature of the airflow through the airway. With a clear airway and a low gas flow rate, flow is laminar (streamlined) and airway resistance is also low, but obstruction or a high flow velocity will give rise to turbulence and a greatly increased resistance. The many branches of the tracheobronchial tree tend to cause turbulent flow patterns, especially where there are irregularities in the bronchial tubes (blebs of mucus, foreign bodies, *Filaroides* nodules, etc.) and the effect will be greater at high gas flow rates. Thus, during IPPV, attempts to produce large gas flows to minimize the duration of inspiration may necessitate the use of high driving pressures but, of course, the airway resistance will normally prevent the direct transmission of these pressures to the alveoli.

Anaesthetic apparatus may afford resistance which is considerably higher than that offered by the animal's respiratory tract. It is difficult to say at what level this apparatus resistance becomes intolerable because a healthy anaesthetized animal seems able to compensate for quite high external resistances to breathing. Nevertheless, common sense would seem to suggest that apparatus resistance should be kept as low as possible. Purchase [2, 7] studied the resistance afforded by four closed circuits used in horses and cattle and in three, all of which had internal bores of 5 cm, found it to be in the order of 1 cmH$_2$O (0.1 kPa) per 100 l/min at flow rates of 600 l/min, which seems acceptable. He also found that the resistance of endotracheal tube connectors was relatively high in comparison with that of the rest of the apparatus.

Mean intrathoracic pressure may be above or below atmospheric pressure as a result of apparatus resistance. For example, if the expiratory flow through a piece of apparatus with a high resistance is great enough to produce turbulence whilst the inspiratory rate is lower (as it often seems to be in horses) so that the flow is laminar, the mean intrathoracic pressure will be above atmospheric. Conversely, if the inspiratory flow rate is greater there may be a subatmospheric mean intrathoracic pressure. Mean intrathoracic pressures above atmospheric pressure may cause cardiovascular failure in hypovolaemic states [8]. High subatmospheric mean pressures may be equally dangerous, perhaps by producing pulmonary oedema, but probably more importantly by reducing lung volume. Trapping of gas in the lungs occurs more readily at low lung volumes [9] and in man, for example, an alveolar pressure of 5 cmH$_2$O (0.5 kPa) below atmospheric produces widespread airway obstruction with quite serious impairment of respiratory function.

Differences between IPPV and spontaneous respiration

In a spontaneously breathing animal active contraction of the inspiratory muscles lowers the normally subatmospheric intrapleural pressure still further by enlarging the thoracic cavity. The decrease in intrapleural pressure lowers the alveolar pressure so that a pressure gradient or driving force is set up between the exterior and the alveoli to overcome the airway resistance. Air flows into the alveoli until at the end of inspiration the alveolar pressure becomes equal to the atmospheric pressure. During expiration the pressure gradient is reversed and air flows out of the alveoli.

The pressure gradient between the pleural cavity and the exterior is largely taken up in overcoming the

retractive forces of the lungs and provided the airway is clear, the remaining small alveolar–exterior pressure gradient set up during inspiration is quite adequate to overcome the airway resistance and produce airflow into the lungs. The concept of intrapleural pressure is, however, difficult to explain. The pleural cavity is under the influence of gravity and if two bubbles of air are introduced into it, one some distance above the other, the pressure which can be measured in them will not be the same — the pressure in the lower bubble will be found to be greater. In man, according to Agostoni and Mead [10], the pressure of the pleural fluid facing the lowest part of the lungs is probably about −5 cmH$_2$O (−0.5 kPa), or just enough to keep the lung expanded and hence equal to the pleural surface pressure. The pressure in the upper part of the pleural cavity should be much more below atmospheric, but it is not at all certain how uniform the pressure on the pleural surface of the lung really is; the hilar forces, the buoyancy of the lung in the pleural cavity and the different shapes of the lung and chest wall are all possible sources of local pressure differences [11]. Because, therefore, there is no one intrapleural pressure it is now customary to measure the intra-oesophageal pressure instead. The changes in intrapleural (oesophageal) pressure in relation to changes in upper airway (mouth) pressure during spontaneous breathing and IPPV are compared and contrasted in Fig. 8.3.

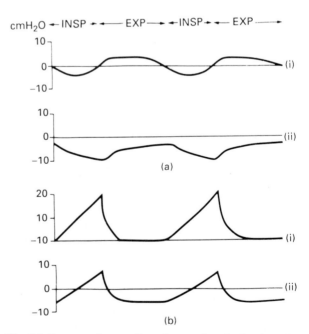

Fig. 8.3 Pressure changes (i) at the mouth end of endotracheal tube and (ii) in the thoracic oesophagus during (a) spontaneous breathing and (b) during IPPV. (After Mushin *et al.* [6], with values obtained from a 420 kg horse ventilated after paralysis with 120 mg *d*-tubocurarine.)

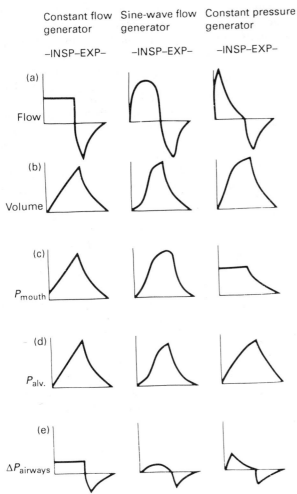

Constant flow generator — Sine-wave flow generator — Constant pressure generator

–INSP–EXP–   –INSP–EXP–   –INSP–EXP–

(a) Flow

(b) Volume

(c) P_{mouth}

(d) $P_{alv.}$

(e) $\Delta P_{airways}$

Fig. 8.4 Characteristics of three types of lung ventilator. (a) Flow pattern; (b) volume change in the lung; (c) pressure change at the mouth; (d) pressure changes in the alveoli; (e) pressure gradient across the airway. (After a diagram in *Automatic Ventilation of the Lungs* by W. W. Mushin *et al.*, Blackwell Scientific, Oxford.)

Possible harmful effects of controlled respiration

From the above considerations it is obvious that IPPV can involve considerable interference with the physiological processes concerned in normal breathing.

Perhaps the most obvious effect of IPPV is on the circulatory system. During spontaneous breathing, inspiration, by lowering intrathoracic pressure, augments the venous return to the heart and in many animals, as can often be seen on a tracing of continuously recorded blood pressure, there are indications that an increase in stroke volume is produced. During controlled respiration, however, the intrathoracic pressure rises during inspiration, blood is dammed back from the thorax, venous return and stroke volume decrease; blood flows freely into the thoracic vessels during the expiratory period. Fortunately, this damming back of blood during inspiration by causing distension of veins produces a reflex increase in venous tone which in normal animals appears to compensate for the changed intrathoracic conditions during the inspiratory period and restores the venous return towards normality. Obviously, the extent to which an increase in venous tone can compensate will depend on the degree of venomotor integrity (which can probably be affected by drugs), on the blood volume, the magnitude of the intrathoracic pressure rise and its duration.

The magnitude and duration of the increased pressure within the thorax during the inspiratory phase of IPPV are critical and are reflected in the 'mean intrathoracic pressure'. This mean pressure, like the mean arterial blood pressure, is not the simple arithmetical mean between the highest and lowest pressures reached in the system and its calculation is not always easy for the non-mathematician. It is clearly important to keep this mean pressure as low as possible during the respiratory cycle and this can be attempted in a variety of ways:

1. *Short application of positive pressure.* The shorter the inspiratory period during IPPV the lower the resulting mean intrathoracic pressure will be for any given applied pressure. Theoretically, it might seem that the peak pressure should never be maintained — expiration should commence as soon as the peak pressure is achieved — or the circulation will suffer. However, the short application of a positive pressure to the airway may not result in very good distribution of fresh gas within the lungs. In man, Watson [12] demonstrated that very short inspiratory periods have the effect of increasing the physiological dead-space (see p. 46) while Hall *et al.* [13] found a decrease in the physiological dead-space/tidal volume ratio in horses ventilated with the ventilator designed by Fowler *et al.* [14] which has a relatively long inspiratory phase. A compromise seems to be necessary here, but exactly what it is likely to be for any one animal of any one species remains pure speculation.

2. *Rapid gas flow rate.* If the necessary tidal volume of gas is to be delivered to the lungs in a short inspiratory period it is clear that the flow rate will need to be high. The rate at which gas can flow into the lungs, however, is largely dictated by the resistance offered by:
   (a) The apparatus used
   (b) The airway resistance
   Here it must be recalled that the airway resistance

to the various regions of the lung may not be uniform. For example, a bleb of mucus may partially obstruct a small bronchus and greatly increase the resistance to gas flow through it. A high gas flow rate through a neighbouring, unobstructed bronchus may result in overdistension of the alveoli supplied by it in an interval of time so short that the alveoli supplied by the partially obstructed bronchus will not have time for more than minimal expansion. Theoretically, it would seem that under these circumstances alveolar rupture might occur, but in practice this complication seems rare. It may well be that sufficiently high flow rates are not generated during the methods of IPPV which are currently used in veterinary anaesthesia.

3. *Low expiratory resistance.* Because any resistance to the air flow created by the passive expiratory phase of IPPV will delay the fall in intrathoracic pressure it will result in an increase in the mean intrathoracic pressure and possibly in circulatory embarrassment. However, Comroe *et al.* [1] point out that in patients with obstructive emphysema the use of expiratory resistance will result in a more orderly emptying of the alveoli and an increase in FRC with consequent widening of the airways. Thus, at least in some circumstances, a higher expiratory resistance may in fact be advantageous to an animal.

4. *Subatmospheric pressure during the expiratory phase.* If a subatmospheric pressure is applied to the airway during the expiratory part of the IPPV cycle the inspiratory pressure will be applied to the airway from a lower baseline. Hence the pressure gradient necessary to produce the required volume change in the lungs can be achieved with a lower peak pressure. A subatmospheric phase in the cycle may therefore help to maintain cardiac output, but the changes in arterial pressure and cardiac output are proportional to the duration of the increased airway pressure and not necessarily simply to the peak pressures reached [15] so that merely decreasing the peak pressure may have only little effect if the inspiratory phase is long. Such studies as have been performed to investigate the effects of a subatmospheric phase on the cardiac output have produced equivocal results and many of the published reports do not contain enough details of the physical characteristics of the subatmospheric phase to make their comparison possible. Clinical experience in dogs with Manley ventilators suggests that the beneficial effects resulting from the use of a subatmospheric expiratory phase, if they exist, are difficult to appreciate. Certainly, during thoracotomy its application will cause the lungs to collapse so completely that re-

expansion may be difficult, and in animals suffering from emphysema where air trapping occurs, its use will result in further impairment of the expiratory gas flow.

It might be expected that most of the potentially harmful effects of IPPV on the circulatory system would be absent during thoracotomy. An opening in the chest wall should prevent compression of pulmonary capillaries when positive pressure is applied to the airway, leading to less interference with blood flow through the lungs. Nevertheless, it has been demonstrated in dogs that thoracotomy reduces the cardiac output to below levels which might be expected from the application of IPPV alone [16, 17], apparently by causing a further reduction in venous return to the heart.

In practice, as far as avoidance of circulatory disturbance is concerned, quite satisfactory results are obtained by the anaesthetist ensuring that only minimal pressures are applied to produce the desired degree of lung expansion smoothly and in as short a time as seems reasonable in relation to the length of the expiratory period. It is difficult to describe exactly how this is done in any particular case and its successful accomplishment remains, at the moment, part of the art of veterinary anaesthesia.

The effects of IPPV on pulmonary ventilation are, of course, in the main clearly beneficial, or the procedure would not have found such extensive use in the treatment of respiratory failure. Rupture of lung tissue is no more likely to occur during properly applied IPPV than during the ordinary activities of life. Very high intrapulmonary pressures develop during such activities as coughing, or straining at parturition or defaecation. It has been found in dogs that pressures above 100 mmHg (13.3 kPa) will produce fatal air embolism, while during thoracotomy pressures above 70 mmHg (9.3 kPa) can produce mediastinal emphysema [18] but pressures of this order are most unlikely to be encountered during normal IPPV where it is seldom possible to create pressures above 60 cmH$_2$O (6 kPa) by compression of the reservoir bag. Care is needed when ventilators are used, for, in some, sticking of valves may expose the patient's airway directly to the high pressures at which gases are delivered from the anaesthetic machine to the ventilator. As already mentioned, uneven inflation of alveoli is a distinct possibility during IPPV but the surrounding tissues seem to provide sufficient support to prevent rupture of the relatively overinflated alveoli.

Any uneven distribution of gas must have the effect of disturbing the normal ventilation/perfusion relationships within the lungs. It appears that these are often upset by anaesthesia itself and if IPPV produces more uneven gas distribution, it will probably fail to affect any improvement in the alveolar–arterial oxygen tension gradient found during anaesthesia, in spite of any improvement in tidal exchange which it may produce. For example, in laterally recumbent horses it is possible that the gravitational force gradient from the top to the bottom of the lungs acting on the low-pressure pulmonary circulation may, by reducing the circulation to the upper lung, cause this lung to be overventilated in relation to its perfusion. Due to the weight of the horse's abdominal viscera acting on the lower cone of the diaphragm, IPPV is more successful in inflating the upper than the lower lung and hence the upper lung receives an even more disproportionately large part of the ventilation to the further detriment of its ventilation/perfusion relationships. Certainly, in the laterally recumbent horse controlled ventilation appears to produce very little improvement in the alveolar–arterial oxygen tension gradient found during general anaesthesia. Other situations in which the normal relationships between ventilation and perfusion may be upset occur in all animals where the expansion of one lung or part of a lung is limited by surgical procedures such as 'packing-off' and retraction of lung lobes during intrathoracic surgery.

IPPV should remove carbon dioxide from the animal's lungs and it is possible, over a period of time, to remove either too much or too little causing the animal to suffer from either respiratory alkalosis or acidosis. Respiratory acidosis (hypercapnia) is characterized by sympathetic overactivity, cutaneous vasodilatation, a rise in arterial blood pressure and a bounding pulse. Respiratory alkalosis (hypocapnia) may, it has been claimed, lead to cerebral damage from cerebral vasoconstriction because the calibre of the cerebral blood vessels depends on the arterial carbon dioxide tension. However, convincing evidence of cerebral damage due to hypocapnia has yet to be produced. Moreover, although it has been demonstrated that hypocapnia has reduced cardiac output in man [19, 20] and in horses [13], at least in normovolaemic states no disaster appears to result and it seems to be generally agreed that hypocapnia is much less harmful than hypercapnia.

IPPV carried out with a face-mask instead of an endotracheal tube can be harmful unless care is taken to avoid forcing gases down the oesophagus into the stomach. This entails careful limiting of the pressure applied at the mouth and nostrils and observations of the epigastric region to detect any inflation of the stomach. An inflated stomach not only hinders intra-abdominal surgery — if it becomes sufficiently distended with gas regurgitation of gastric fluid is a distinct possibility. Gas accidentally forced into the stomach should be removed as soon as possible by passing a stomach tube.

Positive end-expiratory pressure (PEEP) and continuous positive airway pressure (CPAP)

In many conditions of advanced lung disease the imposition of an expiratory threshold resistance has been shown to have beneficial effects on the $P_{a_{O_2}}$. According to Nunn [21], use of an expiratory resistor during IPPV is known as PEEP (positive end-expiratory pressure) and during spontaneous breathing as CPAP (continuous positive airway pressure).

The respiratory benefits of an expiratory resistor include an overall reduction in airway resistance due to an increase in FRC, movement of the tidal volume to above the airway closing volume, a tendency towards re-expansion of any collapsed lung and, possibly, a reduction in total lung water. The net result is that ventilation/perfusion relationships are improved. However, these advantages are, in some circumstances, counterbalanced by circulatory disadvantages due to the inevitable rise in mean intrathoracic pressure which will impede venous return and decrease cardiac output. Although the venous return can be restored with an α-adrenergic stimulator such as metaraminol [22] or by over-transfusion [23, 24], in clinical practice the situation is more complicated.

Both disease and drugs have profound effects on the circulatory response to a rise in mean intrathoracic pressure due to PEEP (or CPAP). Certain conditions may aggravate the reduction in cardiac output but others actually oppose it and it is in these latter conditions that PEEP or CPAP is likely to be of benefit. In animals with poor lung compliance much of the applied end-expiratory pressure will be opposed by the excessive pulmonary transmural pressure thus minimizing the increase in intrathoracic pressure. Thus, the stiffer the lungs, the safer is the application of PEEP (or CPAP) likely to be.

To summarize, PEEP (and CPAP) may confer respiratory advantages and circulatory disadvantages which interact in a complicated manner rendering it necessary to make direct measurements of the relevant physiological functions to ensure that overall benefit results. In veterinary practice, even in intensive care units, such measurements are seldom possible and the use of expiratory threshold resistors is, therefore, unlikely to gain wide acceptance in the treatment of sick animals. Moreover, the results of PEEP and CPAP during routine anaesthesia are disappointing. In 1965, Nunn *et al.* [25] reported that 5 cmH$_2$O (0.5 kPa) of PEEP did not improve $P_{a_{O_2}}$ in human patients and similar results have been obtained by subsequent investigators. Colgan *et al.* [26] showed that PEEP produced no change in the alveolar–arterial P_{O_2} gradient in anaesthetized dogs.

Hall and Trim [27] failed to demonstrate any benefit from CPAP in anaesthetized horses and broadly similar results were obtained by Beadle *et al.* [28]. These results all probably indicate that there is no reduction in lung compliance in the majority of veterinary patients and there would seem to be no indication for the use of PEEP or CPAP in routine anaesthetic practice.

Management of controlled respiration

Before IPPV can be applied all spontaneous breathing movements have to be abolished if the animal is not to 'fight' the imposed ventilation. This is usually accomplished by:

1. Depressing the respiratory centres by relative overdoses of anaesthetics or agents such as morphine or fentanyl.
2. Paralysis of the respiratory muscles by neuromuscular block.
3. Lowering the carbon dioxide tension in the body by hyperventilation. This may be done by squeezing the reservoir bag at the end of each spontaneous inspiration to force a little more gas into the lungs, or by ventilating between spontaneous breaths.
4. Reflexly inhibiting the respiratory centres by regular rhythmical lung inflation. This inhibition does not depend on changes in blood pH and carbon dioxide tension. For example, in the cat subjected to IPPV it is known that respiratory neuronal activity usually synchronizes with the ventilator cycle within two to three respiratory cycles; this is too rapid for significant changes in the arterial blood gases to occur. It is believed that if the lungs are slightly overdistended at each inspiration afferent impulses from pulmonary receptors inhibit the medullary centres.

When IPPV is carried out by manual squeezing of the reservoir bag this should be done gently and rhythmically. Once the desired degree of lung inflation has been produced the bag should be released and the lungs allowed to empty freely. The rate of lung ventilation should be faster than the normal respiratory rate of the animal and the chest wall movement produced should be more obvious than in normal breathing. During thoracotomy, expansion of the lung beyond the limits of the wound indicates that excessive inflation on the lungs is being produced. Simple observations such as these ensure that ventilation is being carried out in a manner which will result in no harm to the animal.

A survey of the literature reveals wide variations in the recommendations for tidal and minute volumes of respiration when IPPV is used. There are no agreed values for the production of adequate levels of ventilation in horses [29, 30] and even in dogs suggested figures range from 20 to 30 ml/kg (tidal volume) and from 400 to 600 ml/kg (minute volume), so it is clear that any figure can only be regarded as a very rough guide. Ideally, the end-tidal concentration of carbon dioxide may be monitored continuously by a rapid infrared analyser [31] and, once the end-tidal to arterial tension difference has been derived from blood gas analysis, the ventilation may be adjusted to yield a normal P_aCO_2, although it is important to note that the end-tidal to arterial carbon dioxide gradient may change during the course of anaesthesia. In practice, facilities for rapid gas and blood analysis are limited by financial and other constraints and it is usually necessary to perform IPPV without such assistance.

For small animal patients, where non-rebreathing systems can be employed, it is relatively easy to ensure the maintenance of satisfactory blood gas tension by hyperventilating with a gas mixture containing 4% carbon dioxide and at least 30% oxygen. Using such a gas mixture in this way it is only necessary to ensure that large tidal and minute volumes are being imposed and this can be done from observation of the frequency of lung inflation and the amplitude of the chest wall excursions. In large animals, where for reasons of economy in the use of gases it is essential to employ rebreathing systems, it is much less easy to ensure satisfactory blood gas levels and, in the absence of monitoring facilities, the anaesthetist has to rely on experience and aim to err, if at all, on the side of providing a degree of hyperventilation. In general, it is better to ventilate at slower rates with large tidal volumes than to achieve the same minute volumes by faster rates and smaller tidal volumes.

Restoration of spontaneous breathing

It is important to note that while in most animals apnoea may be established with the aid of relaxant drugs, in all cases at the end of operation, apnoea should be mainly due to reflex inhibition of respiration by the rhythmical slight overinflation of the lungs and, possibly, hypocapnia. Thus, prompt resumption of spontaneous breathing usually follows if:

1. The rhythm of lung inflation is broken.
2. Some accumulation of carbon dioxide is allowed by either removing the soda lime canister or, in non-rebreathing systems, adding more carbon dioxide to the inspired gases.

Residual neuromuscular block should be counteracted where appropriate by the intravenous administration of anticholinergic and anticholinesterase drugs. This should be done before any carbon dioxide accumulation is encouraged because anticholinesterases appear to be less likely to produce cardiac irregularities when the arterial carbon dioxide tension is low. When inhalation anaesthetics have been used the anaesthetic mixture should be diluted with oxygen. Provided only minimal central depression by anaesthetic agents is present animals will resume spontaneous breathing at very low arterial carbon dioxide tensions and dogs have been observed to start breathing with carbon dioxide tensions as low as 18–20 mmHg (about 2.2 kPa).

In cases where apnoea is established by the use of centrally acting drugs [32], antagonists such as naloxone may be given at the end of operation to overcome the respiratory depressant effects, but the relatively short action of the drugs commonly used today (e.g. fentanyl) usually make this unnecessary.

VENTILATORS

Because the rhythmical squeezing of a reservoir bag for long periods is both tedious and monotonous, mechanical devices ('ventilators') are commonly used to perform this duty. The use of a ventilator frees the anaesthetist to set up intravenous infusions, keep records, suck out the tracheobronchial tree and otherwise attend to the welfare of the patient. Nevertheless, it should be noted that the manual squeezing of a reservoir bag is not to be despised. Observation of the bag between compressions shows volume changes due to the heartbeat; the anaesthetist can alter the rate, rhythm and character of lung inflation to suit the convenience of the surgeon at any particularly critical stage of an operation, and the presence or absence of respiratory obstruction is immediately obvious. Theoretically, the effort necessary to produce the desired degree of lung inflation should give the anaesthetist information about the level of anaesthesia or degree of relaxation of the respiratory muscles, more difficult inflation meaning waning relaxation or lighter anaesthesia. As relaxation wears off it is undoubtedly necessary to exert a greater pressure to maintain the tidal exchange, as may be observed by anyone using a suitably calibrated ventilator, but the authors have seldom been able to appreciate this while actually squeezing a reservoir bag. There may be such a thing as an 'educated hand' which recognizes every flicker of the diaphragm, or attempted cough, or waning relaxation, but it does not seem to be all that easily acquired.

A description of every available machine is quite outside the scope of this book and for a fully comprehensive review of automatic ventilators, their function and construction, the reader is referred to the text *Automatic Ventilation of the Lungs* by W. W. Mushin *et al.* (Blackwell Scientific, Oxford) [33]. Many of the ventilators described therein are designed for prolonged automatic ventilation of patients in respiratory failure in intensive care units and will be found to satisfy requirements quite different to those of a ventilator for use in operating theatres [34].

The respiratory cycle of a ventilator can be divided into four parts [33]:

1. The inspiratory phase
2. The changeover from the inspiratory to the expiratory phase
3. The expiratory phase
4. The changeover from the expiratory to the inspiratory phase

Very briefly the inspiratory phase can be provided by either flow generators or pressure generators. With flow generators the tidal volume delivered is independent of factors outside the ventilator — if, for example, the patient's airway resistance rises then the inflation pressure increases. The flow is not necessarily constant and can be generated by a bellows compressed by a cam mechanism or by pneumatic compression of the anaesthetic reservoir bag situated in a bottle. Pressure generators maintain a constant pressure during the inspiratory phase of the respiratory cycle, often by a weight acting on a concertina bag (as in the Manley ventilator). The volume delivered by a pressure ventilator will depend on such factors as the airway resistance.

Changeover from inspiration to expiration, i.e. the manner in which the ventilator cycles, may be:

1. Time cycled, in which inspiration is terminated after a preset time
2. Volume cycled, where inspiration is terminated after a preset volume has been delivered
3. Pressure cycled, in which case inspiration ceases once a preset pressure is reached

Not all machines can be classified under this scheme and Mushin *et al.* frequently refer to mixed cycling with hybrid cycling mechanisms. Each type of apparatus has its own advantages and disadvantages and discussion of their relative merits is, again, outside the scope of this book.

In the expiratory phase a machine may act as a flow generator (e.g. an injector) or a pressure generator and the commonest arrangement is to expose the patient's airway to atmospheric pressure. The changeover from the expiratory to the inspiratory phase may be time cycled or patient triggered. In the patient-triggered ventilator a slight inspiratory effort by the patient triggers the changeover to the inspiratory phase.

Ventilator performance in the presence of changed parameters in the patient is extremely complex and Mapleson [35] has presented a detailed account of this subject. However, provided a machine meets the following requirements it should be adequate in most circumstances no matter what its mode of operation or mechanism of cycling may be.

Essential characteristics of an adequate ventilator

For use in cats, dogs, sheep, goats, small calves and small pigs, a ventilator needs to provide tidal volumes up to 1000 ml at a cycling rate of from 8 to about 40 cycles/min. The duration of the inspiratory phase should be variable, independent of the other settings and range from about 0.5 to 3 seconds' duration. Whenever possible the expired volume should be monitored since due to leaks the 'stroke volume' of the ventilator may not represent the tidal volume delivered to the animal.

Difficulty is experienced in using most commercially available ventilators in cats and small dogs. The problems seem to be similar to those encountered in infants and small babies which were reviewed by Mushin *et al.* [36], with high respiratory rates, low tidal volumes and, possibly (although in small animals no information appears to be available), high airway resistance. Adaptation of adult ventilators for infants and small babies has been accomplished by employing a controlled leak [37] or a parallel resistance and compliance used in conjunction with an Ayre's T-piece [38]. However, such systems are complicated and a ventilator designed specifically for the purpose would seem to be a better solution to the problem.

Control of the length of expiratory period should, like that of the inspiratory period, be independent of the other settings. (There is nothing more tiresome than having to adjust all the controls of a ventilator when only one setting needs correction.) It should be possible to obtain inspiratory:expiratory ratios of at least 1:3, the expiratory period beginning immediately the desired tidal volume has been delivered to the lungs. Resistance to expiration should be low although, as already mentioned, in certain circumstances it may be to an animal's advantage if the expiratory resistance can be increased.

A high peak gas flow rate during the inspiratory phase is always desirable if the lungs are to be inflated in a short inspiratory period. It is comparatively easy to adapt a ventilator which gives a high peak flow rate to give a lower flow rate but it is impossible to obtain a high peak flow rate from a machine which is not designed to achieve this.

Provided a ventilator satisfies these general criteria, its method of cycling is unimportant. There are, however, several points which should be taken into account before buying a machine. First, for safety, it is essential that provision is made for change to manual squeezing of a reservoir bag should any mechanical fault develop during the course of an operation. Secondly, if electrically driven, the machine must be electrically safe and explosion proof. Possibly less important, the machinery should not be noisy and if free standing it should occupy the minimum of floor space. In practice, the choice of ventilator is largely one of personal preference, convenience of operation for the particular circumstances in which it is to be used and the financial resources available.

Ventilators designed for use in man have given very satisfactory results when used on smaller animals and there is probably no need to develop special machines except, as already mentioned, for cats and very small dogs. Among the very many commercially available machines which have performed consistently are the Bird, the Manley and the Flowmaster. The three small, inexpensive ventilators (Minivent, Automatic Vent, and Microvent) tested by Hall and Massey [39] are particularly suitable for small animal practice whenever supplies of compressed air or oxygen are available. They are small, simple ventilators which fit onto any continuous flow apparatus and act as minute volume dividers. The distended reservoir bag provides the driving force of inspiration and the compliance of this bag must be low if they are to operate correctly; bags made of Neoprene are much less satisfactory than those made from natural rubber. A bobbin is held against a magnet to prevent gas flowing to the patient except when the pressure of the gas in the reservoir bag forces it away and allows inspiration to result. As the lungs inflate, the pressure in the reservoir bag drops and allows the magnet to pull the bobbin back, thus terminating inspiration.

The basic clinical criteria for ventilators for adult horses, cattle and large pigs are similar to those for the other animals described above. A useful ventilator has a tidal volume of between 2 and 20 litres with a cycling rate of between 4 and 15 cycles/min and an inspiratory phase of 2–3 seconds. It should be capable of sustaining pressures of up to 60 cmH$_2$O (6 kPa) in the upper airway during inspiration while the inspiratory:expiratory ratio should be at least 1:2.

Special machines have had to be developed for use with large animals and, until recently, most workers used machines constructed to their own specifications. Ventilators for adult horses and cattle have been available from commercial sources for only a very few years and proper data on their performance is scarce.

The Bird ventilators developed in the USA may be automatic or patient triggered and various models are available which can be adapted for use in anaesthesia by interposing a 'bag in bottle'. (In small animals use with the Bain breathing circuit avoids many of the problems which have resulted in various complexities of the Bird machine modifications now available.) A Bird ventilator was used by Fowler *et al.* [14] to drive a number of bags contained in a tank for the ventilation of horses.

In the UK the 'Cambridge Ventilator' built by Bowring Engineering uses a hydraulically compressed bellows to drive a bag in a bottle. It is a very powerful machine which is connected in place of the reservoir bag of the anaesthetic circuit. Although rather large and cumbersome it is capable of ventilating the largest of horses with ease. The power source is from the electrical mains.

North American Drager produce a volume-cycled large animal ventilator which appears to be capable of adequately ventilating most horses. It is simple to operate with only three controls, has a preset inspiratory:expiratory ratio and works off a supply pressure of 40–60 lb/in^2 (276–414 kPa); the latest models require an electrical power supply. Respiratory frequency can be varied from 6 to 20 breaths/min.

High-frequency ventilation of the lungs

Ventilation with tidal volumes of less than the anatomical dead-space can provide adequate gas exchange in the lungs. However, the mechanisms of achieving this are not immediately obvious; they have recently been reviewed by Drazen *et al.* [40].

Effective gas exchange in the lung requires fresh gas to be presented to the animal's alveoli and the removal of used gas from the alveoli. The amount of gas required per minute to accomplish this is determined by the size and metabolic rate of the animal. The conventional artificial ventilation described in this chapter uses rates and tidal volumes within the physiological range but using small tidal volumes and higher respiratory frequencies is associated with lower peak inspiratory airway pressures and less fluctuation in intrathoracic pressure.

Small tidal volumes

The transition from the conducting airways, with no gas-exchanging function, to the alveolar sacs where gas exchange takes place, is not sharply demarcated anatomically. The respiratory bronchioles are predominantly conducting passages but do have alveolar sacs opening off them. The alveolar ducts have gas-exchanging epithelium throughout and in addition conduct gas to the alveoli. Thus any gas which penetrates to the respiratory bronchioles by bulk convection from the mouth will take part in gas exchange.

Within the lung, differing regions have different time constants (product of compliance and airway resistance). Some areas of the lung are fast fillers with short time constants, whereas other areas are slow fillers with long time constants. During early inspiration the fast-filling regions become full and during late inspiration are actually emptying into the slow fillers. This is known as 'Pendelluft', and the sum of gas movement within the lung is greater than the gas flow down the trachea; there is gas movement between regions of the lung without gas movement in the trachea. It is, therefore, apparent that when small tidal volumes are delivered at high frequency, a slow filler could still be filling from a fast filler which at the same time is providing gas for expiration up the trachea.

Even with high ventilation frequencies fresh gas presented to the alveoli has ample time to diffuse across the alveolar zone (for this is complete within 10 ms) and thus there is an enhanced potential for molecular diffusion to take a considerably greater role in the movement of gas across the alveoli.

High ventilation frequency

In the conventional model of ventilation a mass of gas under pressure (potential energy) is presented at the airway opening. This potential energy is converted to kinetic energy to allow the gas to flow down the airway. By the end of inspiration this kinetic energy has become zero, for the gas is then static and the energy is stored as potential energy in the distended lungs. The time course for this change is determined by the time constant for the lung and it is known that 95% of change occurs within 3 time constants. It is obvious that with higher frequencies of ventilation there will be insufficient time for inspiration to go to completion, that is, with static gas distending the lung alveoli. It therefore follows that with higher ventilatory frequencies either a reduced tidal volume is delivered to the lung periphery or a higher peak inspiratory pressure is required to force the gas to the lung periphery within the available time.

With high frequencies of ventilation the kinetic energy of the molecules of gas undergoing bulk convection as ventilation cycles from inspiration to expiration becomes increasingly important. As ventilation changes from inspiration to expiration the gas retains its forward kinetic energy and will continue to progress peripherally in the lung until this kinetic energy is dissipated. This inertia of gas molecules is not present with conventional IPPV since end inspiration is a static state.

The pressure–flow relationships at conventional breathing rates are adequately expressed by airways resistance but with higher frequencies airways resistance can no longer be assumed to be constant and inertia makes an increasing contribution. Thus, at higher frequencies airway impedance, which takes inertia into account, must be used to express pressure–flow relationships. It has been shown [41] that by far the largest component of impedance to high-frequency ventilation lies in the endotracheal tube. This impedance is greatest with a wide-bore endotracheal tube and high gas flow rates (large tidal volumes at high frequency).

At normal breathing rates gas distribution within the lung is determined by regional compliance. However, with higher respiratory rates airway resistance and gas inertance have an increasing effect on the distribution of ventilation. Potentially this will result in a change of ventilation from areas of high compliance to areas of low impedance. Since there is no evidence to suggest that regional lung perfusion is altered, high-frequency ventilation must, therefore, result in changes in lung ventilation:perfusion ratios.

Another aspect of high-frequency ventilation is that it involves less time for the bulk convection of gas during inspiration and expiration so that the gas path length must become increasingly important. Thus, in animals such as horses with long tracheas, pressure at the airway opening will progressively distend the major conducting passages, then the nearby fast-filling lung units and finally the peripheral slow-filling units. With a progressive shortening of inspiratory time a situation will rise when there is insufficient time for the tidal volume to get beyond the major conducting passages which will then act in a way analogous to that of an electrical capacitor. The implication of this is that pressure at the airway opening is not transmitted to the lung periphery and hence the pleural space. However, the reverse will also occur in that there will not be enough time for the intra-alveolar pressure to empty the alveoli so that there will be a continuous positive airway pressure in the peripheral lung units. This should, in theory, be beneficial in elderly animals or in those with a reduced functional residual capacity since these are the lung units where small airway closure is most likely to occur in these animals.

Methods for achieving high-frequency ventilation of the lungs

Conventional ventilators deliver a volume of gas during inspiration by occlusion of a relatively wide-bore orifice through which expiration takes place and the device used to occlude the expiratory orifice must function rapidly. The more rapidly this device is made to operate the more likely valve bounce is to occur so that conventional ventilators cannot, in general, operate at frequencies above 2 Hz. Because of this limitation high-frequency ventilation is normally provided by either high-frequency jet ventilation (HFJV) or high frequency oscillation (HFO).

High-frequency jet ventilators. These ventilators allow a high-pressure gas source to flow into the airway during part of the respiratory cycle, usually 20–35% of the cycle time, through a narrow-diameter tube usually at tracheal level. They require no expiratory seal and hence the airway is open to atmospheric pressure throughout the cycle. This potentially results in entrainment of an unknown quantity of ambient gas and thus the volume and composition of the tidal volume are unknown, but the system has the inherent safety advantage that the animal can take a spontaneous breath at any time during the respiratory cycle. A method has been described by which the tidal volume can be measured [42] but it is not suitable for clinical use without modification.

High-frequency oscillators. Oscillator-type ventilators tend to be used for higher frequencies (6–40 Hz). A piston driven by a motor or an electronically driven diaphragm at the airway opening generates a to-and-fro motion of gas within the airway. The tidal volume results from displacement of the piston or diaphragm and a subatmospheric airway pressure is generated during the expiratory half of the respiratory cycle. Fresh gas is fed in at the airway opening and a low-pass filter exhaust port allows gas to exit the system. The low-pass filter offers a high impedance to high frequencies which are thus able to direct the tidal volume down the airway which has a lower impedance rather than be lost through the exhaust port.

Carbon dioxide elimination and oxygen delivery

On theoretical grounds it might be expected that with a constant tidal volume there should be a linear relationship between carbon dioxide removal and ventilatory frequency until such a time as the duration of inspiration is insufficient to permit the gas to penetrate the conducting airways to the gas exchanging regions of the lung. In practice this seems to be the case and there is a critical frequency at which carbon dioxide elimination reaches a peak. Above this frequency carbon dioxide elimination becomes a function of tidal volume and independent of ventilatory frequency. The critical frequency is dependent on the anatomy of the lung and is certainly higher in dogs than in horses.

One of the original hopes for high-frequency ventilation was that a change from compliance/airway resistance distribution of ventilation to one determined by airway resistance/gas inertia would result in improved distribution of gas within the lung and improvement in ventilation. However, it is now generally accepted that, at equivalent tidal volumes, neither HFJV nor HFO produce improvement in arterial oxygen tension over that which can be attained by conventional ventilation techniques.

Use in veterinary anaesthesia

High-frequency ventilation of the lungs is undoubtedly an interesting technique and one which, on theoretical grounds, may be particularly useful in horses and other large animals. However, the necessary apparatus is costly and much more work needs to be done to show whether this method will have clinical value. Reports to date of its use in horses [43–45] and dogs [46] are not encouraging. It has been aptly described as 'a technique looking for an application'!

REFERENCES

1. Comroe, J. H., Forster, R. E., Dubois, A. B., Briscoe, W. A. and Carlsen, E. (1962) *The Lung*, 2nd edn. Chicago: Year Book Medical.
2. Purchase, I. F. H. (1965) *Veterinary Record* 77, 913.
3. Gillespie, J. R. and Tyler, W. S. (1969) *Advances in Veterinary Science*, vol. 13. New York: Academic Press.
4. Gillespie, J. R., Tyler, W. S. and Eberly, V. E. (1966) *Journal of Applied Physiology* 21, 416.
5. Campbell, E. J. M. (1957) *Journal of Physiology* 136, 556.
6. Mushin, W. W., Rendell-Baker, L., Thompson, P. and Mapleson, W. W. (1969) *Automatic Ventilation of the Lungs*. Oxford: Blackwell Scientific.
7. Purchase, I. F. H. (1965) *Veterinary Record* 77, 859.
8. Beecher, H. K., Burnett, H. and Bassett, D. I. (1943) *Anesthesiology* 4, 612.
9. Butler, J. and Smith, B. H. (1957) *Clinical Science* 19, 55.
10. Agostoni, E. and Mead, J. (1964) *Handbook of Physiology*, sect. 3, Respiration, vol. 1, chapt. 13. Washington, DC: American Physiological Society.
11. Mead, J. (1961) *Physiological Reviews* 41, 281.
12. Watson, W. E. (1962) *British Journal of Anaesthesia* 134, 502.
13. Hall, L. W., Gillespie, J. R. and Tyler, W. S. (1968) *British Journal of Anaesthesia* 40, 560.
14. Fowler, M. E., Parker, E. E., McLaughlin, R. F. and Tyler, W. S. (1963) *Journal of the American Veterinary Medical Association* 143, 272.
15. Carl, D. T. and Essex, H. E. (1946) *American Heart Journal* 31, 53.
16. Finlayson, K. J., Luria, M. N. and Yu, P. N. (1961) *Circulation Research* 9, 862.
17. Caldini, P., Ho, C. and Zingg, W. (1962) *Journal of Thoracic and Cardiovascular Surgery* 44, 104.
18. Taylor, G. and Gerbode, F. (1948) *Surgery* 30, 316.
19. Kelman, G. R., Nunn, J. F., Prys-Roberts, C. and Greenbaum, R. (1967) *British Journal of Anaesthesia* 39, 450.
20. Prys-Roberts, C., Kelman, G. R. and Greenbaum, R. (1967) *Anaesthesia* 22, 257.
21. Nunn, J. F. (1977) *Applied Respiratory Physiology*, p. 128. London: Butterworths.
22. Braunwald, E., Binion, J. T. and Morgan, W. L. (1957) *Circulation Research* 5, 670.
23. Sykes, M. K., Adams, A. P., Finlay, W. E. I., McCormick, P. W. and Economider, A. (1970) *British Journal of Anaesthesia* 42, 669.
24. Qvist, J., Pontoppidan, H., Wilson, R. S., Lowenstein, R. and Laver, M. B. (1975) *Anesthesiology* 42, 45.
25. Nunn, J. F., Bergman, N. A. and Coleman, A. J. (1965) *British Journal of Anaesthesia* 37, 898.
26. Colgan, F. J., Barrow, R. E. and Fanning, G. (1971) *Anesthesiology* 34, 145.
27. Hall, L. W. and Trim, C. M. (1975) *British Journal of Anaesthesia* 47, 819.
28. Beadle, R. E., Robinson, N. E. and Sorensen, P. R. (1975) *American Journal of Veterinary Research* 36, 1435.
29. Weaver, B. M. Q. and Walley, R. (1975) *Equine Veterinary Journal* 7, 9.
30. Schatzman, U. (1978) *Journal of Equine Medicine and Surgery* 2, 453.
31. Moens, Y. and de Moor, A. (1981) *Equine Veterinary Journal* 13, 229.
32. Foldes, F. F. (1957) *American Journal of Medical Science* 233, 1.
33. Mushin, W. W., Rendell-Baker, L., Thompson, P. and Mapleson, W. W. (1969) *Automatic Ventilation of the Lungs*. Oxford: Blackwell Scientific.
34. Robinson, J. S. (1967) *Modern Trends in Anaesthesia* (eds F. T. Evans and T. C. Grey). London: Butterworths.
35. Mapleson, W. W. (1962) *Anaesthesia* 17, 300.
36. Mushin, W. W., Mapleson, W. W. and Lunn, J. N. (1962) *British Journal of Anaesthesia* 34, 514.
37. Doctor, N. H. (1946) *British Journal of Anaesthesia* 36, 259.
38. Inkster, J. S. and Lunn, J. N. (1964) *British Journal of Anaesthesia* 36, 381.
39. Hall, L. W. and Massey, G. M. (1969) *Veterinary Record* 85, 432.
40. Drazen, J. M., Kamm, R. D. and Slutsky, A. S. (1984) *Physiological Review* 64, 505.
41. Gavriely, N., Solway, S., Loring, S. H., Butler, J. P., Slutsky, A. S. and Drazen, J. M. (1985) *Journal of Applied Physiology* 59, 3.
42. Young, J. D. and Sykes, M. K. (1988) *British Journal of Anaesthesia* 61, 601.
43. Wilson, D. V., Soma, L. R. and Klein, L. V. (1985) *Proceedings of the 2nd International Congress of Veterinary Anaesthesia*, Sacramento, p. 188.
44. Dunlop, C. I. and Hodgson, D. S. (1984) *Federation Proceedings* 43, 507.
45. Dunlop, C. I., Steffey, E. P., Daunt, D., Kock, N. and Hodgson, D. S. (1985) *Proceedings of the 2nd International Congress of Veterinary Anaesthesia*, Sacramento, p. 190.
46. Bednarski, R. M. and Muir, W. W. (1989) *American Journal of Veterinary Research* 50, 1106.

CHAPTER 9

APPARATUS FOR THE ADMINISTRATION OF ANAESTHETICS

ADMINISTRATION OF INTRAVENOUS AGENTS

For agents which are intended to reach the central nervous system and produce narcosis or anaesthesia the intravenous route is obviously more direct than one through the respiratory tract. But it must always be borne in mind that unlike the respiratory pathway the intravenous one does not provide an exit as well as an entrance and, for this reason, apparatus used for the administration of intravenous agents must be designed to allow accurate control of the amount given, for once injected it canot be recovered from the animal's body.

Although any superficial vein may be used, in veterinary practice injections are usually made into the external jugular vein, the cephalic vein or the recurrent tarsal vein. The choice of vein does not influence the apparatus which may be used and detailed descriptions of the techniques of venepuncture will be found in the chapters concerned with anaesthesia of the various species of animal.

Syringes, needles and catheters

The largest syringe which can be handled conveniently is one of 50–60 ml capacity and all those of greater capacity than 2 ml should have eccentrically placed nozzles. All-glass syringes are easy to sterilize but have plungers which tend to stick during injection and, although the best in which to collect samples of blood for blood gas analysis, for all other purposes they have been replaced by the disposable plastic variety.

Needles must be sharp and their points should, preferably, have a short bevel to reduce the risk of transfixing the vein. Good quality disposable needles are always sharp and their use is now almost universal.

The administration of intermittent small doses of a drug, or its constant infusion, requires that a catheter be kept in the vein and free from blood clot. Methods in which a needle is left in the vein and an attached, loaded syringe strapped to the patient are rarely

satisfactory because movement between the skin and the vein, or of the patient, results in the displacement of the needle. Unless this mishap is noticed it may lead to haematoma formation and/or the extravascular injection of drugs, some of which may be highly irritant to the surrounding tissues. Where anaesthesia is to be supervised by nursing staff it is particularly important for the surgeon–anaesthetist to ensure there is a secure open venous line before commencing surgery. An open vein may be ensured with a plastic catheter. Proprietary catheters for this purpose are supplied sterile: they usually consist of a nylon, polythene or Teflon catheter fitted with a hollow metal needle, the point of which projects just beyond the end of the catheter. The catheter is inserted into the vein with the trocar needle in position and the needle is withdrawn when blood flows from its proximal end. The needle hub is then held firmly while the blunt-ended catheter is advanced well up the vein and secured in position with adhesive tape or a stitch. Because of the blunt end of the catheter it does not transfix the vein and a long length can be threaded into the vein so it is much less apt to be displaced than is a needle.

If an attempt is made to insert one of these plastic catheters directly through the skin it usually results in the end of the plastic portion opening out into a bell-mouth which is almost impossible to introduce into the vein, so that they should be inserted through a small skin incision. Should venepuncture be found to be unsuccessful, even if the needle has only been partially withdrawn from the catheter, it must not be reinserted unless the catheter is completely removed from the tissues because it may penetrate the side of the plastic catheter and sheer off the distal portion.

There is a large variety of plastic catheters with internal needles, and more than 25 different catheters are commercially available in the UK alone. There is some variation on their general shape and some have small handles to aid insertion. Most have plastic

149

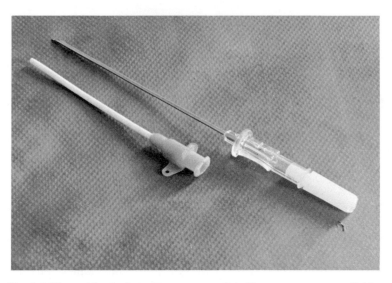

Fig. 9.1 Disposable plastic 'catheter over-needle'. Many patterns are available.

needle hubs which allow the operator to see the blood which runs back when the needle punctures the vein. Three important factors govern the choice of catheter. First, it should be no longer than strictly necessary. The length of most catheters (up to 7 cm) is always adequate and there is no need for the larger diameters to be longer. However, exceptions to this rule occur where the need to ensure that the catheter remains in the vein at all costs (e.g. when administering guaiphenesin to a horse) outweighs the effect of the increased length on resistance to flow. The second important feature is the wall thickness. It is the external diameter which largely determines the size chosen in any given situation and catheters with thinner walls obviously permit more rapid infusions. The third factor is that the external shape should be as smooth as possible, for catheters with smooth contours are the easiest to insert (Fig. 9.1).

Longer catheters are available for special purposes such as measurement of the central venous pressure (see Chapter 2). Although it is possible to obtain some sizes of the catheters described above up to 5.25 inches (13.3 cm) in length (which may be adequate for central venous pressure measurement in cats and small dogs), the longer catheters are generally not provided with introducing needles. These long catheters may be introduced into the vein through a large-bore needle but this method of placing a catheter can be dangerous, as the end of the catheter may be severed by the point of the needle. Such catheters should, therefore, be placed by cutting down surgically on to the vein or else passed through short, large-bore catheters previously introduced into the vessel for this purpose. Indeed, some long catheters (e.g. Abbotts Drum Reel) are supplied with an additional

short, wider-bore catheter of the 'over-needle pattern' that is introduced into the vein so that the longer one can be threaded through it.

A slightly different design of long catheter which is particularly easy to introduce is the E-Z Cath (Deseret Ltd). A needle lies inside the tip of the catheter to assist introduction; it is attached to a wire which passes through the length of the catheter. A split inserting handle attached to a protective sleeve surrounds the catheter, and the catheter can be worked up the vein by advancing it with the inserter, using one hand, and holding it inside its protective sleeve with the other hand.

The number of proprietary catheters of various lengths is now bewilderingly large and choice is difficult. Because the wrong choice is made intravenous infusions which appear to run smoothly when originally set up with electrolyte solutions may prove infuriatingly slow when blood has to be given. Such a disadvantage may cost an animal its life. Consideration of some of the factors influencing fluid flow makes the choice of catheter more rational and less dependent on the information given on the packet by the manufacturers of any particular appliance.

The flow through a tube is proportional to the driving pressure, which is equal to the pressure difference between the two ends of the tube, multiplied by a constant, $\pi/8$. Flow is also inversely proportional to the viscosity of the fluid, since the more viscous it is the harder it will be to force it through the tube. The final factor governing the flow is the size of the tube, flow being directly proportional to the fourth power of the radius, and inversely proportional to the length of the bore. Thus, for maximum flow of any given fluid at any given

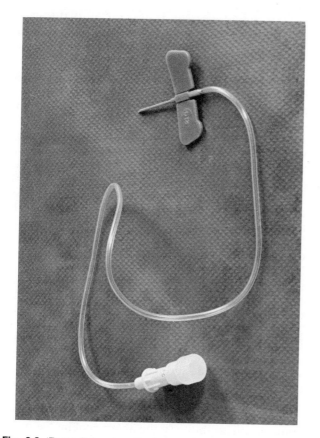

Fig. 9.2 'Butterfly' or 'small-vein set' or 'infant scalp-vein set'. Many types are available but all have lengths of plastic tubing attached and most have winged needles to aid insertion and subsequent fixation to the patient.

pressure, the tube should be as short, and the diameter as large, as possible. It must be noted that a small change in diameter has a large effect on flow.

At very high flows it may be found that the resistance is disproportionately high. There is a critical flow velocity at which the flow changes from streamline to turbulent. During turbulence the driving pressure is largely used up in creating the kinetic energy of the turbulent eddies. The flow no longer depends on the viscosity of the fluid but on its density. However, the critical velocity at which turbulence occurs depends mainly on the viscosity and density of the fluid as well as the radius of the bore of the tube through which it is flowing. In an intravenous infusion system the critical velocity is likely to be exceeded at very high flow rates and also at local points in the apparatus at which, because of sudden change in internal configuration, the velocity of flow momentarily rises. Thus, at points at which the internal diameter changes suddenly, turbulence will occur.

The viscosity of blood is considerably greater than that of water, mainly because of the presence of erythrocytes. It increases with the haematocrit and above about 60% haematocrit blood hardly behaves as a fluid. Viscosity is also increased by a drop in temperature, and the viscosity of blood at 0°C is about 2.5 times as great as at 37°C. Blood-warming coils are, therefore, justified on grounds of increasing the speed of transfusion as well as of preventing the development of hypothermia in the recipient.

An alternative to a catheter for very small veins is a needle attached to a hub by a length of plastic tubing. There are at least nine types of 'small-vein' needles currently available (Fig. 9.2). Some have winged handles to aid insertion and subsequent fixation to the patient. The flow performance of most of the 'small-vein sets' (often called 'infant scalp-vein sets' or 'butterflies') is surprisingly poor, and it is usually best to choose one with the shortest length of tubing attached.

Infusion apparatus

Where, as in the larger farm animals and horses, large-volume infusions are to be given rapidly, simple apparatus may be used. However, if a fairly accurate control of flow rate is needed, or the infusion is to be given slowly as may be necessary in small animal patients, then a system giving a greater degree of control is essential. Proprietary disposable plastic 'giving sets' or 'administration sets' are convenient for these purposes and can be obtained in a variety of patterns.

Essentially, a 'giving set' consists of an outlet tube which may or may not incorporate a filter depending on whether the set is for blood and blood products or crystalloid fluids alone, a drip chamber and a long length of plastic delivery tubing which can be occluded by some form of clamp. If it is intended for use with *bottles* of fluid an air inlet with a filter is incorporated. All plastic sets include a short piece of rubber tubing towards the needle mount end of the delivery tube so that injections can be made into the infusion fluid while administration proceeds. Injections are made through a fine-bore needle whilst the tubing is pinched between the finger and thumb on the drip chamber side of the injection site to prevent the pressure created by the injection from damming back fluid in the drip chamber. The flow rate is controlled by means of the clamp and can be estimated by counting the number of drops which pass through the drip chamber in 1 minute. For example, with most sets 40 drops/min means the administration of approximately 500 ml in 4 hours. Much more accurate control of infusion rate can be obtained by the use of drip rate controllers between the fluid container and the patient. These are electronic devices which monitor the drip rate with a sensor attached to the drip chamber and, by changing the effective cross-sectional area of a section of the standard administration set tubing, maintain a constant drip rate. The automatic control eliminates the need for frequent adjustment of the drip rate. However, drip rate controllers are expensive and cannot compensate for variations in drop size.

Drip rate pumps are similar in cost and appearance to drop rate controllers and most operate satisfactorily with standard administration sets. They generate a pressure by peristaltic fingers or rollers acting on deformable tubing to give a constant infusion rate. As with drip rate controllers the actual volumes delivered depend on drop size.

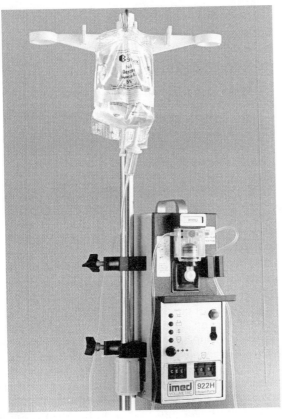

Fig. 9.3 Volumetric or constant-infusion pump. Types such as this drive a disposable pump unit and the need to refill the barrel of the pump means that the infusion rate is not actually constant. They will, however, maintain a reliable infusion rate. Most have devices which warn of the presence of air in the infusion line or occlusion of the line.

Volumetric pumps (Fig. 9.3) are designed to avoid problems associated with variations in drop size. Very good volumetric accuracy is obtained with either a reciprocating-piston-type pump or by peristaltic pumping on an accurately made tube which

forms part of the administration set. With the piston-type pump no fluid is delivered to the patient during the refilling stage of the cycle so that at low flow rates significant fluctuations in delivery rate occur. The need for a dedicated infusion set adds to the cost of each infusion and the volume of fluid required to prime these sets can also be in the region of 20 ml which may give rise to significant wastage of expensive solutions. These pumps are, however, particularly valuable for longer procedures where the solution can be withdrawn from a large container such as a 3 litre plastic bag.

Electrically driven syringe drivers (Fig. 9.4) overcome many of the problems associated with the administration of relatively small volumes of fluid (e.g. to cats, or the continuous administration of drugs during anaesthesia). They are usually calibrated for a particular type and size of syringe. The delivery rate control alters the rate of plunger travel, and hence the cross-sectional area of the syringe barrel is critical in ensuring that the delivery rate is correct. The syringe can be filled from a large container of fluid and connected to the intravenous catheter with a simple administration extension set so that the priming volume is minimal. Syringe drivers are generally less expensive than volumetric pumps or drip rate pumps or controllers as well as being more portable. Further developments include the use of microprocessor control with an ability (if the pharmacokinetics of the infused substance are known) to deliver a changing infusion rate such that a steady state of blood concentrations can be achieved and maintained.

Most infusion pumps monitor line pressure by detecting changes in the motor current needed for driving and to avoid frequent false alarms the pressure at which an occlusion is indicated is usually set well above the anticipated line pressure. This means that occlusion alarms on infusion pumps have little value in indicating that the fluid is being injected into the tissues rather than into a vein. With low flow rates, the time required for a significant increase in interstitial, and subsequently line pressure, will be long and substantial amounts of the fluid will have been injected before any warning is given.

Pharmaceutical companies now provide intravenous fluids in plastic disposable bag containers and some provide bags with an integral giving set. Because such bags are collapsible, no air inlet is necessary, air embolism cannot occur and infusions can be left running unattended — a considerable advantage for veterinary use. When bottles of fluid are used, there is always the possibility of air embolism should the bottle empty unobserved, as air has to enter the bottle before fluid can leave.

When fluids are administered under the influence of gravity the speed of infusion depends more on the

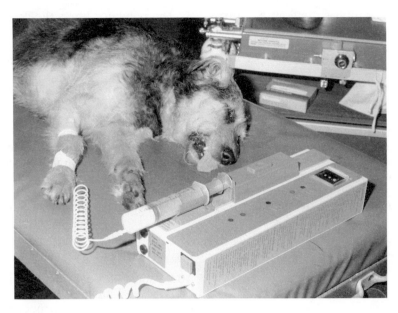

Fig. 9.4 Syringe driver. Many different types of electrically driven syringe drivers are available. Some must be used with one specified size of syringe, others can be used with a variety of syringes.

bore of the needle or catheter than on the pressure (i.e. the height above the needle or catheter at which the container is held). It has been shown that doubling the diameter of the needle or catheter gives a 16-fold increase in the rate of flow, whereas a four-fold increase in the pressure is required to double the rate. However, in the case of the 'flutter-valve' apparatus, traditional and so popular in veterinary practice, the vertical distance between the needle and the air inlet opening determines the rate at which air enters the system; increasing this distance increases the rate of air entry and hence the speed of infusion. The 'flutter valve' is unreliable and there is no real justification for its continued use in veterinary practice.

In circumstances where the maximum size of the needle or catheter is limited, the maximum rate of flow of fluid can be increased by pressurizing the system. Where bottles are in use, they can be pressurized by pumping air under pressure through the air inlet. This procedure carries a high risk of producing air embolism if the supply of fluid runs out, so it should be used with caution and the infusion never left unattended. More safely, pressure can be applied to plastic bags of fluid by placing them in a second pressurized bag or container for there is then no danger of air embolism.

ADMINISTRATION OF INHALATION AGENTS

The administration of an inhalation anaesthetic requires:

1. A source of oxygen (which may be air)
2. A vaporizer or a source of anaesthetic gas
3. A 'patient' or 'breathing' circuit

In its simplest form modern anaesthetic apparatus consists of an oxygen cylinder, with a pressure gauge, pressure regulator and flowmeter, delivering oxygen to a suitable patient breathing circuit. A vaporizer for an inhalation anaesthetic agent may be included inside or outside the patient breathing circuit. Such a simple apparatus is not as versatile as more elaborate equipment but it is adequate for most veterinary purposes.

Oxygen cylinders

For medical use oxygen is obtained compressed at high pressure (138 atm or 2000 lb/in^2) in metal cylinders ('tanks') or as liquid oxygen in special containers. For veterinary purposes cylinders are usually used; in the UK they are colour-coded black with a white top. When delivered, all cylinders have a plastic seal over their outlet to exclude dust and this seal should be removed only immediately before use. There are two types of cylinder outlet. Some cylinders fit into a yoke over pins which are indexed for different gases so as to make it impossible to attach an incorrect cylinder. A small washer termed a 'Bodcock seal' is needed around the inlet on the yoke of these pin-indexed fittings. Other cylinders utilize 'bull-nose' fittings which screw into place and require no sealing washer.

Pressure gauge

It is essential for the anaesthetist to know that there is an adequate supply of oxygen in the cylinder so when in use they are coupled to a pressure gauge to register the pressure inside and, therefore, the quantity of oxygen available. These gauges are most commonly of the Bourdon type (see Fig. 9.5), consisting of a metal tube, the end of which is attached to a pointer. The application of pressure to the inside of the tube causes it to straighten and moves the pointer over a scale.

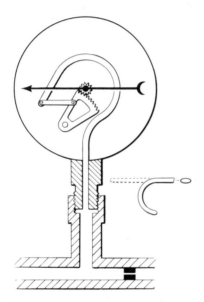

Fig. 9.5 Bourdon gauge. These are used for measuring gas pressure and, placed before an orifice, for gas-flow measurement.

Reducing valves or regulators

A pressure reducing valve is necessary for three reasons:

1. Once the flow has been set for any particular level, frequent readjustment of the flowmeter control, which would be necessary as the pressure in the cylinder fell off, is obviated. Because the reducing valve exerts this automatic control it is often referred to as a 'regulator'.
2. By supplying a low gas pressure to the control valve spindle small variations in the gas flow can be made easily. When a high-pressure cylinder is controlled directly by a simple needle-type valve large changes in flow rate result from very small movements of the control valve spindle.

3. The regulator limits the pressure within the connecting tubing to a low level and the likelihood of bursting the connecting tube when the flow is shut off by the flowmeter control is very much reduced.

The regulators in common use in anaesthesia usually reduce the pressure at which oxygen is delivered to below 13.8 atm (200 lb/in^2) and many modern anaesthetic machines incorporate the valve into the block featuring the cylinder pin index so that on superficial inspection of the machine they may be difficult to identify. Further details of these regulators can be obtained from such texts as *Anaesthetic Equipment* by C. S. Ward (2nd edn, 1985, Baillière Tindall, London) and will not be considered here.

Flowmeters

Today most of the flowmeters used in anaesthesia in the UK are known as 'rotameters' (Fig. 9.6). They make use of the interdependence of flow rate, size of orifice and pressure difference on either side of an orifice. The rotameter consists of a glass tube inside which a rotating bobbin is free to move. The bore of the tube gradually increases from below upwards. The bobbin floats up and down the tube, allowing gas to flow around it. The higher the bobbin in the tube the wider the annular space between the tube and bobbin (orifice) and the greater the flow rate through it. The bobbin, usually made of aluminium, has an upper rim which is of a diameter slightly greater than that of the body, and in which specially shaped channels are cut. As the gas enters the rotameter tube it impinges on the bobbin and causes it to rise and to spin because the rim with its set of channels acts like a set of vanes. The result is that the bobbin rides on a

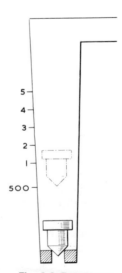

Fig. 9.6 Rotameter.

cushion of gas thereby eliminating errors due to friction between the tube and bobbin. The gas flow rate is read from the top of the bobbin against a scale etched on the outside of the glass tube. If the tube is mounted in a truly upright position these meters are capable of readings of an accuracy of ±2% but only for the gas for which they have been calibrated.

The Heidbrink flowmeter, commonly used in the USA, has a metal tube, the inside of which is tapered in the same way as a rotameter tube. The bobbin is replaced by a rod, the top of which is visible through a glass tube fitted at the top of the metal tube, a scale is fitted to the side of the glass tube and the gas flow rate can be read off from the position of the tip of the metal rod against this scale. In the UK this type of meter is mostly found on oxygen therapy apparatus.

Ball float meters, like the rotameter and Heidbrink, have a tapering bore and are, therefore, variable orifice meters. The bobbin or rod is replaced by a special ball and if the tube is mounted on an inclined plane one ball is sufficient, but if the tube is vertical the ball tends to oscillate; this is overcome by using two ball floats. The reading is taken from the centre of the ball or, in two ball types, the point of contact between the balls. The Connell flowmeter has two ball floats in contact in an inclined tube. With all inclined tube meters it is important that they are set at the correct angle or inaccuracies will occur.

A much more crude flowmeter utilizes a Bourdon pressure gauge (Fig. 9.5). The gas flowing from the cylinder issues from the reducing valve and is made to pass through a small orifice. A pressure builds up proximal to the constriction and this pressure is transmitted to the flexible metal, oval cross-section, Bourdon tube. The tube tends to straighten, the degree of straightening depending on the pressure within it which, in turn, depends on the rate of flow of gas through the orifice. The tip of the Bourdon tube is linked by a simple mechanism to an indicator needle which moves over a scale calibrated in terms of rate of gas flow through the constriction. In fact, in this meter the gauge indicates the pressure difference between the proximal side of the orifice and the atmosphere. This is virtually equivalent to measuring the pressure gradient across the orifice since in anaesthetic practice the pressure on the distal side of the orifice approximates very closely to atmospheric.

The Bourdon type of flowmeter is not satisfactory for measuring small rates of gas flow. Owing to the pressure necessary to cause the Bourdon tube to straighten out, a very small orifice must be used to provide the resistance to gas flow. If this orifice becomes partially blocked by dirt the meter reading increases, whereas the actual flow of gas is decreased; if the orifice becomes completely blocked the meter reading suggests that the flow is being maintained. On the other hand, if the orifice is enlarged due to wear, the gas flow will be increased while the decreased resistance to gas flow will lead to a low meter reading.

Pipeline systems

Where large quantities of oxygen (or other gases) are used, it is more convenient and more economical to utilize larger cylinders. As these are awkward to handle they are kept outside the operating theatre and the gas is supplied to the anaesthetic machine through a pipeline. The central depot has a number of large cylinders connected to a manifold so that gas is taken from all the cylinders in the bank. Warning devices are included so that the manifold can be changed to a second bank of cylinders when the supply pressure drops, or, with more complex apparatus where there are two or more manifolds, the change to the bank of fresh cylinders takes place automatically. If extremely large quantities of oxygen are used daily the cylinder bank may be replaced by a liquid oxygen container but this is most unlikely to be necessary for veterinary practice.

The outlets from the pipelines in the theatre are colour coded and indexed so that, at least in theory, pipes from the anaesthetic machine cannot be connected to the wrong outlet. Oxygen is delivered at a low pressure to the anaesthetic machine and does not need a reducing valve or pressure regulator so the piped supply is fed directly to the flowmeter. However, most pipeline machines also carry a small oxygen cylinder and an associated pressure regulator for emergency use in the event of a failure in the pipeline supply.

Oxygen failure warning devices

Devices which warn the anaesthetist that the pressure of the oxygen supply is low have been very neglected in veterinary anaesthesia, yet it is in this field, when often there is minimal assistance available to monitor the oxygen delivery, where they should be considered an essential feature of the anaesthetic machine. Some types depend on a second source of gas, usually nitrous oxide, for their operation. When the oxygen pressure falls a diaphragm moves to allow the second gas to pass through a whistle and an easily audible warning note is emitted. In other types a valve opens as the oxygen pressure drops and the remaining oxygen passes through the whistle; the whistling noise ceases as the oxygen pressure falls to atmospheric pressure.

Gases other than oxygen

Gases other than oxygen which are commonly found on anaesthetic machines include nitrous oxide (in the

UK cylinders are colour-coded blue), carbon dioxide (grey cylinder) and cyclopropane (orange cylinder). All these gases are compressed into the cylinders under a pressure which liquefies them at ordinary room temperatures. The amount of gas present in the cylinder can only be found by weighing (all these cylinders have their full and empty weights stamped on them) since the pressure of gas above the liquid remains almost constant as long as any liquid remains. Thus, a pressure gauge at the cylinder outlet will register only a small fall during the time the gas is being drawn off due to cooling causing a fall in the saturated vapour pressure, but this will rise again as the cylinder warms and the pressure registered will not drop rapidly until all the liquid has been vaporized and the residual gas is being drawn off.

Nitrous oxide and carbon dioxide cylinders need to be fitted with reducing valves ('pressure regulators') but cyclopropane liquefies at such a low pressure that this is unnecessary.

It is now possible to mix two gases using a monitored dial mixer unit instead of by setting their individual flow rates before delivery into a final common pathway. This type of system (Quantiflex) has been used for nitrous oxide/oxygen mixtures in any proportions from 21 to 100% oxygen at flow rates of 1–20 l/min. The system is costly, but it has the advantage that it can be more convenient and mistakes are less likely. It is inherently safe because hypoxic gas mixtures cannot be delivered.

When an oxygen flow is being mixed with a nitrous oxide flow without the aid of a Quantiflex mixer, failure of the oxygen supply is disastrous because the machine will then deliver 100% nitrous oxide. Oxygen warning devices such as those described above reduce the chance of this happening without the knowledge of the anaesthetist, but many modern machines incorporate a cut-off device so that should the oxygen flow cease the nitrous oxide flow is also cut off. This cut-off device may prevent the machine from being fitted with some types of oxygen failure alarm.

Vaporizers

The ideal vaporizer is one that delivers a suitable and accurately known quantity of a volatile anaesthetic agent at all times and under all conditions of use. Unfortunately many factors which vary during the course of administration influence vaporization and only the most modern of expensive, sophisticated pieces of apparatus approach anywhere near this ideal.

Factors which have most influence on the vaporization of volatile anaesthetics include temperature, gas flow rate through the vaporizer, and back pressure transmitted during IPPV. A low resistance to gas flow

may also be important if the vaporizer is to be used in the breathing circuit (p. 166).

Uncalibrated vaporizers

If a liquid anaesthetic is contained in a bottle it is possible to bubble gas from a cylinder through it or to allow the gas to flow over its surface. This arrangement is sometimes known as a 'plenum vaporizer' because gas is being forced into a chamber and a 'plenum' is a chamber or container inside which the pressure is greater than outside it.

In Britain and the Commonwealth, Boyle-pattern vaporizers are still encountered. In these the method of varying the concentration of anaesthetic vapour utilizes a permanent partition to prevent the direct passage of gases from the flowmeters to the patient. When the control lever is in the 'off' position all gases are diverted around the partition but away from the bottle. With the tap in the 'on' position all gases pass through the bottle containing the liquid anaesthetic agent. The control tap can be placed in any intermediate position and this determines how much of the total gas flow passes through the bottle. A further means of controlling the vapour concentration is also provided. The gases are made to pass through a J-shaped tube before emerging into the space above the liquid anaesthetic in the bottle. The open end of the J-tube is covered by a metal hood which can be positioned as required by moving the rod attached to it up or down. As the hood is pushed downwards, the gas is deflected nearer and nearer to the surface of the liquid and finally, when the open end of the hood is pushed below the surface of the liquid, gases are made to bubble through the liquid anaesthetic. When the tap is in the 'on' position and the hood, or cowl, fully depressed, the whole of the gas flow is made to bubble through the liquid and the maximum concentration of the anaesthetic vapour is picked up. Boyle-pattern vaporizers for potent agents such as halothane have a single, straight inlet tube with a side port and no cowl arrangement.

When air or other gas flows over the surface of a liquid, the vapour of the liquid is carried away, and is replaced by fresh vapour. This continuous process of vaporization is accompanied by a corresponding loss of heat, the magnitude of which is determined by the rate at which the vapour is removed and by the latent heat of vaporization of the liquid. The loss of heat results in a fall in the temperature of the liquid unless heat is conducted to the liquid from some outside source. With a fall in the temperature of the liquid there is a corresponding decrease in the speed of vaporization and, if the gas flow remains constant, the concentration of anaesthetic vapour in the gas stream from a Boyle-pattern vaporizer decreases with time until the heat loss due to vaporization is balanced by the conduction of heat through the glass of the bottle from the surrounding atmosphere to the liquid anaesthetic.

Calibrated vaporizers

There are today many precision vaporizers on the market, all designed to deliver an accurately known concentration of volatile anaesthetic agents over a wide range of gas flow rates. Among the best known of these are the various 'tecs' (e.g. Fluotec, etc., Cyprane Ltd) and the Vapor (Drager). All these consist of a vaporizing chamber and a bypass. The fresh gas stream flowing into the vaporizer is divided into two portions, the larger of which passes straight through the bypass. The smaller portion is ducted through the vaporizing chamber, where it becomes saturated with the vapour, and this ensures that:

1. There is no sudden burst of high vapour concentration when the vaporizer is first switched on
2. The output of the vaporizer is unaffected by shaking

As already pointed out, the vaporization of the liquid anaesthetic results in the removal of heat from a liquid with a resultant fall in its temperature. If this fall is not checked the rate of vaporization will fail and the output concentration of the vaporizer decreases with time. In various 'tecs' (e.g. Fluotec for halothane) temperature compensation is achieved by means of a bimetallic strip valve. This valve is arranged to act as a control of the volume of gas passing through the vaporizing chamber. As the temperature of the liquid falls, the bimetallic strip opens the valve further, allowing more gas to pass through the chamber. In the Vapor, the vaporizer is constructed from a large mass of copper. The high thermal conductivity of this metal allows heat to pass into the liquid from the room and this, together with the high thermal capacity of its mass, supplies the necessary heat for vaporization, holding the liquid temperature constant. In the 'tec' and Vapor vaporizers temperature compensation is automatic and the only control to set is the output concentration.

A major problem in vaporizer design lies in the design of the splitting valves. In the earlier 'tec' vaporizers it proved impossible to ensure that the flow division ratio of this valve remained constant over a wide range of flow rates, and the vaporizers were supplied with graphs which needed to be consulted when the vaporizers were used with gas flow rates below 4 l/min. In current models (e.g. Mark III Fluotec) this problem has been overcome and it is claimed that they are accurate at flow rates above 500 ml/min.

Pressure fluctuations produced by IPPV may have a considerable effect on the output concentration of vaporizers [1]. This 'pumping effect' can result in doubling the output concentration at low fresh gas flow rates and modern vaporizers incorporate a non-return valve to overcome this.

All the vaporizers described so far have a high resistance to gas flow, which is unimportant when the carrier gas is pushed through them by the power of the compressed gases in their cylinders. If the vaporizer is to be used in the breathing circuit, where the gas flow is powered by the respiratory efforts of the animal, then a low-resistance vaporizer is essential.

Low-resistance vaporizers

Vaporizers offering a low resistance to gas flow are usually of a simple type with wide-bore entry and exit ports and no wicks to impede the flow of gases. A simple low efficiency vaporizer of this type often used in dental surgery is the Goldman (Fig. 9.7).

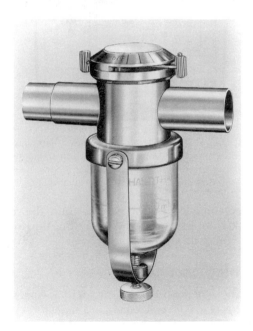

Fig. 9.7 Goldman vaporizer for halothane. This is a simple low-resistance vaporizer which may be placed in the inspiratory limb of circle breathing systems.

The EMO vaporizer (Epstein–Macintosh–Oxford) (Fig. 9.8) was specifically designed for the use of ether and is generally recognized as the best of this type of vaporizer. It is portable, has a temperature-compensating device and is employed in a non-rebreathing system. Its place in small animal anaesthesia was assessed by Hall [2] who concluded that ether/air anaesthesia administered from it met criteria

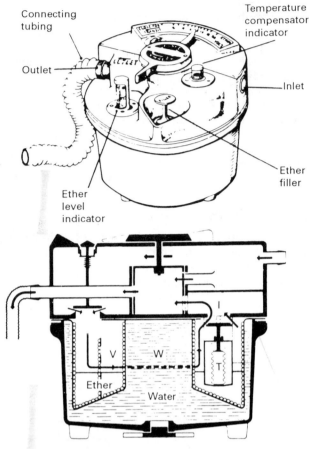

Fig. 9.8 The EMO vaporizer for ether. This draw-over, temperature-compensated unit may be used in situations where supplies of oxygen are not readily available and, consequently, it is very popular in developing countries.

for acceptability in general practice where the veterinarian may be assisted in the operating theatre by a nurse or may be entirely alone.

Breathing circuits

The purpose of the breathing circuit of an anaesthetic apparatus is to convey oxygen and anaesthetic to the patient, and to ensure the removal of carbon dioxide produced by the patient. It does not seem possible to classify all the ways in which this can be done in a completely logical manner and as yet there is no universally agreed system. A system of classification formerly in common use in the UK was:

1. The open method
2. The semi-open method
3. (a) The closed method with carbon dioxide absorption
   (b) The semi-closed method with carbon dioxide absorption
4. The semi-closed method without carbon dioxide absorption

This classification has been criticized on the grounds that it is impractical and does not fit all systems. A more clinically useful definition of circuits is based on the two methods by which carbon dioxide is removed from the circuit. Either the circuit is designed so that the expired gases are vented to the atmosphere and cannot be rebreathed (non-rebreathing circuits) or the expired gases are passed through an absorber which contains soda lime to remove the carbon dioxide (rebreathing circuits).

The open and semi-open methods were used to volatilize agents such as chloroform and ether. The methods are often referred to as 'rag and bottle anaesthesia' and they survived through over a 100 years of anaesthetic history. In the semi-open or 'perhalation' method all the inspired air was made to pass through a mask on which the vaporization of the agent occurred. In horses and cattle, special masks (Fig. 9.9) were often used for the semi-open administration of chloroform. These masks were cylinders of leather and canvas applied over either the upper or both jaws. Chloroform was applied to a sponge inserted in the open end of the cylinder. In the cruder types of mask the sponge was actually in contact with the nostrils, but in more refined patterns a wire mesh partition prevented this direct contact.

Today, the open and semi-open methods of administration are seldom used. The anaesthetic agents are diluted to an unknown extent by air and this dilution is greatest when the minute volume of breathing is large so the inspiratory gas flow rate is

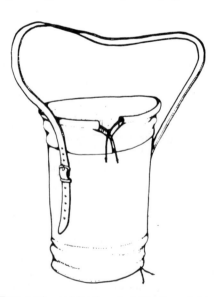

Fig. 9.9 Face-mask used for the administration of chloroform to horses and cattle.

high. The greater the ventilation (and, hence, the dilution of the anaesthetic inhaled), the closer the alveolar concentration of the anaesthetic will approach zero, and anaesthesia lightens as ventilation increases. On the other hand, depression of breathing decreases the air dilution and thereby increases the concentration of anaesthetic inspired. Under these circumstances, unless there is an increase in the uptake of the anaesthetic by the body, the alveolar concentration of the anaesthetic must rise. A rise in the alveolar concentration produces deeper unconsciousness and further respiratory depression. In addition, deepening anaesthesia reduces the cardiac output and hence the uptake of anaesthetic by the body, thus adding still further to the rise in the alveolar concentration. If this process is allowed to proceed unchecked, unconsciousness deepens until the ventilation becomes inadequate. In other words, with the open and semi-open methods of administration, animals which become more lightly anaesthetized tend to continue awakening and animals which become more deeply anaesthetized tend to continue becoming more depressed and nearer to death.

Non-rebreathing circuits

The general principle behind non-rebreathing circuits is that fresh gases flow from the anaesthetic machine into a reservoir from which the patient inhales and the exhaled gases are spilled, usually through an expiratory valve, to the atmosphere. Carbon dioxide removal depends on the fresh gas flow rate, and on the minute and tidal volumes of respiration of the patient. Many circuits have been devised but, in general, they are all variations of those classified by Mapleson [3] (Fig. 9.10). The performance of many of these circuits has been reviewed by Sykes [4]. In veterinary anaesthesia the most commonly used semi-closed non-rebreathing circuits are the Magill circuit (Mapleson A), the T-piece (Mapleson E) and coaxial circuits (variations of Mapleson A and D).

The Magill circuit. The Magill attachment, which incorporates a reservoir bag, wide-bore corrugated tubing and a spring-loaded expiratory valve (Fig. 9.11), is probably the most generally useful of all the non-rebreathing systems for small animal patients. With this system rebreathing is prevented by maintaining the total gas flow rate from the cylinders slightly in excess of the patient's respiratory minute volume. The animal inhales from the bag and wide-bore tubing; the exhaled mixture passes back up the tubing displacing the gas in it back into the bag until it is full. The exhaled gases never reach the bag because the capacity of the tube is too great and once the bag is distended the build up of pressure inside the system

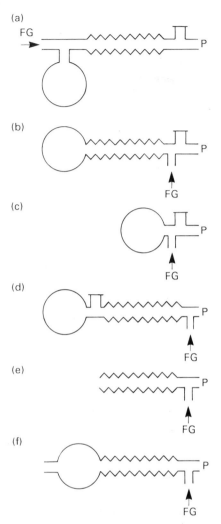

Fig. 9.10 The Mapleson classification of patient breathing circuits. This is a most comprehensive classification. Note that system (a) = Magill and Lack circuits; (e) = T-piece circuit (FG = fresh gas flow, P = patient).

causes the expiratory valve to open so that the terminal part of the expiration (rich in carbon dioxide) passes out of the valve into the atmosphere. During the pause which follows expiration and before the next inspiration fresh gas from the anaesthetic apparatus sweeps the first part of the exhaled gases from the corrugated tube out through the expiratory valve.

To ensure minimal rebreathing of the expired gases the fresh gas flow rate should be equal to, or greater than, the minute volume of respiration of the patient. However, as the system leads to the preferential removal of alveolar gas, a lower fresh gas flow rate (equal to the alveolar ventilation) may be adequate and, in man, Kain and Nunn [5] have shown that in spontaneously breathing patients significant

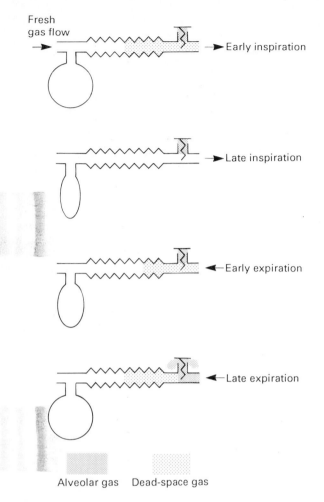

Fig. 9.11 The Magill circuit (spontaneous breathing) showing mode of operation to prevent rebreathing of exhaled gas.

rebreathing does not occur until the fresh gas flow rate falls below 70% of the patient's minute volume. If, however, IPPV is applied by compression of the reservoir bag, then very much higher fresh gas flow rates are needed to prevent rebreathing because under these circumstances the fresh gas is spilled through the expiratory valve at the end of inspiration.

Various non-return valves (Ryan's valve, Ruben's valve, Emerson's valve, Hewer's valve and, in veterinary anaesthesia, Weaver's valve) have been incorporated in the Magill system in place of the simple spring-loaded expiratory valve. All these valves prevent any rebreathing of the exhaled gases other than those contained in the 'dead-space' of the valve itself and its connections. Where they are used the gas flow rates from the apparatus require frequent adjustment, for any alteration in the rate or depth of the patient's breathing affects the degree of distension of the reservoir bag. If the gas flow rate is constant, deep or rapid breathing empties the bag quickly, while slow

or shallow breathing allows the bag to become overdistended. These non-return valves can, therefore, be used to measure the minute volume of respiration, for if the gas flow rates are adjusted to maintain the bag at a constant average size at the end of expiration the total gas flow rate as read at the flowmeters will equal the respiratory minute volume. In practice, to avoid the necessity for repeated adjustments of the total gas flow rate, an excessive flow is employed and a spill valve is incorporated in the circuit between the reservoir bag and the non-return valve.

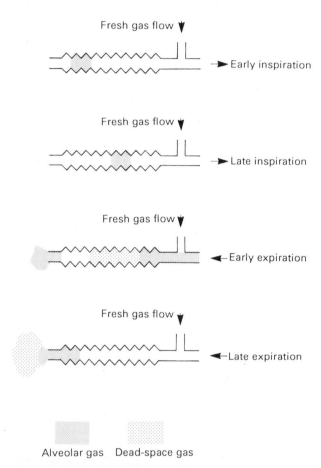

Fig. 9.12 Mode of operation of the T-piece circuit in preventing rebreathing provided the fresh gas flow exceeds about twice the patient's minute volume.

T-piece systems. The low resistance and small dead-space make the T-piece system, first described by Ayre [6], very suitable for use with cats and small dogs.

As shown in Fig. 9.12 an open tube acts as a reservoir and there are no valves. The exhaled gases are swept out of the open end of the reservoir tube by fresh gases flowing in from the anaesthetic apparatus during the expiratory phase. Unless the capacity of the reservoir tube is at least equal to the tidal volume of the animal the terminal part of the inspired gases will be air but if this will only enter the dead-space no dilution of the anaesthetic gases will take place.

The modifications of the T-piece system can be divided into three types. In the first there is no expiratory limb, in the second the capacity of the expiratory limb is greater than the tidal volume, and in the third the capacity of the expiratory limb is less than the tidal volume. On the basis of previous mathematical and laboratory investigations by other authors, Harrison [7] discussed these three types with reference to resistance to respiration, the minimum fresh gas flow required to prevent rebreathing and air dilution during both spontaneous and controlled ventilation. The resistance and fresh gas requirements are obviously related to the expiratory flow rates and respiratory flow patterns which occur in patients of any particular size. Harrison concluded that the most convenient system is one in which the expiratory limb volume is greater than the tidal volume and which has an open-ended bag attached to the distal end of the expiratory limb (Jackson–Rees modification of the T-piece, see below). With such an arrangement fresh gas flows of up to 2.5–3 times the minute volume of respiration are required to eliminate rebreathing.

Using the basic T-piece system IPPV may be applied by intermittently blocking the open end of the reservoir tube thus directing the fresh gas into the animal's lungs. However, the inflation pressure, being that supplied by the anaesthetic machine, may be so high as to cause massive pulmonary damage if overinflation is allowed to occur. Ventilation may be controlled more safely by squeezing a bag attached to the end of the expiratory limb — the Jackson–Rees modification [8] — because this bag has an open tail, the orifice of which can be controlled between the finger and thumb of the anaesthetist and the inflation pressure adjusted to suit the circumstances.

Coaxial systems. The desirability of controlling atmospheric pollution in operating theatres has led to an interest in the use of coaxial circuits because it is relatively easy to duct the waste gases from them to the atmosphere by valves placed at the anaesthetic machine and well away from the patient. Two types of coaxial circuits — the Bain system (Fig. 9.13) and the Lack system (Fig. 9.14) — are in use.

In the Bain type of circuit fresh gas passes up the central tube and expired gas through the outer sleeve. It can be seen that this arrangement is basically that of the T-piece circuit and, therefore, in general, the same gas flow considerations will apply. However, higher gas flow rates are needed to prevent significant rebreathing of expired gases during spontaneous respiration and the pattern of respiration is important.

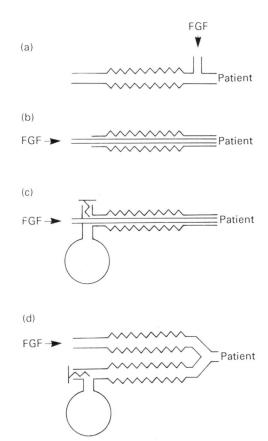

Fig. 9.13 The T-piece circuit (a) compared to the original Bain coaxial circuit (b), the modified Bain coaxial circuit (c) and the modified, parallel Bain circuit (d). It is important to note that in the modified circuits the bag is on the *expiratory* limb. (FFG = fresh gas flow.)

An animal which breathes slowly with a long expiratory pause will make more efficient use of the fresh gas inflow than an animal with a rapid, shallow respiratory pattern.

The Lack circuit uses the alternative arrangement in which the fresh gas flows up the outer sleeve and expiration takes place down the inner tube. This arrangement was designed to aid scavenging of expired gas and is more satisfactory than the conventional Mapleson A system in this respect. The Lack circuit cannot be used with controlled ventilation in the same way as the Bain circuit without excessive rebreathing so its use is restricted to spontaneously breathing animals.

The modified Bain circuit (Penlon Ltd, Fig. 9.13) has proved reasonably satisfactory for use in dogs over 10 kg body weight and was the circuit used with very good results for IPPV in dogs over 20 kg body weight [9, 10].

Use of these circuits in veterinary anaesthesia has revealed a number of problems. In some cases the

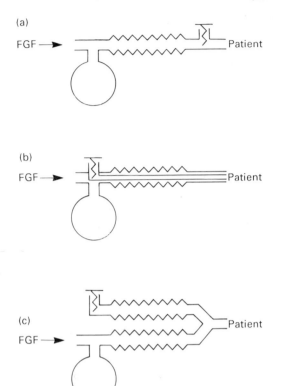

(a) FGF → Patient

(b) FGF → Patient

(c) FGF → Patient

Fig. 9.14 The Lack coaxial circuit (b) compared to the standard Magill circuit (a) and the parallel Lack circuit (c). In all these circuits there is a reservoir bag on the *inspiratory* limb of the circuit (FGF = fresh gas flow.)

internal or external tubing has been of too small a bore so that excessive demands were made on the animal's inspiratory or expiratory efforts. More serious, perhaps, the inner tube has become detached from the anaesthetic machine or patient, resulting in a very large dead-space.

The potential for a large increase in dead-space if the inner tube of a coaxial system becomes detached at the end nearest the anaesthetic machine has been appreciated in respect of the Bain system for some considerable time and it is most important that this circuit is tested immediately before use. Testing may be done by connecting it to the common gas outlet of the anaesthetic machine and passing a flow of at least 6 l/min of oxygen through the inner tube of the system. The distal (patient) end of this inner tube is then occluded (with the finger or the plunger of a 5 ml syringe) and the oxygen flowmeter bobbin should be seen to dip and the machine pressure relief valve heard blowing off, indicating that all is well.

Modifications of non-rebreathing systems. The Enclosed Magill Anaesthetic Breathing System devised by Voss [11] is an interesting modification of a

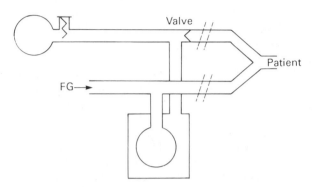

Fig. 9.15 The enclosed Magill circuit, an interesting variation of the Mapleson A breathing system. The fresh gas flow (FGF) passes into the bag on the inspiratory limb enclosed within the box. The expiratory limb of the system leads back to the box and there is a one-way valve proximal to its entry into the box. The expiratory limb is continuous with the interior of the box and has a Heidbrink valve and rebreathing bag or open reservoir placed distally. For IPPV the Heidbrink valve is partially closed and the rebreathing bag squeezed; because of the one-way valve this compresses the reservoir bag in the box and the patient's lungs are inflated with fresh gas. A ventilator can be attached in place of the rebreathing bag and the Heidbrink valve completely closed. Expired gases then spill through the ventilator instead of the Heidbrink valve. During spontaneous breathing, fresh gas flowing into the inspiratory limb limits the reflux of exhaled gas, but the majority of the early expired gas potentially able to reflux should be dead-space gas. The initial dead-space gas is conserved provided the one-way valve remains closed until the enclosed reservoir bag is filled.

Mapleson A (Magill) breathing system (Fig. 9.15). In this configuration the fresh gas flow needed for normocapnia is similar in both spontaneous and controlled ventilation modes. The fresh gas flow passes into a bag, the enclosed reservoir, on the inspiratory limb of the system. This bag is enclosed in a rigid, transparent-walled bottle. The expiratory tube leads back to this bottle and there is a one-way valve proximal to its entrance into the bottle. The expiratory limb is thus continuous with the bottle and there is a Heidbrink valve and an open reservoir bag, situated distally.

During spontaneous breathing, the animal inspires from the enclosed reservoir bag on the inspiratory limb and is prevented from breathing gas from the expiratory limb by the closure of the one-way valve. On expiration, the one-way valve opens, allowing spillage of the expired gas. Fresh gas flowing into the reservoir bag of the inspiratory limb from the anaesthetic machine limits expiration into the inspiratory limb, but the majority of the early expired gas should be dead-space gas. In this respect the system performs as a Mapleson A with the expiratory valve distal from the animal. This is similar to the configuration of either the Lack or Magill system.

Controlled ventilation with this system is undertaken

either with a ventilator or manually by squeezing the reservoir bag placed at the distal part of the expiratory limb. Expired gases spill through either the ventilator or the Heidbrink valve. For inspiration, pressure exerted at the distal end of the expiratory limb closes the one-way valve and increases the pressure in the bottle thereby squeezing the enclosed reservoir bag. This forces fresh gas into the animal. On expiration, expired gas passes into both limbs of the system. Fresh gas inflow limits the passage of expired gas into the inspiratory limb, but fresh gas from the animal's dead-space is conserved. The one-way valve opens and expired alveolar gas is vented into the expiratory limb and out into the atmosphere through either the ventilator or the Heidbrink valve, depending on the mode of controlled ventilation.

Humphrey's 'ADE' system is designed to facilitate changing from a Mapleson D or E configuration during controlled ventilation to a Mapleson A mode for spontaneous ventilation [12] and is another, perhaps more commonly used, modification of an earlier system. It is not very efficient in conserving anaesthetic gases — the Bain system is 24% better [13].

Parallel circuits which operate in the same manner as the Bain and Lack circuits have two tubes running alongside one another rather than one inside the other (Figs 9.13 and 9.14).

Rebreathing circuits

Anaesthetic gases and vapours are said to be more or less physiologically 'indifferent', in that they are largely exhaled from the body unchanged, but when exhaled they are mixed with carbon dioxide. The exhaled gas can be directed into a closed bag and if the carbon dioxide is removed, and sufficient oxygen added to satisfy the metabolic requirements of the animal, the same gas or vapour can be rebreathed continuously from the bag. This is the principle of closed-circuit anaesthetic administration. The same circuits may also be employed as 'low-flow' systems if slightly higher gas flow rates are fed in and the excess gases allowed to escape through an overflow valve.

In anaesthesia, the carbon dioxide is usually removed by directing the exhaled mixture over the surface of soda lime. This is a mixture of 90% calcium hydroxide and 5% sodium hydroxide together with 5% of silicate and water to prevent powdering. It is used in a granular form, the granules being 4–8 mesh in size, and is packed into a canister so that, ideally, the space between the granules is at least equal to the tidal volume of the animal. Some brands of soda lime contain an indicator dye which changes colour when the carbon dioxide absorbing capacity is exhausted. Absence of visible colour change is no guarantee that

the soda lime is capable of absorbing more carbon dioxide — a small quantity should be wrapped in gauze and a brisk flow of carbon dioxide directed through it. When this is done active soda lime becomes very hot but exhausted absorbent remains cool.

Theoretically, during closed-circuit administration, once anaesthesia has been induced and a state of equilibrium established, all that the animal requires from the apparatus is a continuous stream of oxygen just sufficient to satisfy its metabolic requirements, and efficient absorption of carbon dioxide. In practice, however, most periods of anaesthesia are too short to allow a state of equilibrium to be reached and the body continues to take up the anaesthetic agent throughout the administration, so that the agent has to be given all the time in order to maintain the alveolar concentration.

The closed method of administration is simple, and much less anaesthetic is used than in non-rebreathing methods because there is no wastage to the atmosphere. The chief disadvantage of closed-circuit anaesthesia is the resistance to respiration due to the packed soda lime. This resistance is sufficiently great to render the method unsuitable for cats, puppies and very small adult dogs. Another disadvantage is that the conservation of heat and water vapour afforded by the method may give rise to heat stroke in dogs and sheep.

There are two systems in use for carbon dioxide absorption techniques in anaesthesia:

1. The 'to-and-fro' system
2. The 'circle system'

The 'to-and-fro' system. A canister full of soda lime is interposed between the animal and the rebreathing bag, fresh gases being fed into the system as close to the animal as possible to effect changes in the mixture rapidly (Fig. 9.16). This system is simple and efficient but has several drawbacks. It is difficult to maintain the heavy, awkward apparatus in a gas-tight condition and the inspired gases become undesirably hot due to the chemical action between the soda lime and the carbon dioxide. Furthermore, irritating dust may be inhaled from the soda lime and give rise to a bronchitis. Nevertheless the system is the one most commonly used in veterinary anaesthesia for the necessary apparatus is relatively inexpensive and may be improvised.

For small animal anaesthesia (dogs, sheep and goats, young calves, young foals and small pigs) the standard soda lime canisters used in man, which are known as Water's canisters after their designer, are quite satisfactory. They are available in various sizes and one canister to contain about 0.5 kg and a second

(a)

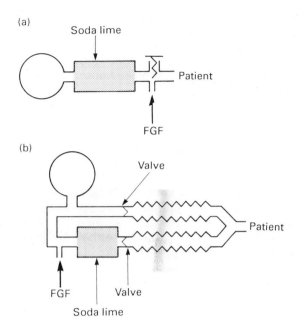

Fig. 9.16 To-and-fro (a) and circle absorber systems (b) (FGF = fresh gas flow).

one to contain about 0.3 kg of soda lime are adequate for most veterinary purposes. These canisters are used horizontally and unless the soda lime is tightly packed when the canister is filled it tends to settle, leaving a channel along the top through which gases pass without being subjected to the action of the soda lime. Robson and Pask [14] suggested that in the larger canisters a domestic nylon pot scrubber may be used to pack the soda lime. The canister is filled and shaken down as well as possible and the nylon scrubber inserted so as to leave about half of it to be compressed by the wire gauze in the lid of the canister when the cap is screwed on.

Adult horses, cattle and large pigs need much larger soda lime canisters. They are designed on the principle that for efficient absorption of carbon dioxide the whole of the animal's tidal volume should be accommodated in the spaces between the soda lime granules. A canister used in the Cambridge Veterinary School for over 35 years has been found to be reasonably efficient yet not too awkward or cumbersome. It measures approximately 20 cm in length and 81 cm in diameter (internal measurements) and contains about 4.5 kg of soda lime. The connections to the rebreathing bag and to the expiratory mount are of 5 cm internal diameter. Because of the difficulty experienced in packing this canister sufficiently tightly with soda lime, special to-and-fro canisters have been designed and developed for large animals. The vertical position of these soda lime canisters means that tight packing is not necessary,

and their cross-sectional area is large to ensure that the respired gases move through the absorbent slowly.

For adult horses and cattle a rebreathing bag having a capacity of about 15 litres is used.

The to-and-fro systems can never be really efficient absorbers of carbon dioxide. The exhaled gases all come into contact with the soda lime at the end of the canister nearest to the patient and the absorbent in this region is quickly exhausted. Thus, as this occurs, the gases have to travel further and further into the canister before carbon dioxide is absorbed or, in other words, the apparatus dead-space steadily increases during anaesthesia.

Purchase [15] investigated the performance of two large to-and-fro absorbers with regard to resistance to breathing and carbon dioxide absorption, using a mechanical analogue of a horse's lung. Both absorbers were found to offer a resistance to breathing of approximately 1.2 cmH$_2$O (0.12 kPa) per 100 l/min at a flow of 600 l/min (a flow rate of the order of that encountered during the respiratory cycle in horses), and both provided a similar mean inspired carbon dioxide concentration. Their dead-space increased steadily as the proximal soda lime became exhausted, but starting with a fresh charge of absorbent in a large animal to-and-fro absorber the mean inspired carbon dioxide concentration should not, in practice, exceed 3% for over 4 hours.

The 'circle' system. The circle system for carbon dioxide absorption incorporates an inspiratory and an expiratory tube with unidirectional valves to ensure a one-way flow of gases; the rebreathing bag and soda lime canister are placed between these tubes. The valves and tubing offer an appreciable resistance to breathing and unless the apparatus is carefully designed with regard to the diameter of airways in relation to flow rates, breathing through the apparatus can impose a considerable strain on the animal. Circle-type absorber units are not, as a general rule, suitable for cats and small dogs of less than about 15 kg body weight because of the resistance offered by even the best-designed units and because of the inevitable degree of rebreathing which occurs at the T-piece connection to the patient. This rebreathing can be prevented by placing the unidirectional valves at the face-piece or connection to the endotracheal tube, but it is difficult to design robust, competent valves for use in this situation. In the majority of modern circle-type units the unidirectional valves are of the turret type; some, however, employ rubber flaps. The turret type is robust and competent but it has the disadvantage that it must be kept upright and of necessity, therefore, has to be mounted on the apparatus at some distance away from the animal.

Circle absorber units (Fig. 9.16) are more efficient

absorbers of carbon dioxide than are to-and-fro units because their dead-space is constant since all the charge of soda lime is available to the respired gases. Exhaustion of soda lime is noticed more suddenly than in to-and-fro absorbers and once it occurs the inspired carbon dioxide concentration may soon become excessive.

To avoid this sudden exhaustion of the soda lime and for economy in its use, canisters are now often made with two compartments. The compartment of the canister which first receives the inspired gases and, therefore, whose soda lime is first used, can be refilled and the position of the canister reversed, so that the expired gases pass through the remaining partially used soda lime, using this to complete exhaustion before reaching the newly filled compartment.

Standard circle absorbers designed for man are satisfactory for young foals, young calves, sheep, goats, most pigs, and dogs over 15 kg body weight. Circle absorbers for large animal patients are now commercially available but there are few reports of their efficiency in terms of carbon dioxide absorbing capacity or resistance to breathing. In North America, circle absorbers designed for small dogs (and even cats) are widely used but they have never found favour in the UK where non-rebreathing systems are preferred for patients of this size.

All circle absorption systems for large animals are relatively cumbersome and expensive and are only likely to find favour for use in hospitals. For general practice a large animal to-and-fro system, in spite of its limitations, is much more convenient.

Practical problems involved in the use of closed rebreathing circuits. All anaesthetists using closed rebreathing circuits must fully understand how the concentrations of gases which the animal breathes from the reservoir bag are altered by the uptake, utilization and elimination of gases and vapours by the patient.

When anaesthesia is first induced with an inhalation anaesthetic the animal takes up the anaesthetic and the expired gases contain a lower concentration of the anaesthetic than the inspired gases. Thus, the concentration of anaesthetic in a completely closed circuit will become diluted. The speed of uptake of the anaesthetic depends on many factors (Chapter 6), but obviously the larger the animal, the greater the dilution, and the longer the time before equilibrium is attained. Also, during induction, nitrogen from the patient accumulates in the anaesthetic circuit and decreases the concentration of oxygn therein.

The problems of denitrogenation and of maintaining an adequate concentration of anaesthetic for the induction of anaesthesia are best overcome by in-creasing the fresh gas flow rate, opening overspill valves, frequently emptying the rebreathing bag ('dumping') and thus converting the system to a semi-closed circuit for the duration of the induction period.

The problems involved in rapidly decreasing the depth of anaesthesia are similar to those of induction but the gases exhaled by the patient will contain anaesthetic in higher concentrations than the inspired gas, so that the concentration of anaesthetic in the circuit will tend to increase, and the depth of anaesthesia will only lighten very slowly. Again, this can be overcome by increasing the gas inflow rates and emptying the rebreathing bag at frequent intervals.

Maintenance of a stable depth of anaesthesia also poses problems when a completely closed rebreathing circuit is employed. Theoretically, all that is required is a fresh gas flow containing exactly the oxygen requirements of the animal, together with low concentrations of anaesthetic just sufficient to replenish that being absorbed by the patient or lost from the wound surfaces, etc. In large animals, where the oxygen requirement exceeds 1 l/min, the completely closed system often works very well and can be used throughout the anaesthetic maintenance period. In small animals, however, it often proves very difficult to maintain stable, smooth anaesthesia without extreme care being paid by the anaesthetist to every aspect of administration. This is because these small animals have very low basal metabolic requirements of oxygen and the vaporizers used to deliver volatile anaesthetics are often very inefficient at low gas flow rates. Even modern vaporizers are only accurate with carrier gas flow rates of more than 0.5 l/min and stable anaesthesia can only be achieved by increasing the fresh gas flow rate to a level at which the vaporizer will deliver an accurately known concentration of anaesthetic, and allowing the excess to escape from an overflow valve. Some veterinarians attempt to overcome these problems by filling the circuit intermittently with high fresh gas flow rates but this results in fluctuating levels of anaesthesia.

A second method of overcoming the problem of vaporization of the anaesthetic at low fresh gas flow rates is to place the vaporizer inside the breathing circuit. If the vaporizer is placed in the fresh gas supply line outside the breathing circuit the circuit receives a steady supply of anaesthetic. When the vaporizer is placed in the breathing circuit, however, the flow through it depends on the respiratory efforts of the patient so that vaporization of the anaesthetic depends on this rather than the fresh gas flow rate.

The influence of the location of the vaporizer on the inspired tension of the anaesthetic agent has been considered in some detail by workers in the Welsh National School of Medicine, Cardiff [16–18]. These workers concluded that each system has its own advantages and disadvantages, but that in the hands of an experienced anaesthetist either arrangement is equally safe (or unsafe). The inexperienced anaesthetist is advised, especially with potent anaesthetics such as halothane, to use a calibrated and preferably thermostatically controlled vaporizer placed outside the breathing circuit. All anaesthetists using vaporizers inside the breathing circuit must understand clearly the way in which the alveolar concentration, and hence the depth of anaesthesia, is dependent on the factors of ventilation, fresh gas flow and vaporizer characteristics.

In general, when the vaporizer is in the breathing circuit:

1. If anaesthesia is too light surgical stimulation will lead to an increase in ventilation and a deepening of unconsciousness.
2. If the vaporizer setting is too high, deepening anaesthesia depresses the ventilation and reduces vaporization. This acts to some extent as a built-in safety factor.
3. If the animal stops breathing no fresh vapour enters the circuit.
4. The smaller the fresh gas flow the greater the economy in the use of the volatile agent.
5. A simple, low-efficiency vaporizer is all that is required (e.g. The Goldman vaporizer for halothane which limits the concentration delivered to less than 3% by volume whatever the gas flow through it).
6. A sudden increase in ventilation and, therefore, of inspired concentration may be dangerous.
7. The fact that respired gases pass through the vaporizer introduce problems of resistance to breathing.

There is wide concern among anaesthetists that inadvertent high flows through the vaporizer may lead to undesirably high concentrations of the volatile agent accumulating in the circuit during assisted lung ventilation with consequent danger from overdose. However, used cautiously with, preferably, monitoring of the circuit concentrations of the volatile agent the method can be very satisfactory.

When the vaporizer is outside the breathing circuit:

1. Ventilation has no effect on vaporization. Assisted or controlled respiration by IPPV has little effect on the depth of anaesthesia and is therefore much safer than is the case when the vaporizer is in the breathing circuit.
2. In most instances for any particular setting of the vaporizer control the smaller the fresh gas flow, the lower is the inspired concentration.
3. Too deep anaesthesia with respiratory depression does not have the built-in safety factor found when the vaporizer is in the breathing circuit and the animal is breathing spontaneously.

Because of the difficulties with both in-circuit and out-of-circuit vaporizer positions many workers have adopted the simpler procedure of injecting the liquid volatile agent directly into the system. Vaporization takes place inside the tubing of the system and a metal sleeve with or without some gauze may be used to aid vaporization [19]. Drip feeds of liquid anaesthetics into anaesthetic system were common in the past but current interest arises chiefly from the work of Lowe and colleagues in the USA [20]. The injection of liquid anaesthetic into the system can be carried out using an electrically driven syringe pump which greatly facilitates automatic control. Using a monitoring device such as the Engstrom Emma anaesthetic gas monitor in the inspiratory limb it is possible to set up a computer-assisted system to maintain a constant inspired concentration of the anaesthetic agent. The closed-circuit system also lends itself to various methods of automatically controlling gas flow into the system. One sophisticated approach uses a concertina bellows in the circuit as a volume transducer which is attached to a linear transducer which control the inflow of oxygen and nitrous oxide [21]. In this system the gas flows can be electrically controlled to produce any desired flow rate from 50 to 1000 ml/min with an accuracy of $\pm 1\%$, an oxygen sensor controlling the oxygen flow to maintain a predetermined concentration and the nitrous oxide to maintain the volume. Work with such systems for veterinary use has been reported by Moens [22].

DEFINITION OF ANAESTHETIC CIRCUITS

There have been many multiple and inconsistent definitions in British and US literature and, as already mentioned, as yet there is no universal nomenclature. The summary in Table 9.1 may serve to illustrate some of the differences between British and US usage of terms.

From this summary it is apparent that the present systems of terminology consist of 'closed' and 'open'

themes with variations, but that this terminology is now of very little value. Moreover, these systems attempt to use rebreathing as the distinguishing factor. No one would deny that rebreathing is an extremely important variable, yet it is impossible to describe accurately variations which occur in the degree of rebreathing by the use of such terms as semi-closed, semi-closed with absorption, partial

Table 9.1 US and British definitions of terms

	Reservoir bag	Rebreathing	Examples
US nomenclature			
Open	No	No	Open drop
			Insufflation
			T-piece
Semi-open	Yes	No	T-piece with bag
			Magill
			Non-rebreathing valves
Semi-closed	Yes	Partial }	Carbon dioxide
Closed	Yes	Complete }	absorbers
British nomenclature			
Open	No	No	Open drop
			Draw over system with non-breathing valves
Semi-open	No	Partial	Open-drop+occlusive packing
Semi-closed without absorption	Yes	Partial	Magill. T-piece
			T-piece with bag
with absorption	Yes	Partial	Carbon dioxide absorbers
Closed	Yes	Complete	Carbon dioxide absorbers

rebreathing, etc. For example, it appears to be agreed upon by most workers that semi-closed refers to partial rebreathing techniques. Thus, a system which has nearly complete rebreathing of the expired gases might have the same label as a system which has almost no rebreathing. When considering the effect of rebreathing and variation in degrees thereof upon the constitution of the inspired gases, it is unwise to use terms which give incomplete and inaccurate information concerning this important variable. Gas, inspired by an animal being anaesthetized, is a mixture of fresh and previously expired gas. When previously expired gas is excluded, a non-rebreathing system results. With such a system, inspired gas tensions may be held constant, and reasonably accurately defined, by calibrated vaporizers and flowmeters. Changes of flow or vaporizer setting produce rapid changes in inspired concentrations. On the other hand, maximal rebreathing occurs when oxygen is added to a system in amounts just sufficient to satisfy the animal's metabolic requirements, and anaesthetic agent in amounts just sufficient to satisfy its uptake by the animal. In this system changes in inspired tensions are very gradual. This inspired tension is seldom, if ever, constant. All degrees of variation may occur between these two extremes of rebreathing. For example, a semi-closed system with absorption might be used with fresh gas added only

just in excess of absolute minimal requirements, or it might be used with very high fresh gas flow rates. In the first instance the inspired gases would consist mainly of previously expired gases; in the second, the inspired volume would consist mainly of fresh gas. Some gas would have to escape in each case, and although there would be rebreathing in both instances it would be complete in neither. It is variations such as this which are incompletely described by the use of current nomenclature.

Variations in the degree of rebreathing are particularly important when it is intended to follow some particular method described in the literature, for unless a degree of rebreathing is known it may be impossible, at first, to repeat the results obtained by the author of the article. Various degrees of rebreathing will affect the rate of nitrogen elimination and rise in inspired oxygen tension in an inhalation system connected to an animal which was previously breathing room air. Moreover, these rates will also be affected by the rate of fresh gas flow into the system.

The introduction of agents such as halothane into anaesthetic practice has further emphasized this need for more accurate nomenclature. Vaporizers have been constructed which deliver an accurately known concentration of halothane and other agents. However, since such wide variations in the degree of rebreathing are possible, the inspired tension of the agent will be constantly changing even with a known amount of agent being added to the system. In addition, the inspired concentration will be influenced by the volume of fresh gas being added to the circuit. Clearly the present system of nomenclature may allow erroneous concepts concerning the actual inspired concentration or tension of any inhalation anaesthetic.

In order to clarify matters so that any reader of an article can obtain an exact picture of what has actually been performed on any occasion, regardless of variations of teaching, practice and geographical location, it is only necessary for an author to give two simple pieces of information [23]. First, the actual equipment used needs to be described, e.g. circle absorber, to-and-fro absorber, T-piece, etc., and, secondly, the fresh gas flow rate should be stated. These two basic items of information need only be supplemented to provide complete data under certain, special circumstances. For example, in certain communications it might be necessary to give such details as exact apparatus dead-space volume, types of valves, type and location of vaporizer (in or out of breathing circuit), etc. For the majority of communications this might well be unnecessary and simply stating the apparatus used and the flow rate of gases would be quite adequate. It is to be hoped that authors will adopt this simple expedient so that the easy exchange of accurate information so vital to patient's welfare, teaching and research, will become a possibility in veterinary anaesthesia.

FACE-MASKS AND ENDOTRACHEAL TUBES

Anaesthetics given by the closed- and semi-closed-circuit methods must be delivered to the animal through a well-fitting face-mask or endotracheal tube otherwise the anaesthetic agent will be diluted and inhaled with an unknown quantity of air.

Anaesthetic face-masks

In domestic animals there are wide variations in the configuration and size of the face, so that it is difficult to obtain an accurate airtight fit between the face and the mask. However, this difficulty can be overcome by the use of malleable latex rubber masks (Fig. 9.17) which can be moulded around the face and held in position with a simple headstrap. The lower jaw must be pushed forward into the mask for if it is displaced backwards the airway may become obstructed by the base of the tongue coming into contact with the posterior wall of the pharynx.

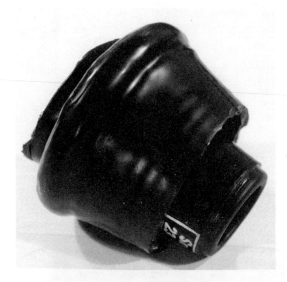

Fig. 9.18 Modification of face-masks for cats and small brachycephalic dogs. Commercially available face-masks are not suitable for cats or small, short-nosed dogs because of excessive dead-space. These masks should be cut in two and the smaller diameter half cemented inside the other. This telescoping produces a more rigid mask with a much smaller dead-space.

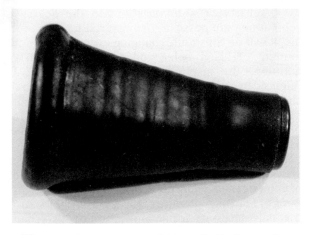

Fig. 9.17 Commercially available malleable face-mask.

After use these masks should be thoroughly washed with soap and hot water and then disinfected.

Whenever a face-mask is used care must be taken not to cause damage to the eyes and, in species of animal that breathe through the nose rather than the mouth, it is most important to ensure that the nostrils are not obstructed by coming into contact with the mask. Some patterns of face-mask are made of transparent material to allow the anaesthetist to observe the position of the mouth and nostrils.

Endotracheal intubation

The history of endotracheal intubation in animals is older than that of anaesthesia. In 1542 Vesalius passed a tube into the trachea of an animal and inflated the lungs by means of a bellows to keep the animal alive while the anatomy of its thoracic cavity was demonstrated. Similar demonstrations were given before the Fellows of the Royal Society by Robert Hook in 1667.

There are two methods by which inhalation anaesthetics can be administered through an endotracheal tube, and the first to be used was that of 'insufflation' in which the anaesthetic agents are blown through a narrow-bore tube, the distal end which lies in the trachea near to the carina. Respiration and the return flow of gases and vapours takes place around the tube. The insufflation technique is said to render respiratory movements unnecessary but has the great disadvantage of causing a considerable loss of heat and water vapour from the body. It has fallen into disuse but has given rise to the technique of intermittent entrainment of air to produce ventilation of the lungs of small animal patients during bronchoscopy

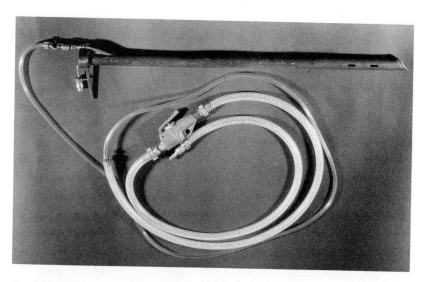

Fig. 9.19 Entrainer on rigid bronchoscope to allow ventilation of the lungs of the apnoeic patient during bronchoscopy.

under general anaesthesia with muscle relaxants. A fine-bore tube (usually an 18 s.w.g. needle) mounted at the eyepiece end of a rigid bronchoscope has oxygen or a mixture of oxygen and nitrous oxide (Entonox) blown through it intermittently. The jet of gas entrains air and generates enough pressure to inflate the animal's lungs which deflate as soon as the gas flow through the fine-bore tube is stopped (Fig. 9.19). In the second endotracheal method to-and-fro respiration takes place through one large-bore tube.

The standard endotracheal tubes used in man in the UK were designed by Magill and two kinds ('oral' and 'nasal') are available. The 'oral' tubes have comparatively thick walls and are intended for intubation through the mouth, while the 'nasal' tubes, designed for passage through the nostril into the trachea, have comparatively thin walls. The tubes are obtainable in red rubber, plastic, or silicone rubber. The oral tubes may be either plain, or fitted with a cuff which can be inflated with air after the tube has been passed into the trachea. The inflated cuff provides an airtight seal between the wall of the trachea and the tube so that all the respired gases must pass through the lumen of the tube. A good seal between the trachea and cuffs reduces the danger of inhalation of foreign material, but overinflation must be avoided as this may result either in pressure damage to the mucous membrane of the trachea or to respiratory obstruction by pressing the wall of the tube into its lumen (Fig. 9.20). Some of these problems may be overcome by the use of tubes which have high-volume, low-pressure cuffs but, in general, their introduction through the larynx may be difficult. On all cuffed tubes a pilot balloon

connected to the cuff gives some guidance to the degree of inflation but does not show when an airtight seal has been obtained. The cuff should be inflated with air until compression of the reservoir bag of the anaesthetic circuit to which the patient is connected no longer causes an audible leak of gas around the tube.

Intracuff and 'leak-past' pressures of various types of tube have been measured by Shah and Mapleson [24] who showed that air diffused out of the cuff irrespective of the material being red rubber, silicone or PVC. The material of the cuff 'crept' under stress, increasing cuff volume. The study showed that the 'leak-past' pressure decreased with red rubber and silicone tubes but increased with PVC tubes for at least 75 minutes. Pressure changes within the cuff may be caused by diffusion of gases — the most important gas is oxygen and when the respired gases contain 30% oxygen the pressure in the cuff can increase by 90 mmHg (12 kPa) [25]. Ideally, the pressure inside the cuff should be monitored to prevent damage to the tracheal mucosa.

Length of endotracheal tubes

An endotracheal tube which is too long may be inadvertently introduced into one or other of the main bronchi, and the lung on the non-intubated side will then act as a venous–arterial shunt. This may give rise to persistent cyanosis and endobronchial intubation should always be suspected if an animal shows cyanosis when breathing an oxygen-rich mixture through an endotracheal tube.

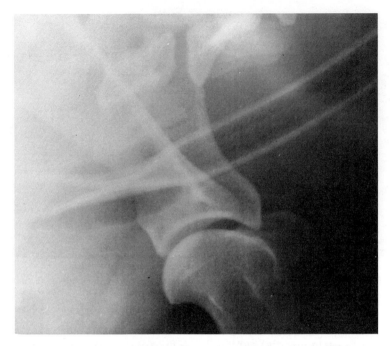

Fig. 9.20 Radiograph showing occlusion of an endotracheal tube due to over-distension of the inflatable cuff.

All new Magill tubes must be cut to the correct length both to ensure that endobronchial intubation is impossible and to minimize the respiratory dead-space. They should be cut so that when their bevelled tip lies in the trachea about midway between the larynx and carina their cut end is immediately below the nostrils. Also, the connecting piece between the tube and any closed or semi-closed anaesthetic apparatus should be as short as possible.

Reinforced endotracheal tubes

Frequent use, with the associated cleaning and sterilizing processes, makes red-rubber endotracheal tubes soft, and plastic tubes may soften when warmed to body temperature Soft tubes flatten out when bent, and are easily compressed by pressure. Obliteration of the lumen from either of these causes may give rise to serious obstruction of the airway. Patency of the airway, when the animal has to be placed in any position which may cause flattening or kinking of the tube, can be assured by the use of an armoured, or reinforced, endotracheal tube. These special tubes are made of silicone rubber and incorporate a wire or nylon spiral in their walls. They are more expensive than the standard tubes, and because there are not many occasions when their use is desirable, most veterinary anaesthetists consider their purchase to be unjustified. On the occasions when compression or

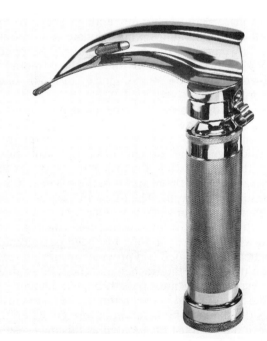

Fig. 9.21 Laryngoscope with Macintosh blade. Laryngoscopes such as the one illustrated have detachable blades and a wide variety of patterns of blade are available.

kinking of the endotracheal tube is likely to be encountered (see Fig. 20.1), the use of a new red-rubber tube is usually quite satisfactory.

Laryngoscopes

Although not strictly essential, a laryngoscope greatly facilitates the process of intubation in many animals and is a piece of equipment which is most desirable if endotracheal intubation is to be widely practised. A suitable laryngoscope is one which holds a dry electric battery in the handle and has a detachable blade in order that blades of different sizes can be fitted to the instrument. The blades should be designed so as to enable the passage of a large-bore endotracheal tube to be made as easily as possible. For veterinary purposes one standard human adult and one child-size 'Magill pattern' blades and one special blade are the minimum requirements. The special blade should be of the Macintosh pattern, ¾ inch (1.9 cm) wide, and between 9 and 12 inches (23 and 30 cm) long. The blades should be separate from the lamp and its electrical connections so that they can be sterilized by boiling without risk of damage to the electrical system. Various types are available and one suitable instrument is shown in Fig. 9.21.

For small animal use, a modified penlight torch can provide an inexpensive light source which, although less satisfactory than a laryngoscope, may prove adequate in an emergency. For large animals, special laryngoscope blades are required and the Rowson blade has greatly simplified the intubation of cattle, sheep and large pigs [26]. Wide-bore tubes may be introduced into the trachea in various ways and the method to be adopted in any particular case is decided by the skill and experience of the anaesthetist and the kind of animal in which the tube is to be passed. In the chapters on anaesthesia for the various species of animals, descriptions will be found of techniques which undergraduate students and anaesthetists in training have found relatively easy to master.

CLEANING AND STERILIZATION OF ANAESTHETIC EQUIPMENT

Anaesthetic equipment is obviously a potential source of cross-infection from one patient to the next; ideally, all parts of the breathing circuits should be sterilized between each use. Unfortunately, this is not very practical as parts of the apparatus do not tolerate many of the possible methods of sterilization and, where they do, most of the methods shorten their life. The nearer the part of the circuit to the patient, the greater the risk of cross-infection from organisms associated with the previous patient. The compromise usually adopted with anaesthetic equipment is, therefore, to sterilize the components close to the patient such as endotracheal tubes or face-masks, whilst the rest of the equipment is only regularly cleaned. This equipment is sterilized periodically, or following its use on a patient thought or known to be suffering from an infectious disease.

Whatever method of sterilization is to be employed, the apparatus must first be thoroughly cleaned by washing in hot water with a detergent or soap. Many parts of the breathing circuit may be damaged if subjected to autoclaving. Heat sterilization by boiling may be used for endotracheal tubes although regular treatment of this nature does shorten their life. The various means of chemical sterilization rarely damage equipment but when they are used the apparatus must be thoroughly washed afterwards because traces of chemical, particularly if remaining on face-masks or endotracheal tubes, may prove very irritant indeed to the next patient. The use of ethylene oxide gas is now a practical method of sterilization in veterinary practice and although it causes no damage to anaesthetic equipment a sufficient time (up to 7 days) must be allowed to elapse before the equipment is used again in order to allow all traces of gas to disappear. Also, it must be remembered that some plastics which have been previously sterilized by γ irradiation produce an extremely toxic substance, ethylene chlorohydrin, when subjected to ethylene oxide gas so they should never be resterilized by exposure to this agent [27].

REFERENCES

1. Hill, D. W. and Lowe, H. H. (1962) *Anesthesiology* **23**, 291.
2. Hall, L. W. (1978) *Journal of Small Animal Practice* **19**, 385.
3. Mapleson, W. W. (1954) *British Journal of Anaesthesia* **26**, 323.
4. Sykes, M. K. (1968) *British Journal of Anaesthesia* **40**, 666.
5. Kain, M. K. and Nunn, J. F. (1968) *Anesthesiology* **29**, 964.
6. Ayre, P. (1937) *Current Research in Anesthesia and Analgesia* **16**, 330.
7. Harrison, G. A. (1964) *British Journal of Anaesthesia* **36**, 115.
8. Rees, G. J. (1950) *British Medical Journal* **ii**, 1419.
9. Hird, J. F. R. and Carlucci, F. (1978) *Proceedings of the Association of Anaesthetists of GB and Ireland* **8**, 10.
10. Waterman, A. E. (1986) *Journal of Small Animal Practice* **27**, 591.
11. Voss, T. J. V. (1985) *Anesthesia and Intensive Care* **1**, 98.
12. Humphrey, D. (1983) *Anaesthesia* **38**, 361.
13. Shah, N. K., Loughlin, C. J. and Bedford, R. F. (1989) *British Journal of Anaesthesia* **62**, 150.
14. Robson, J. G. and Pask, E. A. (1954) *British Journal of Anaesthesia* **26**, 333.

15. Purchase, I. H. F. (1965) *Veterinary Record* **77**, 913.
16. Mapleson, W. W. (1960) *British Journal of Anaesthesia* **32**, 298.
17. Mushin, W. W. and Galloon, S. (1960) *British Journal of Anaesthesia* **32**, 324.
18. Galloon, S. (1960) *British Journal of Anaesthesia* **32**, 310.
19. Wolfson, B. (1962) *British Journal of Anaesthesia* **34**, 733.
20. Lowe, H. J. and Ernst, E. A. (1981) *The Quantitative Practice of Anesthesia*. Baltimore: Williams and Wilkins.
21. Westenkow, D. R., Jordan, W. S. and Gehmlich, D. S. (1979) *Low Flow and Closed System Anesthesia* (Eds Aldrete, Lowe and Virtue). New York: Grune and Stratton.
22. Moens, Y. (1985) *Proceedings of the 2nd International Congress of Veterinary Anaesthesia*, Sacremento, p. 57.
23. Hamilton, W. K. (1964) *Anesthesiology* **25**, 3.
24. Shah, M. V. and Mapleson, W. W. (1986) *British Journal of Anaesthesia* **58**, 103.
25. Chandler, M. (1986) *Anaesthesia* **41**, 287.
26. Rowson, L. E. A. (1965) *Veterinary Record* **77**, 1465.
27. Dorsch, J. A. and Dorsch, S. E. (1975) *Understanding Anaesthetic Equipment*. Baltimore: Williams and Wilkins.

CHAPTER 10

GENERAL PRINCIPLES OF LOCAL ANALGESIA

Many surgical procedures can be satisfactorily performed under local analgesia. Whether or not sedation is employed as an adjunct will depend on the species, temperament and health of the animal, and on the magnitude of the procedure. In adult cattle, many operations are performed on standing animals and since sedation may induce the animal to lie down, it is better avoided. In other animals sedation should be adopted since efficient surgery is greatly facilitated by the reduction of fear and liability to sudden movement. Local analgesics may exert a sedative action when they are absorbed from sites of injection and for surgery on the standing animal the dose of any sedative drug must be reduced to allow for this.

There are several features of local analgesia which render it particularly useful in veterinary practice. It enables protracted operations to be performed on standing animals, and in large animals this avoids the dangers associated with prolonged recumbency. The surgeon can induce local analgesia and operate without the assistance of an anaesthetist. The techniques of local analgesia are not difficult to learn and do not involve the use of expensive or complicated equipment.

ANATOMY AND FUNCTION OF THE NERVE FIBRE

The unit of nervous tissue consists of the nerve cell and its processes, the dendrites and the axon. The processes are dependent upon the intact connection with the nerve cell for survival and nutrition. Conventional theories of nerve function have long been based on the assumption that the surface membrane of nerve fibres and cells exists as a differentially permeable interface between tissue fluid and the liquid phase of the neuronal cytoplasm. However, modern cytological studies render it very unlikely that external surfaces of nerve cells and fibres are bathed directly by tissue fluid, for it now appears that most neurones are entirely, or almost entirely, covered by supporting cells applied directly to their external surfaces. Thus, the diffusion barrier surrounding neurones must be considered to involve these supporting cells and their membranes. The larger nerve fibres are surrounded by a coat of fatty material — the myelin sheath. The thickness of this sheath increases with the diameter of the axon it encloses, and it is composed of a number of lipoprotein lamellae which, in the case of peripheral nerve fibres, are laid down from the Schwann cells that enclose the axons. The myelin lamellae are not continuous along the entire length of the fibre, being interrupted at more or less regular intervals (the nodes of Ranvier) to leave short segments of the axon covered by the Schwann cells. Thus the axon is always separated from the surrounding tissue fluid by the thickness of the Schwann cell in which it is embedded, throughout the length of the unmyelinated fibres and at the nodes of Ranvier in myelinated fibres; and, in the internodal segments of the latter, by the myelin lamellae also. Peripheral nerves are composed of fibres of many different diameters, the finest of which usually have no myelin within their Schwann cells, while the larger fibres are surrounded by increasing numbers of myelin lamellae. There is some correlation between fibre size and function, and the fibres in the spinal peripheral nerves may be classified into three broad groups in terms of diameter ranges, each of these groups mediating particular functions. Such an arbitrary division does, of course, give rise to some overlap (Table 10.1).

The action of local analgesics is one of stabilization of the active membrane which surrounds the nerve fibre, and in the case of myelinated fibres, the inhibitory effect on the membrane occurs only at the node of Ranvier. All, including motor nerves, may be blocked and transmission at the neuromuscular junction at the autonomic ganglia may be affected by a similar mechanism.

When a peripheral nerve is exposed to a local analgesic, conduction in its constituent fibres is blocked at a rate that is inversely proportional to their

Table 10.1 Relationship between nerve fibre size and function

Group	Fibre diameter range (μm)	Functions
I	15–25 (myelinated)	Somatic motor efferents Proprioceptive afferents
II	5–15 (myelinated)	Cutaneous afferents (except pain)
	2–5 (myelinated)	Pain efferents γ–motor efferents
III	<5 { < 2 (unmyelinated)	Pain afferents Postganglionic sympathetic efferents

The divisions are not absolute and there is a varying degree of overlap from one diameter group to the other.

diameters. If a pool of local analgesic solution surrounds a peripheral nerve, function fails first in the unmyelinated fibres then in the smaller, followed by the larger, myelinated fibres. This sequence is due to the fact that Schwann cells containing myelin are relatively impervious to local analgesic solutions compared to those which contain little or no myelin. Therefore, once a drug has penetrated through the connective tissues of the nerve into the endoneural fluid, it can act upon the entire length of any unmyelinated fibres but only on the short segments of

myelinated fibres at the nodes of Ranvier. As the number of nodes per unit length of an axon is greater in fine fibres than in thick ones, there will be more of such segments within the pool of solution in the finer fibres than in the thicker ones. For this reason also, local blockade of nerve fibres becomes more rapid and effective the greater the length of the fibres exposed to the action of the drug. An alternative to employing an increased concentration of drug to accelerate local analgesic is, therefore, to infiltrate along a greater length of the nerve with a more dilute solution.

MECHANISM OF NERVE BLOCK

Most of the clinically useful local analgesics are weakly basic tertiary amines which exist in a charged (ionic) or uncharged (free base) form. The greater the alkalinity of the solution the more uncharged or free base form is present. The pK_a (the pH at which the solution contains equal proportions of charged and uncharged molecules) of currently used compounds lies between 7.7 and 8.5 and commercially available solutions are always acid so that they contain more charged molecules. It seems that both the unionized base (B) and the ionized cationic form (BH^+) are important for actual local blocking activity. The more lipid soluble the analgesic compound, the more potent it is and protein binding is believed to determine the duration of the block produced.

It can be shown by voltage-clamp experiments that local analgesics block conduction in excitable tissues by diminished entry of sodium ions during the generation of the action potential. As the local concentration of the drug is increased this results in a progressive fall in the rate of rise of the spike potential causing a corresponding slowing of conduction velocity. This is because the less intense the depolarization at any point, the shorter the range of the local circuits produced. Finally, there is inability to reach the threshold potential, resulting in conduction block. Although higher concentrations of drug can decrease the exit of potassium ions this is irrelevant to the local blocking action which can occur without any change in resting potential.

CLINICALLY USEFUL LOCAL ANALGESIC DRUGS

Clinically useful local analgesics have a common chemical pattern of aromatic group–intermediate chain–amine group (Table 10.2). The aromatic group confers lipophilic properties, while the amine group is hydrophilic. The intermediate chain is usually either an ester or an amide. The ester linkage can be hydrolysed by esterases, while the amide group can only be broken down by liver enzymes. Some compounds lack the hydrophilic tail (e.g. benzocaine) and

are nearly insoluble in water so that they are unsuitable for injection but they can be applied to mucosal surfaces.

Modification of the chemical structure alters activity and the physical properties of the molecule. Lengthening of the intermediate chain or addition of carbon atoms to the aromatic or amino groups results in an increase in potency up to a certain maximum beyond which any further increase in molecular weight is

Table 10.2 Chemical structures and properties of some commonly used local analgesics

	Chemical structure			Lipid solubility	Anaesthetic duration	Onset time
	Aromatic end	Intermediate chain	Amine end			
Amino esters						
Procaine	H_2N—⬡—	$COOCH_2CH_2$	—N(C_2H_5)(C_2H_5)	1	Short	Slow
2-Chloroprocaine	H_2N—⬡(Cl)—	$COOCH_2CH_2$	—N(C_2H_5)(C_2H_5)	1	Short	Fast
Tetracaine	H_9C_4\N(H)—⬡—	$COOCH_2CH_2$	—N(CH_3)(CH_3)	80	Long	Slow
Amino amides						
Lignocaine	⬡(CH_3)(CH_3)---	$NHCOCH_2$	—N(C_2H_5)(C_2H_5)	4	Moderate	Fast
Prilocaine	⬡(CH_3)---	$NHCOCH$	—N(C_3H_7)(H)	1.5	Moderate	Fast
Etidocaine	⬡(CH_3)(CH_3)---	$NHCOCH$(CH_3)(C_2H_5)	—N(C_2H_5)(C_3H_7)	140	Long	Fast
Mepivacaine	⬡(CH_3)(CH_3)---	$NHCO$	N—CH_3 (piperidine)	1	Moderate	Fast
Bupivacaine	⬡(CH_3)(CH_3)---	$NHCO$	N—C_4H_9 (piperidine)	30	Long	Moderate

followed by a decrease in activity. The addition of a butyl group to the aromatic end of the procaine molecule increases lipid solubility and gives a 10-fold increase in protein binding with an increased duration of local analgesic activity and systemic toxicity. Similarly, the substitution of a butyl group for the methyl group of the amine of mepivacaine gives greater potency and a more prolonged duration of activity. Once again there is an increase in lipid solubility and a greater degree of protein binding.

Cocaine

Cocaine is an alkaloid obtained from the leaves of *Erythroxylum coca*, a South American plant. It was first introduced into surgery by Koller in 1884, some 38 years after the introduction of general anaesthesia.

Sir Frederick Hobday popularized its use in veterinary surgery towards the end of the last century.

The toxic actions of cocaine and its addictive properties in man led to a search for synthetic substitutes and reference to it has now become largely historical for it has become almost entirely replaced by compounds which do not suffer from these disadvantages to the same extent. Its one remaining use is for surgery in the nasal chambers where its property of producing intense vasoconstriction shrinks the mucous membrane and aids haemostasis.

Procaine

Procaine was introduced in 1905 under the trade name of Novocain, and largely replaced cocaine as a local analgesic. Compared to cocaine its power of penetration of mucous membranes is poor and following injection block is slow in onset.

Amethocaine

Amethocaine is a member of the procaine series of compounds which is particularly useful for the desensitization of mucous membranes. A 1% solution is used for instillation into the eye, and a 2% solution is used for the pharynx, larynx and nasal mucous membranes.

Cinchocaine

This was first introduced as Percaine by Uhlmann in 1929. It is known as 'Nupercaine', a name which prevents confusion with procaine, and in the USA as 'Dibucaine'. The drug is quite different from either cocaine or procaine, being a quinoline derivative — butyloxycinchoninic acid diethyl ethylene diamide. It is readily soluble in water and solutions may be boiled repeatedly for sterilization. It is very readily decomposed by alkali, and for this reason traces of hydrochloric acid are added to solutions which are to be stored. For the same reason Nupercaine must always be kept in alkali-free glass containers. The drug is much more toxic than procaine, but this is counterbalanced by the smaller quantities used, for its minimal effective concentration is about one-fortieth that of procaine. In addition, the analgesia it produces lasts for very much longer. Nupercaine has been used for every type of local analgesia, but has been found to be most effective for surface and spinal analgesia.

Lignocaine

Since its introduction into veterinary clinical practice in 1944 this compound has proved itself as a very effective local analgesic and has replaced procaine (and indeed most other compounds) in every field where local analgesia is used. Chemically, lignocaine is *N*-diethylaminoacetyl-2,6-xylidine hydrochloride and as it is not an ester it is unaffected by pseudocholinesterase (procainesterase). It is extremely stable in solution and can be boiled with strong acids or alkalis for several hours without decomposing. This extraordinary stability places the compound in a class by itself, for solutions can be stored and resterilized almost indefinitely, without fear of toxic changes or loss of potency. Compared with procaine, lignocaine has a far shorter period of onset, a more intense action, and a longer duration of action. Spread through the tissues is much greater with lignocaine than with procaine, and injections made in the neighbourhood of a nerve trunk penetrate more

effectively. This facility for tissue penetration has some important practical applications. It is unnecessary to add hyaluronidase to solutions of lignocaine for infiltration or nerve-blocking purposes (as is often recommended with other agents) since the inherent spreading power of this agent is already adequate. Probably as another result of its tissue-penetrating properties, lignocaine also has marked local analgesic activity when applied to the surface of mucous membranes or the cornea. Its activity on mucous membranes is similar to that of cocaine, while on the cornea 4% solution of lignocaine is approximately equivalent to a 2% solution of cocaine.

The drug is rapidly absorbed from tissues and mucous surfaces. In dogs, after subcutaneous or intramuscular injection, the concentration of lignocaine in the blood reaches a maximum in about 30 minutes. The addition of adrenaline to the injected solution approximately doubles the time required for complete absorption. Ten per cent or less of an injected dose of lignocaine is excreted unchanged in the urine and the metabolism of lignocaine has, therefore, been the subject of much investigation. Liver is the only tissue which has been shown to metabolize lignocaine in significant quantities.

The approximate maximum dose by infiltration before toxic signs become apparent is not known with any certainty but is thought to be of the order of 10 mg/kg.

Prilocaine

This substance is closely related to lignocaine and possesses the same pK_a and onset time of the block in isolated nerves. However, *in vivo*, prilocaine nerve blocks do not develop as rapidly as lignocaine blocks. It is popular in equine surgery because it is said to produce less tissue reaction than lignocaine. It is the most rapidly metabolized amide and its metabolism releases *o*-toluidine which causes methaemoglobinaemia.

Mepivacaine

This compound (Carbocaine) closely resembles lignocaine hydrochloride but is slightly less toxic. It has been found to be especially useful for the nerve blocks used in the diagnosis of equine lameness because there is less postinjection oedema than with lignocaine.

Bupivacaine

Bupivacaine (Marcain) is *dl*-1-butyl-2',6'-pipecoloxylidide hydrochloride, a remarkably stable compound which is resistant to boiling with strong acid or alkali and shows no change on repeated autoclaving. It possesses, to greater or lesser degrees, the most desirable general properties of a local analgesic drug.

The local analgesic effect of bupivacaine is similar in rate of onset and depth to that of lignocaine and mepivacaine, but is of much longer duration. The addition of adrenaline in low concentration has been shown to increase both the speed of onset and the duration of analgesia so that all solutions of bupivacaine available for clinical use contain adrenaline.

Bupivacaine is approximately four times as potent as lignocaine; hence a 0.5% solution is equivalent in nerve-blocking activity to a 2% solution of lignocaine. It is generally agreed that bupivacaine provides a period of analgesia at least twice as long as that of lignocaine, and that it is exceptionally well tolerated by all tissues.

PHARMACOKINETICS OF LOCAL ANALGESIC DRUGS

The concentration of local analgesics in the blood is determined by the rate of absorption from the site of injection or application, the rate of tissue distribution and the rate of metabolism and excretion of the particular compound. The physiological disposition and resultant blood concentration will also depend on the age of the animal, its cardiovascular status and hepatic function.

Absorption

Factors which influence the systemic absorption and potential toxicity of local analgesics are:

1. The site of injection
2. The dosage
3. The addition of a vasoconstrictor agent
4. The pharmacological profile of the agent itself

Multiple injections (e.g. intercostal nerve blocks) may expose the agent to a great vascular area, resulting in a greater rate and degree of absorption. The same dose of the agent injected in one site results in a much lower maximum blood level. Topical application of local analgesics at various sites also results in differences in absorption and toxicity. In general, absorption occurs most rapidly after intra-tracheal spray for the agent is dispersed over a wide surface area, promoting vascular absorption. The rate of absorption is less after intranasal instillation, and administration into the urethra and urinary bladder. The use of ointments or gels to apply local analgesic drugs to the mucous membranes tends to delay absorption.

The absorption and subsequent blood levels of local analgesic agents is related to the *total* dose of drug administered regardless of the site or route of administration. For most agents there is a linear relationship between the amount of drug given and the resultant peak blood level.

Local analgesic solutions frequently contain a vaso-constrictor agent, usually adrenaline, in concentrations varying from 5 to 20 µg/ml, to delay the absorption and prolong the action of the agent.

Although other vasoconstrictors such as phenylephrine and noradrenaline have been employed with local analgesic drugs neither seems to be as effective as adrenaline in a concentration of 1:200 000.

The pharmacological characteristics of the specific local analgesic agent also influence the rate and degree of vascular absorption. For example, ligno-caine and mepivacaine are absorbed more rapidly than prilocaine from the epidural space, while bupi-vacaine is absorbed more rapidly than etidocaine. These differences are probably a reflection of differences in both the vasodilator activity and lipid solubility of the agents.

Local analgesic drigs distribute themselves throughout the total body water. Their rate of disappearance from the blood (tissue redistribution), the volume of distribution and the relative uptake by the various tissues are related to their physicochemical properties. The distribution can be described by a two- or three-compartment model. The rapid disappearance (α) phase is believed to be related to uptake by rapidly equilibrating tissues (i.e. those with a high vascular perfusion). The slower (β) phase of disappearance from blood is mainly a function of distribution to slowly equilibrating tissues and the metabolism and excretion of the compound. This secondary phase may also be subdivided into a β phase (distribution to slowly perfused tissue) and a γ phase (metabolism and excretion). A comparison of the three amide drugs (lignocaine, mepivacaine and prilocaine) reveals that prilocaine is redistributed at a significantly greater rate from blood to tissues than is lignocaine or mepivacaine (which have similar rates of tissue redistribution). In addition, the β disappearance phase from blood also occurs more rapidly with prilocaine, suggesting a more rapid rate of metabolism.

Local analgesics become distributed throughout all body tissues, but the relative concentration in the different tissues varies. In general the more highly perfused organs show a greater concentration of local analgesic drugs than less well-perfused organs. The highest fraction of an injected dose is found in the skeletal muscles since their mass makes them the largest reservoir but they have no specific affinity for these drugs.

The pattern of metabolism of the local analgesic agents varies according to their chemical composition. Plasma pseudocholinesterase hydrolyses the ester-class agents. Chloroprocaine is hydrolysed more rapidly than procaine and tetracaine and the toxicity of these agents is directly related to their rate of degradation. Less than 2% of unchanged procaine is found in the urine but 90% of *p*-aminobenzoic acid, its primary metabolite, is excreted in urine. The amide class of local analgesics undergoes enzymatic degradation primarily in the liver. The rate of hepatic degradation may vary between compounds which, in turn, may influence the toxicity of the specific agent. Prilocaine undergoes the most rapid rate of hepatic metabolism and is the least toxic of the amide-type agents. Lignocaine is metabolized more rapidly than is mepivacaine. Some degradation of these amide compounds may take place in tissues other than the liver and their metabolism is more complex than that of the ester compounds. The metabolites of local analgesics are of clinical importance since they may exert both pharmacological and toxicological effects similar to those of their parent compounds.

The excretion of amide-type compounds occurs through the kidneys. Less than about 5% of the drug is excreted unchanged. The major fraction appears in the urine in the form of various metabolites, some as yet unidentified. The renal clearance of the amide-type drugs appears to be inversely related to their protein-binding abilities. Renal clearance is also inversely proportional to urinary pH, suggesting that urinary excretion occurs by non-ionic diffusion.

In animals with a pathologically low hepatic blood flow, or advanced hepatic disease, significantly higher blood concentrations of the amide agents may be expected. This is important for the disappearance of lignocaine from the blood may be markedly prolonged in animals with congestive heart failure.

SYSTEMIC AND TOXIC EFFECTS OF LOCAL ANALGESIC DRUGS

Local analgesics affect not only the nerve fibres but all types of excitable tissue including skeletal, smooth and cardiac muscle. Side-effects occur when they enter the systemic circulation and the most severe usually follow from inadvertent intravascular injection, but absorption from tissue depots can also be responsible if the rate of absorption exceeds the rate of metabolism or elimination from the body. Cardiovascular, respiratory and central nervous disturbances are the common side-effects but allergic reactions occasionally occur with the ester-type agents.

Central nervous system

Local analgesics have a complex effect on the central nervous system. Usually, sedation is the first obvious sign but a further increase in the brain concentration of the drug produces grand mal tonic–clonic seizures. The explanation given for this is that local analgesics stabilize cell membranes even at low concentrations but as the concentration increases more and more of the cells having inhibitory functions are affected and as the inhibitory pathways become blocked facilitatory neurones are released to act unopposed, thus giving rise to excitation and convulsions. As the concentration of the drug in the brain rises still higher, however, depression of both inhibitory and facilitatory systems occurs with overall loss of central nervous activity. For this explanation to be valid it would seem that there must be certain predilection sites of activity in the brain but evidence for their precise location is conflicting.

Lignocaine and other agents have anticonvulsant activity as well as the ability to produce seizures. In general, the dose giving rise to anticonvulsant activity is less than that associated with convulsions and a marked antiepileptic effect is observed. It seems probable that this antiepileptic activity is due to depression of specific hyperexcitable cortical neurones.

Seizures induced by local analgesics may be managed in several different ways but it should be remembered that many are self-limiting due to rapid redistribution of the drug from the brain to other tissues. Grand mal seizures increase the cerebral oxygen consumption yet interfere with normal pulmonary function, while hypercapnia potentiates the effect of local analgesics on the brain. Thus, whatever else is done, measures to protect the airway and ensure adequate alveolar ventilation must be taken immediately. If the seizures continue for more than 1–2 minutes, diazepam (0.1 mg/kg) or thiopentone (5 mg/kg) should be given by intravenous injection. It has been suggested that diazepam has a specific antagonist effect against the excitatory effects of local analgesics on the limbic brain, and that it gives rise to fewer side-effects than thiopentone, but the barbiturate has a shorter duration of action and in many situations this short action may be desirable.

The stimulant action of local analgesics on the brain has led to their abuse by human subjects seeking to achieve the preseizure aura without using sufficient of the drug to produce a generalized seizure, and in the horse-racing industry where they have been given to enhance performance.

Cardiovascular system

Local analgesics have both direct and indirect effects on the cardiovascular system. More is known about the cardiovascular effects of lignocaine than of any other local analgesic. In experiments on isolated cardiac muscle preparations with concentrations of lignocaine known to control arrhythmias but not toxic it has been shown that automaticity is strongly suppressed. The duration of the action potential and of the effective refractory period is shortened in both Purkinje fibres and ventricular muscle and it has been suggested that these effects are responsible for the stabilizing action which lignocaine has on cardiac irregularities. Toxic concentrations of lignocaine are associated with a decrease in the maximum rate of depolarization on Purkinje fibres and ventricular muscle, a reduction in amplitude of the action potential, and a marked decrease in conduction velocity. On the electrocardiogram there is an increase in the P-R interval and in duration of the QRS complex. Sinus bradycardia may proceed to cardiac arrest at high lignocaine concentrations. At concentrations of lignocaine sufficient to control arrhythmias there is no reduction in cardiac output or myocardial contractility. Lignocaine is particularly useful for controlling ventricular arrhythmias perhaps because it enhances the efflux of potassium from ventricular muscle and Purkinje fibres but not from atrial tissue.

The usual doses of lignocaine and other local analgesics used for regional analgesia do not give rise to blood levels which are associated with cardio-depressant effects. Accidental intravascular injection of excessive doses may, however, give rise to concentrations which result in significant decreases in myocardial contractility and cardiac output or even in cardiac arrest.

Cocaine itself is the only one of these agents which produces vasoconstriction and it is believed that this results from uptake of catecholamines into tissue-binding sites. Most other agents have a dose-related effect; low concentrations stimulate smooth muscle producing vasoconstriction, while high concentrations cause vasodilatation.

Secondary effects independent of the direct actions of whatever agent is used can occur due to the regional nature of the block produced. Systemic hypotension frequently accompanies epidural block due to sympathetic blockade. For the heart to be able to compensate for falls in arterial pressure the cardio-accelerator fibres in the first two thoracic nerves must be unaffected and if the block reaches this level vasodilatation will occur in the fore-limbs and peripheral resistance will decrease so that hypotension will be very severe. If the block affects the posterior nerves only the hypotension is less profound because of compensatory vasoconstriction in the anterior part of the body.

Renal and hepatic blood flow may also decrease secondary to the effects of the drugs on the central nervous system and this will result in a decrease in both renal excretion and liver metabolism of the local analgesics belonging to the amide group.

Respiratory system

At subtoxic doses bronchial smooth muscle is relaxed and some respiratory depression may occur from central nervous activity of the drugs.

Local toxic effects

Large doses of local analgesics cause local damage to tissues such as nerves and skeletal muscles and the use of excessive amounts together with a vasoconstrictors in wound areas may delay healing. Cytotoxicity is correlated with potency — the more potent the drug the greater its cytotoxic activity.

Methaemoglobinaemia has been reported in dogs following the topical application of large amounts of benzocaine for the relief of pruritis.

Local analgesics must always be treated with respect and it is important that in practice only minimal, accurately placed quantities are used if toxic effects are to be avoided.

INTERACTION WITH OTHER DRUGS

The duration of nerve block can be increased, and the potential risk of systemic toxicity can be reduced, by combining vasoconstrictor drugs with local analgesics so as to delay absorption from the injection site. As already mentioned, it is probable that adrenaline in concentrations between 1:100 000 and 1:200 000 is the most generally useful drug for this purpose. Dilute solutions of adrenaline tend to be unstable and for this reason most commercially available solutions of local analgesics contain rather more — usually about 1:80 000 — to allow for deterioration in strength during shelf-life. Although less convenient, it is better practice to purchase solutions of local analgesics which do not contain vasoconstrictors and to add the correct amount of adrenaline immediately before use.

Local analgesics can enhance the duration of action of both depolarizing and non-depolarizing muscle relaxants, and agents such as the phenothiazine derivatives and pethidine may lower the threshold at which the convulsant actions of local analgesics are encountered.

METHODS OF PRODUCING LOCAL ANALGESIA

Surface analgesia

Agents which cause freezing of the superficial layers of the skin are sometimes used for analgesia. Ice is the simplest but, generally, volatile substances which cause freezing by the rapid volatilization from the surface of the skin are used. Ethyl chloride spray, ether spray and carbonic acid snow are examples. Their action is very superficial and transient, and their use is limited to the simplest forms of surgical interference, such as the incision of small superficial abscesses. Used too freely, they may cause considerable necrosis. In man, the thawing out after their use is known to be painful. Decicaine and lignocaine are sometimes incorporated in ointments and applied with friction to the skin. Some slight absorption occurs producing a local numbing which is useful for the relief of pruritis. Aqueous solutions of 2% lignocaine or 4% procaine may be applied topically for the relief of pain from superficial abraded or eczematous areas. The application is made by soaking a piece of absorbent wool or gauze in the solution and placing it on the affected area for about 5 minutes.

For analgesia of the mucous membrane of the glans penis and the vulva, solutions of lignocaine may be applied in a similar manner. However, perhaps the most satisfactory agent to use on the glans penis and vulva is the preparation of lignocaine made for use in the urethra — a sterile carboxymethylcellulose gel containing 2% of the analgesic agent. (This gel possesses very good lubricating properties and is an excellent lubricant for urethral catheters.)

For procedures in the nasal chambers of the horse, or the transnasal passage of a stomach tube in dogs, spraying with 4% lignocaine provides satisfactory analgesia. In ophthalmic surgery 4% lignocaine is quite safe in the eye but perhaps the agent of choice for topical analgesia of the cornea is proxymetacaine hydrochloride (2-diethylaminoethyl-3-amino-4-propoxybenzoate hydrochloride), known by the trade name 'Ophthaine'. The commercial preparation is a 0.5% solution which contains 2.45% glycerin as a stabilizer, and 0.2% chlorobutanol together with 1:10 000 benzalkonium chloride as preservatives. Using a single drop, the onset of corneal analgesia occurs in about 15 seconds and persists for about 15 minutes [1]. This compound does not produce pupillary dilatation and is non-irritant, but its solution is rather unstable, having a shelf-life of only 12 months.

Intrasynovial analgesia

Surface analgesia is also employed for the relief of pain arising from pathological processes involving joints and tendon sheaths. A solution of local analgesic is injected into the synovial cavity and then dispersed throughout the cavity by manipulation of the limb. If the synovial cavity is distended with fluid, it is first drained to ensure that the injected solution is not excessively diluted. Analgesia develops within 5–10 minutes after injection and persists for about 1 hour. The injection renders the synovial membrane insensitive but it is not known whether the nerve endings in the underlying structures are affected.

The use of intra-articular injections of local analgesics in connection with the diagnosis of lameness was first introduced by Forssell at the Royal Veterinary College, Stockholm, in 1921, and his techniques, with only slight modifications, are still in use today. Clearly, almost every joint and tendon sheath in the body can be treated in this way [2].

A needle can be introduced into synovial sheaths quite easily when they are distended with synovial fluid, but entry into a normal sheath is not easy. When searching for a synovial sheath the exploring needle should be connected to a syringe containing local analgesic solution and a slight pressure maintained on the syringe plunger. As soon as the needle enters the sheath the resistance to injection disappears and some of the solution enters the synovial cavity, lifting its wall away from the underlying tendon.

Infiltration analgesia

By this method the nerve endings are affected at the actual site of operation. Most minor surgical procedures not involving the digits or teats can be performed under infiltration analgesia and the technique is also useful, in conjunction with light basal narcosis, for major operations in animals which are bad operative risks. Infiltration should, however, never be carried out through, or into, infected or inflamed tissues.

Suitable concentrations of lignocaine are 0.2–0.5%, and stronger solutions than 0.5% should never be necessary. It is usual to add adrenaline

(1:400 000–1:200 000) to the solution, but this vaso-constrictor should be omitted when there are circumstances present which may interfere with healing, e.g. damaged tissue, possible contamination.

A hypodermic syringe and needle is all the apparatus necessary for the administration of local infiltration analgesia.

The limits of the area to be infiltrated are conveniently defined and marked for subsequent recognition by the use of intradermal weals. To produce an intradermal weal a short needle is held almost parallel to the skin surface with the bevel of its point uppermost away from the skin. The needle is thrust into the skin until the bevel is no longer visible and by exerting considerable pressure on the plunger of the syringe 0.5–1 ml of local analgesic solution is injected. The resulting weal is insensitive as soon as it is formed and if punctures are repeatedly made at the periphery of such weals, a continuous weal can be produced along the proposed line of incision without an animal feeling more than the initial needle prick. Such intradermal infiltration is only easily performed in thick-skinned animals; in horses and cattle it is usual to simply mark the proposed line of infiltration by raising a weal at either end of the line.

Subcutaneous tissues are infiltrated by introducing a needle through the skin at the site of an intradermal weal. For infiltration of a straight-line incision a needle about 10 cm long is introduced almost parallel to the skin surface and pushed through the subcutaneous tissue along the proposed line. Before injecting any local analgesic solution, aspiration is attempted to ascertain that the needle point has not entered a blood vessel. If blood is aspirated back into the syringe, the needle is partially withdrawn and reinserted in a slightly different direction. If no blood is aspirated, injection of the local analgesic is carried out as the needle is slowly drawn out of the tissues so that a stream of solution is deposited subcutaneously. About 1 ml of solution is required for every centimetre of incision. If the proposed incision is longer than the needle it may be infiltrated from its middle through one puncture site, the needle being introduced first in one direction and then in the opposite direction. Very long incisions will necessitate more than one puncture, but the needle may be reinserted through the extremity of an area which has already been infiltrated so that the animal only suffers the sensation of one needle puncture. Care should be taken to infiltrate an adequate area at the outset, so that there is no necessity for further infiltration as the operation proceeds. It is always better to overdo local infiltration than to apply it inadequately and to use more of a dilute, rather than less of a concentrated, solution of local analgesic.

To infiltrate several layers of tissue, the procedure

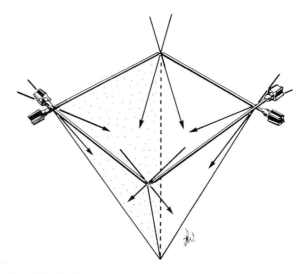

Fig. 10.1 Technique of infiltrating a 'cup' of tissue to include the operation site.

is to inject, from one puncture site, first the subcutaneous tissue and then, in succession by further advancing the needle, the deeper tissues.

Field block consists of making walls of analgesia enclosing the operation field. It is accomplished by making fanwise injections in certain planes of the body so as to soak all the nerves which cross these planes on their way to the operation field, but no attempt is made to pick out the nerves individually. Usually the entire thickness of the soft tissue in which the nerves run is involved. Generally, walls of analgesia are created obliquely to the skin surface, involving only part of the tissues around the region, but meeting below so that the operation area is held in a sort of cup of infiltrated tissue (Fig. 10.1).

If a vasoconstrictor is incorporated in the solution of local analgesia the principal advantages of field block are:

1. Absence of distortion of the anatomical features in the line of incision
2. Ischaemia of the tissues within the blocked area
3. Muscular relaxation
4. Absence of interference with the healing of the wound which is often claimed to be the chief objection to direct local infiltration analgesia

The field block most commonly used in veterinary practice is probably that for rumenotomy and this block differs from the type of field block described above. Because of the course and distribution of the nerves supplying the operation site (see p. 245) it can be accomplished by two linear infiltrations of the whole thickness of the body wall, one anterior to, and one above, the line of incision (Fig. 10.2). Up to 200 ml of local analgesic solution may be required for this block.

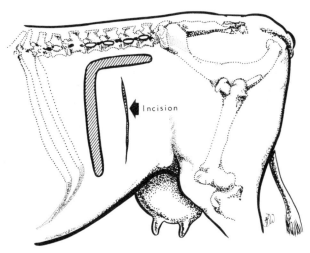

Incision

Fig. 10.2 The L-block often used for flank coeliotomy in cattle. This technique is effective but cumbersome and, if properly carried out, time consuming.

Ring block of an extremity is another special type of field block in which a transverse plane through the whole extremity is infiltrated with local analgesic solution and particular attention is given to the sites of large nerve trunks. The technique is more effective when the injection is made distal to a tourniquet. It is a type of block which is particularly useful for amputation of digits in cattle and may also be used for operations on cows' teats. Vasoconstrictors should not be added to solutions used to produce ring block in teats, for prolonged vasoconstriction may result in ischaemic necrosis of the end of the teat.

Regional analgesia

Regional analgesia is brought about by blocking conduction in the sensory nerve or nerves innervating the region where an operation is to be performed. The operative field itself is not touched while its sensitivity is being abolished and good analgesia results from the use of small quantities of local analgesic solution. The solution must, however, be brought into the closest possible contact with the nerve which is to be blocked, and special care must be taken to ensure that there is no sheet of fascia between the nerve and the site of deposition of the solution since solutions do not diffuse through fascial sheets. Success in regional analgesia comes only from practice, as does success in other techniques, but clearly it requires a thorough knowledge of the topographical anatomy of the nerves and the sites of injection. Moreover, no description, however long and detailed, or however well illustrated, can ever be more than a poor substitute for demonstration and tuition by an experienced practitioner.

It is quite beyond the scope of this book to give a complete account of all the nerve blocks that can be carried out, but in the following chapters various techniques will be described, arranged more or less on a regional basis. Selection presents difficulty in a book of limited scope and must be rather arbitrary, but two considerations have been borne in mind. First, the methods described are, with one or two exceptions, comparatively easy to carry out and may be attempted without apprehension. Secondly, they are all useful techniques which are suitable for inclusion in a general textbook of anaesthesia.

Intravenous regional analgesia

In 1908 Bier reported a technique of 'venous anaesthesia' and recorded 134 cases, but his technique seems to have been largely forgotten until it was revived [3]. It has since been widely used in many parts of the world. After suitable modification it has been employed in canine and bovine surgery with gratifying results [4–6].

A small needle or catheter is inserted into a vein at the distal extremity of a limb. The limb is exsanguinated, usually with an Esmarch bandage, a tourniquet is inflated or tied to occlude the arterial blood supply at the top of the limb and local analgesic solution is injected via the needle or catheter. Analgesia of the limb up to the lower limit of the tourniquet comes on rapidly, and when the tourniquet is released it wears off with almost equal rapidity.

The mode of action of this technique is unclear but it seems to be both safe and simple for operations on the digits, especially in ruminant animals and in dogs unfit for general anaesthesia because of a full stomach or intercurrent disease. The good analgesia and the bloodless field are appreciated by the surgeon.

Local analgesia for fractures

A technique which does not fit readily into any system of classification, but which must be mentioned, is that of local analgesia for the relief of pain arising from fractured bones. The injection is made directly into the haematoma at the site of the fracture and deposition of the solution in the correct place is essential for success. The needle should be inserted as far into the haematoma and as near the bone ends as possible. The position of the needle should be verified by aspiration, when blood or blood clot should be drawn into the syringe. Lignocaine hydrochloride (1% solution without adrenaline) is the best agent to use. In small animal patients, 2–5 ml, and in large animals, 10–15 ml of solution are required. Analgesia follows 5–10 minutes after injection. Scrupulous asepsis must be observed when injecting into a fracture site as the consequences of infection are serious.

This technique is particularly suitable as a first-aid measure and in the relief of pain arising from fractured ribs.

Spinal analgesia

Spinal analgesia comprises the injection into some part of the spinal canal of a local analgesic solution, which by coming into contact with the spinal nerves temporarily paralyses them and gives rise to loss of sensation in those parts of the body from which the sensory portion of the nerves carries impulses, and motor paralysis of those parts supplied by the motor fibres. The method was first suggested by Corning in 1885, who found that the injection of cocaine solutions into the spinal canal of the dog was followed by paralysis of the animal's hind-limbs and loss of sensation in them. This observation received very little attention until 1899, when Bier published his observations in the injection of cocaine solutions into the subarachnoid space in man.

Spinal analgesia is divided into two distinct types:

1. Subarachnoid injection, in which the needle penetrates the dura mater and the arachnoid mater and the analgesic solution is introduced into the cerebrospinal fluid.
2. Epi- (extra-) dural injection, in which the needle enters the spinal canal but does not penetrate the meninges, and the injected solution penetrates along the canal outside the dura mater.

In veterinary practice subarachnoid injections were first performed in France by Cuille and Sendrail in 1901. They demonstrated the method in the horse, ox and dog, but consequent upon its difficulties and dangers, particularly in the larger species of animal, it has fallen into disuse and has been replaced by epidural injection.

Epidural injection was introduced into Britain by Brook in 1930 [7], and this same worker contributed an extensive review of the subject [8].

Anatomical considerations

The spinal cord is covered by three membranes, the dense dura mater, the arachnoid mater and the delicate pia mater, and lies within the spinal canal. The wall of the spinal canal is formed by the vertebral arches and bodies, the intervertebral discs and the intervertebral ligaments. The tube-like canal is somewhat flattened dorsoventrally and has two enlargements, one in the posterior cervical region, the other in the posterior lumbar region. The spinal cord and dura mater end at the lumbar enlargement and the

canal itself tapers off behind this enlargement to end in the fourth or fifth coccygeal vertebra. In each vertebral segment the canal has lateral openings between the vertebral arches, the 'intervertebral foramina', through which pass blood vessels and the spinal nerves.

In the cranial cavity the dura mater is arranged in two layers, the 'periosteal' and 'investing' layers, which are firmly adherent except where they split to enclose venous sinuses. The outer layer forms the periosteum of the inner surface of the cranial bones and in the spine acts as the periosteum lining the vertebral canal. The investing layer is continued from the cranium into the spinal canal but at the foramen magnum is firmly adherent to the margins of the foramen where it blends with the outer or periosteal layer. Between the two layers in the spinal canal is the extra- or epidural space, which anatomically would be better termed the 'interdural' space. Because of the adhesion between the investing layer and the periosteum at the foramen magnum, solutions deposited correctly in the spinal epidural space cannot enter the cranial cavity or produce nerve block more cranial than the first cervical nerves.

The dorsal and ventral nerve roots issuing from the spinal cord penetrate the investing layer of dura and carry tubular prolongations (dural cuffs, 'ink cuffs') which blend with the perineurium of the mixed spinal nerve.

The spinal arachnoid mater is a continuation of the cerebral arachnoid. An incomplete and inconsistent septum divides the spinal subarachnoid space along the midline of the dorsal surface of the cord.

In the spinal canal the pia mater is closely applied to the cord and extends into the ventral median fissure. The blood vessels going to the spinal cord lie in the subarachnoid space before piercing the pia mater. They carry with them into the spinal cord a double sleeve of meninges.

The formation of the epidural space by the splitting of the two layers of the dura has already been described. The venous plexuses of the spinal canal lie in the epidural space and receive tributaries from the adjacent bony structures and the spinal cord. Although they form a network they can be subdivided into:

1. A pair of ventral venous plexuses which lie on either side of the dorsal longitudinal ligament of the vertebra, into which the basivertebral veins drain.
2. A single dorsal venous plexus which connects with the dorsal external veins.

Both types connect with the intervertebral veins, and although they are divisible into anatomical groups, all interconnect with one another and form a series of venous rings at the level of each vertebra. The accidental injection of local analgesic solutions into these veins may occur during the performance of an epidural block and be responsible for toxic manifestations.

In addition to the venous plexuses, branches from the vertebral, ascending cervical, deep cervical, intercostal, lumbar and iliolumbar arteries enter the intervertebral foramina and anastomose with one another, chiefly in the lateral parts of the epidural space.

The spaces between the nerves, arteries and veins in the epidural space are filled with fatty tissue, the amount of which corresponds with the adiposity of the subject.

The phenomena which accompany paralysis of the spinal nerves are more complex than is the case with peripheral perineural injection, because of the varying types of fibre which enter into the formation of a spinal nerve. Sensory fibres are paralysed more readily and more rapidly than are motor fibres. While sympathetic fibres are still more susceptible.

Each spinal nerve results from the union of two roots — a dorsal, ganglionic or sensory root and a ventral motor root. In the horse these roots perforate the dura mater separately and converge towards the intervertebral foramina, where they join, immediately external to the point where the dorsal root has the ganglion placed upon it. In the cervical, dorsal and cranial lumbar regions the bundles of both roots pass through separate openings in the dura mater in linear series before uniting into a root proper, but further caudally the bundles of each root unite within the dura mater. In the dog, union is effected within the intervertebral foramina, except in the lumbar and coccygeal regions, where it takes place within the vertebral canal. The point regarding the site of fusion of the two roots is of practical significance — at any rate, in the small animals in which epidural anaesthesia is induced. It is the dorsal root which it is desired chiefly to influence, and thus when injecting volumes likely to permeate in front of the cranial lumbar region it is an advantage to place the animal on its back after injection in order to reduce the extent of the complicating factors which result from paralysis of the vasomotor fibres emerging with the ventral root.

Since epidural injection is generally made near the termination of the vertebral canal, the area in which analgesia and motor paralysis supervene will extend progressively cranially according to the quantity of solution injected, the distribution of the spinal nerves should always be reviewed from behind forwards.

Autonomic effects of spinal analgesia

The phenomena which accompany spinal nerve block are not entirely due to paralysis of sensory and motor nerve fibres, since many of the spinal nerves which may be involved contain fibres of the autonomic nervous system. The autonomic nervous system is merely a convenient designation for a multitude of different types of efferent fibres which transmit impulses from centres in the brain to such structures as the blood vessels and the viscera. If these fibres are cut, most of the structures supplied are capable of autonomic activity independent of any central control. The function of these nerve fibres varies according to the site at which they leave the spinal cord. The cranial and sacral outflow (parasympathetic) is, in general, concerned with vegetative functions such as digestion and excretion, whereas the thoracic and lumbar outflow (sympathetic) is more closely concerned with protective reflex activity.

The anaesthetist is more concerned with the sympathetic nervous system and there are two cell stations in this system. The first is in the lateral horn of the spinal cord and the second is in one of the sympathetic ganglia which lie outside the cord. The axon which passes from the lateral horn cell to its sympathetic ganglion is termed the 'preganglionic fibre' and that which passes from the ganglion to the structure innervated is termed the 'postganglionic fibre'. The ganglia are situated on either side of the vertebral column. The fibres from the lateral horn cells at first join with the central ramus of the mixed spinal nerve and pass to the periphery. However, very soon after joining they leave the ventral ramus and pass to the ganglia in a white rami communicantes. The white rami are, therefore, connector fibres feeding the ganglia and they may synapse in the first ganglia they encounter, or they may run up or down the sympathetic chain to synapse in some distant ganglion. A few of the fibres do not synapse in these ganglia but pass on into the splanchnic nerves. From the ganglia in the sympathetic chain postganglionic fibres run in the grey rami communicantes back to the spinal nerve.

Distinct from the sympathetic nervous system but running with it are afferent fibres from the viscera. These visceral afferent fibres travel with the postganglionic fibres, but run in the opposite direction, passing through the ganglia, up the white rami and into the dorsal root of the spinal nerve. Their cell bodies are located in the dorsal root ganglia and an axon passes to a synapse in the lateral horn of the spinal cord. These fibres must not be confused with the postganglionic autonomic fibres (vasoconstrictor and vasodilator fibres) which also follow the dorsal root but whose cell bodies have not yet been precisely located.

The postganglionic fibres to a limb mainly pass with the spinal nerves to reach the cutaneous blood vessels, and the sweat and sebaceous glands in its distal four-fifths. The proximal one-fifth of the limb in the groin and axilla is supplied by fibres passing directly from the ganglia without joining the spinal nerves. Since the spinal nerve always carries sympathetic fibres, a peripheral nerve block always produces vasodilation in the distal part of the limb.

To the anaesthetist probably the most important components of the sympathetic system are the vasoconstrictor fibres. The largest vasomotor nerves in the body are the splanchnic, which pass to the abdominal viscera. The area supplied by them is so great that their paralysis causes a fall in blood pressure. It is probable that this fall is most marked in herbivores, in which the abdominal viscera are large and their blood supply correspondingly great. It will thus be apparent that when the lumbar and thoracic nerves are blocked a marked fall in blood pressure may occur.

Spread of solutions in the epidural space

The extent of neural blockade after injection of an analgesia solution into the epidural space is determined by a number of variables. Some of these variables are intrinsic to the animal, and some are extrinsic — variations of technique and drugs employed.

The intrinsic variables governing the spread of solutions in the epidural space are perhaps best understood if the space is considered to be a cylindrical reservoir, the volume of the reservoir being determined by factors such as the length and diameter of the cylinder and the size of the structures which it contains. Draining the reservoir are certain escape channels through which seepage and absorption of injected materials can take place. The rate of disappearance of solutions from the reservoir will depend on the patency and efficiency of the escape routes. The most important of these are the intervertebral foramina and the extradural venous plexuses, and any consideration of the spread of analgesic solutions must take account of any factors which affect these structures. Clearly, the extent of neural blockade will be governed, at least in part, by the speed at which nerves are blocked in relation to the rate at which the analgesic solution is removed from their vicinity. If this removal is fast compared with the speed of block, solutions may be removed so rapidly that there is no chance for them to spread and so produce widespread blockade. On the other hand, if absorption is slow there will be an opportunity for more prolonged contact between solution and nerves, so that the extent and intensity of spread is likely to be greater. The space in the epidural 'reservoir' is taken up by:

1. Spinal cord and nerves, and cerebrospinal fluid, contained in their meninges.
2. Fat and blood vessels, including the extradural venous plexuses which adjust alteration in venous pressure throughout the body, and which can undergo considerable distension in doing so.

The reservoir's exits through which injected solutions can escape are:

1. The intervertebral foramina.
2. The blood vessels and lymphatics which can absorb and remove drugs from the space. These vessels thus have a dual function, acting simultaneously both as space-occupying structures and as escape routes.
3. Possibly the dura mater, which may act as a partially permeable membrane, allowing some passages of solutions and drugs into the cerebrospinal fluid [9]. The 'ink-cuff' area surrounding the spinal nerve trunks is particularly important in this respect [10].
4. Solution and diffusion in the epidural fat.

Solutions which are injected into the epidural space spread up and down within to an extent determined by these opposing factors. The larger the space-occupying structures, the less space remains to be filled and so the further a given volume will travel. Relatively little spread will take place, on the other hand, if the escape routes are patent and efficient, since solutions will pass out of the epidural space through these exits rather like water through holes in a bucket.

Age has an influence on the spreading of solutions in the epidural space. In young animals the capacity of the space is small, but increases steadily to a maximum as the animal reaches maturity. In early adult life the size of the space and the patency of the escape routes are both maximal. The neurovascular bundles pass freely through widely patent intervertebral foramina and both venous and lymphatic drainage are maximal with all the adjustments of venous pressure which accompany active or violent behaviour. With advancing years the ageing process becomes apparent and conditions change. Blood flow becomes less brisk and opercula of fibrous tissue obstruct the intervertebral foramina, and, as the animal becomes more sedentary in habits, major adjustments of venous pressure become less frequent.

The length of the vertebral canal is, of course, an important factor governing the volume of the epidural space. Workers such as Harthoorn and Brass [11] relate the dosage of local analgesic solutions to the occiput–tail root measurement. Gravity also plays a part in the spread of solutions injected into the epidural space [12], although not all workers recognise its effects [13].

Once an initial injection has created a solid area of analgesia, succeeding but much smaller injections given at the same site as the first injection produce an extension of the area of analgesia. This is difficult to understand since on consideration it would seem that the succeeding, smaller injections should be lost through the exits from the epidural space while still contained well within the area of spread of the first injection. However, the fact that these succeeding small injections do extend the area of block cannot be denied. A well-recognized and commonly used method for exposing the penis in bulls makes use of this phenomenon. An initial injection is given and if after a wait of 15–20 minutes, the penis is not extruded, further increments of 2–3 ml are injected into the epidural space at the site of the initial injection until the desired result is obtained. These succeeding injections seem to track along in the wake of the original 'path-finding' dose and pass onwards to extend the neural block.

It is well recognized that epidural block has a tendency to spread widely during pregnancy [14], at least at term and when labour has begun. The reasons for this marked decrease in dose requirements at term still remain obscure. According to Bromage [12] several factors are probably involved. One of the most important is the space-occupying and massaging effects of the distended venous plexuses in the epidural space, causing rhythmic pressure waves which tend to disperse solutions lying around them.

Increased vascularity of the meninges and changes in the cerebrospinal fluid have been invoked as an additional explanation for altered response to epidural injections in pregnancy [15]. It is quite possible that changes of this nature may contribute to the enhanced spread for, if the coverings of the nerve roots are more permeable than usual, analgesic solutions will have a greater chance to penetrate the nerves within them.

Brook [8] quotes the assertion of several practitioners that, in cattle, the concentration of the solution employed affects the extent of the block. Similar observations have been made in man [12, 16]. This is difficult to understand. Why, for example, should 2–3 ml of 5% lignocaine injected into the caudal epidural space of a cow block as many segments as 10–12 ml of 2.0% lignocaine? As suggested by Bonica *et al.* [16], the explanation must be that there is a heightened tissue penetration when the more concentrated solution is employed.

Increased diffusion across the meninges into the cerebrospinal fluid was one of the first possibilities considered by Bromage [12], but injection into the caudal epidural space in cows will not come into contact with the meninges until they reach the junction of the third and fourth sacral segments. Moreover, the observations of Foldes *et al.* [17] also suggest that diffusion across the meninges is unimportant. These workers took samples of cerebrospinal fluid at the onset of analgesia, and then at intervals until the block disappeared. They found that when the block had disappeared, the concentration of the drug in the cerebrospinal fluid was three times as high as when the block was first fully developed. From these results Foldes *et al.* concluded that the site of action of analgesics injected into the epidural space is primarily outside the dura-arachnoid and the spinal canal, involving the mixed nerves in the paravertebral spaces. However, there is strong circumstantial evidence against this conclusion. The volume of solution available for each paravertebral space after epidural injection is too small to account for the prolonged effective block which follows, and studies with radiopaque materials suggest that the solution never reaches the paravertebral spaces in many instances [18].

In 1962, Bromage [12] proposed an explanation for one of the main pathways and sites of action of epidural analgesia which appears to reconcile all the clinical and experimental evidence which is available at present. The explanation was suggested by the work of Brierley and Field [10, 19, 20] on the passage of viruses into the central nervous system. They showed that the neighbourhood of the dural 'ink-cuffs' where the dorsal and ventral roots fuse is permeable to quite large particles, 0.5 μm in size, and that material can diffuse readily between the subarachnoid, subdural and epidural spaces in this region. Moreover, they showed that extremely small quantities of radioactive substances, introduced without pressure into the subperineural spaces of the sciatic nerve, could enter the spinal cord, brain stem, and even the basal ganglia, in significant amounts after a short time. On the other hand, passage into the cerebrospinal fluid was slow, and maximum concentrations were not revealed until 50–60 minutes after injection (i.e. about the same time that elapsed before maximum concentration of chloroprocaine appeared in the cerebrospinal fluid in experiments of Foldes *et al.*). The similarity of the time relations in these two series of experiments is very suggestive of an underlying mechanism common to both.

Moore *et al.* [21] also carried out injection studies, using an oily solution of a local analgesic with methylene blue, on the peripheral nerves of monkeys. They too found very rapid spread from the peripheral nerves into the subpial spaces of the spinal cord.

Bromage [12] suggested that this portal of entry into the neuraxis appears to be the key to the problems of unexpected variations in epidural spread.

All earlier discussion and tentative explanations about the site of block in epidural analgesia had been dominated by the assumption that passage into the cerebrospinal fluid precedes neural fixation and blockade. Bromage contended that if this assumption is dropped in favour of the idea that passage into the cerebrospinal fluid follows or accompanies neural involvement after subdural and subpial spread, then all the available clinical and experimental findings fall into place. Analgesic solutions can reach the subperineural spaces by diffusion around the capillary and lymphatic channels of the vasa nervorum, at and beyond the dural 'ink-cuff' areas. Once inside the endoneural spaces, longitudinal capillary networks provide tissue interfaces along which the analgesia solutions can track up the spinal routes and into the subpial spaces of the cord itself. From there the concentration gradient allows a gradual diffusion out into the cerebrospinal fluid — but nerve block has already taken place.

It is clear that on this basis spread from the site of an epidural injection depends upon:

1. *Spread within the epidural space itself.* This is dependent on such factors as the volume of solution injected, the speed of injection, the patency of the intervertebral foramina, the posture of the animal, gravity and vascular absorption.
2. *Spread in the subdural and subpial spaces.* The amount of drug which reaches the subpial spaces will be proportional to the amount which is able to diffuse through the perineurium into the subperineural spaces. This, of course, is governed by the physical laws which affect diffusion, such as the area of contact, the concentration gradient and the duration of contact. Thus, ultimately, segmental spread is dependent on the mass of analgesic drug available for transneural diffusion in the epidural space. The appropriate mass of drug can be delivered in the form of a large volume of dilute solution (when it will travel widely in the epidural space but diffuse relatively poorly), or as a small volume of concentrated solution (when epidural spread will be small, but the concentration gradient for diffusion, steep).

The outcome of an epidural injection may, therefore, be regarded as dependent on the action of many different forces. If any of these are unusually weak, or strong, the result will not be as expected. Thus, epidural block can never be claimed to be a very precise technique, and the ability to achieve consistent results will depend on the ability to choose the appropriate dose of local analgesic drug for each occasion with intelligent anticipation.

The addition of a vasoconstrictor drug to the analgesic solution constricts the epidural blood vessels and reduces the blood flow through the epidural space. This, in turn, reduces the blood stream absorption of the analgesic drug. Roberts [22] found that using procaine hydrochloride alone for caudal epidural block in cattle, the average duration of the blockage was 1.9 hours, whereas when adrenaline was added to the analgesic solution the average duration was increased to 2.4 hours.

Epidural and caudal block

It is now customary to classify analgesia as epidural (formerly referred to as 'anterior' or 'high') and caudal (formerly 'posterior' or 'low'), according to the distance forward the analgesic solution spreads and thus the extent of the area in which sensory and motor paralysis subsequently develop. This will depend chiefly on the volume of solution injected, although, as has been pointed out above, the concentration and diffusibility of the drug and the rate of absorption from the space also play a part.

If the motor control of the hind-limbs is uninfluenced the block is referred to as a 'caudal block'. Skin analgesia develops over the tail and croup as far as the mid-sacral region; the anus, vulva, perineum and the caudal aspect of the thigh lose sensation. Paralysis of motor fibres will cause the anal sphincter to relax and the posterior part of the rectum to balloon. Defaecation will be suspended and stretching of the vulva will provoke no response. The vagina will dilate and in animals at parturition 'straining' or 'bearing-down' ceases while uterine contractions are uninfluenced.

'Epidural block' implies that some degree of interference with the control of the hind-limbs is present. The motor nerve fibres need not be blocked, for block of the afferent fibres alone will suffice to destroy temporarily the integrity of the reflex arcs involved in the maintenance of muscle tone. If the lumbar and thoracic segments are blocked, the sympathetic outflow will be affected and hypotension may result. Block of cardiac accelerator nerves prevents the operation of the normal compensatory mechanism (increase in the heart rate) and the hypotension associated with epidural analgesia is then unaccompanied by tachycardia. Clinical experience would appear to indicate that in healthy animals the hypotension which may be produced by epidural blocks results in no harm, and indeed is often helpful since it tends to reduce haemorrhage at the operation site. Nevertheless, during any epidural block careful attention should be paid to the state of the circulation, for death can occur from a quite small loss of blood from the operation site since the animal cannot compensate for reductions in the volume of circulating blood.

REFERENCES

1. Formston, C. (1964). *Veterinary Record* **76**, 384.
2. Westhues, M. and Fritsch, R. (1960). *Die Narkose der Tiere*, vol. 1, Lokalanesthesia. Berlin: Paul Parey (English edn (1964) Edinburgh: Oliver and Boyd).
3. Holmes, C. McK. (1963). *Lancet* **i**, 245.
4. Hall, L. W. (1971). *Wright's Veterinary Anaesthesia and Analgesia*, 7th edn. London: Baillière Tindall.
5. Weaver, A. D. (1972). *Journal of the American Veterinary Medical Association* **128**, 238.
6. Jones, R. S. and Prentice, D. E. (1974). *Proceedings of the Association of Veterinary Anaesthesia of Great Britain and Ireland* **5**, 13.
7. Brook, G. B. (1930). *Veterinary Record* **10**, 30.
8. Brook, G. B. (1935). *Veterinary Record* **15**, 549.
9. Frunin, M. J., Schwartz, M., Burns, J. JH., Brodie, B. B and Papper, E. M. (1953). *Journal of Pharmacology* **109**, 102.
10. Brierley, J. B. and Field, E. J. (1949). *Journal of Neurology, Neurosurgery and Psychiatry* **12**, 89.
11. Harthoorn, A. M. and Brass, W. (1954). *Veterinary Record* **66**, 117.
12. Bromage, P. R. (1962). *British Journal of Anaesthesia* **34**, 161, (c)418.
13. Nishimura, N., Kitahara, T. and Kusakabe, T. (1959). *Anesthesiology* **20**, 758.
14. Tufvesson, G. (1963). *Local Anaesthesia in Veterinary Medicine* p. 44. Stockholm: Astra.
15. Marx, G. F., Zermaitis, M. T. and Orkin, R. R. (1961). *Anesthesiology* **22**, 348.
16. Bonica, J. J., Backup, P. H., Anderson, C. E., Hadfield, D., Creeps, W. F. and Monk, B. F. (1957). *Anesthesiology* **18**, 723.
17. Foldes, F. F., Colavincenzo, J. W. and Birch, J. H. (1956). *Current Researches in Anesthesia and Analgesia* **35**, 33.
18. Bromage, P. R. (1954). *Spinal Epidural Analgesia*. Edinburgh: Livingstone.
19. Field, E. J. (1948). *Journal of Anatomy (London)* **82**, 153.
20. Brierley, J. B. (1950). *Journal of Anatomy (London)* **82**, 1007.
21. Moore, D. C., Hain, R. H., Ward, A. and Bridenbaugh, L. D. (1954). *Journal of the American Veterinary Medical Association* **156**, 1050.
22. Roberts, S. J. (1952). *Journal of the American Veterinary Medical Association* **82**, 336.

PART II

ANAESTHESIA OF THE SPECIES

CHAPTER 11

ANAESTHESIA OF THE HORSE

Probably no other species of animal presents as many special problems to the veterinary anaesthetist as the horse. In spite of the fact that general anaesthesia is one of the major factors involved in mortality and morbidity, the majority of equine surgeons are reluctant, for a variety of reasons, to operate on heavily sedated standing horses under local analgesia. The veterinary anaesthetist is, therefore, faced with the numerous disturbances of cardiopulmonary and skeletal muscle function associated with general anaesthesia in equine patients. These are only very incompletely understood

and their certain prevention is currently impossible. Moreover, it is unfortunate that in equine anaesthesia measures designed to overcome one problem often only result in exacerbation of another. For example, recovery to the standing position needs to be as rapid as is consistent with absence of excitement, floundering on trying to arise and ataxia once standing. Although it is now possible to control emergence excitement with various drugs, their use may lengthen the time for recovery to standing and may result in greater ataxia after the standing position is achieved.

ANALGESIA AND SEDATION OF THE STANDING HORSE

It is frequently necessary to sedate horses to enable clinical and other procedures to be carried out easily and safely. Horses are not good subjects for sedation for if they experience a feeling of muscle weakness or ataxia they may panic in a violent manner. Historically the most effective sedative was, for many years, chloral hydrate, but its use required the administration of large volumes of solution and panic responses to ataxia produced by it were occasionally encountered. Other drugs used included bulbocapnine, bromides, cannabis and pentobarbitone [1–3]. The introduction of the mood-altering 'neuroleptic' agents, followed in 1969 by xylazine [4], and more recently other similar α_2-adrenoceptor agonists, revolutionized sedation of standing horses but even with them the sedated horse must be handled with caution for the animal may be aroused by stimulation and when disturbed can respond with a very well aimed kick.

Mood-altering drugs

Drugs previously termed 'tranquillizers' and now classified as 'mood-altering' agents have been extensively used in horses. *Reserpine* has been employed for its prolonged calming action, but has many side-effects and does not give the type of sedation allowing veterinary procedures to be carried out easily [5, 6]. The phenothiazine derivatives are utilized for both mood-altering and sedative actions; of these agents

acepromazine is the most widely used. In horses it has an elimination half-life of approximately 3 hours [7]. In intravenous doses of 0.02 mg/kg or in intramuscular doses of 0.05 mg/kg it exerts a calming effect. Obvious sedation is limited to about 60% of the subjects and the shape of the dose–response curve is such that increasing the dose only increases the duration of effect. However, even when apparent sedation is limited the horse is easier to handle. When used for premedication, acepromazine lengthens the duration of effect of many anaesthetic drugs. Acepromazine has little effect on ventilation [8] but causes hypotension through vasodilatation [9] and hypovolaemic horses may faint if given the drug. Tachycardia is the usual resonse to acepromazine but occasionally first-degree atrioventricular block is seen.

In male animals effective sedation with the phenothiazine derivatives is associated with protrusion of the flaccid penis from the prepuce and care must be taken to avoid physical damage to this organ. In the vast majority of animals the penis retracts spontaneously as sedation wears off; in a very small proportion, prolonged prolapse or even priapism occurs. Treatment of this complication is by manual massage, compression bandage and replacement in the prepuce followed by suture of the prepucial orifice. Treatment must not be delayed, because failure to reduce the prolapse may necessitate surgical amputation of the penis. It is the opinion of the authors that the incidence of this complication is too low to afford a good reason for contraindicating the use of the phenothiazine derivatives in stallions or geldings when alternative agents confer no substantial advantage.

Benzodiazepines

The anxiolytic properties of *diazepam* are not obvious in horses and the drug should not be used on its own as it gives rise to ataxia, possibly through its muscle-relaxing properties [10]. Another benzodiazepine, climazolam, has been found to have similar properties in horses [11]. The ataxia may in turn result in what appears to be a state of panic. Although not useful as a sedative, diazepam has been incorporated into anaesthetic regimes used in horses.

Chloral hydrate

Chloral hydrate was a popular sedative for horses but it has largely fallen into disuse because its administration poses problems and sedation is accompanied by ataxia. However, it is still a useful component in mixtures used in equine anaesthesia.

α_2-Adrenoceptor agonists

Following the introduction of *xylazine* as a sedative agent for the horse [4, 12] it rapidly gained in popularity because of the reliable sedation it produces. Intravenous doses of 0.5–1 mg/kg are followed within 2 minutes by obvious signs of effect. The horse's head is lowered, the eyelids and lower lip droop [4, 12, 13]. Although the horse may sway on its feet and some cross their hind legs or knuckle on a foreleg, it will remain on its feet and show no panic. Sedation is maximal after about 5 minutes and lasts 30–60 minutes depending on the dose. Intramuscular injection at doses of 2–3 mg/kg give similar effects, maximal sedation being reached 20 minutes after injection. Transient mild local tissue reaction occurs after intramuscular injection of a 10% solution. Xylazine has marked analgesic properties [14, 15], particularly in colic [16] and in colic cases analgesia is associated with the marked reduction in gut movement caused by drugs of this class. Despite the evidence for analgesia, horses sedated with xylazine appear very sensitive to touch [4, 12, 17] and the apparently well-sedated horse may, if disturbed, respond with a very sudden accurate kick.

The cardiovascular effects of xylazine in horses have been well investigated [4, 18–20]. Intravenous injection is followed by a transient rise in arterial blood pressure which peaks 1–2 minutes after injection; the pressure then slowly falls to below resting values

and remains depressed for at least 1 hour. Concurrent with the hypertensive phase there is profound bradycardia coupled with both atrioventricular and sino-atrial heart block. The heart block is most intense in the first few minutes and disappears as the heart rate increases. Changes in arterial pressure and heart rate are dose dependent in intensity and duration and following intramuscular injection the changes are similar but less marked. Cardiac output is significantly reduced, intravenous doses of 1.1 mg/kg causing falls of 20–40% below the normal resting values [13, 20]. At doses of up to 1.1 mg/kg xylazine does not cause severe respiratory depression [20, 21] although there may be a small rise in P_aCO_2 and slight decrease in P_aO_2. However, the authors' experience agrees with that of Muir [17] in that xylazine does appear to cause some upper airway obstruction. Other side-effects include sweating, which mainly occurs as sedation is waning, hyperglycaemia [22] and diuresis, these latter effects being typical α_2-adrenoceptor agonist actions. Changes in insulin production and hyperglycaemia do not appear to be a feature of xylazine action in neonatal foals [23].

Detomidine, a more recently introduced, very potent α_2-adrenoceptor agonist, was first used as a sedative and analgesic agent by Alitalo and Vainio in 1982, and since its introduction has gained great popularity for sedation of all types of horse [24–27]. Initially, very high doses (up to 160 μg/kg) were employed, but it soon became obvious that maximal sedative effects were obtained by intravenous doses of 20 μg/kg and that higher doses simply increased the duration rather than depth of sedation [19, 27–29]. For intramuscular use higher doses, approximately twice those given intravenously, are required to produce the same effect [26, 28, 29]. Slightly higher doses are needed to produce analgesia.

Both xylazine and detomidine give excellent analgesia in equine colic [30, 31] and, in fact, may mask pain in cases which should undergo surgery. For this reason it is best to use relatively small doses (0.5 mg/kg xylazine or 10–20 μg detomidine intravenously) and these may be repeated as required. Where these drugs are used their effect in reducing heart rate and gut movement must be considered in diagnosis.

The effects of detomidine can be reversed with atipamezole [32] but where only small doses of sedative are used reversal is unlikely to be necessary.

The type of sedation produced by detomidine is identical to that produced by xylazine (K. W. Clarke and G. C. W. England, unpublished observations), doses of 20 μg/kg of detomidine being equivalent to 1 mg/kg of xylazine. Detomidine does, however, have a slightly longer action, giving deep sedation for about 1 hour. As with xylazine, horses under detomidine sedation are very sensitive to touch and may kick

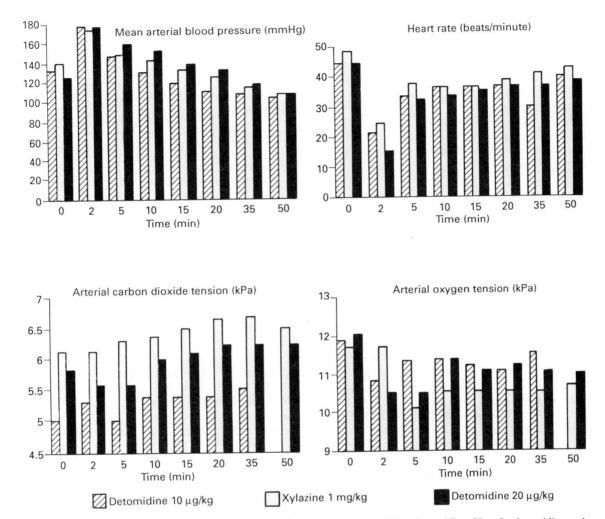

Fig. 11.1 Comparison of the cardiopulmonary effects of intravenous doses of 10 μg detomidine, 20 μg/kg detomidine and 1 mg/kg xylazine. Data from five ponies. Standard error bars omitted for sake of clarity. (From K. W. Clarke (1988) D. Vet. Med. Thesis, University of London.)

[25, 33]. Lower doses of detomidine do not always result in maximal sedation but may prove useful where a short period of action is particularly required [25]. Detomidine does not appear to be irritant when given by intramuscular injection, it has some effect when injected subcutaneously and is also absorbed through mucous membranes. The latter property has been utilized by administering the drug on sugar lumps, peppermint sweets or even (more reliably) squirting under the tongue. This property of easy absorption across mucous membranes must, for reasons of personal safety, be taken into account when handling the drug.

The pharmacological properties of detomidine are typical of those of an α2-adrenoceptor agonist. Following the intravenous injection of doses of 10–20 μg/kg, cardiovascular changes are very similar to those following xylazine (Fig. 11.1), there being a marked bradycardia with heart block, coupled with arterial hypertension followed by hypotension. However, with higher doses the hypertensive phase is considerably more prolonged [19, 34]. Whether this hypertension is then followed by prolonged hypotension has not been investigated. At clinically used doses respiration is slowed but P_aO_2 is only slightly decreased [34]. Some horses snore — presumably from congestion of the nasal mucous membranes. The authors have noted occasional horses (usually those suffering from toxaemic conditions) hyperventilating for some 10–15 minutes after the administration of detomidine and a similar reaction has been observed after the use of xylazine (J. N. Moore, personal communication). Other effects include reduction in gut motility, hyperglycaemia, sweating and an increase in urination. With doses of above 60 μg/kg there have been reports of swelling of the head; this problem appears to be associated with the prolonged head droop and can be prevented by propping the head up in a more normal position. Occasionally, skin manifestations of an anaphylactoid nature have been noted. Detomidine is claimed to be safe in pregnancy and many mares have received multiple doses throughout gestation without any maternal or fetal harm resulting. Katila and Oijala [35] have reported abortion in a pony mare after the administration of detomidine but this was probably from other causes.

Opioid analgesics

Opioid analgesics are now widely used in the horse to provide analgesia during and after surgery, as well as in combination with sedative agents for restraint. As in all other species of animal, they cause a dose-related respiratory depression, and in the horse the cardiovascular effects include tachycardia and arterial hypertension, although at clinical dose rates such responses are minimal [36]. At one time opioids were rarely used in horses as it was considered that the danger of them producing an excitement response was too great, but it is now realized that this is a manifestation of dosage and whether or not the horse is in pain at the time of their administration. Nevertheless, excitement can occur following their use, being shown in various ways from muzzle twitching, muscular spasms, ataxia, snatching at food, uncontrollable walking through to violent excitement. Tobin and coworkers [37] developed a 'step-counting' method of measuring the walking or locomotor response and obtained dose–response curves very similar to those obtained for analgesia. It is probable that many of these responses are due to stimulation of μ receptors since a pure κ agonist has been found to cause no excitement.

The assessment of analgesic activity is very difficult. Drugs may affect different types of pain in different ways and despite a variety of experimental methods of assessment [16, 17, 38, 39] it is not easy to be certain of the most effective dose in any clinical circumstance. Table 11.1 lists suggested doses for some opioids but it must be remembered that the response obtained (both of analgesia and side-effects such as excitement) will depend on many factors such as the presence or absence of pre-existing pain and the presence of sedative or anaesthetic drugs.

Of the agonist drugs, *morphine* is still to be regarded as an excellent postoperative analgesic, but again there is controversy as to the most effective dose. Classically, a suitable dose is said to be 0.1 mg/kg. Muir considered that even this dose caused dysphoria, but Combie *et al.* [40, 41] found that doses of up to 0.3 mg/kg produced minimal

Table 11.1 Suggested doses for analgesia with some opioids in horses

Buprenorphine	0.006 mg/kg i.v. or i.m.
Butorphanol	0.1 mg/kg i.v. or i.m.
Morphine	0.05–0.1 mg/kg i.v. or up to 0.25 mg/kg i.m.
Methadone	0.05–0.1 mg/kg i.v. or i.m.
Pethidine	1–2 mg/kg i.m.

behavioural effects, although they did comment that any locomotor response was delayed. *Methadone* has also been widely used but equipotent analgesic doses appear to cause more ataxia and incoordination than does morphine [42]. *Pethidine* has been one of the most widely used opioids in horses [40, 43] especially for spasmodic colic as it is claimed to have an antispasmodic action on the gut. Doses of up to 2 mg/kg have been recommended. Despite its wide use pethidine does have several drawbacks. It is comparatively short acting [44] and analgesia rarely lasts more than 2 hours. Following its intravenous use excitement reactions are common [41–44] and, more important, a small but significant number of horses appear to suffer anaphylactoid reactions [45], manifest by severe sweating, shaking and even collapse. Such anaphylactoid reactions are less common and less severe when pethidine is given by intramuscular injection; excitement is also less common and so this route should be considered the one of choice. *Etorphine* is a very potent μ agonist which is used for anaesthesia in the preparation 'Immobilon'.

The advantage of the partial agonist opioid drugs is that they are often less addictive in man and therefore subject to less control regulations than are the pure agonist drugs. Again, there is often controversy concerning their most suitable doses for horses. This may be because dose–response effects occur in which higher doses antagonize analgesia already produced (see p. 66) so if, in clinical use, analgesia is not obtained with such drugs it is inadvisable to increase the dose, and another analgesic should be used. *Pentazocine* has been used in horses in North America but dose recommendations are very variable, ranging from 0.9 to 2.2 mg/kg. *Butorphanol* is now more popular for analgesia in premedication, during surgery, postoperative analgesia and in sedative/opioid combinations. Again, dose recommendations vary widely. Doses of 0.022 mg/kg have been claimed to produce effective analgesia in equine colic for up to 2 hours, whilst experimental studies indicate that the minimal analgesic dose is 0.1 mg/kg and that even then analgesia is transient, higher doses being required for longer effective pain relief [46, 47]. Cardiovascular effects appear to be minimal [12] but all studies of its use in pain-free animals found it to produce behavioural effects — ataxia, shivering and restlessness — at doses as low as 0.1 mg/kg. Differences may be due to whether or not the horse is in pain but, in the authors' experience of the use of this drug alone as an analgesic, intravenous doses of 0.1 mg/kg to horses with mild colic pain cause the horse to walk constantly around the box for 1 hour (a locomotor response), and such a response could be disastrous in postoperative orthopaedic cases. *Buprenorphine*, another partial agonist, gives analgesia for about 8 hours although it must be remembered that the onset of analgesia requires at least 15 minutes even after intravenous injection. There are no publications relating to its use as an analgesic in horses, but the authors have found in clinical practice that doses of 0.006 mg/kg i.m. or i.v. to the horse in pain apparently give good analgesia for several hours.

Drug mixtures

In the search for a completely reliable, safe method of producing sedation in standing horses a number of mixtures of drugs have been used. Appropriate doses of many of these have proved to have a more certain and profound effect than can be regularly obtained from the use of any single drug. However, the possibility of untoward reactions and the appearance of as yet unrecognized drug interactions must always be considered when these mixtures are employed. Moreover, the rationale behind several of the combinations which are currently used is not at all clear. The most popular drug combinations in use at the present time include those shown in Table 11.2.

Table 11.2 Drug combinations used by intravenous injection to sedate horses

Drug mixture	Dose of components (mg/kg)
Xylazine	0.6
Methadone	0.1
Xylazine	1.0
Morphine	0.1–0.2
Xylazine	0.6
Buprenorphine	0.004
Acepromazine	0.04
Xylazine	0.2
Buprenorphine	0.006
Detomidine	0.01–0.02
Butorphanol	0.03–0.05

Acepromazine/α₂-adrenoceptor agonist combinations

Acepromazine (0.02 mg/kg) and xylazine (0.5 mg/kg) have often been used together for sedating horses. Originally the combination was used in an attempt to reduce the dose of the costly xylazine but it was soon realized that the prolonged calming action of acepromazine could be exploited in a variety of circumstances where the α₂-adrenoceptor agonists were used, particularly for premedication and in combination with opioids. However, many North American sources now state that acepromazine and the α₂-adrenoceptor agonists should not be used together [48]. Short [49] comments that there is a danger that if high doses of both agents are given to a horse it may collapse, but considers that carefully administered low doses may be safe. The pharmacological reasoning behind the suggestion that the two drugs should not be given together rests on the fact that acepromazine causes hypotension through α-blocking action and xylazine causes bradycardia. However, it must be noted that maximal bradycardia occurs 1–2 minutes after the intravenous injection of xylazine and at this time is accompanied by hypertension [50]. If detomidine is given to horses already sedated with acepromazine, there is still a hypertensive response, albeit starting from a lower base. The authors have administered xylazine or detomidine to over 2000 horses already sedated with acepromazine with no ill effects and agree with Short that providing both drugs are given at suitable doses there is no reason why the combination cannot be used.

Sedative/opioid combinations

The pharmacological basis for the combination of sedatives with opioids has already been discussed (Chapter 4). Their use in the horse is not new [51, 52] and a very large number of such combinations have been investigated and advocated for use in this species of animal [17, 50–56]. The addition of the opioid, even at subanalgesic doses, appears to enhance sedation dramatically and, in particular, diminishes the response to touch, thus reducing the likelihood of provoking well-directed kicks from the sedated horse. The disadvantage is that ataxia is also increased (particularly with combinations involving methadone or butorphanol). Also, opioid excitement reactions such as aimless walking may occur when sedation becomes inadequate and it is irrational to combine a short-acting sedative such as xylazine with opioids with long actions such as buprenorphine or high doses of morphine. Acepromazine has a very long action so problems are less when this is part of the combination. The chance of the opioid-induced excitement occurring early on can be reduced by administering the sedatives first followed by the opioid once sedation is apparent, although if the opioid concerned is one which has a delayed onset of action (e.g. buprenorphine) this is neither necessary nor desirable.

Table 11.2 lists some of the sedative/opioid combinations that have been satisfactorily used. Morphine has been given in much higher doses than recommended here [52, 53] but although generally satisfactory a few animals show marked bradycardia and respiratory depression and the doses given in Table 11.2 are safer and generally adequate. The advantage of drug mixtures using butorphanol or buprenorphine is that they are not subject to such strict control regulations as the pure agonists and in the UK the combination of intravenous detomidine (15 μg/kg) and butorphanol (0.03 mg/kg) has proved very successful, particularly for clipping fractious horses.

LOCAL ANALGESIA

The many techniques of nerve block used in horses for purely diagnostic purposes and the methods for producing intrasynovial desensitization will not be considered here. Details of these techniques can be obtained from surgical textbooks or from *Die Narkose der Tiere*, volume 1, *Lokalanasthesie*, by Westhues and Fritsch [57]. Those to be described here are only the ones which the authors have found useful in operative surgery or for giving pain relief.

Infraorbital nerve block

The infraorbital nerve is the continuation of the maxillary division of the fifth cranial nerve after it crosses the pterygopalatine fossa and enters the infraorbital canal. The nerve emerges on the face as a flat band about 1 cm broad, through the infraorbital foramen, where it is partly covered by the levator nasolabialis muscle. It is entirely sensory. During its course along the infraorbital canal it supplies branches to the upper molar, canine and incisor teeth on that side, and their alveoli and contiguous gum. The nerves supplying the first and second molars (PM1 and 2), the canine and incisors, arise within the canal about 2.5 cm from the infraorbital foramen and pass forwards in the maxilla and premaxilla to the teeth. The nerves to cheek teeth three to six (PM3, M1, 2 and 3) pass directly from the parent nerve trunk in the upper parts of the canal. After emerging from the foramen the nerve supplies sensory fibres to the upper lip and cheek, the nostrils and lower parts of the face.

It may be approached at two sites:

1. At its point of emergence from the infraorbital foramen: the area desensitized will comprise the skin of the lip, nostril and face on that side up to the level of the foramen.
2. Within the canal, via the infraorbital foramen, when in addition the first and second premolars, the canine and incisor teeth with their alveoli and gum, and the skin as high as the level of the inner canthus of the eye, will be influenced.

The lip of the infraorbital foramen can be detected readily as a bony ridge lying beneath the edge of the flat levator nasolabialis muscle. When it is desired to block the nerve within the canal it is necessary to pass the needle up the canal about 2.5 cm. To do this the needle must be inserted through the skin about 2 cm in front of the foramen after reflecting the edge of the muscle upwards. An insensitive skin weal is an advantage. For the perineural injection a needle 19 gauge (1.1 mm), 5 cm long, is suitable. The quantity of local analgesic solution required will vary from 4 to 5 ml. For blocking the nerve at its point of emergence from the canal, the needle is introduced until its point can be felt beneath the bony lip of the foramen.

From 4 to 5 ml of 1% mepivacaine is injected, withdrawing the needle slightly as injection proceeds. Loss of sensation should follow in 15–20 minutes and last a further 30–40 minutes if the solution injected contains a vasoconstrictor.

Injections at site 1 may be employed for interferences about the lips and nostrils, such as the suturing of wounds, removal of polypi, etc. Extraction of the canine or incisor teeth is seldom required in horses, and for extraction of molar teeth general anaesthesia is much to be preferred. For trephining the facial sinuses, local infiltration analgesia offers a good alternative.

Mandibular nerve block

The alveolar branch of the mandibular division of the fifth cranial nerve enters the mandibular foramen on

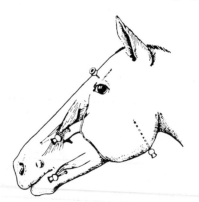

Fig. 11.2 Sites for insertion of the needle to block the supraorbital, infraorbital, mental and mandibular nerves.

the medial aspect of the vertical ramus of the mandible under cover of the medial pterygoid muscle. It traverses the mandibular canal, giving off dental and alveolar branches on that side, and emerges from the bone through the mental foramen. From this point it is styled the mental nerve. The nerves supplying the canine and incisor teeth arise from the parent trunk within the canal 3–5 cm behind the mental foramen, and pass to the teeth within the bone.

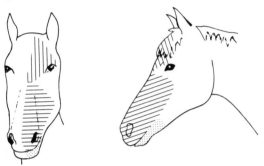

Fig. 11.3 Area of skin desensitization after blocking: the infraorbital nerve within the canal (transverse lines); the supraorbital nerve (vertical lines); the mental nerve (spotted).

If the mandibular alveolar nerve is injected at its point of entry into the mandibular canal at the mandibular foramen, practically the whole of the lower jaw and all the teeth and alveoli on that side will become desensitized. The technique is difficult and uncertain, for the nerve enters the canal high up on the medial aspect of the vertical ramus. The foramen lies practically opposite the point of intersection of a line passing vertically downwards from the lateral canthus of the eye, and one extending backwards from the tables of the mandibular molar teeth.

A point is selected on the caudal border of the mandible about 3 cm below the temporomandibular articulation. After penetrating the skin the needle is allowed to lie in the depression between the wing of the atlas and the base of the ear. The needle is advanced as its point is depressed until it passes deep to the medial border of the ramus. It is then advanced further in the direction of the point of intersection of the previously mentioned lines, keeping as close as possible to the medial surface of the mandible but, as the nerve lies medial to the accompanying artery and vein, the needle does not need to follow the bone closely. Following this method the needle should lie parallel with the nerve for a distance of 3–4 cm. About 5 ml of analgesic solution is injected along this length. German writers describe a modification. The foramen is approached from the ventral border of the ramus, just in front of the angle. The point of the needle must penetrate a distance of 10–15 cm to reach the foramen.

The chief indications are molar dental interferences in the lower jaw, but most surgeons today prefer to carry out all dental surgery under general anaesthesia and this nerve block will only be used when, for some reason, general anaesthesia is impracticable.

Mental nerve block

Suturing of wounds of the lower lip may be conveniently carried out under mental nerve block. The nerve can be injected as it emerges from the mental foramen and analgesia of the lower lip on that side will ensue. Attempts may be made to pass the needle along a canal a distance of 3–5 cm (in which case the canine and incisor teeth will also be desensitized) but this is not easily performed.

The mental foramen is situated on the lateral aspect of the ramus in the middle of the interdental space. It can be palpated after deflecting upwards the pencil-like tendon of the depressor labii inferioris muscle. The nerve may be detected as an emerging thick straw-like structure. From this point the technique is the same as that outlined for the infraorbital nerve.

Supraorbital nerve block

Suturing of wounds involving only the upper eyelid is easily possible after block of the supraorbital nerve.

Anatomical considerations

The supraorbital (frontal) nerve is one of the terminal branches of the ophthalmic division of the fifth cranial nerve. It emerges from the orbit accompanied by the artery through the supraorbital foramen in the supraorbital process. It supplies sensory fibres to the upper eyelid and, in part, to the skin of the forehead. The nerve is injected within the supraorbital foramen.

The upper and lower borders of the supraorbital process, close to its junction with the main mass of the frontal bone, are palpated with the fingers. The foramen is recognized as a pit-like depression midway between the two borders. The skin is prepared and an insensitive weal produced. A needle, 19 gauge (1.1 mm), 2.2 cm long, is passed into the foramen to a depth of 0.5–1 cm and 5 ml of analgesic solution injected.

Auriculopalpebral nerve block

The auriculopalpebral nerve is a terminal branch of the facial division of the trigeminal (fifth) cranial nerve innervating the orbicularis oculi muscles. Blocking this nerve prevents voluntary closure of the eyelids but does not in any way desensitize them. In conjunction with topical analgesia of the conjunctiva it is most useful for examination of the eye, as well as for the removal of foreign bodies from the cornea and other minor eye surgery. It may be blocked by placing 5 ml of 2% mepivacaine solution subfascially at the most dorsal point of the zygomatic arch. A 2.5 cm, 22 gauge (0.7 mm) needle is a convenient size for this injection.

Palmar/plantar nerve block

These are the most common nerve blocks employed in veterinary practice. The nerves confer sensibility to the digit. The medial palmar nerve of the fore-limb is one of the terminal branches of the median nerve. Beginning at a variable point above the carpus, it passes within the deep palmar arch in close company with the large medial palmar artery, both resting on the side of the deep flexor tendon. Here the nerve crosses beneath the artery, to place itself behind it. Throughout the metacarpal region the same relationship is preserved, the nerve lying immediately behind the artery, in front of which is the medial palmar vein. Just above the metacarpophalangeal joint the artery sinks in somewhat more deeply than the vein and nerve, and thereby allows these to approach each other. About the middle of the metacarpus it gives off a considerable branch, which winds obliquely downwards and outwards behind the flexor tendons, to join the lateral palmar nerve 2.5 cm or more above the button of the fourth metacarpal bone. At the level of the proximal sesamoid bones the trunk of the nerve divides into three digital branches, which are distinguished as dorsal, middle and palmar. The palmar is much the largest. The middle is the smallest and most irregular, and all three branches are in close relationship with the digital vessels. The dorsal branch in front of the vein distributes cutaneous branches to the front of the digit, and terminates in the coronary cushion. The middle branch, which is small and irregular, descends between the artery and vein. It is generally formed by the union of several smaller branches which cross forwards over the artery before uniting, and it terminates in the sensitive laminae and the coronary cushion. The palmar branch lies close behind the artery, except at the metacarpophalangeal joint, where the nerve is almost superposed to the artery. It accompanies the digital artery in the hoof, and passes with the palmar branch of that vessel to be distributed to the distal phalanx and sensitive laminae.

The lateral palmar nerve is formed by the fusion of the termination of the ulnar nerve with one of the terminal branches of the median. These two branches unite at the upper border of the accessory carpal bone, beneath the flexor carpi ulnaris. Behind the carpus the nerve inclines downwards and outwards,

in the texture of the annular ligament that completes the carpal sheath. In the metacarpal region it occupies, on the outside of the limb, a position on the flexor tendons analogous to that of the medial palmar nerve on the inside. Unlike the latter nerve, however, it is accompanied by only a single vessel — the lateral palmar vein — which lies in front of it. (A small artery — the lateral palmar metacarpal artery — accompanies the nerve and vein from the carpus to the metacarpophalangeal joint on the lateral aspect of the limb.) At the level of the sesamoid bones it divides into three digital branches exactly as does the medial palmar nerve already described.

In the hind-limb, plantar nerves result from the bifurcation of the tibial nerve when it gains the back of the tarsus. They accompany the deep digital flexor tendon in the tarsal sheath and, diverging from one another, they descend in the metatarsal region, one at each side of the deep digital flexor tendon. Each is accompanied in the metatarsus by the metatarsal vein of that side, and by a slender artery from the vascular arch at the back of the tarsus. A little below the middle of the metatarsus the medial nerve detaches a considerable branch that winds obliquely downwards and outwards behind the flexor tendons to join the lateral plantar nerve about the level of the button of the fourth metarsal bone. At the metarsophalangeal joint, each nerve, coming into relation with the digital vessels, resolves itself into three branches for the supply of the digit.

In the hind-limb the main artery — the dorsal metatarsal artery — passes downwards on the dorso-lateral aspect of the limb in a groove formed on the outer side of the metatarsus by the junction of the large and outer small metatarsal bones. It passes to the back of the metatarsus by dipping under the free end of the fourth metarsal bone, and finally bifurcates above the fetlock, between the two divisions of the suspensory ligament, to form the digital arteries. In the pastern region the disposition of the nerves and vessels is the same as in the fore-limb. Plantar nerve block does not give the same results as palmar block in the fore-limb. The skin and deeper tissues on the dorsal aspect of the hind fetlock and pastern are innervated by terminal branches of the fibular nerve. This may be important from a surgical standpoint although less important from a diagnostic point of view (S. Dyson, personal communication).

Technique for palmar/plantar (abaxial sesamoid) injection

Injection in both the fore- and hind-limbs is where the nerves course just proximal to the metacarpophalangeal/metatarsophalangeal joint. Although the nerves divide up into three branches at about this point the

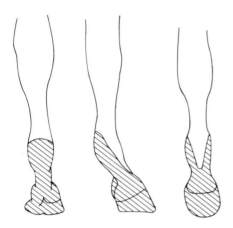

Fig. 11.4 Area of skin desensitization after bilateral plantar or palmar nerve block.

injection of 2–3 ml of local analgesic solution medially and laterally still produces complete desensitization of the entire foot. An advantage of this site is that when the limb is held up and the joint flexed, the nerves and their associated vessels can be palpated so their accurate location is easy.

A strict aseptic technique must be practised and the lateral and medial sites should be clipped and prepared as for an operation. In thin-skinned horses a 25 gauge (0.5 mm), 2.5 cm long needle is used; disposable needles can usually be introduced through the skin without the horse showing resentment. In restless animals the application of a twitch may be necessary.

After the injections have been completed, the twitch, if used, is removed, and the animal is allowed to stand quietly for 10–15 minutes. At the end of this time the limb is tested for sensation by tapping on the skin with a blunt-ended spike on the end of a short pole. This is a better way of detecting loss of deep sensation than pricking with a needle. Any response to tapping around the coronet and heel indicates failure to block the nerve on that side. One indication of sensation is sufficient to prove this, and successive trials only serve to agitate the animal. It may be necessary to cover the animal's eye to prevent it seeing the approach of the test instrument.

Technique of palmar/plantar metacarpal/metatarsal injection

An alternative site for blocking the palmar/plantar digital nerves is from 5 to 7 cm proximal to the metacarpophalangeal/metarsophalangeal joint at the level of the distal enlargements of the second and fourth metacarpal or metatarsal bones. This ensures that the analgesic solution is in contact with the nerve proximal to its point of division. The local analgesic is injected into the groove between the deep digital flexor tendon and the suspensory ligament. The nerve lies deep to the subcutaneous fascia immediately in front of the deep flexor tendon. A 25 gauge (0.5 mm) needle 1.2 cm long is used. The skin over the site is clipped and cleansed and, if necessary, a twitch applied to the animal. If it is considered advisable, in addition to the twitch, the opposite forelimb may be raised, although this is not usually necessary.

In the great majority of cases the needle can be inserted without movement on the part of the animal. With the animal standing on the limb, the skin and subcutaneous fascia are tense, and it is easy to penetrate the latter and thus ensure that the subsequent injection is in direct contact with the nerve. If the limb is held raised during insertion of the needle, the flaccidity of the skin may cause the point to enter the subcutaneous connective tissue and the method will fail. If blood escapes from the needle, it indicates that the vein (or possibly the artery) has been penetrated: the point of the needle was inserted to the correct depth, but its position was slightly wrong. It should be partially withdrawn, redirected and reinserted. When dealing with coarse-limbed animals it may be decided, first, to provoke an insensitive skin weal, and then pass the needle through this at the appropriate angle until its point lies beneath the fascia. When it is intended to block both sides of the limb supplied by these nerves, the opposite side of the leg is similarly dealt with. When dealing with the medial nerve it is necessary to work 'around' the opposite leg. With the horse standing squarely, the operator passes one hand around the front of the adjacent leg for inserting the needle, while the other is passed behind the limb for holding the syringe to the needle.

The most likely cause of failure is that the solution was injected into the subcutaneous connective tissue, and not beneath the fascia. Fortunately the skin at the site is now desensitized and a second and deeper injection can be made without restraint.

About 2.5–5 ml of 1% mepivacaine or 0.5% bupivacaine solution is commonly injected around each nerve. The average hunter is given 3 ml over each nerve.

In the hind-limb the technique is similar, except that the procedure exposes the operator to a greater risk of injury, especially when dealing with a nervous animal. Thus not only must the animal be twitched, but the fore-limb raised in addition if the operation is to be carried out with the animal standing on the affected limb. Should the operator feel indisposed to make the injection with the hind-leg free, it may be raised by an assistant, but the needle must be inserted sufficiently deeply to penetrate the fascia.

Technique of blocking palmar terminal digital nerves

The terminal divisions of the palmar and plantar nerves may be subjected to medial and lateral perineural injection in the pastern region. The site for injection is midway between the fetlock joint and the coronet. The palmar or volar border of the first phalanx is located, and the dorsal edge of the (at this point flattened) deep digital flexor tendon is palpated. The nerve lies immediately dorsal to the tendon. About 2 ml of 1% mepivacaine or 0.5% bupivacaine solution is injected subcutaneously just proximal to the collateral cartilages. The area desensitized is limited to the palmar or volar part of the foot and heel on that side.

Indications for palmar/plantar block

Palmar/plantar block is commonly used to aid diagnosis of the site of lameness, particularly of the forelimb, in those cases in which visual and manipulative examination fail to reveal it, or when doubt exists as to the significance of some obvious lesion.

Apart from their use in the location of the site of lameness, these nerve blocks may be used to relieve pain and allow rest. Palmar and plantar blocks are particularly useful in the treatment of acutely painful lesions about the foot, for, by the relief of pain even if only for a few hours, the animal experiences much-needed rest. The practice may be repeated daily for a few days in severe cases. Longest pain relief is obtained by using bupivacaine with a vasoconstrictor such as adrenaline at a concentration of 1:200 000.

The nerve blocks may also allow the painless performance of palmar and plantar neurectomy and of operations about the foot, coronet and heel, such as exposure of a corn or gathered nail track, partial operations for quittor and sandcrack. In fact, many operations about the horse's foot are more conveniently performed with the animal standing. However, even when operations about the foot are performed under general anaesthesia, palmar and plantar blocks are useful in that if performed at the end of the operation they can provide analgesia in the recovery period and thus control emergence excitement due to pain. The desensitization of the foot which they produce does not seem to be an obstacle to the animal regaining its feet after general anaesthesia or to contribute to ataxia immediately afterwards.

The complete desensitization of the fore-limb below the carpus

Simultaneous block of the median, ulnar and musculocutaneous (cutaneous branch) nerves desensitize the entire manus.

Median nerve

The best site at which to inject the median nerve is the one used for the operation of median neurectomy — that is, the point on the medial aspect of the limb about 5 cm distal to the elbow joint, where the nerve lies immediately caudal to the radius and cranial to the muscular belly of the internal flexor of the metacarpus, deep to the caudal superficial pectoral muscle and the deep fascia.

With the animal standing squarely, the administrator stoops adjacent to and slightly behind the opposite fore-limb. The caudal border of the radius where it meets the distal edge of the caudal superficial pectoral muscle is located with a finger. The point of insertion of the needle is immediately proximal to the finger. A needle, 19 gauge (1.1 mm), 2.5–3 cm long, is suitable. It is directed proximally and axially at an angle of 20° to the vertical, to ensure penetration of the pectoral muscle and the deep fascia; 7.5–10 ml of local analgesic solution are injected. To facilitate insertion of the needle to the proper depth it is best first to induce an insensitive skin weal.

The indications for blocking the median nerve alone are limited, for the surface area desensitized is little more than that obtained with medial palmar block (see Figs 11.4 and 11.5).

Ulnar nerve

This nerve may be blocked by the injection of 10 ml of local analgesic solution in the centre of the caudal aspect of the limb about 10 cm proximal to the accessory carpal bone, in the groove between the tendons of the ulnaris lateralis and flexor carpi ulnaris, and beneath the deep fascia.

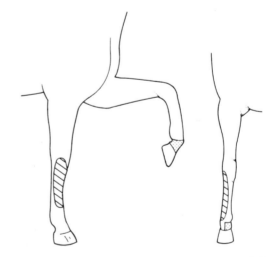

Fig. 11.5 Area of skin desensitization after block of the ulnar (shaded) and medial nerves (spotted). (S. Dyson, personal communication.)

Musculocutaneous nerve

This nerve is blocked on the medial aspect of the limb where it lies on the surface of the radius halfway between the elbow and carpus, immediately adjacent to the cephalic vein. At this site, it can easily be palpated just cranial to the cephalic vein and blocked by the injection of 10 ml of local analgesic solution.

The complete desensitization of the distal hind-limb

The technique of nerve block of the hind-limb sometimes works extremely well but is unreliable, especially for removal of cutaneous sensation. Westhues and Fritsch [57] described techniques for blocking the tibial and peroneal (fibular) nerves.

Tibial nerve

Injection is made about 10–15 cm above the point of the tarsus, in the groove between the gastrocnemius tendon and the deep digital flexor tendon. Palpation of the nerve at this site is facilitated by holding up the foot and slightly flexing the leg although the injection is best made with the limb bearing weight. Care must be taken to inject deep to the subcutaneous fascia or only the superficial branch of the nerve will be affected. Some 20 ml of local analgesic solution should be injected at this site through a 2.5 cm, 20 gauge (0.9 mm) needle that has been placed beneath the fascia.

Peroneal (fibular) nerve

The superficial and deep branches of this nerve are best blocked simultaneously in the groove between the tendons of the long and lateral digital extensors about 10 cm proximal to the lateral malleolus of the tibia. First a 3.75 cm, 22 gauge (0.7 mm) needle is introduced subcutaneously and 10 ml of the local analgesic solution injected through it to block the superficial nerve. The needle must then be inserted another 2–3 cm to penetrate the deep fascia and about 10–15 ml of local analgesic solution injected (Fig. 11.6) around the deep branch.

Saphenous nerve

The deposition of 5 ml of local analgesic solution on the dorsal aspect of the median saphenous vein proximal to the tibiotarsal joint will effectively block the saphenous nerve.

Block of the tibial nerve above the hock, and of the deep peroneal (fibular) nerve, desensitizes the plantar metatarsus, the medial and lateral aspects of the fetlock and whole digit. To produce a complete block distal to the hock, these two nerves must be injected together with the saphenous nerve, the superficial peroneal (fibular) nerve and the caudal cutaneous nerve (a branch of the tibial nerve).

Today, with the general demise of firing in the treatment of lameness — for which complete desensitization of the limb was often used — the various nerve blocks needed for complete desensitization are seldom employed to allow any surgical operations to be performed. They are only likely to be indicated when for some reason general anaesthesia is impracticable.

Accidents and complications

Sudden movement by the animal, while inserting the needle or during injection, may cause the shaft of the needle to break from the hub. The accident is especially liable to occur if an attempt is made to carry out the operation without twitching a nervous or fractious animal. A sufficient length of needle may remain exposed for it to be gripped with forceps and withdrawn. Removal will be facilitated by raising the limb, and thus easing the tension of the skin. Should the needle be completely buried, it is necessary to insert another needle into the subcutaneous connective tissue, provoke an insensitive weal, and make an incision 1 cm or so long, directly over the broken needle to expose it.

Although horses can perform fast work after surgical neurectomy care should be taken that a horse under the influence of palmar/plantar block is not exercised vigorously, for incoordinate movement after the acute loss of sensation may result in bone fracture. (Cases involving the proximal and distal phalanges were reported by J. G. Wright in the 1st edition of this book.)

Local analgesia for castration

There are three methods in common use for desensitizing the scrotum, testicle and spermatic cord by injection of local analgesics but for all of them it is essential that the animal is properly restrained or sedated if the operator is not to be injured when carrying them out on the standing animal. The animal is placed with its right side against a wall or partition and if not sedated a twitch is applied to its upper lip. After preparation of the skin of the scrotum, prepuce and medial aspect of the thighs, the operator stands with his left shoulder pressed lightly against the caudal part of the animal's left chest wall. The neck of the scrotum on the right side is gripped with the left hand and the testicle drawn well down until the skin of the scrotum is tense.

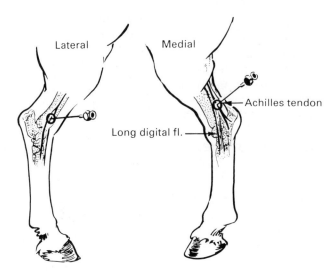

Fig. 11.6 Sites for injection about the peroneal nerve on the lateral aspect
and the tibial nerve on the medial aspect of the horse's hind-limb.

Method 1

A 19 gauge (1.1 mm) needle is quickly thrust into the
substance of the testicle to a depth of 3–4 cm and
30–35 ml of 2% lignocaine injected. When an adequate amount of lignocaine has been injected the
testicle feels firm. The procedure is repeated for the
left testicle, and local analgesic solution is injected
along the median raphe of the scrotum. Castration
can then be carried out painlessly after about 10
minutes has elapsed.

Method 2

The spermatic cord is grasped with the fingers just
above the testicle and a 5 cm 19 gauge (1.1 mm)
needle thrust into the subcutaneous tissues of that
region. The needle is kept stationary to avoid penetration of blood vessels and about 20 ml of 2%
lignocaine injected around each spermatic cord. The
scrotal skin is injected along the line of the proposed
incisions. This method does not seem as effective as
the one described above.

Method 3

A long (12–15 cm) 19 gauge (1.1 mm) needle is thrust
through the testicle and directed into the spermatic
cord while 20–25 ml 2% lignocaine are being injected.
After treatment of both spermatic cords the scrotal
skin is infiltrated.

To infiltrate the scrotal skin it is important that
the direction of the needle shall be almost parallel to
the skin to ensure that its point lies in the subcutaneous connective tissue, for if it enters the dartos
or the substance of the testicle itself, difficulty
may be experienced in injecting the solution and,
what is more important, the skin does not become
analgesic. The animal usually moves as the needle
is inserted and the operator must be prepared for
this.

Some right-handed operators prefer to stand on
the right side of the horse, with the left hand holding
the scrotum or spermatic cord, so that the left arm
is against the stifle and affords some measure of
protection against a kick. The person holding
the twitch should stand on the same side as the
operator.

It is interesting to note that many equine practitioners assert that a twitch applied around the upper
lip appears to produce some measure of analgesia and
is not simply a distraction or 'counter-irritant'. It may
be relevant that the midpoint in the midline between
the upper lip and the nose is, in fact, a well-
recognized acupuncture point.

CAUDAL (EPIDURAL) ANALGESIA

In horses the caudal block is performed by entering
between the first and second coccygeal vertebrae
(Fig. 11.7); the spinal cord and its meninges ending in
the midsacral region. The depression between the
first and second coccygeal dorsal spinous processes
can usually be felt with the finger when the tail is

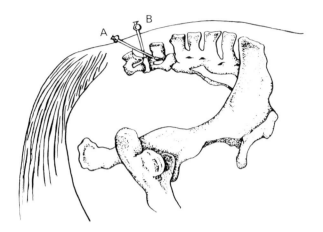

Fig. 11.7 Caudal block in the horse. The needle may be inserted at right angles to the skin surface between the first and second caudal vertebrae or it may be introduced further caudally over the cranial border of the second coccygeal vertebra and inclined at an angle of about 30° to the horizontal to run up the neural canal.

raised, even in the heavy breeds, about 2.5 cm cranial to the commencement of the tail hairs although in fat animals it may be impossible to detect any of the sacral or coccygeal dorsal spinous processes. Upward flexion at the sacrococcygeal articulation is seldom discernible; in fact, in many animals this joint is fused. A line drawn over the back joining the two coxofemoral joints crosses the midline at the level of the sacrococcygeal joint. Immediately behind this may be palpated the dorsal spinous process of the first coccygeal bone, and the site for insertion of the needle is the space immediately caudal to this. The interarcual space is smaller than in the ox and may be more difficult to locate with the needle, particularly in well-developed or fat animals in which the root of the tail is well covered by muscle or fat. Sometimes it is possible to detect a 'popping' sensation as the interarcual ligament is penetrated. The surest evidence, however, that the canal has been entered is the almost complete absence of resistance to injection of the local analgesic solution.

Most anaesthetists introduce the needle at right angles to the general contour of the croup until the floor of the neural canal is struck, but Browne [58] advised a different method. In Browne's method the point of the needle is inserted at the caudal part of the intercoccygeal depression and directed cranioventrally at an angle of 30° from the horizontal so that its point will glide along the floor of the neural canal and the needle can be inserted to its full length (the steep cranioventral direction of the canal at this point allows this). It is probable, however, that the first method, whereby the needle is inserted at a 60° angle from the horizontal, is easier to perform.

A small weal of local analgesic solution injected

into the skin with a 25 gauge (0.5 mm) needle will prevent any painful reaction to the epidural (3–5 cm, 19 gauge or 1.1 mm) needle.

Ten millilitres of 2% lignocaine or 5 ml of 2% mepivacine, with or without a vasoconstrictor, is usually sufficient to produce caudal block in the largest of horses. Tufvesson [59] states that 12 ml can be injected in large horses without the risk of hind-limb incoordination. Analgesia takes much longer to develop than in cattle and unless allowance is made for this it may be erroneously concluded that injection was not made correctly. Analgesia will usually be present after about 20 minutes and persists for 35–50 minutes depending on whether or not the solution used contained a vasoconstrictor.

Indications

General

For amputation of the tail (an operation which in the UK may only be performed for surgical reasons), and for operations about the anus, perineum and vulva: suture of wounds, operation for prolapsed rectum, Caslick's operation for vaginal wind sucking.

Obstetrical

To overcome straining during manipulative correction of the simpler forms of malpresentation of the fetus, and for partial embryotomy.

Use of other agents

It would obviously be advantageous to use a drug that induced blockade of sensory fibres without affecting autonomic or lower motor neurones. Clonidine has been found to be effective for this in man and hence it is probable that the other α_2-adrenoceptor agonists more commonly used in veterinary anaesthesia, xylazine and detomidine, will exhibit similar useful properties. Indeed LeBlanc *et al.* [60] have shown that caudal epidural administration of 0.17 mg/kg of xylazine in 10 ml of normal saline produces safe, effective perineal analgesia of 2.5 hours' duration in horses without apparent side-effects. Increasing the xylazine dose produced mild ataxia.

There is likely to be further interest in the use of adrenoceptor agonists and other drugs by epidural injection. It may well be found that combinations of the adrenoceptor agonists with opioids will have advantages, but caution should be exercised in using solutions of any drug prepared for intramuscular or intravenous use for epidural injection; only preservative-free solutions should be used.

EPIDURAL BLOCK

Because the risk of injury during recovery is so great, there is probably no place for extending the block cranially in horses, but Tufvesson [59] recorded that for analgesia up to the level of the costal arch at least 100–150 ml of 2% lignocaine must be injected through a needle placed as for caudal block. Should signs of hypotension develop with a block up to this level, rapid transfusion of large quantities of fluid, or the use of vasopressors, is indicated.

In most cases for which it might be indicated general anaesthesia is to be preferred.

GENERAL ANAESTHESIA

General anaesthesia in horses appears beset with more problems than are encountered in any other anaesthetized domestic animal. In particular, cardio-pulmonary dysfunction and ischaemic muscle damage appear more pronounced and more difficult to avoid. The problems are related and seem to follow directly from the actions of the anaesthetic agents themselves, or from interference with mechanisms existing in conscious horses to compensate for respiratory or cardiovascular changes induced by recumbency.

Young foals of all breeds and small ponies are relatively easy to restrain so that anaesthesia can be induced with inhalation agents given through a face-mask or nasal endotracheal tube; large adults generally need to be heavily sedated or actually anaesthetized with an intravenous agent before inhalation anaesthesia is possible. Apparatus designed for inhalation anaesthesia in man may be adequate for foals and small ponies but for other horses will offer too much resistance to breathing.

Breed is often allied to temperament and must not be ignored in the selection of an anaesthetic technique for any particular case. A phlegmatic heavy horse, or a trotter or quarter horse, may be restrained alongside a vertical table top for the intravenous induction of anaesthesia without previous heavy sedation, but a very excitable young thoroughbred may require heavy sedation before even simple venepuncture can be performed. Similarly, some horses will stand quietly after little or no sedation while anaesthesia is induced by a slow intravenous injection given over several minutes; with excitable breeds or nervous youngsters it may be wiser to choose an agent which can be injected within a few seconds and minimize the time in which the animal can interfere with the procedure.

The sheer weight and bulk of a large horse makes it difficult to handle, transport or position for surgery without adequate manpower or mechanical aids. Many unconscious horses are transported for short distances (e.g. from the operating table to recovery box) suspended in a net or their hobbled legs from an overhead hoist. Some workers claim that suspension by the legs can ruin orthopaedic results but with care this is avoidable and suspension in nets can cause difficulty in breathing.

Disturbances of cardiopulmonary function have long been recognized in anaesthetized horses but, in spite of much research, their cause remains uncertain. Because general anaesthesia necessarily involves recumbency there has been some debate as to the relative importance of the roles of recumbency and of anaesthetic agents in their genesis. In conscious experimental animals the cardiopulmonary disturbances produced by lateral recumbency have been found to be minimal [61, 62]. However, all these experiments were carried out in animals weighing up to 350 kg and greater changes might be found in heavier horses since more marked changes were found in the heavier experimental animals. The effects of posture cannot be ignored for disturbances are more severe in supine than in laterally recumbent anaesthetized horses but it is probable that while various postures may magnify the effects they do not initiate them.

From the evidence available today it seems likely that any disturbances resulting from recumbency are minimized in conscious animals by the operation of compensatory mechanisms that fail or become depressed when an anaesthetic is administered. Their failure or depression is manifested in several ways but probably the three most important results which affect equine anaesthetic morbidity and mortality are postanaesthetic myositis, cardiovascular depression and the development of a large alveolar–arterial oxygen tension gradient, $(A-a)P_{O_2}$.

Postanaesthetic rhabdomyolysis (myositis)

The weight of a horse or of one of its limbs can compress veins while patent arteries allow blood to flow into muscle capillaries until these are engorged and vascular stasis results, or, the arteries themselves may be compressed, shutting off the blood supply to muscle masses. It has been suggested [63–66] that postanaesthetic rhabdomyolysis may be the result of such ischaemia. Decreased muscle capillary blood

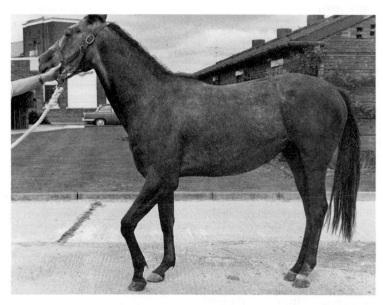

Fig. 11.8 Postanaesthetic rhabdomyolysis shown in the fore-limb. Characteristic posture of pain with the head thrown back and up when made to walk. In this case there was hard swelling of the shoulder muscles and triceps. The posture due to pain varies with the muscles involved.

flow has been found in anaesthetized horses [68, 69], while Lindsay and colleagues [66] demonstrated increased intracompartmental pressure in the compressed triceps brachii muscle of the laterally recumbent horse sufficient to compromise capillary blood flow. Prolonged halothane-induced arterial hypotension is more likely to be followed by muscular dysfunction than prolonged normotensive halothane anaesthesia [70].

The simple muscle ischaemia suggestion cannot explain why clinically apparent postanaesthetic rhabdomyolysis only occurs in a sporadic manner. The condition has many similarities to equine azoturia ('paralytic myoglobinuria', 'tying up', 'set-fast', 'Monday morning disease'), a non-traumatic myopathy which, as far as is known, does not involve muscle ischaemia or local hypoxia. Moreover, in man intramuscular pressures of over 240 mmHg (32 kPa) can cause traumatic rhabdomyolysis initially independent of ischaemia [71] so it is possible that the syndrome is more directly related to pressure on, or stretching of, muscles. There are many more theories than facts relating to the predisposing and triggering factors as well as the biochemical causes of equine rhabdomyolyis and the same is true for the postanaesthetic condition. It is possible that the nutritional status of the animal at the time of anaesthesia is important. Waldron-Mease [72] from a limited study suggested that rhabdomyolysis may be secondary to hypothyroidism and further work is indicated to see if

postanaesthetic myositis occurs more frequently in animals with clinically unrecognized hypothyroidism. The condition also seems to occur more frequently in fit horses on high-protein diets and it may be that the intracellular pH at the time of anaesthesia is another factor involved.

It is likely that this type of muscle damage is multifactorial in origin. Following anaesthesia it is most serious because, although lameness due to it usually disappears in 24–48 hours, the horse may experience great difficulty in regaining the standing position and postanaesthetic recumbency is prolonged. Also, muscle wasting due to replacement of necrotic fibres by fibrous tissue is permanent and can seriously affect athletic performance.

Until its aetiology is definitely established all that can be done to minimize its occurrence would seem to be the adoption of measures designed to relieve pressure on muscles and blood vessels. The most popular suggestion for prevention of the myositis is the use of a soft surface to offer widespread support of the recumbent animal and although many workers doubt this to be the complete answer, Lindsay *et al*. [67] did produce evidence that a soft mattress or water bed results in lower intracompartmental pressures in the lowermost muscles than does a hard surface. However, there is no conclusive proof that softer supporting surfaces decrease the incidence of the condition.

Cardiopulmonary effects

Several studies have shown that halothane depresses the equine heart [73–75]. Accommodation occurs and at a given end-tidal concentration cardiac output and heart rate rise as anaesthesia progresses, probably due to the release of catecholamines although the cause of this release remains uncertain. Accommodation is more pronounced in spontaneously breathing animals [76, 77]. Enflurane and isoflurane also cause circulatory depression [78] and intravenous agents such as the anaesthetic cocktail of xylazine/guaiphenesin/ketamine have been found to decrease cardiac output [78].

Vasodilatation, which may have particularly disastrous consequences in hypovolaemic animals, is a usual result of general anaesthesia except, possibly, when ketamine is given.

A major problem encountered in equine anaesthesia is that the arterial oxygen tension is always much lower than might be expected from the inspired oxygen tensions, i.e. there is a large $(A–a)PO_2$. A normal $(A–a)PO_2$ of about 18 mmHg (2.4 kPa) in standing horses breathing air is doubled in anaesthetized, laterally recumbent animals. Most investigations concerned with $(A–a)PO_2$ gradients have been carried out under halothane/oxygen anaesthesia but similar differences have been found during general anaesthesia with other agents. The increased $(A–a)PO_2$ may be the result of a combination of several factors and these have been the subject of many investigations in recent years.

The arterial oxygen tension depends on the size of the animal and its position during anaesthesia [80], but it is relatively unaffected by the degree of respiratory depression produced by the anaesthetic agent. Schatzmann *et al.* [81] demonstrated that horses lying in lateral recumbency under the influence of guaiphenesin were able to maintain normal P_aCO_2s but were still hypoxaemic; others have reported relative or absolute decreases in P_aO_2 with or without increased P_aCO_2 levels [79–85]. Moreover, there has been shown to be no statistically significant difference in $(A–a)PO_2$s in a series of animals anaesthetized once with spontaneous breathing and on another occasion with IPPV to normocapnia [74]. One notable feature is that the $(A–a)PO_2$ gradient does not increase significantly with time [86].

When a horse is disconnected from a breathing circuit containing an oxygen-rich mixture of gases or vapours and allowed to breathe air, P_aO_2s around 50 mmHg (6.5 kPa) are common [87]. This may represent a blood O_2 saturation of around 90% but the steep part of the dissociation curve starts about here and any accident such as temporary obstruction of the airway can have very serious consequences. It is not uncommon for frank cyanosis to be observed in the recovery period if oxygen is not administered but it must be remembered that the P_aO_2 may fall to 40 mmHg (5.3 kPa) without cyanosis becoming apparent if the blood flow to the mucous membranes is adequate. To improve the situation oxygen must be insufflated at a minimum rate of 15 l/min [88]. It has been suggested that an oxygen demand valve may be used to administer oxygen during the recovery period [89] but others have found this rather unsuitable [90]. The P_aO_2 apparently recovers to normal levels as soon as the animal regains its feet.

Factors other than hypoventilation which may contribute to the large $(A–a)PO_2$s include diffusion defects in the lungs, right-to-left intrapulmonary vascular shunts, mismatching of ventilation and perfusion in the lungs, atelectasis and a fall in cardiac output without a corresponding fall in tissue oxygen consumption.

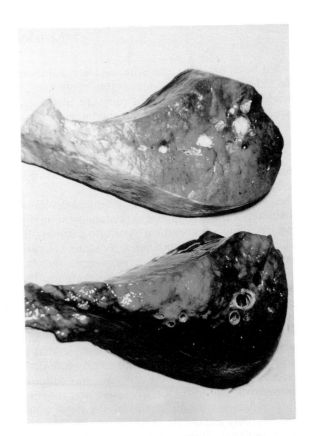

Fig. 11.9 Slices of the lungs of a large horse killed after about 30 minutes of anaesthesia in lateral decubitus. The dependent lung (lower picture) shows a large region of total collapse, while even in the lung which was uppermost during anaesthesia there are areas of collapse around the hilar region.

Diffusion impairment

There is no evidence that diffusion impairment occurs so this must be regarded as an unlikely cause of hypoxaemia.

Atelectasis

Progressive atelectasis is unlikely because in horses the $(A–a)P_{O_2}$ develops very soon after the induction of anaesthesia and thereafter remains relatively constant. There is no doubt, however, that atelectasis does occur for total collapse of regions of the dependent lung is commonly seen at autopsy of horses dying while anaesthetized (Fig. 11.9). This collapse is presumably due to compression of the lung by overlying abdominal and thoracic viscera. A totally collapsed lung acts as a venous–arterial shunt and can cause marked arterial hypoxaemia. A shunt of 15% of the total pulmonary blood flow has been found in laterally recumbent horses under halothane anaesthesia, compared with about 5% in the standing animal [86]. Decrease in lung volume short of collapse may not have all that an adverse effect on alveolar ventilation for the alveolar compliance curve predicts that a small alveolus will expand proportionally more for any given change in intra-alveolar pressure.

Examination of lung tissue quickly frozen *in situ* demonstrated that the upper lung of the laterally recumbent anaesthetized animal was well expanded while atelectasis and large engorged capillaries were seen in the lower lung [91]. Pulmonary oedema was not seen, suggesting that the radiopacity of the lower lung reported by McDonell *et al.* [92] (Fig. 11.10) is caused by atelectasis and pulmonary capillary congestion rather than increased lung water.

Venous admixture

It would seem unlikely that total collapse of lung regions resulting in right-to-left vascular shunting accounts for all the venous admixture which occurs in anaesthetized horses. A substantial amount must be due to the occurrence of gross mismatching of ventilation and perfusion in the lungs. Some indication of this may be obtained from the physiological dead-space:tidal volume ratio. In most mammals this ratio is about 0.3 but in anaesthetized horses it is over 0.5 [74]. Gravitational forces affect the relationship between ventilation and blood flow so that because of their large vertical dimension much of the upper part of the horse's lung can be relatively underperfused for the prevailing ventilation [93]. This effect can be expected to apply to the upper lung of the laterally recumbent anaesthetized horse. Moreover, because of this gravitational effect, the lower lung regions may

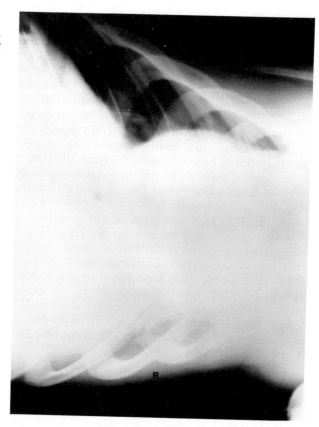

Fig. 11.10 Opacity of the lower lung seen in a radiograph taken at full expiration after 20 minutes of halothane anaesthesia in right decubitus. (From W. N. McDonell, L. W. Hall and L. B. Jeffcott (1979) *Equine Veterinary Journal* **11**, 24, with permission).

receive more blood flow than can be oxygenated by the prevailing ventilation for, unlike the situation in spontaneously breathing laterally recumbent human beings, ventilation of the lower lung of the laterally recumbent horse is restricted by limitation of diaphragmatic and rib cage movement. The net result is a scatter of ventilation:perfusion ratios throughout the lungs from the extremes of ventilation without perfusion to perfusion without ventilation.

The large physiological dead-space:tidal volume ratio probably explains why IPPV is relatively ineffective in decreasing the $(A–a)P_{O_2}$ in horses. The augmented tidal volume resulting from IPPV merely increases ventilation to those regions of the lung which are already overventilated in relation to their perfusion — i.e. those contributing to the physiological dead-space. While even in horses the increased ventilation will remove carbon dioxide from the lungs and keep the $P_{a}CO_2$ within normal limits it will not greatly increase the $P_{a}O_2$.

Reduction in cardiac output

Cardiac output is usually reduced under anaesthesia but tissue oxygen consumption may remain substantially unchanged. The resulting arterio-mixed venous oxygen tension difference, $(A-V)P_{O_2}$, thus increases and venous blood passing through anatomical shunts or regions of lung collapse has a greater effect on the P_aO_2. It is important to note here that the magnitude of the reduction in cardiac output cannot be inferred from the arterial blood pressure and that IPPV may reduce cardiac output. Indeed, the oxygen tension of mixed venous blood from the pulmonary artery (P_vO_2) is lower when IPPV is used despite a slight increase in P_aO_2, presumably because of an increased extraction of oxygen from the blood by the tissues necessitated by the reduced cardiac output — and hence rate of tissue perfusion. Because the right-to-left intrapulmonary shunt increases from the normal 5% in the standing, awake horse to about 15% under halothane anaesthesia [86], the effect of the shunted blood of lower than normal P_{O_2} will be to produce a noticeable reduction in the mixed P_{O_2} of the blood in the left atrium (P_aO_2).

Lung volume

The larger the lung the greater the stretch across the airways and the less tendency for closure to occur on expiration. The lung volume at which airway closure starts to occur ('the closing volume') is important, for, if airways close, gas trapped distal to the point of closure soon becomes depleted of oxygen and the blood perfusing the region gets through unoxygenated to join the blood from other regions and reduces the mixed P_aO_2. McDonell's studies [94] strongly suggest that during general anaesthesia the horse's lung volume is reduced to a level at which airway closure may occur. He also demonstrated that the reduction in lung volume in the laterally recumbent horse was not equally distributed between the lower and upper lungs. In both right and left lateral decubitus there was a greater reduction in the volume of the lower lung, and pulling the legs together in hobbles reduced lung volume still further.

The effect of airway closure on P_aO_2 might be at least partially mitigated by collateral ventilation from neighbouring alveoli but although anatomical studies [95] indicate that this is possible, it is unlikely to do so in horses [96].

On the basis of studies with thiopentone sodium, McDonell [94] concluded that recumbency rather than anaesthesia was responsible for the reduction of lung volume found in anaesthetized ponies but more recent work has shown that halothane and enflurane reduce lung volume in ponies already recumbent under intravenous anaesthesia and relaxed with pancuronium, while isoflurane increases it [97].

Confirmation of serious impairment of expansion of the lowermost lung has been obtained from histological examination of very rapidly frozen lung regions. Also, from the histological appearances it would seem that a reduction of the tethering effect of lung parenchyma on extra-alveolar vessels might well be responsible for the increased resistance to blood flow in this lung [98].

Radiographic studies [92] and blood samples drawn from pulmonary veins through implanted catheters in conscious and anaesthetized animals in lateral decubitus [98, 99] have afforded further confirmation of the impairment of function in the lower lung. Radiographic appearances cannot be correlated with P_aO_2 but are suggestive of a greatly reduced volume of the lower lung in laterally recumbent animals [92]. When a horse lies on its side a diffuse radiographic opacity of the lower lung develops within 20 minutes and may be due to alveolar collapse, regional pulmonary congestion and/or interstitial oedema. Spontaneous deep breaths or forced expansion of the lung by compression of an anaesthetic reservoir bag, both of which might be expected to re-expand collapsed alveoli, fail to alter the radiological appearance. Stolk [100] demonstrated no significant increase in the water content of the lower lung and considered that the radiographic opacity must be due to an increased blood content. The opacity persists for some time after the horse is turned over and this raises the possibility that venous congestion may kink pulmonary veins and hinder the prompt drainage of blood from the affected lung.

It might be thought that increasing the airway pressure to above atmospheric pressure (positive end-expiratory pressure or PEEP) will, by increasing the lung volume to an amount equal to the product of the total compliance and the pressure, decrease the tendency for airways to close and thus raise the P_aO_2. However, the imposition of a 10 and 20 cmH_2O (1 and 2 kPa) expiratory resistances by the insertion of a water trap in the expiratory limb of a circle absorber fails to improve the P_aO_2 in horses breathing spontaneously under halothane/oxygen anaesthesia [101]. Moreover, imposition of this resistance usually produced immediate respiratory arrest of many seconds duration. Broadly similar results were obtained in horses under barbiturate/guaiphenesin anaesthesia [102], but in both studies arterial oxygen saturation was always over 95% and it is possible that some beneficial effect of expiratory resistance might be found where arterial oxygen saturation is reduced by pulmonary disease. It seems likely, however, that because of its dome-like shape, only the upper part of the horse's diaphragm is susceptible to displacement by end-expiratory pressure, and thus lung volume will only increase in regions which are already well ventilated. The indiscriminate use of end-expiratory pressure certainly has no place in routine equine anaesthesia and, by reducing cardiac output, it may even be harmful in some circumstances.

PREPARATION FOR GENERAL ANAESTHESIA

The preanaesthetic examination and the general principles of preparation prior to anaesthesia described in Chapter 1 are, of course, applicable to horses, but there are some aspects of preanaesthetic preparation of these animals which warrant further consideration.

To preserve the largest oxygen store in the body and to minimize gas trapping in the lungs, the FRC needs to be maintained at the highest possible level. Many of the factors which tend to reduce the FRC are beyond the anaesthetist's control but, except in emergencies, it is always possible to ensure that the animal is fasted before anaesthesia. Fasting for more than 18 hours may result in acidosis and is probably inadvisable, but McDonell [94] found that starvation for this period increased the FRC by up to 30% presumably due to a reduction in the bulk of the abdominal contents through loss of ingesta and reduced gas content.

Extremely fit horses on high levels of nutrition, fed on grain-rich diets, and horses entirely grass fed seem particularly difficult to manage. They often develop abdominal distension during anaesthesia even after careful fasting and there is a clinical impression, unsupported by investigational data, that they are more prone to develop circulatory and other problems. Some anaesthetists believe that they show a higher than usual incidence of postanaesthetic rhabdomyolysis and implicate the diet in its aetiology. Although there appears to be little scientific justification for it, many experienced anaesthetists and equine surgeons are firm believers in the old practice of 'letting down' an animal before subjecting it to anaesthesia and operation, i.e. reducing the protein and energy content of its diet for some 7–10 days before anaesthesia. In the authors' opinion, to postpone all but the most urgent of operations until a horse which is in full training has lost the peak of its fitness from being fed a less rich diet certainly does no harm and may have much to commend it. Unfortunately, economic considerations often demand that horses be returned to full work with the minimum of delay and this period of therapeutic inactivity is not well received by many owners.

The recent advancs in equine anaesthesia and the better understanding of fluid balance disturbances have encouraged equine surgeons to undertake more ambitious surgical procedures and many cases which only a few years ago would have been regarded as hopeless are now being saved. Most of this recent expansion of surgical capability has been in the fields of emergency abdominal and thoracic surgery and it is in these fields that proper preanaesthetic preparation and management are of paramount importance. Elective abdominal or thoracic surgery on reasonably healthy animals presents few problems provided the basic principles of anaesthesia are observed but, in contrast, general anaesthesia for emergencies can present a major challenge.

Most acute thoracic crises are the result of trauma and horses suffering from chest injuries may be agitated or restless (presumably due to pain and/or cerebral hypoxia), dyspnoeic, cyanosed, hypovolaemic and showing signs of shock. When shock is advanced the horse is usually dull and apathetic so the handling presents few problems, but a violent or restless injured horse must be given an analgesic both for its sake and to reduce the risk of injury to attendants. Provided excessive doses are not used, the potential ability of analgesics to produce respiratory depression can be completely ignored. Treatment of pneumothorax by the insertion of a chest drain may be carried out under local infiltration or intercostal block and the drain connected to a one-way (Heimlich) valve before general anaesthesia is induced. Hypovolaemia also needs to be corrected before induction of anaesthesia and is best treated by transfusion of blood or plasma but if these are not available the rather expensive plasma substitutes such as the dextrans, starches or gelatins can be used. Polyionic intravenous solutions are much less effective in that they need to be given in much larger quantities but are considerably less expensive.

Most cases of colic presented for surgical treatment have already been treated medically and it is important to consider the drugs used, their route of administration, doses and time of dosing, for they can influence the response to subsequent anaesthesia. Pain is usually indicative of gastric and/or intestinal distension and of acute ischaemia. Its severity may make the horse unmanageable until it becomes utterly exhausted and pain must be controlled, although this is not always easy. Many anaesthetists favour pethidine given intramuscularly in large doses but it is not always effective in doses which do not cause hypotension. Xylazine and detomidine are often surprisingly effective and may be used in comparatively small doses. The effect of these agents on gut motility is probably unimportant. The sudden disappearance of pain in an unmedicated horse is an omnious sign for it is usually associated with rupture of a distended viscus. Acepromazine, being an α-adrenergic blocker, will contribute to hypotension in dehydrated or shocked animals and has no more than a very limited place in the treatment of colic pains.

The main problem in the preanaesthetic preparation of most colic cases is the replacement of fluids in the dehydrated and possibly shocked animal. Medical treatment usually relies on conservative supportive therapy but fluid replacement is extremely urgent in surgical cases if any consistent measure of success is to be obtained. Unfortunately, diagnosis is very imprecise, and there is an understandable reluctance on the part of both owners and veterinarians to spend a considerable sum of money and time on cases which may at laparotomy prove to be inoperable. To overcome this reluctance some acceptable routine which does not involve replacement of the major part of the fluid deficit prior to anaesthesia is clearly desirable. Such a routine may be obtainable, for experience of cases in which tympany or violent intractable pain allowed only minimal preparation indicates that if really vigorous replacement is carried out once the surgeon has confirmed that surgical treatment is possible, a successful outcome is quite as likely as in cases treated before the induction of anaesthesia. Moreover, in cases of intestinal obstruction many are of the opinion that massive preoperative infusions are better avoided since much of the fluid infused accumulates in the obstructed intestine, making operation more difficult and time consuming because of the greater need for decompression of the bowel. Thus, it is possible that 'minimal' preparation can be justified on both surgical and economic grounds but it must be emphasized that for success it must be carried out in a rational manner.

Whenever possible anaesthesia should not be induced in a colic case until hypovolaemia has been improved and the packed cell volume (PCV) decreased. Tachycardia may persist, due to pain or toxaemia, even after the blood volume has been restored to normal. Hypovolaemia is best treated by the transfusion of plasma but plasma substitutes are acceptable, if expensive, alternatives. Polyionic solutions having a composition similar to that of equine extracellular fluid (e.g. lactated Ringer's solution) can be used but, because they diffuse so readily from the circulation, much larger quantities will be needed. These large quantities may have to be infused at rates of 20–30 l/h to produce a measurable effect on the central venous pressure. Acid-base disturbances are seldom a problem in the preoperative period and there is no need to administer bicarbonate at this stage. Even in cases which are thought to be complicated by septic shock, the routine administration of very expensive glucocorticoids before operation has been shown to be of doubtful value. Non-steroidal antiflammatory drugs (NSAIDs) such as flunixin have been claimed to be of benefit but it has never been shown that their use affects the survival rate.

Regardless of whether preoperative fluids are to be given to a colic case, at least one reliable intravenous line must be introduced into the jugular vein and retained in position with a suture. When not in use these catheters may be capped or sealed with a stopcock after being filled with heparinized saline (10 units of heparin per millilitre of saline). A stomach tube should be passed through one nostril before the horse is anaesthetized and the stomach decompressed. It should be withdrawn into the oesophagus before the induction of anaesthesia because if left in the stomach it seems to encourage regurgitation, but it should not be completely removed for once the horse is recumbent under anaesthesia it is almost impossible to pass a tube down the oesophagus to the stomach. Gastric decompression will minimize the likelihood of the stomach rupturing during induction. Whenever possible the surgical site should be clipped and prepared while the animal is conscious and standing, for the duration of the anaesthetic period needs to be kept to a minimum in these very ill animals.

Mares suckling foals should not be separated from their offspring in the preanaesthetic period. If it is necessary to operate on the mare, the need for sedation is greatly reduced if anaesthesia is induced in the presence of the foal. Similarly, the presence of a foal's tranquillized mother contributes to the smooth induction of anaesthesia in the foal.

Shoes should be removed before anaesthesia, or at least covered with adhesive plaster, to prevent damage to flooring or the animal itself in the recovery period.

ANAESTHETIC TECHNIQUES

Intravenous technique

In horses intravenous injections are usually made into the jugular vein about half-way down the neck. The horse should be handled quietly and the use of a twitch is to be avoided, for its application often tends to provoke rather than prevent head movement. Many horses will tense their neck muscles and obscure the jugular furrow whenever a twitch is applied. With the usual aseptic precautions 1 or 2 ml of local analgesic solution are injected through a short, fine needle into the dermis and subcutaneous tissue to produce an insensitive area over the jugular furrow. The importance of this cannot be over-emphasized for the insertion of a stout intravenous needle or catheter through the skin which has not been desensitized may be associated with such pain that young or nervous animals will become uncontrollable. When local analgesia has developed, the intravenous needle (about 6–7 cm long and 2.1 mm bore or 14 gauge) or a 5 cm, 2.4 mm bore (13 gauge) over-needle catheter is thrust through the skin over the vein with its point directed towards the head.

Catheters need to be introduced through a small skin incision made in the weal of local analgesic solution. The vein is distended by the application of pressure which is best applied by pressing the thumb into the jugular furrow just below the site of venepuncture (Fig. 11.11). This tenses the skin and the distended vein is easily palpable. The point of the needle or catheter is directed towards the vein and thrust into it. It is important that a good length of needle or catheter shall be introduced into the vein otherwise there is a risk that as the vein subsides, on the release of pressure, it will retract away from the needle or catheter whose position is fixed by the skin. Moreover, unless about 2–3 cm of the needle or catheter is in the lumen of the vein, the slightest movement is likely to cause it to leave the vessel. A free flow of blood indicates that it is well placed in the lumen of the vein. If only a few drops of blood fall

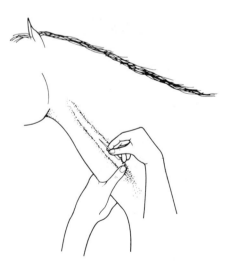

Fig. 11.11 Injection into the jugular vein of the horse. The vein is easily raised with simple digital pressure and 'neck ropes' should never be employed for this purpose because they invariably displace the skin, resulting in withdrawal of the needle or catheter when their compression is released.

it may be concluded that either (1) the needle or catheter is in a perivascular haematoma or (2) the needle or catheter is in the vein but its lumen is partially blocked. Once it is certain that a catheter is in the vein to its maximum length it should be secured in position with a partial skin thickness stitch of nylon or linen thread, and a stopcock attached. The catheter may be kept patent for many hours if its lumen is periodically flushed with heparin saline solution (10 units/ml). The skin suture should be laid before venepuncture is attempted so that it may be tied securely around the catheter without risk of displacing this from the vein.

A needle used for intravenous injections should be held and pressed gently and continuously against the animal's neck during any injection so that should the animal move its neck the hand (and needle) will move with it and thus overcome any tendency for the needle to be pulled out of the vein.

When irritant substances (such as guaiphenesin) are being given by slow intravenous injection over a period of several minutes, restive animals frequently move so that a needle may be pulled out of the vein during the course of the injection. In such circumstances the risk of perivascular deposition of the solution is high and greater certainty of correct intravenous injection is obtained when catheters are used instead of needles. There are today numerous types of disposable intravenous catheters which may be bought sterile, in packets, ready for immediate use. Up to 10 inches (25 cm) of catheter may be introduced into the lumen of the vein and the risk of complete dislodgement during the course of injection is slight.

There is no advantage to be gained from introducing a needle or catheter into the vein in a downwards direction away from the head except, possibly, for the infusion of large volumes of solutions such as guaiphenesin. Indeed, technical errors are much more likely to arise if attempts are made to perform venepuncture in this manner. The operation is more awkward; it is more difficult to assess the depth to which the needle is being inserted and if the animal moves its neck the direction of movement will be against the point of the needle thus tending to transfix the vein. Care must be taken to avoid air embolism when a needle or catheter is directed downwards since its tip will be at a lower pressure than its hub, predisposing to the aspiration of air if the hub is not closed off with a stopcock whenever an injection is not being made.

Endotracheal intubation

In horses the passage of a Magill-type endotracheal tube presents no great problem. With the anaesthetized

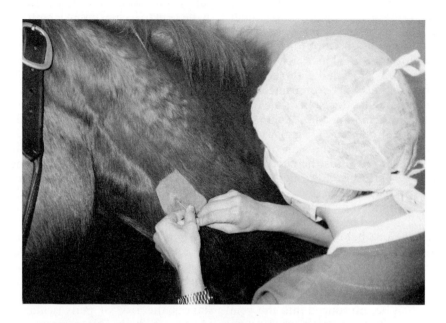

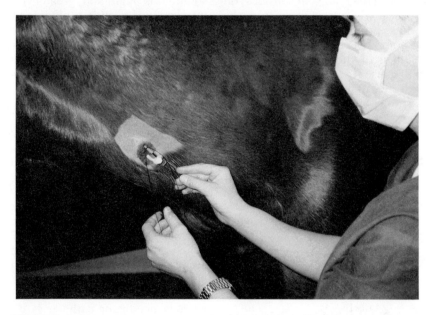

Fig. 11.12 Introduction of a catheter into the jugular vein. In (a) a catheter of the 'over-needle' variety is being introduced through an insensitive skin weal produced by the intradermal injection of 1 ml of 2% lignocaine. Depending on the particular type of catheter being introduced it may be necessary to make a small skin incision in the centre of the weal to prevent 'belling out' of the catheter tip or the catheter being pushed back along its introducing needle as the skin is penetrated. After penetration of the skin the vein is distended by digital pressure and the catheter advanced well into the vein. In (b) the catheter and its occluding tap are being fixed in position with partial skin thickness sutures. (It is advisable to lay these sutures before introducing the catheter but this was avoided here for the sake of clarity.)

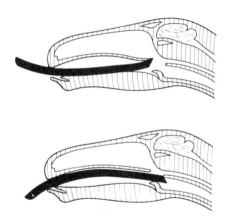

Fig. 11.13 Passage of an oral endotracheal tube in a horse.

horse in lateral recumbency the head is moderately extended on the neck, and the mouth opened and the tongue pulled forward. The tube, lubricated on its outside with a suitable lubricant (K–Y Jelly, Johnson and Johnson), is introduced into the mouth with the concave side of its curve directed towards the hard palate and advanced, keeping to the midline, until its tip is in the pharynx. It is then rotated so that the concavity of its curve is towards the tongue (Fig. 11.13) and at the next inspiration it is pushed rapidly on into the trachea. The rotation of the tube when its tip is in the pharynx ensures that it does not become impacted on the epiglottis. Failure of the tube to enter the trachea indicates that the alignment of the

head and neck is incorrect. Straight tubes or those with only a shallow curvature are more difficult to introduce and the head needs to be more extended on the neck than is needed for Magill-type tubes (which are now manufactured in the UK to British Standards specifications).

Intubation through the mouth permits the use of the largest tube which will comfortably fit the trachea. A 16.0 mm tube is suitable for ponies up to about 150 kg body weight, while a 30 mm tube is adequate for most thoroughbreds. Heavy hunters often take surprisingly large tubes. Endotracheal tubes can be passed through the inferior nasal meatus but this limits the size of the tube to that which can be accommodated by the nostril. Such tubes are often too small to allow free unobstructed respiration and their introduction and removal entails the risk of damaging the turbinate bones. In young foals, however, where the nasal passages are relatively much larger than in adults, tubes of adequate size can be introduced through the nostril. If local analgesic gel is used for lubrication, a tube can be passed without difficulty in conscious foals and anaesthesia may then be induced with an inhalation agent given through the tube without the foal being aware of the smell of the anaesthetic.

The cuffs of endotracheal tubes are often damaged by contact with the horse's teeth even when a reliable mouth-gag is used to keep the mouth open during intubation and extubation. Cuffed tubes made of red rubber for use in horses are very expensive and

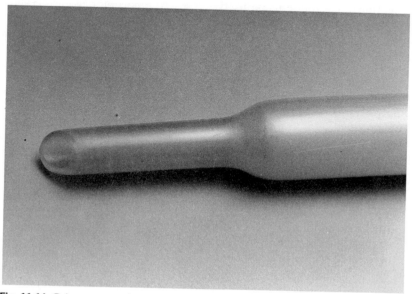

Fig. 11.14 Cole-pattern endotracheal tube for the horse. (Photograph by courtesy of Dr C. M. Trim, College of Veterinary Medicine, University of Georgia, Athens, Georgia, USA.)

because of the relatively short life attempts have been made to produce them in much less expensive plastics. So far these have met with only partial success; either the plastic is so hard that atraumatic intubation is difficult or, when they reach body temperature they soften so much that they become obstructed when the head is flexed on the neck, or from compression due to the air in the cuff. Due to the high price of new red-rubber tubes and the difficulties experienced in getting damaged tubes properly recuffed, some anaesthetists have allowed the use of tubes which have had punctured cuffs repaired with patches which have not been vulcanized on. This is a potentially dangerous practice for these patches may become detached during anaesthesia and lodge in one of the smaller air passages with disastrous results.

The Cole-pattern tube (Fig. 11.14), which has no inflatable cuff, has been used in horses but these tubes have to be of the exact size needed for any given animal and accurately placed in the larynx if they are to provide an atraumatic seal which is sufficiently gas tight for IPPV to be carried out without gross leakage of anaesthetic gases. They must be used with care in young animals having soft laryngeal cartilages for in them forcible dilatation with these tubes can seriously damage the larynx. They have been reported in association with acute laryngeal oedema in two adult horses although whether they were in fact the cause was not established [103]. Siliconized latex rubber cuffed tubes do not conform to British Standards specifications, have less curvature and are more difficult to introduce but are otherwise satisfactory.

PREMEDICATION

Premedication is an integral part of the anaesthetic technique and can never be considered in isolation. The choice and dose of any premedicant drug will depend on the physical condition of the horse, the likely duration of the proposed examination or operation and the nature of the anaesthetic technique to be employed. Heavy premedication will enable smaller doses of the maintenance anaesthetic agent to be used and recovery need not be prolonged. In many respects, the relative importance given to the premedicant drugs or the anaesthetic agents is a matter of personal preference. Some anaesthetists favour heavy sedative premedication which decreases the quantities of the potentially more dangerous anaesthetic to be used, while others habitually use light premedication and more of the anaesthetic. In the hands of their exponents both regimens appear to produce similar results.

Anticholinergic drugs (atropine, glycopyrrolate) have no place in the routine premedication of horses but should be used in surgery likely to provoke vagal reflexes. Horses do not produce copious quantities of saliva, laryngeal spasm and reflex effects from laryngeal stimulation do not present problems, and these drugs may be given intravenously on the infrequent occasions when bradycardia from vagal reflexes develops during anaesthesia. Their routine use may lead to bronchial secretions becoming more viscid and more likely to obstruct the smaller airways with subsequent collapse of distal alveoli. The effects of atropine on the eye may interfere with vision, thus making some horses more difficult to control, while its effects on the gut may decrease intestinal mobility and contribute towards intestinal distension and ileus in colic cases. In horses, glycopyrrolate is probably better than atropine, for it does not readily cross the

blood–brain barrier and is thus unlikely to give rise to central excitatory effects.

Premedication with acepromazine has been used in horses for many years to lessen, or to prevent, excitement during recovery from barbiturate anaesthesia, and to reduce the quantity of anaesthetic needed for maintenance (but not for induction) of anaesthesia. It may be given by intramuscular injection in doses of 0.03–0.05 mg/kg about 1 hour before anaesthesia is to be induced, or it may be given intravenously at half this dose rate. After intravenous injection it is necessary to allow 5–20 minutes to elapse to ensure it is producing its full effects.

α_2-Adrenoceptor agonists (xylazine and detomidine) are much more versatile agents for premedication. They contribute markedly to the anaesthetic and reduce the dose of both intravenous and inhalation anaesthetic agents. Xylazine may be given in a 10% solution by intramuscular injection in doses of 2 mg/kg about 15–20 minutes before induction of anaesthesia. Alternatively, it may be given by intravenous injection in doses of 1 mg/kg about 2–4 minutes beforehand. Detomidine may be used in a similar manner, the appropriate doses being 20–40 µg/kg and 10–20 µg/kg, respectively. After premedication with these agents horses are reluctant to walk so whenever possible the drug should be administered in the place where anaesthesia is to be induced.

Mixtures of α_2-adrenoceptor agonists with narcotic analgesics which are used for sedating standing horses (see Table 11.2) can also be employed, in half the sedative doses, for premedication. Full doses may be needed in difficult horses but then it may be possible to reduce greatly the dose of induction agent.

INDUCTION OF ANAESTHESIA

General anaesthesia of horses should produce a state of recumbency and unconsciousness for as long as may be necessary, followed by a rapid, excitement-free recovery to the standing position, without damage or danger to the animal, personnel or surroundings. The past 40 years have seen great improvements in equine anaesthesia but this target still cannot be achieved with anything like certainty in each case, and a routine method suitable for every situation has yet to be discovered. The anaesthetist must choose a suitable method with regard to the size, health and temperament of the individual horse, the cost of the procedure and the facilities available.

It is always safer if the weight of the animal is known and it should be determined by actual weighing, for visual appraisal, even with experience, is too inaccurate. Under field conditions it is improbable that weighing facilities will be available, and the average figures given in Table 11.3 then constitute a useful guide. The weight of a horse may also be estimated with acceptable accuracy from the formula:

$$\text{Weight (kg)} = \frac{\text{Girth (inches)}^2 \times \text{Length (inches)}}{660}$$

The girth is measured just behind the elbow and the length is from the point of the shoulder to the line of the ischial tuberosity. Both are more conveniently measured in inches than in centimetres, but if the metric scale is used these measurements may be converted to inches by dividing each by 2.5. Jones *et al.* [104] reviewed the accuracy of prediction of the liveweight of horses from body measurements and concluded that the best overall prediction is (umbilical girth in centimetres)$^{1.78}$ × (length of body from tuber ischii to elbow in centimetres)$^{0.97}$/3011 and gave a nomogram based on this equation. It is claimed that use of this involves an acceptable error of 5% and thus for a true 450 kg horse this would give an estimated weight of between 472.5 and 427.5 kg (a range of nearly 50 kg). However, there may be an observer bias for M. Down and L. Gray (personal communication) weighed 400 horses of all ages, including geldings, stallions and mares admitted to the Cambridge Veterinary School over a 3 year period and found that the formula given above always estimated the weight to within 25 kg of the true weight.

If anaesthesia is induced in a loose box or barn, a thick straw bed must be provided to prevent injury to the horse when it falls unconscious. No bedding need be provided if anaesthesia is induced in a grassy field, but some protection of the undermost eye is essential.

Table 11.3 Ranges in weight for various types of animal

	Weight (kg)
Children's ponies	150–300
Donkeys	150–200
Thoroughbred	
yearlings	300–350
2 year old	300–400
3 year old	400–450
adults	450–550
Hunters	
mares	450–550
geldings	500–675
Cart	
yearlings	350–450
2 year old	450–525
Draught Cross	550–625
Heavy Draught	650–850

Some anaesthetists consider that the best protection against injury at induction is to pad the horse rather than try to provide a cushioning bed. A. Messervy (personal communication) designed padded head gear and a padded horse blanket split along the back and joined with quick-release lacing, which proved very satisfactory at the Bristol Veterinary School.

In some equine hospitals (mostly in North America) horses may be positioned for the induction of anaesthesia alongside a table top tilted to the vertical position; the adequately premedicated or quiet animal is restrained against the table top by straps (Fig. 11.15). As the horse loses consciousness during the induction process it is brought smoothly into lateral recumbency by restoring the table top to its normal horizontal position. The method usually works very well but it is only possible where an adequate number of trained personnel are available and trouble can result if a fault develops in the table mechanism at a critical stage of induction. In some hospitals the horse may be allowed to recover on the horizontal table top and placed on its feet as soon as it is judged able to stand by rotating the top to vertical; in most centres, however, the horse is transferred to a padded room for recovery from anaesthesia.

In the majority of equine hospitals in Britain and elsewhere it is now customary to induce general anaesthesia in a special, padded room. Often, a padded bar hinged to one wall is incorporated to enable the horse to be confined in one place in the room and to assist it in assuming recumbency in a gentle, controlled manner. A part of the flooring of this area may be mounted on wheels so that the unconscious horse can be positioned on it for

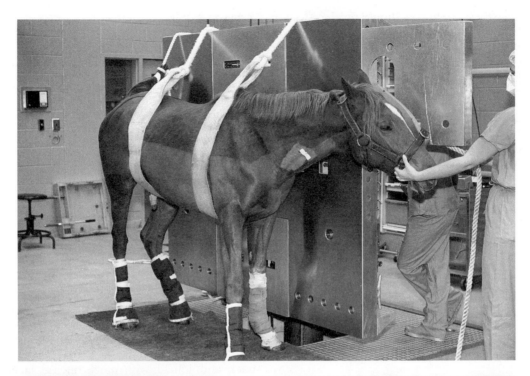

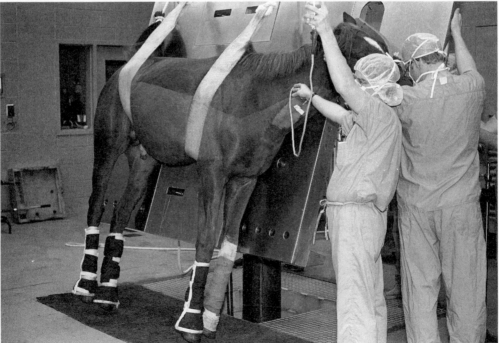

Fig. 11.15 Induction of anaesthesia using a tilting table top. The sedated horse is restrained against the table which is rotated to the horizontal position as the animal becomes unconscious and relaxed. Usually, induction of anaesthesia is with guaiphenesin/thiopentone and four to six people are involved in manipulation of the table and animal. (Photographs by kind permission of Dr C. M. Trim, College of Veterinary Medicine, University of Georgia, Athens, Georgia, USA.)

transport to the operating theatre. In the theatre the wheeled trolley may become the top of the operating table, or the horse may have to be transferred from it to the table. An electrically operated overhead hoist is most helpful both for this and for maintaining the position of the animal on the table during surgery. This system can be operated with minimal, even relatively untrained assistants and mechanical failures are unlikely to be disastrous.

Induction agents

General anaesthesia may be induced with either inhalation anaesthetics or intravenous agents but in most cases the intravenous route is used. The ease of induction with inhalation anaesthetics and the dose of intravenous agents needed are dependent on the sedation produced by premedication. Toxaemia and hypoproteinaemia also reduce the quantity of anaesthetic agent required.

Thiopentone

Thiopentone, at a dose of 10 mg/kg given as a bolus by intravenous injection into the jugular vein, has been found to be very satisfactory for the induction of anaesthesia in horses premedicated with 0.03–0.04 mg/kg of acepromazine 30–40 minutes previously. Unconsciousness is produced and the horse becomes recumbent 25–30 seconds after the thiopentone injection. For many years it has been the practice of some anaesthetists to inject a bolus dose of suxamethonium (0.12 mg/kg) immediately after the thiopentone to smooth the transition to an inhalation agent when anaesthesia is to be maintained for long periods. The use of intravenous xylaxine (1 mg/kg) or detomidine (15–20 µg/kg) premedication 4–5 minutes prior to induction reduces the dose of thiopentone to about 5.5 mg/kg and the use of suxamethonium to ease the induction of continuation inhalation anaesthesia is unnecessary. Premedication with the α_2-adrenoceptor agonists slows the circulation and the onset of unconsciousness is delayed for 40 or more seconds after completion of the thiopentone injection. The horse may make paddling or galloping movements when it first becomes recumbent; these movements disappear within 10–20 seconds as unconsciousness deepens but if at this stage attempts are made to control them with forcible restraint, the animal may not become sufficiently unconscious for endotracheal intubation to be performed.

Thiopentone can also be used with guaiphenesin to induce anaesthesia in horses after premedication with acepromazine. Guaiphenesin is used in concentrations of 5–15% (depending on the personal preferences of the anaesthetist and the preparations available) and

infused into the jugular vein until the horse shows marked ataxia. A bolus intravenous dose of about 5 mg/kg of thiopentone then produces recumbency and apparent unconsciousness. Panic due to muscle weakness may be seen if guaiphenesin is infused without prior administration of a sedative. It is also possible to combine guaiphenesin and thiopentone solutions for infusion into the jugular vein to produce recumbency but there is much less control over anaesthesia when this is done and profound respiratory depression can be produced.

Methohexitone

After heavy premedication with intravenous xylazine (1 mg/kg) or detomidine (15 µg/kg) anaesthesia can be induced some 4–5 minutes later with 2.8 mg/kg of methohexitone given intravenously as a bolus dose. Lateral recumbency follows 40 or more seconds after completion of the injection and the breathing rhythm is often abnormal, three deep breaths being succeeded by 30–40 seconds without any sign of respiratory activity. This breathing pattern does not produce any significant increase in $P_a\text{CO}_2$, but $P_a\text{O}_2$ decreases as in any recumbent horse. Similar breathing patterns occur in horses with other anaesthetic agents but the clinical impression is that they are more common during anaesthesia involving methohexitone. Anaesthesia lasts for about 5 minutes and the horse usually stands up about 25 minutes later. Recovery is usually quiet and uneventful.

Ketamine

In horses, the use of ketamine on its own results in stimulation rather than depression of the central nervous system, with poor muscle relaxation, tremors and even convulsions. Many drugs have been used in attempts to suppress these most undesirable effects but only the benzodiazepines and the α_2-adrenoceptor agonists have proved to be of any real value.

A combination of an α_2-adrenoceptor agonist premedication and injection of a ketamine bolus will produce an excellent induction of anaesthesia followed by a spectacularly rapid, but usually very quiet, recovery. It appears to be safe, and possesses certain advantages over α_2-adrenoceptor agonists/thiopentone or methohexitone combinations. However, if consistently good results are to be obtained a very strict adherence to a set procedure is essential. This procedure has evolved by trial and error and almost all the possible variations of it which have been tried have been found to be less consistently successful. In detail the method is as follows:

Xylazine (1 mg/kg) over a 2 minute period or detomidine (20 µg/kg) as a bolus is given by intravenous injection and its effects observed for 5 minutes. This should produce a marked reluctance to move, hanging of the head, adoption of a wide-based stance, mild ataxia and, in males, a slight protrusion of the penis from the prepuce. If these effects do not follow the injection of these doses of xylazine or detomidine more is administered until they are observed. It is seldom necessary to exceed 1.4 mg/kg of xylazine in horses but in donkeys up to 1.8 mg/kg may be necessary. It is imperative that an α_2-adrenoceptor agonist is administered in quiet surroundings; loud noises must be avoided and even talking in the vicinity should be discouraged. An interval of 2–3 minutes is allowed after the injection of these drugs to enable their full effects to be obtained before the administration of the ketamine. Noise at this stage may provoke excitement and the desired deep sedation will not develop. When maximum sedation has developed, ketamine (2.2 mg/kg) is given by rapid intravenous injection. Lateral recumbency is assumed in 85 ± 30 seconds after the ketamine injection.

The manner in which the horse lies down is completely different from that following the rapid intravenous injection of barbiturates such as thiopentone or methohexitone. It is a much more gradual process, the animal often taking a step or two sideways or backwards before sitting back on its haunches and sinking to its brisket. It then rolls gently over on to its side and may make one or two quite vigorous limb movements before becoming still. Once recumbent, the animal settles much more quickly and the onset of unconsciousness is more rapid when no attempt is made forcibly to restrain the head. As judged by the gradual disappearance of eye movements, anaesthesia continues to deepen for 1–2 minutes after the horse becomes recumbent, and even when eye movements cease, relaxation of the jaw muscles is not always good. It may be necessary to prise the mouth open for the passage of an endotracheal tube but intubation presents no problems once the mouth is open. Respiratory depression is minimal so that a smooth transition to inhalation anaesthesia is easily achieved. The classical signs and stages of anaesthesia are not recognizable and the surest guide to the depth of anaesthesia is the presence or absence of response to surgical stimulation. Nystagmus and tear formation may be observed but the eye is usually closed at depths suitable for surgery.

When no other anaesthetic is given, depending on the degree of surgical stimulation, horses first raise their heads 10–30 minutes after the ketamine injection, roll into sternal recumbency some minutes later and stand 5 or 6 minutes after this. Termination of surgical anaesthesia is very abrupt but recovery is remarkably free from excitement and horses usually stand at the first attempt. Once standing there is very little evidence of ataxia.

The method is not without disadvantages. The very abrupt end of surgical anaesthesia when no other anaesthetics are given can lead to difficulties where anaesthesia has to be induced by the surgeon and there is no other skilled person available to monitor its course. Horses require very different handling from that used when anaesthesia is induced with the barbiturates, and xylazine, detomidine and ketamine are expensive drugs. However, the method appears to be a very safe way of producing short periods of anaesthesia. Cardiovascular parameters are well maintained, respiration is adequate and continuation of anaesthesia with an inhalation agent presents no problems.

In North America the method is sometimes modified by the inclusion of guaiphenesin. For example, xylazine (2.2 mg/kg) is given by intramuscular injection 20 minutes before 55 mg/kg of guaiphenesin is infused as a 5% solution in 5% dextrose into the jugular vein. This is followed by the intravenous injection of 1.7 mg/kg of ketamine [77]. It is probable that the inclusion of guaiphenesin does little more than ensure the absence of muscle tremors or rigidity due to ketamine when the dose of xylazine is inadequate or where the surroundings are not peaceful enough for it to produce the sedation needed.

Tiletamine–zolazepam

This combination has been administered to six horses after xylazine premedication [105]. Although it produced 'reasonably safe' short-term anaesthesia of a little longer duration than that seen after xylazine/ketamine it offered very little other advantage.

Etorphine

Etorphine is used in horses as 'Large Animal Immobilon', a yellow solution containing 2.45 mg etorphine hydrochloride with 10 mg acepromazine maleate per millilitre. The minimum dose for horses is 0.5 ml of the solution per 50 kg injected intravenously or intramuscularly. Half the intramuscular dose may be used in donkeys. The intramuscular route should only be used in dire emergencies since it results in a period of marked excitement before sedation and anaesthesia ensue. Animals made recumbent with Immobilon are very stiff, with muscle tremors, severe respiratory depression, cyanosis, tachycardia and hypertension. In male animals priapism is not uncommon. Transfer to inhalation anaesthesia is usually not required because the effects of Immobilon last about 45 minutes.

Because of the marked effects in the body, Immobilon is not recommended for use in horses with cardiac problems or liver damage. Animals should not be slaughtered for consumption either by humans or by other animals until 7 days have elapsed.

The actions of Immobilon may be antagonized by the injection of Revivon, a blue solution containing 3 mg/ml of diprenorphine hydrochloride. A quantity of Revivon equal to the total volume of Immobilon injected should be given intravenously as soon as possible after the required period of restraint is complete. Most horses regain their feet within a few minutes of this injection. Injection of Revivon antagonizes only the actions of etorphine, hence analgesia is lost but sedation due to the acepromazine is unaffected. Undesirable hyperexcitability may be associated with the injection of the antagonist and enterohepatic cycling may occur, causing excitement and apparently compulsive walking 6–8 hours after remobilization. Should these delayed effects be observed a further half dose of Revivon must be given.

Combinations of etorphine with other agents such as xylazine and azaperone have proved no more satisfactory in practice than Immobilon, and the attempts of some clinicians to obtain greater muscle relaxation by combining α_2-adrenoceptor agonists with Immobilon are unwise in view of the respiratory and circulatory disturbances which result.

The use of Immobilon is associated both with a degree of risk to the life of even healthy horses and to that of the anaesthetist. Large Animal Immobilon is an extremely potent neuroleptanalgesic which is highly toxic to man. In man it causes dizziness, nausea, pinpoint pupils, respiratory depression, cyanosis, hypotension, loss of consciousness and death. In the event of accidental injection, spillage on the skin or immediate clothing, or splashing into the eyes or mouth, immediate treatment is essential. Any veterinarian contemplating the use of Immobilon should be thoroughly familiar with the latest treatment measures set out in the data sheet and ensure that adequate supplies of (in date) naloxone are to hand. If it is considered for any reason that the use of Immobilon is absolutely essential, it is clearly most unwise to use it unless another qualified person is present.

Metomidate and etomidate

The results obtained in pharmacologically oriented trials of metomidate following azaperone premedication did not encourage clinical use of this drug in horses. However, metomidate (2.25 mg/kg) following premedication with detomidine (10 μg/kg) produces excellent induction prior to maintenance of anaesthesia with halothane since significant apnoea does not occur. This method of induction of anaesthesia when not followed by subsequent halothane administration is associated with a prolonged and ataxic recovery.

Etomidate has apparently not been used in horses.

Inhalation agents

Under field conditions anaesthesia may have to be induced in the open. The weather may be cold, giving rise to difficulty in volatilizing anaesthetic liquids, or it may be so hot as to cause dangerous concentrations of volatile anaesthetics to be delivered from simple types of vaporizers.

Many veterinarians in the UK still induce anaesthesia in even large horses with chloroform, using methods described in detail in earlier editions of this book. However, in view of the ease with which anaesthesia can now be more safely induced with injectable drugs it is difficult, today, to justify this practice except, possibly, on grounds of cost. Induction of anaesthesia with chloroform is unnecessary even in very needle shy horses, for detomidine can be administered by mouth (see p. 76, 193) to produce good sedation and render the animal manageable by other means.

Thus, today, it is customary to induce anaesthesia in adult animals by the use of intravenous agents and inhalation induction is confined to young foals which may not have the hepatic detoxicating mechanisms fully developed and which are easily managed with the minimum of assistance. A head collar is put on the standing foal and the inhalation anaesthetic (halothane, enflurane or isoflurane volatilized in a stream of oxygen or nitrous oxide/oxygen) administered through a face-mask applied lightly over both nostrils whilst assistants stand at each shoulder and grasp the head collar. The volatile agent is introduced gradually, its concentration being increased every three or four breaths up to a maximum of 4 × MAC until consciousness is lost. As the foal loses consciousness the attendants lower it gently to the ground, the mask is removed, an endotracheal tube passed through the mouth in the usual manner and the anaesthetic continued through this tube. Alternatively, instead of using a face-mask an endotracheal tube may be passed into the trachea via one nostril, its cuff inflated and the anaesthetic administered through it. The best endotracheal tubes for this purpose are those made of silicone rubber and they should be about 55 cm long. The nasal passages are relatively larger in foals than in adults and surprisingly large tubes can be passed through the ventral nasal meatus without difficulty. Neonatal thoroughbred foals can accommodate tubes of 7–9 mm internal diameter and in 6 week old foals 11 mm tubes can be passed with ease. Passage of the tube is greatly facilitated by prior preparation of the ventral nasal mucosa with lignocaine ointment or gel and lubrication of the tube with the same preparation. If the foal persistently prevents the tube from entering the trachea by swallowing when its tip is in the pharynx, 2–5 ml of lignocaine solution may be instilled through the lumen of the tube into the pharynx. After a short pause there is then generally no difficulty in advancing the tube to the tracheal lumen. Obviously, when anaesthesia has been induced through a nasal endotracheal tube the administration can be continued through the same tube for as long as is necessary. The possible complications of this technique have been well reviewed by Webb [106] but with care they are rare. Anaesthetic apparatus designed for use in adult human subjects is adequate for foals up to 2–3 months of age.

MAINTENANCE OF ANAESTHESIA

No matter what method is used to maintain anaesthesia, precautions have to be taken to ensure that the horse is not injured accidentally while anaesthetized. Many complications may be avoided if careful attention is given to positioning the animal for radiology or surgery and surgical convenience may have to be sacrificed for the benefit of the horse.

During general anaesthesia the weight of the horse compresses blood vessels so that tissues become ischaemic; in the lateral position the brachial nerves and vessels may be trapped between the humerus and the rib cage, while venous congestion of the upper hind-limb can result from its weight causing adduction to obstruct veins in the groin. It is not entirely certain that postanaesthetic lameness can be prevented by careful positioning of the horse during anaesthesia. The same horse may be anaesthetized under apparently similar conditions for the same length of time and develop lameness on one occasion and not on another. However, raising the limbs by a hoist so that the shoulder region is clear of the table or ground surface and the upper hind-limb does not adduct appears to reduce its incidence after periods of lateral recumbency. Similarly, partial suspension by the legs in conjunction with the use of a V-shaped back support (Fig. 11.16) seems to diminish the risk of serious damage to the back muscles. Under field conditions, where these facilities are not available, a horse lying on its side may have adduction of the upper limbs prevented by supporting them on straw bales, and the undermost fore-leg may be drawn as far forward as possible to minimize pressure on the brachial vessels and nerves.

To avoid damage to the masseter muscle and eyes

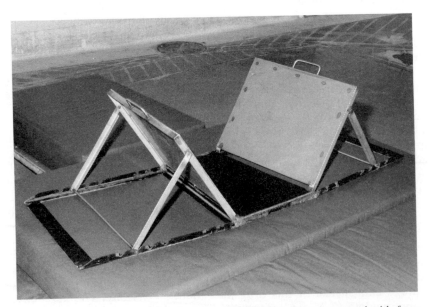

Fig. 11.16 Back support for supine horse. In use the support is covered with foam padding 3 inches (7.5 cm) thick. The weight of the horse is taken by the dorsal spines and the spines of the scapulae, thus avoiding pressure on the back muscles.

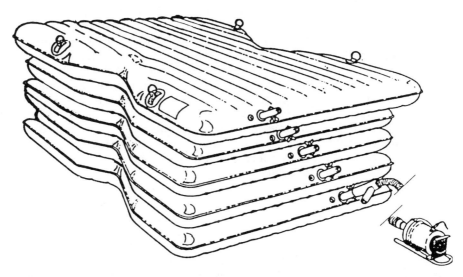

Fig. 11.17 The Snell Infla-table. This is an extremely portable, pneumatically raised table comprising of five stacked chambers for use in the field. The top chamber provides the working surface and should not be fully inflated. The lower four provide support and height adjustment. It is placed in its deflated condition alongside the anaesthetized horse which is then rolled on to it. The table is inflated to the desired working height using an electrically powered air pump. At the conclusion of the operation the table is deflated and the horse slid off to recover from anaesthesia. The complete kit weighs about 60 kg and packs into a space of 1600 × 540 × 210 mm. (Manufactured by Snell-Wessex Ltd, Fosters Farm, Boyshill, Holnest, Sherborne, Dorset DT9 5PJ, UK.)

care must be taken to ensure that the face is not allowed to remain in contact with sharp edges of halters, head collars or the table top. The head should not be restrained in a position of opisthotonus, nor rotated on the neck. If possible the head should be slightly raised during anaesthesia to ensure good venous drainage. When the anaesthetized horse has to be moved the head should be supported in a normal position in relation to the neck. Failure to observe these points may be followed by intense vascular congestion of the nasal passages leading to gross upper respiratory obstruction after extubation.

It was hoped that positioning the recumbent horse on a water mattress, or partially inflated air bed (Fig. 11.17), might overcome problems of post-anaesthetic myopathy associated with recumbency, but the results of many attempts have been disappointing. Certainly, operating on a horse which is lying on a water bed is not conducive to the performance of any delicate surgery. The use of a ripple mattress or a rigid body shell has yet to be extensively tried.

To prevent burns, the earthing plate-electrode of diathermy machines must be in good contact with the skin. It should be placed on a hairless region of the skin or the hairs between it and the skin kept wet with saline or conducting jelly. Rope burns from the overbrisk withdrawal of ropes from beneath the horse are entirely avoidable.

Agents for the maintenance of anaesthesia

Intravenous agents

The advantages associated with the use of intravenous agents for the maintenance of anaesthesia are obvious. They are easy to administer using only the simplest of apparatus, there is no difficulty in instructing nursing staff or others to give controlled doses as needed during anaesthesia, and they do not pollute the atmosphere. Unfortunately, in the past the agents available had such a long duration of action and great toxicity that their use in horses was very restricted; it was these disadvantages which gave impetus to the development of inhalation anaesthesia for equine surgery. Today, drugs which are rapidly metabolized and eliminated from the body are being introduced and there is evidence of renewed interest in intravenous anaesthesia for horses. The duration of recovery after the use of some of the more recently introduced, relatively non-toxic, agents is no longer than after anaesthesia with halothane. Also, reassessment of some of the older agents has shown that many of their disadvantages can be overcome by using them in different ways (often in combination with other parenterally administered drugs). It seems certain that over the next few years there will be further developments in intravenous anaesthesia for horses but it is difficult to predict what they will be.

To ensure adequate oxygenation during intravenous anaesthesia oxygen must be administered through a face-mask, endotracheal tube or nasopharyngeal catheter. If apnoea follows the injection of an overdose of anaesthetic, IPPV must be performed and the necessary apparatus must, therefore, be available whenever a horse is anaesthetized.

Chloral hydrate. Today, few anaesthetists would consider using chloral hydrate as an intravenous anaesthetic. The use of chloral hydrate is usually restricted to producing deep sedation of the standing horse before anaesthesia is induced with a barbiturate. When given in this way it provides a useful background depression on which the effects of other agents may be superimposed. It is usually necessary to infuse about 80 mg/kg to produce marked ataxia before thiopentone (5.5 mg/kg) is given as a bolus dose to induce anaesthesia.

Pentobarbitone sodium. Although horses metabolize pentobarbitone sodium relatively rapidly the drug must be considered to be an unsuitable anaesthetic for horses. In spite of the rapid metabolism the recovery period is long and associated with marked narcotic excitement and struggling. In the past it was used for continuation of anaesthesia induced with chloral hydrate. It was claimed that up to 4 g could be given to an adult horse during the course of an operation without prolonging the duration of the recovery period beyond the 1½ hours which would, in any case, have followed from the chloral hydrate induction.

Thiopentone sodium. Although thiopentone is a reasonably satisfactory agent for the induction of anaesthesia of up to about 10 minutes' duration, it is unwise to prolong thiopentone anaesthesia for longer than about 20 minutes by the injection of repeated doses or constant infusions. The speed and quality of recovery depend on the total dose of thiopentone used and, therefore, the low doses used after sedative premedication permit more increments to be given than is possible if the induction dose of 10 mg/kg is given initially.

While the drug cannot be regarded as an agent which is suitable for both inducing and maintaining anaesthesia in a horse, small doses (0.5–1.0 mg/kg) may be given during anaesthesia maintained by other agents at any time when the animal awakens unexpectedly and needs to be brought under control

with the minimum of delay. Thiopentone has also proved to be a useful agent during halothane anaesthesia in horses following induction with xylazine/ketamine when the animal cannot be prevented from moving except by the administration of such high concentrations of halothane that severe hypotension is produced. In this situation the intravenous injection over 20–30 seconds of 0.5–1.0 mg/kg of thiopentone has been found to abolish limb movements and allow much lower concentrations of halothane to be used.

Methohexitone sodium. The apparently rapid metabolism and elimination of methohexitone might suggest that it may be given to horses by constant infusion or injected intermittently to maintain anaesthesia. However, limited trials have shown that maintenance of surgically useful levels is associated with marked respiratory depression. Recovery is usually violent and the need to control this with other drugs makes it unacceptably long. Cautiously given in large horses, intravenous doses of 100 mg have been found useful in prolonging anaesthesia induced with xylazine/ketamine, and subsequent recovery has been rapid, quiet and uneventful.

Ketamine hydrochloride. There seems to be general agreement that attempts to prolong anaesthesia induced with α_2-adrenoceptor agonists/ketamine mixtures with additional ketamine may encounter undesirable excitatory effects. In a limited series of 10 horses Short [107] found that administration of half the initial dose of both xylazine and ketamine at 20 minute intervals produced satisfactory anaesthesia in nine of the 10 animals; the other horse developed severe respiratory depression. In view of the good induction and invariably quiet, rapid recovery after xylazine/ketamine there is clearly a need for further investigation and it may be found that a separate, controlled infusion of each drug will be satisfactory.

Propofol. Propofol has undergone preliminary trials in horses. Following intravenous premedication with xylazine (0.5 mg/kg) it has been found to produce a smooth induction of anaesthesia when given intravenously in doses of 2.0 mg/kg. Intravenous infusion of 0.2 mg/(kg min) has then maintained apparently satisfactory anaesthesia with a quiet recovery to the standing position about 15 minutes after termination of the infusion. Although these results are encouraging, much more work needs to be done to assess the potential value of this agent in equine anaesthesia.

Mixtures. Methods of producing anaesthesia by the combination of agents have been described.

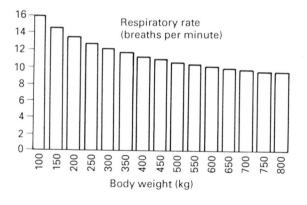

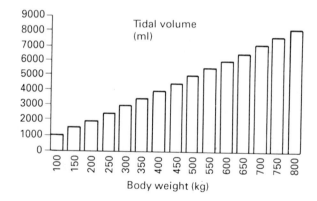

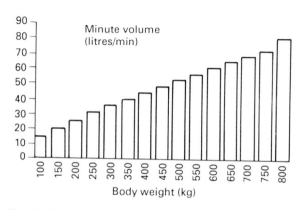

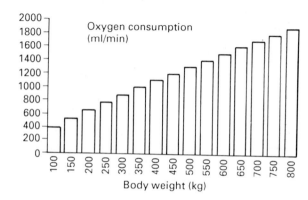

Fig. 11.18 Respiratory variables for the conscious, standing horse. These values only offer a guide as to what might reasonably be expected and are calculated from the allometric equations in *Scaling* by K. Schmidt-Nielsen (1984) Cambridge University Press, Cambridge.

Green *et al.* [108] described the use of intravenous xylazine (1.1 mg/kg) followed by ketamine 2.2 mg/kg and maintained with an intravenous infusion of 2.75 ml/kg/h) of a guaiphenesin/ketamine/xylazine mixture containing 50 mg guaiphenesin, 1 mg ketamine and 0.5 mg of xylazine per millilitre of 5% dextrose in water. This technique has been used very successfully at the Cambridge Veterinary School for operations of up to 90 minutes of duration. E. Lagerweij (personal communication) has used detomidine (0.01 mg/kg intravenously) for premedication, induced anaesthesia with 50 mg/kg of guaiphenesin followed by 2 mg/kg of ketamine, and maintained it with an infusion of 0.75 ml/(kg h) of guaiphenesin (98 mg/ml), ketamine (1.96 mg/ml) and detomidine (0.0196 mg/ml) with satisfactory results. More recently guaiphenesin has been replaced by diazepam but there are no reports of such combinations being used in large numbers of horses.

Inhalation agents

In the 1950s the difficulties and dangers which were apparently inseparable from the use of the then available intravenous agents in the maintenance of anaesthesia prompted a reappraisal of inhalation techniques. Development of more refined methods for their administration and the advent of halothane were probably the most significant factors in this resurgence of interest which led to the present-day popularity of inhalation methods in equine anaesthesia. Although modern inhalation anaesthesia involves the use of bulky, expensive, specialized equipment, it is the safest and most effective means of restraining horses for prolonged diagnostic and surgical procedures.

Halothane. Following its introduction in 1957 [109] halothane rapidly became the inhalation agent of choice for maintenance of anaesthesia in horses. Its special advantages were (and still are) the reasonably rapid induction and recovery, minimal excitement during induction or recovery, adequate reflex suppression and muscle relaxation to allow most surgery to be performed, lack of toxicity and the ease with which anaesthesia can be controlled. The effect of halothane on the cardiovascular system is to cause a dose-dependent fall in arterial blood pressure and cardiac output and a rise in central venous pressure (see p. 106). The fall in cardiac output (which is believed to be largely responsible for the arterial hypotension) is thought to be due to a direct depressant effect of the agent on the myocardium and falls of up to 55% of the non-anaesthetized values have been recorded [74]. There is a marked respiratory acidosis in spontaneously breathing halothane-anaesthetized horses and while this can be overcome by IPPV this causes a further fall in cardiac output [74, 75]. Schatzmann in 1982 [110] showed that hypoxaemia causes a respiratory drive in horses anaesthetized with halothane in air, thus demonstrating that hypoxia can overcome halothane-induced respiratory depression. Halothane is so much of a respiratory depressant that difficulty can be experienced in the transition to anaesthesia with this agent after induction by an intravenous technique. Attempts to hasten the uptake by the administration of high inspired concentrations will usually provoke respiratory arrest after one or two breaths of the concentrated vapour and the horse will not breathe again until redistribution in the body reduces the tension of halothane in the brain. High inspired concentrations will also provoke cardiovascular collapse. The transition phase is especially difficult to manage in horses which have been heavily premedicated before induction with a respiratory depressant such as a barbiturate; it is easier after xylazine/ketamine induction for breathing is less depressed.

In horses it is remarkably difficult to judge the depth of unconsciousness during halothane anaesthesia as hypoxia from any cause results in sympathetic stimulation and signs such as nystagmus, sweating, hyperventilation and even movement [111]. These may be taken as signs of inadequate depth of unconsciousness by the inexperienced anaesthetist with disastrous consequences.

As the MAC value for halothane (p. 104) is known to be about 0.9% it is possible to monitor the depth of halothane by continuous measurement of the end-tidal concentration (p. 34). When oxygen alone is used as the carrier gas, stable maintenance of anaesthesia is usually achieved with end-tidal concentrations of 0.7–1.1% halothane; when nitrous oxide/oxygen mixtures are used end-tidal concentrations of 0.9–1% are usually sufficient. However, because of the shape of the normal distribution curve, some horses will require higher and some lower concentrations to prevent movement in response to surgical stimulation. Also, if heavy premedication has been given before intravenous induction, lower end-tidal concentrations will suffice for maintenance. During halothane anaesthesia there is usually some slowing of the pulse and decrease in blood pressure. Continuous measurement of the arterial blood pressure affords a quite good guide to the depth of halothane anaesthesia.

When halothane is given by low-flow methods after intravenous induction, about 30–35 ml of liquid halothane are required to maintain anaesthesia for 1 hour in horses of about 450 kg body weight. During the second and subsequent hours the uptake decreases and eventually equilibrium is reached between the concentration in the body and the alveolar air (although this may, in fact, take several days).

Horses normally regain their feet within about 30 minutes following the termination of halothane administration after induction with xylazine/ketamine; after acepromazine premedication and thiopentone induction, recovery takes about twice as long. Shivering is often seen during recovery from halothane anaesthesia. The reason is unknown; it does not seem to be related to body or environmental temperature and usually is of no importance. However, by increasing oxygen demands it may be harmful to horses suffering from respiratory and/or cardiovascular diseases which limit oxygen uptake when they are breathing air. Most horses show a measure of incoordination after recovery from halothane and they should not be made to walk (e.g. from recovery to loose box or stall) within 10–15 minutes of standing up.

Enflurane. The MAC value of enflurane (see p. 104) is about 2% and, clinically, end-tidal concentrations of about 2.3% appear to produce reasonably satisfactory surgical anaesthesia after acepromazine premedication and thiobarbiturate induction. Spontaneous breathing stops when the end-tidal concentration is about 4.5% and respiratory arrest is associated with severe arterial hypotension. The use of IPPV to overcome hypercapnia is, under enflurane anaesthesia, associated with more hypotension than is encountered when halothane is used. Induction with xylazine/ketamine is possibly followed by less respiratory and cardiovascular depression than after thiobarbiturate induction.

One of the difficulties encountered in anaesthetizing horses with enflurane has been to obtain a sufficiently high inspired concentration to produce and maintain anaesthesia when using an 'Enflurotec' vaporizer and a circle absorber system which has a large internal volume, without using excessively high, wasteful, fresh gas flow rates. This vaporizer, which can deliver a maximum of 5% enflurane to the breathing circuit, has been used more successfully with a to-and-fro absorber system.

Another problem is that attempts to deepen anaesthesia to prevent movement in response to surgical stimulation may not only produce marked respiratory depression; they may also provoke abnormal twitchings in the muscles of the head, neck and fore-limbs. These twitchings become progressively more pronounced as the end-tidal concentration of enflurane increases, and only cease at about the time complete respiratory arrest is produced. They are associated with seizure-like patterns in the EEG and although they may be abolished by muscle relaxants, these drugs do not suppress the seizure patterns [112].

There is no doubt that recovery from enflurane anaesthesia is very rapid, but it is associated with more shivering and incoordination than is recovery from halothane. Some horses have become excited in the recovery period and although this excitement has been short-lived, it has given rise to some concern after orthopaedic procedures.

It must be admitted that the results of trials of enflurane in equine anaesthesia carried out in this country [113] have been disappointing and reports from North America [112, 114] were not very encouraging. It must be noted that in horses the safety margin is small for Steffey has reported that inhalation of $2 \times$ MAC caused fatal hypotension in his experimental horses [112]. It seems that enflurane cannot be regarded as an agent which is likely to replace halothane in equine anaesthesia.

Isoflurane. Reports from North America where it was first released for use in horses suggest that isoflurane has advantages over halothane as an inhalation anaesthetic for horses [114–116].

The MAC value (see p. 104) is said to be about 1.3% so that at equilibrium, surgical anaesthesia should be produced with end-tidal concentrations of about 1.5%. Dose-related depression of the respiratory and cardiovascular systems by isoflurane is reported to be similar to that caused by halothane. After isoflurane anaesthesia recovery is impressively quick, and was initially thought to be uniformly good but later experience showed this was not always the case. It is now appreciated that, especially when ketamine is used for induction, isoflurane anaesthesia may be associated with poor recovery.

Like halothane, isoflurane produces dose-dependent cardiovascular and respiratory depression but isoflurane causes a smaller fall in cardiac output than does halothane. Unlike halothane, isoflurane causes arterial hypotension mainly from decreased peripheral resistance. Its effects on respiration are more severe [117] than those of halothane and it is advisable to perform IPPV on isoflurane-anaesthetized horses to prevent hypoxia and hypercapnia.

Currently in the UK isoflurane is very much more expensive than halothane and whilst this is the case halothane is likely to remain the volatile agent of choice for the maintenance of anaesthesia in the horse for isoflurane offers no very significant advantages.

Methoxyflurane. Methoxyflurane is an agent with such a low saturated vapour pressure that it can be used safely from relatively simple, inexpensive vaporizers placed in the breathing circuit. However, it is not a very satisfactory agent for horses because its high solubility and low volatility make for sluggish control of depth of anaesthesia coupled with very slow induction and recovery.

Methods of administration. Although theoretically it is possible to use a Magill or coaxial circuit for administering inhalation anaesthetics to horses, their use would require very high (and consequently expensive) gas flow rates. In equine anaesthesia, therefore, for reasonable economy, either a circle or to-and-fro absorption system is used as a low-flow system. There is little practical difference in the administration of halothane and isoflurane in a low-flow system.

A low-flow system can be defined as one in which there is substantial rebreathing of previously expired gas which has passed through a carbon dioxide absorber, usually in a circle system. The fresh gas inflow to the system, however, is greater than the mere consumption of anaesthetic and oxygen by the animal for when these are equal the arrangement becomes a closed system with no spill-over to the atmosphere. For all practical purposes in horses a low-flow system is one in which the fresh gas inflow to the circuit is between 2–4 l/min. If the fresh gas inflow is this low there may be a considerable difference between the concentrations of gases and vapours set on the anaesthetic machine and the inspired concentration available to the animal.

In general, the approach to the use of low-flow systems developed as outlined below is similar to that described by Spence for human subjects [118] and does not call for apparatus to measure the concentration of either gases or vapours and so is quite practical in most situations. In some centres, however, there is insistence that the more gas analysis which is available to the anaesthetist, the better from the point of view of safety. For the most part, the authors agree with Spence that this is probably an abuse of available technology. For example, oxygen analysis is unnecessary if there is known to be no risk of hypoxia, as is the case with oxygen flows of over 2.5 l/min and with concentrations of over 50% oxygen with nitrous oxide. In addition, the clinical signs produced by a potent volatile agent may be more useful than precise measurements of its concentration.

The simplest way to use a low-flow system is to restrict the method to only one gas as the carrier gas — oxygen — and a volatile anaesthetic such as halothane or isoflurane. At the outset the anaesthetic system should be full of air and the animal should have been breathing air. Thus, the animal/system will contain a considerable amount of nitrogen at a concentration of around 80%. This is undesirable and the nitrogen should be eliminated by a fresh gas flow of oxygen sufficient to allow significant spillage through the exhaust valve, although it is not possible to eliminate nitrogen from the system entirely. For practical purposes a concentration of 3–5% nitrogen is acceptable and to produce this a fresh gas flow of above 6 l/min is necessary for the first 10–15 minutes of anaesthesia. Given this high initial gas flow rate a vaporizer placed outside the breathing circuit but in the fresh gas supply line will behave in exactly the same way as it does when used in a circuit in which there is no or virtually no rebreathing, i.e. the concentration set on the vaporizer will be more or less the same as the concentration inspired by the animal. At the end of 10–15 minutes, provided the reservoir bag is filling well and the vaporizer setting has been adjusted in accordance with the clinical needs of the animal, the fresh gas flow can be reduced to about 4 l/min, for while the inspired concentration of the volatile agent may become slightly less than set on the vaporizer the difference for all practical purposes is too small to be significant.

Later on in the course of the anaesthetic the fresh gas flow may be reduced still further (e.g. to 2–2.5 l/min) provided that the reservoir bag continues to fill well at the end of expiration and is not totally collapsed at the end of inspiration. There will now be an important difference between the likely inspired concentration of the volatile agent and the vaporizer setting. The reason for this is simply that the mass of volatile agent delivered to the circuit at this low flow rate is insufficient in the first few hours of the anaesthetic period to make up the net losses from the breathing system to the animal's tissues. A reliable approximate is that the inspired concentration of the volatile agent will be one-half to one-third of that set on the vaporizer. In the case of isoflurane, which is rather less soluble in the tissues than halothane, closer to one-half the vaporizer set concentration will be available as the inspired concentration for the animal. This 'rule of thumb' has been found to be reliable but in any particular case the inspired con-

centration to be aimed at is that which is judged to be appropriate to the clinical need of the animal and this will vary from animal to animal and in the same animal between different phases of the surgical procedure.

The conditions which make the fresh gas/inspired gas concentration differences when the fresh gas flow is low also dictate that an alteration in the inspired concentration in response to a change in vaporizer setting will be slower in becoming effective than is the case with high-flow systems. This disadvantage may be overcome in one of two ways — the vaporizer can be set to its highest setting if anaesthesia becomes inadequate or, alternatively, the fresh gas flow can be increased and the vaporizer setting adjusted as if a non-rebreathing system were in use. To achieve a rapid reduction in inspired concentration it is necessary to increase the fresh gas flow rate while turning the vaporizer off.

When nitrous oxide/oxygen mixtures are used as the carrier gas problems arise from the different rates at which nitrous oxide and oxygen will be consumed from the breathing system. The uptake of gases by the animal obeys the so-called square root of time law — i.e. the amount taken up is proportional to the square root of the elapsed time. At the start of an anaesthetic, nitrous oxide consumption by the tissues is much greater than that of oxygen but, after a variable period of time, it becomes less than that of oxygen, so that the great fear of many anaesthetists is that under these circumstances a state could be reached in a low-flow system in which nitrous oxide accumulation within the system would occur with a serious reduction in the oxygen concentration, leading to severe or fatal hypoxia. While there is no doubt that such a situation could arise during low-flow anaesthesia it is reassuring to note that:

1. If the fresh gas inflow is over 4 l/min, the difference between the proportions of oxygen to nitrous oxide in the fresh gas supply and the inspiratory limb of the circuit are likely to be so small as to be negligible.
2. For the vast majority of animals whose metabolic rate is normal it is quite safe to use a fresh gas flow comprising equal proportions of nitrous oxide and oxygen (e.g. 'Entonox') at flow rates above 4 l/min. To use smaller flows of fresh gases is probably unwise unless the oxygen concentration is increased or the concentration of oxygen in the inspired limb of the circuit is actually monitored.

Treatment of circulatory depression. Arterial hypotension is common in anaesthetized horses but is probably more marked and more often encountered during halothane or isoflurane anaesthesia. Circulatory support may be given in various ways. The simplest is to increase the circulating fluid volume to match the increased volume of the dilated vascular bed and so restore the venous return. This entails the intravenous infusion of 5–20 litres of fluid, depending on the size of the animal, as rapidly as possible immediately after the induction of anaesthesia. Gelatine solutions are expensive and may give rise to oedema so consequently, Hartmann's solution is the fluid most commony used. If this fluid loading fails to restore the arterial blood pressure to an acceptable level (usually taken to be a mean pressure of more than 65–70 mmHg), it must be assumed that hypotension is due to heart weakness and inotropic drugs may be used to improve the cardiac output. Calcium borogluconate, being readily available in veterinary practice, is a common choice. Up to 300 ml of a 40% w/v solution is given by slow intravenous infusion while the arterial blood pressure is carefully monitored. An alternative is the use of hypertonic saline (7.5%) infused intravenously up to a total volume of about 4 ml/kg [119]. Hypertonic saline is believed to enhance myocardial contractility and can be surprisingly effective in raising the arterial blood pressure.

Dopamine and dobutamine are two other agents used to treat hypotension in anaesthetized horses. Dopamine is a naturally occurring precursor of noradrenaline with a predominantly β_1-adrenoceptor agonist action but it also has α-adrenoceptor agonist activity. Dopamine increases cardiac output at doses of 5–10 μg/(kg min) but at these doses lowers total peripheral resistance [120]. Dobutamine is also a β_1-adrenoceptor agonist and a direct agonist of α_1 and β_2 adrenoceptors but it has no α_2-agonistic activity; intravenous infusions of 3μg/kg increase cardiac output without any appreciable effect on total peripheral resistance. Sinus tachycardia with atrioventricular conduction block occurs in some horses given these drugs and when they are infused the ECG should be monitored to avoid the development of potentially fatal cardiac arrhythmias from overdosage. Arrhythmias are more commonly seen in spontaneously breathing horses with hypercapnia and can be dangerous unless the P_aCO_2 is below 50 mmHg (6.6 kPa) because serious arrhythmias may appear suddenly when the P_aCO_2 is higher than this.

USE OF MUSCLE RELAXANTS

Apart from guaiphenesin, all the relaxant drugs used in horses exert their effects at the neuromuscular junction. Doses of guaiphenesin between 3 and 5 g/ 50 kg given to the anaesthetized horse will produce some relaxation of the abdominal muscles without interfering with respiratory activity but this is never as good as can be produced by the proper use of neuromuscular blocking drugs. Guaiphenesin may be useful in situations where inhalation anaesthesia cannot be used or the services of a trained anaesthetist are not available. This drug does, however, appear to have a negative inotropic effect [121] and if this results in arterial hypotension the most rational counter measure would appear to be the intravenous infusion of a positive inotrope such as dobutamine.

It must be very clearly understood that a neuromuscular blocking agent should never be administered unless facilities which enable immediate and sustained artificial respiration to be applied to the horse are available, and it is possible to be certain that the horse will be unconscious throughout the duration of their effect.

There is a wide variation among individuals in the response to a given dose of neuromuscular blocking agent and in the rate of recovery from blockade. For this reason no attempt should be made to administer them in fixed doses; they should always be given so as to produce just the desired effect. An incremental dosage regimen enables this to be done; about one-

half the anticipated full dose is given initially and further increments of half this initial dose are given at 3–5 minute intervals until the desired degree of relaxation is obtained. Only small doses are needed to suppress unwanted muscle movements during general anaesthesia but large doses will be required to produce the nearly complete blockade demanded by some surgical procedures. In every case the aim should be to use only a minimum dose and to ensure a complete recovery of neuromuscular function before the termination of anaesthesia. If unwanted muscle tone is returning towards the end of a surgical procedure it is usually wiser to restore relaxation by a slight deepening of anaesthesia rather than the administration of more relaxant drug. Clinical monitoring of neuromuscular block is facilitated by the use of a peripheral nerve stimulator (Chapter 7) but this apparatus is by no means essential for the proper use of relaxant drugs. When available it may be used on the facial or superficial peroneal nerves and the strength of contraction of the relevant muscles estimated by manual sensing at the muzzle or toe.

In general equine practice, myoneural block may be monitored by careful observation of the breathing and general muscular activity of the anaesthetized horse. Signs of partial blockade include brief, weak inspiratory movements, without holding of inspiration, and feeble, unsustained withdrawal responses to painful stimulation. One extremely simple objective test is measurement of airway pressure with a water manometer when the endotracheal tube is occluded before an inspiratory effort. No significant degree of myoneural block is present if the horse can generate a pressure in the upper airway below the site of occlusion of more than 25 cmH$_2$O (2.5 kPa) below atmospheric pressure. During anaesthetic recovery the horse is unable to stiffen the neck or hold up the head when attempting to sit in sternal recumbency, or it may make brief, weak attempts to stand followed by shaking of the limb muscles and collapse, if a degree of block is present.

Dosage and duration of action of neuromuscular blocking drugs

d-*Tubocurarine chloride*

In halothane-anaesthetized animals with end-tidal concentrations of halothane between 0.8 and 1.0%, doses of the order of 0.22–0.25 mg/kg d-tubocurarine chloride produce good relaxation with respiratory arrest. Unless complete relaxation is achieved horses are extremely difficult to ventilate adequately and the use of high airway pressures to expand the lungs may result in marked circulatory depression. The use of d-tubocurarine in horses suffering from asthma or alveolar emphysema may be associated with the production of bronchospasm, presumably due to histamine release.

It is seldom possible to restore adequate spontaneous breathing by the use of anticholinesterases in less than 35–40 minutes after d-tubocurarine has been given in doses which produce respiratory arrest. Limb movements are not seen during this period unless the depth of anaesthesia is allowed to become inadequate.

Gallamine triethiodide

In halothane-anaesthetized horses doses of gallamine triethiodide of 0.5–1.0 mg/kg produce complete paralysis with apnoea for some 15–20 minutes. Its use is associated with an increase in heart rate and rates below 50 beats/min are seldom seen in horses given this relaxant.

Pancuronium bromide

During light anaesthesia doses of 0.06 mg/kg produce complete relaxation with apnoea of about 20 minutes' duration [122], but it is more usual to give doses of 0.1 mg/kg to be certain of producing apnoea with complete relaxation of the respiratory muscles so that IPPV can be performed with the lowest-possible airway pressures [123]. The delay in achieving maximum effect after intravenous injection is much less

than that of d-tubocurarine chloride and no cases of relapse into neuromuscular block have been encountered after the use of neostigmine. The lack of histamine release makes this drug of value in cases where the administration of d-tubocurarine might be dangerous.

Alcuronium chloride

During light anaesthesia the dose required to produce complete relaxation with respiratory arrest is of the order of 0.1 mg/kg. Intravenous injection produces no change in heart rate, arterial blood pressure or central venous pressure. The return of spontaneous breathing is apparently followed by a prolonged period of partial paresis and reversal with an anticholinesterase is advisable in every case. If only one dose of alcuronium chloride has been given during the course of the operation, the block is readily reversed by neostigmine. However, when more than one dose of alcuronium has been administered, some difficulty has been experienced in antagonizing its effects. It is, therefore, probably advisable to limit its use to anaesthesia for operations which can be completed in 25–30 minutes of relaxation which follows the use of one dose of this drug.

Atracurium

The relatively short duration of action of activity and the lack of cumulative neuromuscular blocking effect make atracurium particularly suitable for use in horses in doses of 0.12–0.2 mg/kg [124, 125]. The authors recommend an initial dose of 0.1 mg/kg followed, if this does not produce the desired degree of relaxation as indicated by train-of-four stimulation, by doses of 0.01 mg/kg at 2 minute intervals until the block is judged to be adequate (reduction of initial twitch height). Edrophonium 0.5–1 mg/kg will antagonize any residual neuromuscular blocking effects at the end of the procedure for which it is given and the prior administration of atropine or glycopyrrolate is unnecessary provided the antagonist is injected slowly over more than 1 minute. Atracurium has also been given by continuous infusion at 0.17 mg/(kg h) after an initial bolus dose of 0.05 mg/kg [126]. Cardiovascular stability is good but there may be some slowing of the heart rate after an initial increase in arterial pressure in response to edrophonium.

Vecuronium

Doses of 0.1 mg/kg produce neuromuscular block of some 20–30 minutes duration in horses lightly anaesthetized with halothane. Although experience with this drug is limited it appears to be well suited for use in horses in that there is no evidence of histamine release and complete antagonism of block is readily obtained about 20 minutes after the attainment of full relaxation with depression of the first twitch height in train-of-four stimulation of the superficial peroneal nerve. There then is no evidence of muscle weakness in the anaesthetic recovery period.

Suxamethonium chloride

The use of suxamethonium for casting and restraint of horses is considered by the vast majority of veterinary anaesthetists to be an extremely inhumane practice. The development of safe and effective tranquillizers, sedatives and other agents has rendered the use of suxamethonium all but unnecessary for the restraint of horses and, in any case, the procedure is now known to be unsafe on pharmacological grounds.

Neal and Wright [127] drew attention to the tachycardia and cardiac arrhythmias encountered in horses submitted to casting with suxamethonium. Tavernor [128] confirmed their findings and reported two cases of cardiac arrest associated with the use of the drug. Larsen [129] reported two deaths in Australia due to rupture of the aorta after the administration of the drug and it seems likely that these resulted from the marked rise in blood pressure produced by suxamethonium in horses. Clearly, too, the rise in blood pressure is more likely to be dangerous if a horse has any parasitic lesions of the blood vessels. There is evidence that in horses, as in other animals, the injection of suxamethonium causes the release of adrenaline from the adrenal medulla and stimulation of postganglionic sympathetic nerves [130]. Since it is generally agreed that production of these effects by any agent can cause cardiac irregularities there is probably no need to postulate any direct effect on the horse's myocardium [131]. It has also been shown that one dose of the drug causes a rise of as much as 3 mmol/l in the serum potassium level [132] and an increase of this magnitude may well be sufficient to embarrass cardiac function or cause cardiac arrest.

In anaesthetized horses doses of 0.12–0.15 mg/kg usually cause paralysis of limb, head and neck muscles without producing diaphragmatic paralysis. In most horses double this dose will cause total paralysis but the exact effect produced in any individual animal will depend on the depth of anaesthesia at the time when the relaxant is administered. After a single dose paralysis lasts from 4 to 5 minutes although limb weakness may persist for several more minutes. In the presence of severe liver disease, cachexia or malnutrition an increased duration of action should be anticipated. Once paralysis is established it can be maintained by the constant infusion of about 2.2 mg/kg/h with uneventful recovery when the infusion is terminated.

Termination of neuromuscular block

There is no effective antidote to suxamethonium, but neostigmine is an efficient antidote to the non-depolarizing relaxants. In horses its use should be preceded by the intravenous injection of 10 mg atropine sulphate or, better, 5 mg glycopyrrolate, and it is then given in incremental doses up to a total dose of 10 mg. A period of 2–3 minutes should be allowed between increments and the effect of each carefully assessed before the next is given. Neostigmine should be given while IPPV is continued so that there is no danger of hypoxia or hypercapnia because if given to hypoxic or hypercapnic animals neostigmine may cause serious arrhythmias. As a general rule, the dose of neostigmine needed to restore full spontaneous breathing should be noted and a further dose of half this amount given to be completely sure of full antagonism of all the effects of the relaxant drug. Care must be taken not to confuse the weakness of respiratory activity due to deep inhalation anaesthesia, hypothermia or metabolic alkalosis from excessive bicarbonate administration, with that due to residual neuromuscular block.

Intermittent positive pressure ventilation (IPPV)

Careful thought is needed before IPPV is used in horses. Since blood gas measurements have become readily available during anaesthesia, many anaesthetists have thought it advisable to institute IPPV whenever the P_aCO_2 increases by about 15 mmHg (2 kPa). Often in these circumstances IPPV is commenced under inhalation anaesthesia without the use of muscle relaxants, the chest wall is stiff due to tone in the intercostal muscles and diaphragm so that compliance is low and high airway pressures are needed to expand the lungs. These high inspiratory pressures raise the mean intrathoracic pressure and can have a most deleterious effect on the circulation. Many anaesthetists have reported much lower arterial blood pressures during IPPV than during spontaneous ventilation but have erroneously attributed them to lowering of the P_aCO_2. A decline in P_aO_2 is frequently observed in anaesthetized horses when muscle tone is returning after the use of muscle relaxants and airway pressures are increased to maintain the respiratory tidal volume. In these cases restoration of the P_aO_2 requires nothing more than the administration of a further dose of the relaxant.

Normally, any increase in mean intrathoracic pressure is countered by peripheral venoconstriction which raises the peripheral venous pressure and restores the pressure gradient to the right atrium. This has the effect of increasing the venous return and hence the cardiac output. In hypovolaemic horses (e.g. many colic cases), and where the inhalation anaesthetic agents block the effect of sympathetic discharge, the peripheral venoconstriction may be inadequate to counter the rise in mean intrathoracic pressure due to IPPV so that venous return falls and the cardiac output declines. Diagnosis of hypovolaemia in horses is not always easy and even when correctly diagnosed there may be insufficient time for full replenishment of the blood volume by transfusion before anaesthesia has to be induced. For these reasons many anaesthetists claim that equine colic cases which may be hypovolaemic fare better if allowed to breathe spontaneously during anaesthesia even if their P_aCO_2 rises to around 60 mmHg (8 kPa). (In this connection it must be noted that there is no evidence that P_aCO_2 increase to these levels is harmful — indeed it may be beneficial by increasing tissue perfusion.) The picture is, however, not quite as simple as this for spontaneous ventilation must produce an adequate tidal volume and many horses with bowel obstruction only ventilate satisfactorily once the abdomen has been surgically decompressed. If there is any delay in this decompression it may be essential to institute IPPV as soon as anaesthesia is induced. IPPV is, of course, essential for thoracotomy or the repair of penetrating wounds of the chest.

Ideally, analysis of arterial blood samples drawn after about 20 minutes after the commencement of IPPV will enable adjustments to be made to the imposed tidal volume and/or rate of ventilation so that an adequate P_aO_2 is maintained with as near as possible normal P_aCO_2. Unfortunately, in many cases facilities for blood gas estimation are not readily available and the setting of the ventilator has to be made from simple clinical observation of the horse. Excursion of the chest wall should be somewhat greater than might be expected in the spontaneously breathing horse, the respiratory frequency should be between 8 and 12 breaths/min, the tidal volume about 10 ml/kg; the airway pressure should be kept as low as is consistent with adequate expansion of the chest wall and the inspiratory time should be between 2 and 3 seconds. Experience is often the only reliable guide to proper pulmonary ventilation in any individual horse. Whenever possible, the arterial blood pressure should be monitored so that any embarrassment of the circulation can be recognized before too much harm results from an unsuitable pattern of lung inflation.

Assisted ventilation, in which the horse triggers the ventilator which then delivers a prescribed tidal volume, cannot be recommended in equine anaesthesia. The horse determines the frequency and hence the minute volume of respiration, so under general anaesthesia alveolar hypoventilation and hypercapnia are to be expected.

ANAESTHETIC RECOVERY PERIOD

It is not always easy to decide whether a horse is likely to recover from anaesthesia smoothly and quietly or whether additional drugs will be required to ensure this. Probably the best course is to wait and see; if signs of excitement do appear it is a simple matter to give an intravenous dose of about 0.1 mg/kg of xylazine, particularly if an intravenous cannula introduced earlier in the anaesthetic is still in place. This dose of xylazine will nearly always ensure a quiet recovery without causing circulatory problems or undue prolongation of recumbency.

After surgery under field conditions a horse may be left to recover in a grassy field or on a thick straw bed; no attempt should be made to induce it to stand before it tries to do so of its own accord. In the field, some anaesthetists apply hobbles and physically restrain the horse for the first 20–30 minutes (which is when excitement is most likely to occur) before allowing it to attempt to stand up, but with the judicious use of the drugs which are available today, this is probably unnecessary. Under hospital conditions most horses are likely to be allowed to recover in a quiet, dimly lit, well-padded room to minimize the chance of serious injury resulting from excitement in the recovery period or staggering after standing up.

As surgery or examination under anaesthesia nears completion the level of anaesthesia should be lightened as much as possible, even to the point where spontaneous movements occur. Horses do not suddenly get up and walk away at the end of anaesthesia and in the majority of cases there is no reason why anaesthesia should be maintained at deep levels while the animal is transported to the recovery area. An animal which has been supine should be placed on its left side in the recovery area, but animals which have been lying on their sides probably should not be turned over to lie on the side which was uppermost during anaesthesia.

Endotracheal tubes which have been passed through the mouth should be removed as soon as the anaesthetic is terminated because the recovering animal may occlude the tube by biting on it. Respiratory obstruction caused in this way can be difficult to relieve and expensive tubes may be ruined. In addition, stimulation of the trachea by the tube has been associated with cardiac arrest, presumably through a vagal mechanism, as anaesthesia lightens. Following prolonged anaesthesia, respiratory obstruction is frequently observed after removal of the endotracheal tube. It is probably due to hypostatic congestion of the nasal and pharyngeal mucous membranes during anaesthesia and the horse makes a characteristic snoring noise. It may be relieved by passing a small-bore endotracheal tube through one nostril and this tube should be secured in place by a transfixing suture tied to the head collar or halter. Unless it is properly secured such a tube may be aspirated into the tracheobronchial tree.

It is probably advisable to administer oxygen to all horses recovering from general anaesthesia, but it is obligatory in critically ill animals. The oxygen should be given through a nasal endotracheal tube or a narrow-bore stomach tube passed into the trachea via the nostril. The endotracheal or stomach tube should be connected to a source of oxygen in such a manner that it will become disconnected if the horse moves or rolls during recovery. To produce any significant improvement of P_aO_2, oxygen must be administered into the trachea at a flow rate of at least 15 l/min.

In general, analgesics should not be given until the horse is standing because if given before this they may prolong recovery. However, doses of intramuscular pethidine of up to 0.5 g or intravenous flunixin (1 mg/kg), do not seem to add to recovery time and may be given at the end of anaesthesia to control pain during the recovery period. Moreover, local nerve blocks given at the end of surgery on the digits for postoperative analgesia do not seem to cause problems for the horse attempting to stand up. Unless catheterized, the bladder of male animals given fluid intravenously during operation may become distended and cause considerable abdominal pain. Catheterization of the bladder produces immediate relief of this pain. This problem does not occur in female animals because urine will seep from the bladder during anaesthesia.

ANAESTHESIA IN THE FIELD

Although horses are most safely anaesthetized under controlled hospital conditions, there are times when it is necessary to perform short operations, such as castration, in the field. As anaesthetic apparatus is unlikely to be available, although some practitioners still use chloroform, anaesthesia is usually both induced and maintained with intravenous agents. Every effort should be made to ensure that a supply of oxygen under pressure is at hand, however, for should respiratory arrest occur IPPV of the lungs can only be satisfactorily provided by the use of a stream of oxygen directed into the trachea for the Venturi effect or by a Hudson valve (see p. 206).

The aims of anaesthesia in the field are much the same as in a hospital — to provide a quiet induction, adequate anaesthetic conditions for surgery (including analgesia and relaxation), an adequate time for the procedure, followed by a quick, calm recovery with minimal ataxia when the animal regains the standing position. In the field it is particularly important that the drugs used do not cause respiratory depression, for under the circumstances prevailing it will be found that this is difficult to manage. Almost any drug or combination of intravenous agents already discussed may be used but as yet there is no perfect combination — hence the multiplicity of methods employed, the number of clinical trials found in the literature and the many literature reviews relating to the subject [133–137].

Chloroform

Chloroform has little place in routine equine anaesthesia but in the field there may be circumstances where its use is justified on grounds of economy. It is chiefly employed for the castration of colts or minor operations on wild, vicious or unbroken animals. Premedication with intramuscular acepromazine (0.3 mg/kg) is very desirable for its antiadrenergic effects. Anaesthesia is best carried out in a field where there is space for the animal to move about before it falls down. A strong, well-fitting head collar, which as a rope 2.4–3 m long attached to the D-piece on each side of the face, is applied to the horse. Each rope is held by one or more assistants who stand about 1.5 m from the horse and slightly behind its head. A Cox-type mask is usually employed and an initial dose of 30–60 ml of chloroform is poured onto the sponge which is then inserted into the mask, and very often the mask is adjusted so that the air intake is curtailed.

The first reaction of most horses is to shake the head in an effort to remove the mask and this is often followed by plunging or rearing. The animal may goose-step or stand with its fore-legs widely separated, swaying but refusing to move. Often it is impossible to get beyond this stage with a single dose. The animal is then either cast with ropes or, more commonly, a second dose is given. The front of the mask is opened and half the initial dose of chloroform is applied to the sponge. This generally provokes more movement and greater incoordination until finally the animal falls to the ground. An assistant must be ready to pull the animal's head to the ground and maintain it there otherwise vigorous attempts to rise with floundering may occur. From this point induction is completed by the further administration of small (5–10 ml) doses of chloroform, *allowing a free air supply*. The anaesthetist must aim at maintaining an even plane of anaesthesia and this is best performed by giving 5–10 ml doses of chloroform whenever anaesthesia shows signs of becoming lighter. On completion of the operation the mask is removed and the nostrils wiped clean. Anaesthesia is followed by hypnosis, the horse lying quietly in a state of sleep which lasts for about 20–30 minutes, and no attempt should be made to induce it to rise during this period. As soon as the horse feels able to do so it will get to its feet — usually in a sluggish manner. There may be considerable incoordination, particularly of the hind-limbs, but provided that the animal has not been made to get up before it was ready to do so, it will be able to maintain the standing position. Very occasionally anaesthesia is followed by a state of vigorous narcotic excitement and if all restraint has been removed the animal may sustain injury. Because of this occasional excitement it is probably wise to maintain control of the head and to continue restraint for 10 minutes after completion of the operation in every case. If no struggling occurs during this period, it may be taken as certain that recovery will be quiet.

Despite its crudeness the method gives fairly satisfactory results.

Table 11.4 Drug combinations useful for colt castration

Premedication	Induction	Maintenance (increments)
Acepromazine i.v. (0.02 mg/kg)	Thiopentone (11 mg/kg)	Thiopentone (1 mg/kg)
Xylazine i.v. (1 mg/kg)	Thiopentone (5.5 mg/kg)	Thiopentone (1 mg/kg)
Xylazine i.v. (1 mg/kg)	Methohexitone (2.5 mg/kg)	Methohexitone (0.5 mg/kg)
Detomidine i.v. (20 µg/kg)	Thiopentone (5.5 mg/kg)	Thiopentone (1 mg/kg)
Acepromazine i.v. (0.03 mg/kg)	Chloral hydrate 10% i.v. until ataxic then thiopentone (5.5 mg/kg)	Thiopentone (1 mg/kg)
Acepromazine i.v. (0.03 mg/kg)	Guaiphenesin until ataxic (about 50 mg/kg) then thiopentone (5 mg/kg)	Thiopentone (1 mg/kg) ± further guaiphenesin
Xylazine i.v. (1 mg/kg)	Ketamine i.v. (2 mg/kg)	Thiopentone (1 mg/kg) or xylazine (0.5 mg/kg) + ketamine (1 mg/kg)
Detomidine (20 µg/kg)	Ketamine (2 mg/kg)	Thiopentone (1 mg/kg) *or* ketamine i.v. (1 mg/kg)
Acepromazine i.v. (0.03–0.05 mg/kg)	Chloroform by mask	Chloroform by mask

Intravenous agents

Table 11.4 gives a summary of the drug combinations and their doses which the authors have found useful for colt castration. Most are based on barbiturates or ketamine.

Thiopentone may be used alone, but recovery tends to be violent. Premedication with acepromazine given an adequate time previously lengthens anaesthesia and recovery although more prolonged (about 40 minutes) tends to be quiet. However, if drugs are used which allow the dose of thiopentone to be reduced to 5–6 mg/kg recovery is even better. For example, following xylazine (1 mg/kg intravenously) or detomidine (20 µg/kg intravenously) the dose of thiopentone can be reduced to a bolus of 5.5 mg/kg 5 minutes later when the horse is well sedated. This usually produces good anaesthesia of approximately 15 minutes' duration and if anaesthesia is inadequate or requires extending a further dose of 1 mg/kg of thiopentone may be given. Occasionally this results in slight awakening before relaxation occurs and it is important to recognize this as such and to allow adequate time for the barbiturate to take full effect (often over 1 minute) before giving further doses as otherwise there is a danger of thiopentone overdose and respiratory arrest. If essential, further 1 mg/kg doses of thiopentone may be given to prolong anaesthesia (they are rarely necessary for a routine castration), but will delay recovery. In general, recovery from both regimes is usually quiet and calm, taking around 30 minutes after xylazine/thiopentone and 45 minutes after detomidine/thiopentone. Chloral hydrate or guaiphenesin may also be used to reduce the dose of thiopentone. Acepromazine premedication may be used in either case if required, and indeed is advised before guaiphenesin.

Chloral hydrate lost favour due to its irritant nature if injected outside the vein and to the fact that if used alone recovery is very slow. However, in combination with the barbiturates it gives good field anaesthesia. It should always be injected through a long intravenous catheter sutured in place to reduce the risk of perivascular injection. A 10% solution is infused until the horse becomes ataxic (after 50–60 mg/kg have been administered) when thiopentone (5 mg/kg) is injected intravenously as a bolus. Surgical anaesthesia may need to be maintained by injection of increments of thiopentone (1 mg/kg). The horse usually stands some 50–60 minutes after the end of the procedure but recovery is usually calm.

Methohexitone (at half the dose of thiopentone) is particularly satisfactory in combination with chloral hydrate but in the authors' experience thiopentone is preferable in other drug combinations.

Guaiphenesin (5–15%) may be infused instead of

chloral hydrate until the horse becomes ataxic; anaesthesia can then be induced with intravenous thiopentone (5 mg/kg). It is not advisable to exceed a dose of 50 mg/kg of guaiphenesin, as otherwise muscle weakness may still be present at a time when the animal attempts to stand.

Ketamine is best combined with the α_2-adrenoceptor agonists in order to reduce its convulsive effects. It is important that the horse is adequately sedated with xylazine (1 mg/kg intravenously) or detomidine (20 µg/kg intravenously) before the ketamine is injected intravenously in a bolus dose of 2 mg/kg. This will give 10–15 minutes of anaesthesia but with xylazine/ketamine combinations recovery can be disconcertingly sudden (particularly if surgery is not complete) but the horse usually regains its feet with minimal ataxia. The longer action of detomidine means that as the effects of ketamine wane the horse is still deeply sedated, thus making it easier to anticipate awakening and administer further drugs in good time. However, if the horse attempts to stand within 25 minutes of the detomidine injection ataxia may result in a violent recovery. With either ketamine combination anaesthesia can be lengthened with further doses of half the initial dose of ketamine (plus more xylazine where this sedative has been used) or with doses of 1 mg/kg of thiopentone, this latter method proving very satisfactory because the effects of ketamine and thiopentone appear synergistic and the barbiturate also improves muscle relaxation. These small doses of thiopentone do not cause respiratory depression and as long as the total dose of thiopentone given does not exceed 5 mg/kg recovery, although longer, is calm. Again, it is essential to allow adequate time for the thiopentone increment to be effective before giving a further dose.

Although xylazine/ketamine mixtures have been used with guaiphenesin, both for induction and by infusion to maintain anaesthesia, management of infusion techniques is not easy under field conditions.

REFERENCES

1. Wright, J. G. (1942) *Veterinary Anaesthesia.* London: Baillière, Tindall and Cox.
2. Amadon, R. S. and Craige, A. H. (1936) *Journal of the American Veterinary Association* **41**, 737.
3. Sweebe, E. E. (1936) *Veterinary Medicine* **31**, 158.
4. Clarke, K. W. and Hall, L. W. (1969) *Veterinary Record* **85**, 512.
5. Earl, A. F. (1976) *Journal of the American Veterinary Medical Association* **129**, 227.
6. Tobin, T. (1978) *Journal of Equine Medicine and Surgery* **2**, 433.
7. Ballard, S., Shults, T., Kownacki, A. A., Blake, J. W. and Tobin, T. (1982) *Journal of Veterinary Pharmacology and Therapeutics* **5**, 21.
8. Muir, W. W. and Hamlin, R. L. (1975) *American Journal of Veterinary Research* **36**, 1439.
9. Kerr, D. D., Jones, E. W., Holbert, M. S. and Higgins, K. (1972) *American Journal of Veterinary Research* **33**, 777.
10. Muir, W. W., Sams, R. A., Huffman, R. H. and Noonan, J. S. (1982) *American Journal of Veterinary Research* **43**, 1756.
11. Rehm, W. F. and Schatzmann, U. (1984) *Proceedings of the Association of Veterinary Anaesthetists* **4**, 93.
12. Tronicke, R. and Vocke, G. (1970) *Veterinary Medica Reviews (Leverkusen)*, p. 247.
13. Kerr, D. D., Jones, E. W., Huggins, K. and Edwards, W. C. (1972) *American Journal of Veterinary Research* **33**, 525.
14. Garner, H. E., Amend, J. F. and Rosborough, J. P. (1972) *Veterinary Medicine/Small Animal Clinician* **66**, 1016.
15. Pippi, N. I. and Lumb, W. V. (1979) *American Journal of Veterinary Research* **40**, 1082.
16. Lowe, J. E. (1978) *Journal of Equine Medicine and Surgery* **2**, 286.
17. Muir, W. W. (1981) *Equine Anesthesia, Veterinary Clinics of North America, Large Animal Practice*, pp. 34, 35.
18. McCashin, F. B. and Gabel, A. A. (1975) *American Journal of Veterinary Research* **36**, 1421.
19. Vainio, O. (1985) Academic Dissertation, Helsinki.
20. Muir, W. W., Skarda, R. T. and Sheenan, W. C. (1979) *American Journal of Veterinary Research* **40**, 1518.
21. Garner, H. E., Amend, J. F. and Rosborough, J. P. (1971) *Veterinary Medicine/Small Animal Clinician* **66**, 921.
22. Thurmon, J. C., Neff-Davis, C., Davis, L. E., Stoker, R. A., Benson, G. J. and Lock, T. F. (1982) *Journal of Veterinary Pharmacology and Therapeutics* **5**, 241.
23. Robertson, S. A., Carter, S. W., Donovan, M. and Steele, C. (1990) *Equine Veterinary Journal* **22**, 43.
24. Alitalo, I. and Vainio, O. (1982) *Proceedings of the Association of Veterinary Anaesthetists*, Suppl. 10, p. 222.
25. Ricketts, S. W. (1986) *Acta Veterinaria Scandinavia*, Suppl. 82, p. 197.
26. Clarke, K. W. and Taylor, P. M. (1986) *Equine Veterinary Journal,* **18**, 366.
27. Alitalo, I. (1986) *Acta Veterinaria Scandinavia*, Suppl. 82, p. 193.
28. Hamm, D. and Jochle, W. (1984) *Proceedings of the American Association of Equine Practitioners* **30**, 235.
29. Jochle, W. and Hamm, D. (1986) *Acta Veterinaria Scandinavia*, Suppl. 82, p. 69.
30. Jochle, W. (1989) *Equine Veterinary Journal*, Suppl. 7 (Equine colic), p. 117.
31. Jochle, W., Moore, J. N., Brown, J., Baker, G. J., Lowe, J. E., Furbin, S., Reeves, M. J., Watkins, J. P. and White, N. A. (1989) *Equine Veterinary Journal*, Suppl. 7 (Equine colic), p. 111.
32. Nilfors, L. and Kuart, C. (1986) *Acta Veterinaria Scandinavia*, Suppl. 82, p. 121.
33. Oijala, M. and Katica, T. (1988) *Equine Veterinary Journal* **20**, 327.

34. Short, C. E., Matthews, N., Tyner, C. L. and Harvey, R. (1984) *Proceedings of the American Association of Equine Practitioners* **30**, 243.
35. Katila, T. and Oijala, M. (1988) *Equine Veterinary Journal* **20**, 323.
36. Muir, W. W., Skarda, R. T. and Sheehan, W. (1978) *American Journal of Veterinary Research* **39**, 1632.
37. Tobin, T. (1978) *Journal of Equine Medicine and Surgery* **9**, 397.
38. Kalpravidh, M., Lumb, W. V., Wright, M. and Heath, R. B. (1984) *American Journal of Veterinary Research* **45**, 211.
39. Brunson, D. B., Majors, L. J. and Brown, C. E. (1985) *Proceedings of the 2nd International Congress of Veterinary Anaesthesia*, Sacremento, p. 158.
40. Combie, J. and Dougherty, J. (1979) *Journal of Equine Medicine and Surgery* **3**, 377.
41. Combie, J., Shults, T., Nugent, E. C., Dougherty, J. and Tobin, T. (1981) *American Journal of Veterinary Research* **42**, 716.
42. Schauffler, A. F. (1969) *Modern Veterinary Practice* **50**, 46.
43. Archer, R. K. (1947) *Veterinary Record* **59**, 401.
44. Alexander, F. and Collett, R. A. (1974) *Research in Veterinary Science* **17**, 136.
45. Clutton, R. E. (1987) *Equine Veterinary Journal* **119**, 72.
46. Kalpravidh, M., Lumb, M. V., Wright, M. and Heath, R. B. (1984) *American Journal of Veterinary Research* **45**, 217.
47. Robertson, J. T., Muir, W. W. and Sams, R. (1981) *American Journal of Veterinary Research* **42**, 41.
48. Paddleford, R. R. (1988) *Manual of Small Animal Anaesthesia*, pp. 13–30. New York: Churchill Livingstone.
49. Short, C. E. (1987) *Principles and Practice of Veterinary Anaesthesia*, p. 272. Baltimore: Williams and Wilkins.
50. Muir, W. W., Skarda, R. T. and Sheehan, W. C. (1979) *American Journal of Veterinary Research* **40**, 1518.
51. Martin, J. E. and Beck, J. D. (1956) *American Journal of Veterinary Research* **17**, 678.
52. Klein, L. V. (1975) *20th World Veterinary Congress*, Thessiloniki. Summaries, vol. 2, p. 739.
53. Muir, W. W., Skarda, R. T. and Sheehan, W. C. (1979) *American Journal of Veterinary Research* **40**, 1417.
54. Nolan, A. M. and Hall, L. W. (1984) *Veterinary Record* **114**, 63.
55. Robertson, J. T., Muir, W. W. (1983) *American Journal of Veterinary Research* **44**, 1667.
56. Clarke, K. W. and Paton, B. S. (1988) *Equine Veterinary Journal* **20**, 331.
57. Westhues, M. and Fristch, R. (1960) *Die Narkose der Tiere*, vol. 1, Lokalanasthesie. Berlin: Paul Darey (English edn (1964) Edinburgh: Oliver and Boyd).
58. Browne, T. G. (1938) *Veterinary Record* **50**, 1617.
59. Tufvesson, G. (1963) *Local Anaesthesia in Veterinary Medicine*, p. 44. Stockholm: Astra.
60. LeBlanc, P. H., Caron, J. P., Patterson, J. S., Brown, M. and Matta, M. A. (1988) *Journal of the American Veterinary Medical Association* **193**, 105.
61. Hall, L. W. (1984) *Equine Veterinary Journal* **16**, 89.
62. Rugh, K. S., Garner, H. E., Hatfiels, D. G. and Herrold, D. (1984) *Equine Veterinary Journal* **16**, 185.
63. Trim, C. M. and Mason, J. (1973) *Equine Veterinary Journal* **5**, 71.
64. Short, C. E. and White, K. (1978) *Proceedings of the American Association of Equine Practitioners* **24**, 107.
65. Lindsay, W. A., McDonell, W. N. and Bignell, W. (1978) *Proceedings of the American Association of Equine Practitioners* **24**, 115.
66. Lindsay, W. A., McDonell, W. N. and Bignell, W. (1980) *American Journal of Veterinary Research* **41**, 1919.
67. Lindsay, W. A., Pascoe, P. J., McDonell, W. N. and Burgess, M. I. F. (1985) *American Journal of Veterinary Research* **46**, 688.
68. Weaver, B. M. Q., Lunn, C. and Staddon, S. (1984) *Equine Veterinary Journal* **16**, 71.
69. Serteyn, D., Mottart, E., Michaux, C., Micheels, J., Philippart, C., Lavergne, L., Guillon, C. and Lamy, M. (1986) *Equine Veterinary Journal* **18**, 391.
70. Grandy, J. L., Steffey, E. P., Hodgson, D. S. and Woliner, M. J. (1987) *American Journal of Veterinary Research* **48**, 192.
71. Better, O. S. and Stein, J. H. (1989) *New England Journal of Medicine* **322**, 825.
72. Waldron-Mease, E. (1979) *Journal of Equine Medicine and Surgery* **3**, 124.
73. Eberley, V. E., Gillespie, J. R., Tyler, W. S. et al. (1968) *American Journal of Veterinary Research* **29**, 305.
74. Hall, L. W., Gillespie, J. R. and Tyler, W. S. (1968) *British Journal of Anaesthesia* **40**, 560.
75. Steffey, E. P. and Howland, D. (1978) *American Journal of Veterinary Research* **39**, 611.
76. Steffey, E. P., Kelly, A. B. and Woliner, M. J. (1987) *American Journal of Veterinary Research* **48**, 952.
77. Dunlop, C. I., Steffey, E. P., Miller, M. F. and Woliner, M. J. (1987) *American Journal of Veterinary Research* **48**, 1250.
78. Steffey, E. P., Dunlop, C. I., Farver, T. B., Woliner, M. J. and Schultz, L. J. (1987) *American Journal of Veterinary Research* **48**, 7.
79. Muir, W. W., Skarda, R. T. and Sheehan, W. (1978) *American Journal of Veterinary Research* **39**, 1274.
80. Hall, L. W. (1968) *Proceedings of the 8th Congress, European Society of Veterinary Surgery*, Bologna, p. 79.
81. Schatzmann, U., Koeli, N., Dundan, F., Rhor, W. and Jones, R. S. (1982) *American Journal of Veterinary Research* **43**, 1003.
82. Tyagi, R. P. S., Arnold, J. P., Usenik, E. A. and Fletchers, T. F. (1964) *Cornell Veterinarian* **54**, 584.
83. Tavernor, W. D. (1970) *Research in Veterinary Science* **11**, 92.
84. Mitchell, B. and Littlejohn, A. (1972) *Proceedings of the Association of Anaesthetists of Great Britain and Ireland*, p. 61.
85. Steffey, E. P., Wheat, J. D., Meagher, D. M., Noris, R. D., McKee, J., Brown, M. and Arnold, J. (1977) *American Journal of Veterinary Research* **38**, 379.
86. Gillespie, J. R., Tyler, W. S. and Hall, L. W. (1969) *American Journal of Veterinary Research* **30**, 61.
87. Mason, D. E., Muir, W. W. and Wade, A. (1978) *Journal of the American Veterinary Medical Association* **190**, 190.
88. DeMoor, A., Desmet, P. and Verschooten, F. (1974) *Zentralblat Veterinaermedicin* **21**, 525.
89. Reibold, T. W., Evans, A. T. and Robinson, N. E. (1980) *Journal of the American Veterinary Medical Association* **176**, 623.
90. Watney, G. C. G., Watkins, S. B. and Hall, L. W. (1985) *Veterinary Record* **117**, 358.
91. Stolk, P. W. (1982) *Proceedings of the Association of Veterinary Anaesthetists of Great Britain and Ireland*, Supplement, p. 119.
92. McDonell, W. N., Hall, L. W. and Jeffcott, L. B. (1979) *Equine Veterinary Journal* **11**, 24.

93. Hall, L. W. (1971) *Equine Veterinary Journal* **3**, 95.
94. McDonell, W. N. (1974) Ph.D. Thesis, University of Cambridge, England.
95. Tyler, W. S., Gillespie, J. R. and Nowell, J. (1971) *Equine Veterinary Journal* **3**, 84.
96. Robinson, N. E. and Sorensen, R. P. (1978) *Journal of Applied Physiology* **44**, 63.
97. Watney, G. C. G., Jordan, C. and Hall, L. W. (1987) *British Journal of Anaesthesia* **59**, 1022.
98. Hall, L. W. (1979) *Equine Veterinary Journal* **11**, 71.
99. Hall, L. W., Senior, J. E. B. and Walker, R. G. (1968) *Research in Veterinary Science* **9**, 487.
100. Stolk, P. W. (1979) Ph.D. Thesis, University of Cambridge, England.
101. Hall, L. W. and Trim, C. M. (1975) *British Journal of Anaesthesia* **47**, 819.
102. Beadle, R. E., Robinson, N. E. and Sorensen, P. R. (1975) *American Journal of Veterinary Research* **36**, 1435.
103. Thurmon, J. C. (1988) *Advances in Veterinary Anaesthesia*, p. 8.
104. Jones, R. S., Lawrence, T. J. L., Veevers, A., Cleave, N. and Hall, J. (1989) *Veterinary Record* **125**, 549.
105. Hubbell, J. A. E., Bednarski, R. M. and Muir, W. W. (1989) *American Journal of Veterinary Research* **501**, 737.
106. Webb, A. I. (1984) *Journal of the American Veterinary Medical Association* **185**, 48.
107. Short, C. E. (1981) *Veterinary Clinics of North America* **3**, 204.
108. Green, S. A., Thurmon, J. C., Tranquilli, W. J. and Benson, G. J. (1986) *American Journal of Veterinary Research* **47**, 2364.
109. Hall, L. W. (1957) *Veterinary Record* **69**, 615.
110. Schatzmann, U. (1982) *Proceedings of the 1st International Congress of Veterinary Anaesthesia*, Cambridge, p. 112.
111. Muir, W. W. (1985) *American Association of Equine Practitioners* **30**, 117.
112. Steffey, E. P., Howland, D., Giri, S. and Eger, E. I. (1977) *American Journal of Veterinary Research* **38**, 1037.
113. Taylor, P. M. and Hall, L. W. (1985) *Equine Veterinary Journal* **17**, 51.
114. Steffey, E. P. (1978) *Journal of the American Veterinary Medical Association* **172**, 367.
115. Auer, J. A., Garner, H. E., Amand, J. F., Hutcheson, D. P. and Salem, C. A. (1978) *Equine Veterinary Journal* **10**, 18.
116. Steffey, E. P. and Howland, D. (1980) *American Journal of Veterinary Research* **41**, 821.
117. Steffey, E. P., Dunlop, C. I., Farver, T. B., Woliner, M. J. and Schultz, L. J. (1987) *American Journal of Veterinary Research* **48**, 7.
118. Spence, A. A. (1986) *Lectures in Anaesthesiology* (ed. J. S. M. Zorab). Oxford: Blackwell Scientific.
119. Dyson, D. H. and Pascoe, P. J. (1990) *American Journal of Veterinary Research* **51**, 17.
120. Swanson, C. R., Muir, W. W., Bednarski, R. M., Skarda, R. T. and Hubbell, J. A. E. (1985) *American Journal of Veterinary Research* **46**, 365.
121. Pascoe, P. J., McDonell, W. N. and Fox, A. E. (1985) *Proceedings of the 2nd International Congress of Veterinary Anaesthesia*, Sacramento, p. 61.
122. Massey, G. M. (1970) Personal communication.
123. Hildebrand, S. V. and Howitt, G. A. (1984) *American Journal of Veterinary Research* **45**, 2441.
124. Hildebrand, S. V., Howitt, G. A. and Arpin, D. (1986) *American Journal of Veterinary Research* **47**, 1096.
125. Hildebrand, S. V., Holland, M., Copland, V. S., Daunt, D. and Brock, N. (1989) *Journal of the American Veterinary Medical Association* **195**, 212.
126. Hildebrand, S. V. and Hill, T. (1989) *American Journal of Veterinary Research* **50**, 2124.
127. Neal, P. A. and Wright, J. G. (1959) *Veterinary Record* **71**, 731.
128. Tavernor, W. D. (1959) *Veterinary Record* **71**, 774.
129. Larsen, L. H. (1958) *New Zealand Veterinary Journal* **6**, 61.
130. Stevenson, D. E. and Hall, L. W. (1959) *Veterinary Record* **71**, 818.
131. Hansson, C. H. (1958) *Nordisk Veterinrmedicin* **10**, 201.
132. Stevenson, D. E. (1960) *British Journal of Anaesthesia* **32**, 364.
133. Brouwer, G. J., Hall, L. W. and Kuchel, T. T. (1980) *Veterinary Record* **107**, 241.
134. Taylor, P. M. (1983) *In Practice* **5**, 112.
135. Clarke, K. W., Taylor, P. M. and Watkins, S. B. (1986) *Acta Veterinaria Scandinavia*, Suppl. 82, p. 167.
136. Watkins, S. B., Watney, G. C. G., Hall, L. W. and Houlton, J. E. F. (1987) *Veterinary Record* **120**, 273.
137. Thurmon, J. C. (1988) *Proceedings of the Association of American Equine Practitioners*, p. 529.

CHAPTER 12

ANAESTHESIA OF THE OX

Cattle are by no means good subjects for any form of general anaesthesia and today the problems involved in the use of general anaesthesia in these animals are well known. Most of them are associated with the danger of regurgitation and inhalation of the contents of the rumen, or the inhalation of saliva. Once a ruminant animal is in lateral or dorsal recumbency, the oesophageal opening is submerged in ruminal content, normal eructation cannot occur, and gas accumulates. The degree of bloat depends on the amount of fermentation of the ingesta and on the length of time that gas is allowed to accumulate. Gross distension of the rumen thus becomes a hazard which may be met if anaesthesia is prolonged. In addition, increased intraruminal pressure may give rise to regurgitation if the tone of the oesophageal sphincter mechanism is inadequate. Furthermore, when the animal is recumbent, the weight of the abdominal viscera and their contents prevents the diaphragm from moving freely on inspiration and respiration tends to become shallow, rapid and in-efficient for the purpose of gaseous exchange in the lungs.

The inhalation agents are, in general, safer in cattle than the intravenous drugs, for their elimination from the body is more rapid and recovery of the righting, swallowing, coughing and eructation reflexes after anaesthesia is, consequently, also more rapid. Experience has shown that provided certain precautions are taken, and that due care is exercised, adult cattle can be subjected, quite safely, to periods of at least 2 hours of inhalation anaesthesia.

The danger of regurgitation and inhalation of ingesta is always present but the likelihood of it occurring can be minimized by:

1. Withholding water for at least 6 hours before anaesthesia.
2. Withholding green foodstuffs and other easily fermentable food for at least 24 hours before anaesthesia.
3. When the animal is to be in lateral recumbency during anaesthesia arranging that the occiput is above the general body level and that the head

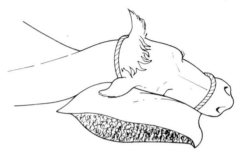

Fig. 12.1 Cow's head inclined over a support to allow saliva to drain out of the mouth.

slopes so that saliva and any regurgitated material runs freely from the mouth (Fig. 12.1).

Regurgitation occurs during both light and deep anaesthesia so that it is probable that two mechanisms are involved in the process. It would appear that during light anaesthesia ingesta may pass up the oesophagus into the pharynx as a result of an active, but uncontrolled, reflex mechanism. It is then a matter of chance whether or not the protective reflexes, e.g. laryngeal closure, coughing, etc., are active, and can or cannot prevent aspiration. The order in which the reflexes of laryngeal closure, coughing, swallowing and regurgitation disappear as anaesthesia is deepened may well differ from one anaesthetic agent to another but the relative safety of the various agents in this respect cannot, at the present moment, be assessed. During deep anaes-thesia, on the other hand, regurgitation is a passive process. The striated muscle of the oesophagus loses its tone and any increase in the intraruminal pressure — whether from pressure on the abdominal wall or from fermentation in the rumen itself — may force ingesta up into the pharynx. The protective reflexes are not active and aspiration occurs all too easily. It has been suggested that for complete safety the following procedure may be adopted to prevent regurgitation and aspiration regardless of the method of general anaesthesia employed.

A narrow-bore stomach tube which has a rubber balloon vulcanized on to its tip so that air blown down the tube inflates the balloon, is passed through one nostril down to the stomach in the fully conscious animal immediately before anaesthesia is induced. The balloon is inflated and the tube withdrawn until the inflated balloon engages in the cardia; it is maintained inflated in this position while anaesthesia is induced. As soon as the animal is anaesthetized it is intubated with a cuffed endotracheal tube, the balloon on the stomach tube is deflated and the stomach tube withdrawn.

Although this procedure may prevent regurgitation during light anaesthesia and overcomes the risk of aspiration during deep anaesthesia there are several reasons why it is not often employed. First, it necessitates the use of oesophageal blockers which are not readily available. Secondly, it is often impossible to maintain the balloon in position at the cardia while anaesthesia is induced. Some anaesthetists attempt to overcome this difficulty by simply inflating the balloon in the oesophagus and making no effort to block the cardia. However, when the balloon in the oesophagus is inflated to a degree sufficient to block the passage of ingesta many animals show the signs of marked discomfort seen in cases of acute oesophageal obstruction. Furthermore, it is perhaps simpler in every case to dispense with the use of the oesophageal blocker. Should regurgitation occur during the induction of anaesthesia after the protective reflexes have been subdued but before endotracheal intubation has been performed, the endotracheal tube may be immediately passed into the oesophagus and its cuff inflated so that the regurgitated material passes down the tube. Aspiration is then impossible and the trachea can be intubated with a second tube.

During general anaesthesia salivation also presents a problem in cattle for the copious flow does not cease when the animal is anaesthetized. Antisialagogues are not of much use for they make the secretion more viscid in nature and do not significantly reduce its production. Obstruction of the airway by large quantities of saliva is not uncommon in anaesthetized ruminant animals. It is important to arrange the head of the anaesthetized animal so that saliva drains from the mouth and does not accumulate in the pharynx. Once again, intubation with a cuffed endotracheal tube is the only certain way of preventing the inhalation of saliva. Long-term loss of saliva may lead to an acidosis but this is unlikely to be a major problem in most anaesthetics.

The restriction of diaphragmatic movement by the heavy abdominal contents may have serious consequences if anaesthesia is prolonged. The anaesthetized ruminant animal should, whenever possible, be placed on an incline so that the viscera fall away from the diaphragm.

The respiratory difficulties of cattle under general anaesthesia can be difficult to alleviate. Oxygen enrichment of inspired gases is always needed and often IPPV may be required to prevent arterial hypoxaemia. Under nitrous oxide/halothane anaesthesia with inspired oxygen concentrations of 50%, spontaneously breathing adult animals have respiratory minute volumes of 0.06 (SD 0.03) 1/min/kg, with frequencies of 38 (SD 10) breaths/min. P_aCO_2s range from 55 to 60 mmHg (7.3–8 kPa) and P_aO_2s from about 120–220 mmHg (16–29.3 kPa). Similar anaesthesia with IPPV to maintain the P_aCO_2 at 35–40 mmHg (4.6–5.3 kPa) after the administration of 0.08 mg/kg alcuronium involves the use of maximum airway pressures of 12–25 mmHg (1.6–3.3 kPa) and has little effect on the P_aO_2 [1].

One feature worthy of note is that under general anaesthesia tissue perfusion is probably much better than it is in horses because arterial blood pressures are much higher. In cattle under halothane anaesthesia arterial systolic pressure is usually between 150 and 250 mmHg and the diastolic pressure between 110 and 135 mmHg. The reason for these high pressures is, as yet, unknown, but the authors agree with Schatzman and his colleagues [1] that they cannot be attributed to hypoxia or hypercapnia.

When all is considered, it is not surprising that the vast majority of bovine clinical surgery is carried out under local analgesia, whenever possible in the standing subject. Its performance is made easier by the use of appropriate sedation and/or restraining 'crushes' or 'chutes'. The design of cattle 'crushes' so that they do not interfere with surgical approaches is not easy and its discussion is outside of the scope of this volume. Because of the difficulty of obtaining satisfactory 'crushes' many surgeons prefer to work on heavily sedated, recumbent animals, but it is always desirable, if surgical considerations permit, to keep such animals in the sternal position during operation and this may not be easy. If the animal is to remain standing throughout an operation, sedation needs to be chosen with care — aseptic surgery is impossible if the animal lies down during the course of the procedure.

SEDATION OF CATTLE

Chloral hydrate

Although some of the more recently introduced agents such as the α_2-adrenoceptor agonist xylazine may have some advantages, chloral hydrate is still a perfectly acceptable, inexpensive sedative for adult cattle. It may be given by mouth or intravenous injection. To obtain a recumbent, very lightly unconscious adult cow, the drug is usually administered by drench, or preferably by stomach tube, in doses of 30–60 g as a 1 in 20 solution in water. Sedation attains its maximum depth in a period of 10–20 minutes and local analgesics may be injected while sedation is developing. As cows can generally be cast and restrained without difficulty, intravenous administration will generally be in this position with the head and neck extended. The external jugular vein can be readily distended by finger pressure and the use of choke cords is unnecessarily distressful for the animal. The dose required is between 80 and 90 mg/kg of a 10% solution and it should be remembered that narcosis will continue to deepen after the intravenous injection is completed. The induction and recovery periods are excitement free.

Young bulls present no particular difficulties provided their temperament is such that they can be effectively restrained for safe drenching or precise intravenous injection. In older bulls the precise intravenous injection of drugs in the standing position may not only be uncertain on account of difficulties in satisfactorily introducing the needle into the vein but sometimes impossible because of movement by the animal.

In many instances the temperament of the bull to be dealt with is such that large doses of chloral hydrate have to be given by the mouth in order to obtain sufficient sedation to allow of the application of casting tackle. The further administration of the drug by intravenous injection after casting gives rise to a danger of fatal overdosage consequent on continued absorption from the stomach. When, without any previous medication, chloral hydrate is given to a bull by intravenous injection at the usual rate, the dose required to induce deep narcosis is the same as for the big cow — about 90–100 mg/kg. When the drug is given by the mouth a dose of 140–200 g (or even more) may be required to induce a degree of sedation whereby the animal may be handled and even after such a quantity the animal may still be able to stand.

The bull which is running free in the yard or a loose-box may be quite dangerous even to approach. In such cases it is advised that drinking water be withheld for 36 hours and that the animal then be offered water containing 90–120 g of chloral hydrate in 12 litres. It is generally taken and the degree of sedation is such that, with care, it can be approached and a leading pole applied.

Xylazine

Because they are so much more convenient to administer the α_2-adrenoceptor agonists have, in the UK almost completely replaced chloral hydrate for the sedation of cattle. The intramuscular injection of 0.05–0.2 mg/kg of xylazine is sufficient to produce deep sedation in most animals and they lie down within 10–20 minutes after the injection. Using xylazine, deep sedation last 30–35 minutes and recovery occurs gradually over the next 7 or more hours. Intravenous injection of these doses produces much more profound sedation which closely resembles deep narcosis induced with chloral hydrate. In cattle, as in all other animals, this agent produces a rise in blood sugar. It is contraindicated in the last trimester of pregnancy as it has a marked ecbolic action; premature birth has been reported after the administration of xylazine to heavily pregnant cows. Although the ability to eructate, cough and swallow is retained during the period of sedation, cattle must be closely watched during the recovery period. It has been found that some animals will get to their feet, walk around and appear fully conscious, then relapse into lateral recumbency and become tympanitic. These recumbent animals must be disturbed so as to provoke eructation. Fortunately, this danger period is of limited duration.

Hepatic glucose production and plasma glucose increase after xylazine administration [2–4]. Although hyperglycaemia contributes to the marked diuresis in the first 2–3 hours after xylazine has been given, most of this diuretic effect is due to suppression of anti-diuretic hormone (ADH) release.

Some reports indicate that xylazine produces analgesia in cattle, and surgical operations have been performed under the sedation produced by this compound on its own. Others have reported an absence of demonstrable analgesia, and have stated that for surgery supplementation with a general anaesthetic or the use of local analgesia was essential to prevent movement in response to painful stimulation. The authors consier that local analgesia is always needed to supplement any analgesic effect of the α_2-adrenoceptor agonist unless it is proposed to proceed to full general anaesthesia with other agents.

Detomidine

Detomidine has not replaced the use of xylazine in cattle, as the doses required are similar to or greater than those for horses, thus making detomidine comparatively more expensive for use in cattle. Doses of 30–150 µg/kg by intramuscular injection were originally recommended from experimental trials, but clinical trials [5] resulted in a recommendation of doses of 30–60 µg/kg, the duration of effect being dose dependent and recovery to normality prolonged. In the authors' experience intravenous doses of 10 µg/kg result in sedation similar to that produced in horses by this dose. The head is lowered and there is marked ataxia but the animal remains standing and sedation is ideal for surgery under local analgesia.

The side-effects of detomidine in cattle are very similar to those of xylazine (bradycardia, hyperglycaemia, salivation and increased urination) but with two major exceptions. Detomidine causes arterial hypertension, which is dose dependent in duration [5] and, more importantly, low doses appear to have negligible effects on the uterus. It has been concluded that detomidine given intravenously to pregnant cows in doses of 20 µg/kg should be safe [6] although the widespread trials needed to confirm this conclusion have not yet been carried out. However, there would seem to be no doubt that the use of detomidine at doses of 20 µg/kg should be preferable to the use of xylazine in heavily pregnant cows.

Medetomidine

In cattle medetomidine is more hypnotic than either xylazine or detomidine. Deep sedation without recumbency is obtained with intravenous doses of 5 µg/kg while 10 µg/kg produces recumbency and sedation equivalent to that obtained with intravenous doses of 0.1–0.2 mg/kg of xylazine (G. C. W. England and K. W. Clarke, unpublished observations). However, the current pricing structure makes it unlikely that medetomidine will be widely used in the larger species of animal, although it may have an application in calves.

Antagonists to the α_2-adrenoceptor agonists

As prolonged recumbency causes so many problems in cattle, the availability of α_2-adrenoceptor antagonists is of particular value. These antagonists not only cause the animal to awaken — they also antagonize the majority of the side-effects of the agonists, including restoring ruminal motility to normal.

Almost all the α_2-adrenoceptor antagonists have been used in cattle sedated with xylazine. Yohimbine (0.125 mg/kg) with aminopyridine (0.3 mg/kg) will awaken cattle sedated with 0.2–0.3 mg/kg of xylazine, but will not restore a normal state of consciousness [7]. Tolozoline at 0.2 mg/kg reverses the suppression of ruminal motility induced by xylazine [8] but higher doses are required for full reversal of sedation. Idazoxan at doses of 0.01–0.1 mg/kg is reported to be particularly effective against xylazine in calves, with no relapse to sedation [9] although it is not clear for how long the calves were observed. Atipamezole in doses of 25 and 50 µg/kg, intravenously or intramuscularly, causes awakening in cows sedated with 0.2 mg/kg of xylazine, with restoration of ruminal motility to normal, but 2 hours later some relapse occurs (A. Mayne, personal communication) although resedation is never so deep as to cause recumbency. Relapse does not occur after intramuscular injection of the antagonist and Mayne has suggested that atipamezole should be given in a dose of 25 µg/kg by both the intravenous and intramuscular routes.

Mayne, England and Clarke also found atipamezole effective against medetomidine when given in similar dose ratios to those used in dogs, i.e. atipamezole dose five times the medetomidine dose. They warned that 25 µg/kg of atipamezole given to unsedated cattle, or as medetomidine sedation is waning, can induce a state of hyperactivity, unrestrained cows galloping around the field, kicking and bucking, yet remaining thoroughly aware of their surroundings and apparently in full self control. (Unlike the opioid excitement reaction.)

Acepromazine

Cattle should not be given acepromazine (or propiopromazine) if a general anaesthetic is to be administered, for it will increase the risk of regurgitation of ruminal contents at the time of induction, and cause a most inconvenient delayed recovery. Acepromazine may be given in doses of 0.1 mg/kg by intramuscular injection about 1 hour before the injection of local analgesics; these doses should not be exceeded if the operation is to be performed on the standing animal.

Pentobarbitone sodium

Toosey [10] used a 20% solution of pentobarbitone injected slowly intravenously for the restraint of nervous or excitable cattle. To make the animal sway slightly on its hind-legs while being able to walk unaided, a dose of between 1 and 2 g is needed for the adult cow. A dose of about 3 g/500 kg usually makes an adult cow recumbent and almost unconscious.

Small doses (15–20 ml of the 6.5% solution, i.e. 1–1.25 g) may be given to prolong basal narcosis which has been induced with chloral hydrate. It is injected intravenously as soon as the chloral hydrate depression becomes inadequate and provided the injection is made slowly and to effect, no harmful effects occur. The period of recumbency is much less than if additional doses of chloral hydrate are administered and recovery is not associated with struggling and excitement. More than one injection of pentobarbitone may be given during the course of long operations.

LOCAL ANALGESIA

Any technique of local infiltration may be used in cattle. Although nerve blocks are simple to perform, many flank laparotomies are still carried out using clumsy, time-consuming and often inefficient L- or T-block infiltration of the abdominal wall (p. 180).

Cornual nerve block

This method was first developed by Emmerson in the USA, and was introduced to British veterinarians by Browne of Dublin [11].

The horn corium and the skin around its base derive their sensory nerve supply from a branch of the ophthalmic division of the fifth cranial nerve. The nerve emerges from the orbit and ascends just behind the lateral ridge of the frontal bone. This latter structure can be readily palpated with the fingers. In the upper third of the ridge the nerve is relatively superficial, being covered only by skin and a thin layer of the frontalis muscle.

The site for injection is the upper third of the temporal ridge, about 2.5 cm below the base of the horn. The needle (19 gauge, 2.5 cm long) is inserted so that its point lies 0.7–1 cm deep, immediately behind the ridge, and 5 ml of local analgesic solution injected. The needle must not be inserted too deeply,

otherwise injection will be made beneath the aponeurosis of the temporal muscle and the method will fail. In large animals with well-developed horns, a second injection should be made about 1 cm behind the first block the posterior division of the nerve (Fig. 12.2). Loss of sensation develops in 10–15 minutes and lasts about 1 hour. This form of nerve block has been widely used for the dishorning of adult cattle but under conditions of practice, it is not invariably successful. Variability in the curvature of the lateral ridge of the frontal bone makes exact determination of the site of the nerve difficult, while in a struggling animal it may be difficult to ensure that the point of the needle is at the correct depth. A third injection may be required in adult cattle with well-developed horns; it is made posterior to the horn base to block cutaneous branches of the second cervical nerve.

Lignocaine hydrochloride, on account of its great power of diffusion in the tissues, has come to be widely used for dishorning, generally as a 2% solution.

Auriculopalpebral nerve block

The nerve supplies motor fibres to the orbicularis oculi muscle. It runs from the base of the ear along the facial crest, past and ventral to the eye, giving off its branches on the way.

The needle is inserted in front of the base of the ear at the end of the zygomatic arch and is introduced until its point lies at the dorsal border of the arch.

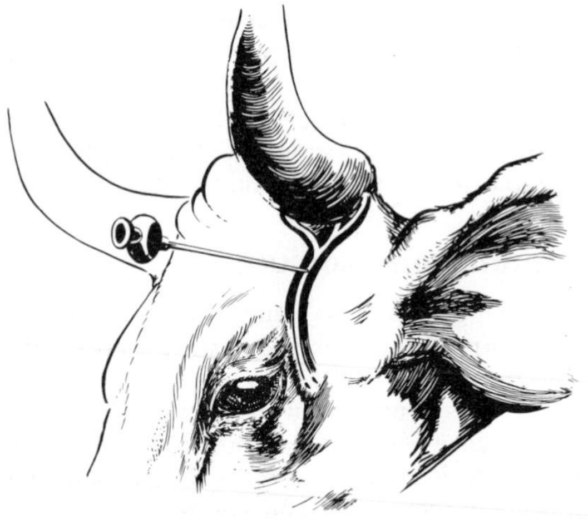

Fig. 12.2 Injection of the nerve to the horn core. In some animals the branch to the caudal part leaves the parent trunk cranial to the normal site for injection.

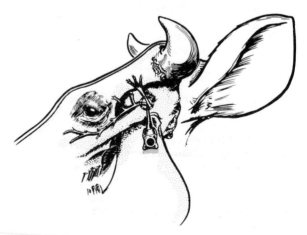

Fig. 12.3 Auriculopalpebral nerve block.

About 10–15 ml of analgesic solution is injected beneath the fascia at this point (Fig. 12.3).

This block is used to prevent eyelid closure during examination of, or interferences on, the eyeball. It does not produce analgesia of the eye or the lids. In conjunction with topical analgesia it is useful for the removal of foreign bodies from the cornea and conjunctival sac.

Retrobulbar block

To block the nerves behind the eyeball a needle is introduced about 2.5 cm lateral to the medial canthus of the eye and pushed along the floor of the orbit until it penetrates the tough periorbita, 20–30 ml of 2% lignocaine solution (or its equivalent) being injected in small increments as the needle is advanced and the bulk of the injection is made beneath the periorbita. Proper deposition of the local analgesic solution produces corneal analgesia, mydriasis and proptosis of the eyeball. The nerves to the ocular muscles are blocked so that paralysis of the eyeball follows.

Peterson [12] described a different technique. A 2.5 cm, 22 gauge needle is used to infiltrate subcutaneously, with about 5 ml of 2% lignocaine solution, the notch formed by the supraorbital process cranially, the zygomatic arch ventrally and the coronoid process of the mandible caudally. A 2.5 cm, 12 or 14 gauge needle placed as far anterior and ventral as possible in the desensitized skin of the notch serves as a cannula and a 10 or 12 cm, 18 gauge needle is introduced through this. The long needle is directed in a horizontal and caudal direction until it strikes the coronoid process of the mandible. It is then redirected towards the pterygopalatine fossa rostral to the orbitorotundum foramen at a depth of about 8–10 cm from the skin and 10–15 ml of 2% lignocaine solution is injected. This blocks the oculomotor, trochlear, abducens and the three branches of the trigeminal nerves as they emerge from the foramen orbitorotundum. The needle is withdrawn to the subcutaneous tissue and redirected caudally and laterally to block the auriculopalpebral nerve on the zygomatic ridge by the injection of another 5–10 ml of the local analgesic solution. The Peterson technique obviously requires more skill to perform than a simple retrobulbar block but is probably safer.

Adverse effects of both the Peterson and retrobulbar blocks result from penetration of blood vessels to produce orbital haemorrhage, direct pressure on the eyeball, damage to the optic nerve and injection of the optic nerve meninges, but clearly most are unimportant when the blocks are used for enucleation. When the block is used for other purposes care must be taken to ensure that the corneal surface does not become dry because of loss of tear formation for several hours.

Digital nerve blocks

The nerve supply of the digits of the ox is much more complex than in the horse and regional analgesia is more difficult to produce. The skin below the carpus and tarsus is tense and the subcutaneous tissue is very fibrous, so that precise location of nerves is not easy. Many workers consider that simple ring block, in which a transverse plane through the whole extremity is infiltrated, is the most reliable way of producing regional analgesia of the digit. However, block of the individual nerves is more elegant.

An excellent description of the course of the nerves in the fore- and hind-limbs has been given by Taylor [13]:

Nerves of the fore foot

The dorsal metacarpal nerve is the continuation of the cutaneous branch of the radial. It runs over the dorso-medial aspect of the metacarpal bone in company with the dorsal metacarpal vein to gain the medial border of the tendon at the extensor digiti tertii (medial digital extensor) half-way down the metacarpus. It then crosses the tendon, runs on that of the common extensor and divides into the axial dorsal nerves of the third and fourth digits just above the fetlock. There are anastomoses between these and the axial volar digital nerves.

At about the middle of the metacarpus the dorsal metacarpal nerve gives off a medial branch. This runs in the groove between the bone and the suspensory ligament, over the inside of the fetlock and down as the abaxial dorsal nerve of the third digit.

The dorsal branch of the ulnar nerve completes the innervation of the dorsal aspect. It runs laterally in the groove between the metacarpal bone and the suspensory ligament and continues into the foot as the abaxial dorsal nerve of the fourth digit. It also supplies the lateral dewclaw, i.e. the fifth digit.

On the palmar aspect the main parent of the digital nerves is the median. It supplies all of the palmar part of the third digit, the axial part of the fourth digit, and contributes to the innervation of the abaxial part of the latter. It runs down the metacarpus somewhat deeply embedded in the local fascia alongside the medial border of the flexor tendons related to the superficial volar metacarpal artery. In the first part of its course it may be deep to the tendon. On reaching the distal third of the metacarpus the nerve divides in a variable manner, typically into medial and lateral branches. These eventually form three palmar digital nerves and part of a fourth.

The medial branch continues the direction of its parent in the groove between suspensory ligament and flexor tendons. It runs over the sesamoid behind the medial digital vein to become the abaxial palmar nerve of the third digit. Just above the fetlock the lateral branch is joined by the palmar ramus of the ulnar nerve and then receives a branch from the medial nerve. On reaching the bifurcation of the flexor tendons it divides into the axial palmar digital nerves of the third and fourth digits. Before it divides the nerve is related to the palmar common digital artery and lies in fat below the strong fibrous plate associated with the dew-claws.

The volar branch of the ulnar nerve runs down laterally in the groove between the suspensory ligament and the flexor tendons. It joins, as already mentioned, the lateral ramus of the median and the abaxial palmar nerve of the fourth digit is thus formed.

According to Taylor, analgesia may be produced in the fore-limb by injection at the sites indicated in Fig. 12.4. The dorsal metacarpal nerve is located by palpation at about the middle of the metacarpus, medial to the extensor tendon. The dorsal branch of the ulnar is blocked about 5 cm above the fetlock on the lateral aspect of the limb, in the groove between the suspensory ligament and the metacarpal bone. At this point the volar branch of the ulnar nerve may also be blocked, the two nerves being respectively situated in front of, and behind, the suspensory ligament. The axial palmar aspect of the digits may be rendered analgesic by a single injection in the midline just above the fetlock. The injection will reach the lateral branch of the median nerve before it divides, or if it has already divided its two branches will still be close to each other. The two branches may also be simultaneously blocked on the midline just below the level of the dew-claws, i.e. after they have passed from below the fibrous plate of the dew-claws. The medial branch of the median nerve is blocked on the medial side of the limb in the groove between the suspensory ligament and the flexor tendons about 5 cm above the fetlock. As practically the whole of the palmar aspect, and a large part of the lateral aspect of the digits is supplied by the median nerve, the obvious point to make the injection is higher up the limb before the nerve divides. Unfortunately, at this point the nerve lies beneath the artery and vein and is not conveniently situated for injection.

To summarize: To block completely the whole of the digits, injections must be made at points A, B, C, D and E (Fig. 12.4). To block the medial digit, injections should be made at points A, D and E. To block the lateral digit, inject at points B, C, D and E.

Pincemin [14] described a technique of six injections about the nerves below the level of the metacarpophalangeal articulations to produce analgesia of the claws alone. However, precise location of the sites for injection is not easy at this level.

Nerves of the hind foot

On the dorsal aspect the superficial peroneal nerve runs downwards on the extensor tendons giving off medial and lateral branches at the middle of the metatarsus though the lateral branch may be given off earlier.

It is accompanied laterally by the dorsal metatarsal vein and at the bifurcation of the long extensor it gives off the axial dorsal nerves of the third and fourth digits. It then turns into the interdigital space to join the deep peroneal nerve and the common truck so formed divides into two branches that run back and deep to join the axial plantar digital nerves. The deep peroneal nerve runs down in the dorsal metatarsal groove, where it is accompanied by the dorsal metatarsal artery. The lateral and medial branches cross obliquely to the respective sides of the metatarsus and enter the grooves between the bone and the edge of the suspensory ligament. They continue over the sesamoids, in front of the digital vein and become the abaxial dorsal nerves of the third and fourth digits. The two branches also supply the dew-claws and give off other nerves that run cutaneously down to digits.

On the plantar aspect the tibial nerve divides into the lateral and medial plantar metatarsal nerves which run down along the respective sides of the flexor tendons. The lateral nerve continues into the foot as the abaxial plantar nerve of the fourth digit. The medial plantar nerves gives off a branch that runs into the foot as abaxial plantar nerve of the third digit and then divides into the axial plantar nerves of the third and fourth digits.

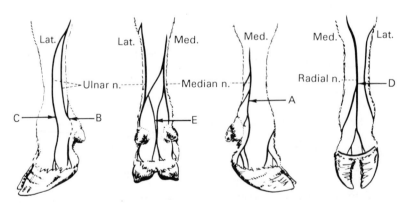

Fig. 12.4 Nerve block of the fore-limb. To block the whole of the digit, injections must be made at A, B, C, D and E. To block the medial digit, inject at A, D and E. To block the lateral digit, inject at points B, C, D and E.

Collin [15] reviewed the methods available for producing analgesia of the digits of the hind-limb and described a technique very similar to that of Brown [16]. This technique involves blocking the tibial and fibular (common peroneal) nerves above the hock. Among the advantages offered by the technique are the following: only two injections are necessary; the injections are made into soft tissues, at a convenient level — this means that they are easily performed, thin needles may be used and they can be carried out in the standing animal with the very minimum of restraint; the position of the nerves is readily determined by reference to definite and palpable landmarks; there is only moderate interference with the nerve supply to muscles — the leg does not become paralysed and bears weight in an almost normal manner, most of the lower limb is rendered analgesic; the complications which may arise from the insertion of needles into diseased tissues of the digits are avoided.

The fibular (peroneal) nerve is blocked immediately behind the caudal edge of the lateral condyle of the tibia, over the fibula and before it dips down between the extensor pedis and flexor metatarsi muscles to divide into the deep and superficial fibular nerves. The bony prominence can easily be palpated in most animals, and in some the nerve itself can be rolled against the bone as it passes superficially, obliquely downwards and cranially, at this point. A narrow gauge needle about 2.5 cm long is inserted through the skin, the subcutaneous tissue and the aponeurotic sheet of the biceps femoris until its point just touches the bony landmark and 20 ml of lignocaine hydrochloride solution (or its equivalent) are injected through it. Analgesia develops after 5–20 minutes. Paralysis of the nerve is shown by a loss of sensation in the exteroceptive area and a paralysis of the extensor muscles of the digit. The signs associated with this motor paralysis are that the animal can walk normally on a level surface but is inclined to stub the toe against obstructions so that the fetlock and phalangeal joints flex [17].

The tibial nerve is blocked about 10–12 cm above the summit of the calcaneus on the medial aspect of the limb, just in front of the Achilles tendon. The Achilles tendon is grasped between the thumb and index finger of one hand while a needle, about 2.5 cm long, is inserted immediately below the thumb until its point can be felt just under the skin by the index finger. About 15–20 ml of local analgesia solution is injected at this site and the block takes 5–15 minutes to develop, depending on the drug used.

When both nerves are blocked (Fig. 12.5), there is complete loss of sensation from the fetlock downwards.

An alternative method for desensitization of the hind-limb below the fetlock joint has been described

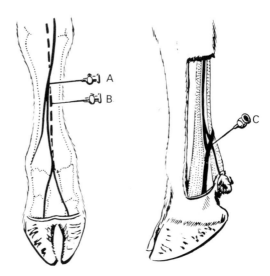

Fig. 12.5 Nerve block of the distal part of the hind-limb using Raker's technique: A, injection of the superficial peroneal nerve; B, injection of the deep peroneal nerve; C, injection of the plantar metarsal nerves.

[18]. The superficial fibular (peroneal) nerve is blocked in the upper third of the metatarsus where it lies subcutaneously over the midline of the dorsal aspect of the metatarsal bone. The deep fibular (peroneal) nerve accompanies the dorsal metatarsal vessels in a groove on the anterior aspect of the metatarsal bone under the cover of the extensor tendons. Injection is made about half-way down the metatarsus beneath the extensor tendons. To facilitate this the needle is inserted from the lateral aspect of the bone and its point directed beneath the edge of the tendon. The plantar metatarsal nerves are blocked at the sites so familiar in the horse, i.e. in the depression on the medial and lateral sides of the limb between the suspensory ligament and the flexor tendons some 5 cm proximal to the fetlock joint and deep to the superficial fascia. About 5 ml of local analgesic solution is injected over each nerve (Fig. 12.5).

Pincemin's technique [14] is also applicable to the hind-limb but, as in the fore-limb, gives no analgesia above the claw itself.

Intravenous regional analgesia of the digit

Intravenous regional analgesia (IVRA), is a simple method for the provision of analgesia of the digit which requires no detailed anatomical knowledge, and has now largely superseded other methods for surgery of the bovine foot. It is achieved by injecting local analgesic into any accessible superficial vein in the extremity isolated from the general circulation by an arterial tourniquet. The limb distal to the site of

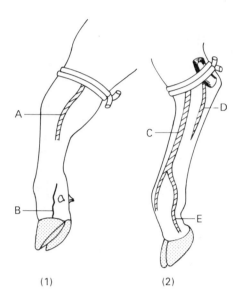

(1)   (2)

Fig. 12.6 Easily recognized veins of the distal parts of the limbs. (1) Medial view of the right fore-leg: A, radial vein; B, medial palmar digital vein. (2) Lateral view of the right hind-leg: C, lateral branch of lateral saphenous vein; D, lateral plantar vein; E, lateral plantar digital vein.

application of the tourniquet becomes analgesic and remains so until the tourniquet is released. Adequate analgesia is provided for the amputation of digits, removal of interdigital hyperplastic lesions and treatment of infections of the foot.

After suitable sedation the animal is cast with ropes and restrained in lateral recumbency. The hair overlying the prominent lateral saphenous or lateral plantar veins of the hind leg, or the radial vein which is accessible on the medial aspect of the carpus and proximal end of the metacarpal bone in the fore-limb, is clipped and the skin prepared for injection. A 19 gauge (1.1 mm) needle, or short catheter, attached to a stopcock is directed proximally or distally into the vein and its lumen kept patent with heparin–saline solution. A tourniquet of stout rubber tubing, or an ordinary sphygmomanometer cuff inflated to a pressure of above 200 mmHg (26.7 kPa), is applied above the hock or carpus to obstruct the arterial inflow. In the hind-limb the efficiency of the tourniquet is improved by including a roll of bandage in the depression between the tibia and the Achilles tendon, or by applying it immediately distal to the hock. In adult cattle, 30 ml of 2% lignocaine hydrochloride (without adrenaline) is then injected into the vein. Complete analgesia distal to the tourniquet occurs within 10 minutes. Once the operation is completed the tourniquet is released and sensation returns within 3–5 minutes of its release.

Complete success can be expected in about 90% of cases or more if the limb is exsanguinated by the use

of an Esmarch bandage before the tourniquet is applied but after insertion of the intravenous needle or catheter. Some failures are inexplicable but the majority are due to the tourniquet being too loose or failure to allow an adequate time for the block to develop. When the block is only partially successful, it is usually found that it is the interdigital region which remains sensitive.

The speed of onset of analgesia is governed by the volume of solution injected because the greater the volume the greater is the intraluminal pressure created and hence the more rapid the diffusion of the analgesic. About 30 ml is, however, the optimum because syringes of greater capacity are not easy to handle and the injection cannot be made so rapidly so the animal has more time to move whilst the injection is made. The duration of analgesia is limited only by the time it is considered safe to leave an arterial tourniquet in place. IVRA is certainly safe for periods of up to $1\frac{1}{4}$ hours [17] and this provides ample time for most surgical procedures on the bovine foot. The safety may be due to continued circulation beneath the tourniquet through only partially occluded vessels.

Initial concern that removal of the tourniquet might be followed by signs of general lignocaine toxicity has proved to be unfounded. The highest systemic venous plasma concentration of lignocaine following the release of the tourniquet found by Bogan and Weaver [19] was 1.5 µg/ml, which is much lower than that generally considered to be toxic [20]. Nevertheless, it is probably advisable to keep a check on pulse and respiratory rates for 10 minutes after release of the tourniquet and to be prepared to treat any signs of toxicity which may appear.

Paravertebral block

By paravertebral block is understood the perineural injection of local analgesic solution about the spinal nerves as they emerge from the vertebral canal through the intervertebral foramina.

Farquharson [21] introduced the method into bovine surgery for the operations of laparotomy and rumenotomy and claimed for it the following advantages over field infiltration: the abdominal wall, including the peritoneum, is completely and uniformly desensitized; excellent muscular relaxation is produced and intra-abdominal pressure is decreased; the method is simple and safe, quicker to effect, and the postsurgical convalescent period is shorter and of no consequence; there is a saving of local analgesic solution. Experience has indicated that Farquharson's claims were fully justified provided the technique of injection was exact and it has now become a most commonly used method for laparotomies in cattle.

The area of the flank bounded cranially by the last

rib, caudally by the angle of the ilium and dorsally by the lumbar transverse processes, is innervated by the thirteenth and first and second lumbar nerves. In addition, the third lumbar nerve, although it does not supply the flank, gives off a cutaneous branch which passes obliquely backwards in front of the ilium. Operations involving the ventral aspect of the abdominal wall will require additional desensitization of the dorsal nerves anterior to the thirteenth. The last dorsal and first lumbar intervertebral foramina in the ox are occasionally double. The last dorsal foramen lies immediately caudal to the head of the last rib and on a level with the base of the transverse process of the first lumbar vertebra. The lumbar foramina are large and are situated between the base of the transverse processes and approximately on the same level. The spinal nerves, after emerging from the foramina, immediately divide into a smaller dorsal and a larger ventral branch. The dorsal branch supplies chiefly the skin and muscles of the loins, but some of its cutaneous branches pass a considerable distance down the flank. The ventral branch passes obliquely ventrally and caudally between the muscles and comprises the main nerve supply to the skin, muscles and peritoneum of the flank. The ventral branch is also connected with the sympathetic system by a ramus communicans. Paralysis of the nerves at their point of emergence from the intervertebral foramina will provoke desensitization of the whole depth of the flank wall and complete muscular relaxation. The effects of blocking the sympathetic fibres through the rami communicantes must be complex and require special study, but according to Farquharson the corresponding abdominal viscera are desensitized and intra-abdominal pressure is reduced.

It is obvious from such factors as the deep situation of the nerves and the lack of absolute precision by which 'landmarks' may be detected that paravertebral block cannot be induced with absolute certainty. The secret of success is an appreciation not only of the depth at which the nerves are situated, but also that they lie beneath the intertransverse ligaments for it is improbable that analgesia will ensue if the solution is injected dorsal to those structures. Fortunately penetration to this depth is not attended by serious risks of injury to subjacent structures, for in the average subject the psoas and quadratus muscles are of considerable bulk. It is probable that blocking of the dorsal branch is automatic if the larger, ventral branch is effectively contacted, but if the dorsal branches only are injected, desensitization of the flank will be incomplete.

The number of nerves to be dealt with will depend on the site and extent of the incision to be made. The areas involved by blocking of the respective nerves

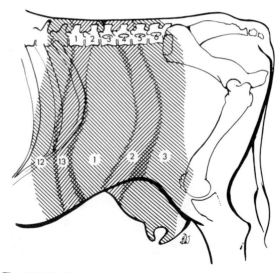

Fig. 12.7 Regions of the flank involved after paravertebral block of the respective nerves.

are illustrated in Fig. 12.7. It will be seen that for rumenotomy, using the customary incision — parallel with and about 7 cm caudal to the last rib — analgesia of the thirteenth thoracic and the first lumbar nerves is adequate, whereas for caesarean section by flank incision it will be necessary to inject the first, second and third lumbar nerves.

Farquharson located the sites for injection as follows: by following the last rib with the index finger, the head of the rib can be felt about 5 cm lateral to the midline. This marks the site for the injection of the thirteenth thoracic nerve. To determine the sites for the lumbar nerves, a transverse line is drawn immediately caudal to the spinous process of the particular vertebra and the needle is inserted at a point on this line 5 cm from the midline. The nerves lie at a depth of about 5 cm.

Adopting Farquharson's method of siting, operators in the UK have had irregular results and alternative sitings have been described. In the Liverpool Veterinary School the most regular results have attended the following method. For injection of the lumbar nerves the point of skin penetration is some 6 cm lateral to the centre point of the corresponding spinous process. Vertical incision of the needle at this point causes it to penetrate the intertransverse ligament just behind the caudal edge of the transverse process and it is in this position that the ventral branch of the nerve lies. Should the needle strike the hinder edge of the transverse process it is redirected a little caudally. Location of the position of the thirteenth thoracic nerve is more difficult because the anatomical features relating to the lumbar nerves do not apply. The point selected as being the most certain is

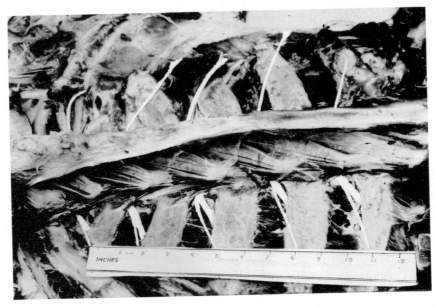

Fig. 12.8 Dissection of the thoracolumbar spine of the ox to show the thirteenth thoracic and first four lumbar nerves. (Dissection by R. G. Walker.)

6 cm from the midline opposite the anterior extremity of the first lumbar spinous process. Inserted at this point the needle strikes the cranial edge of the first lumbar transverse process. It is then redirected a little cranial and deeper just in front of the process, for it is at this point that the thirteenth thoracic nerve which crosses the costotransverse space diagonally attains the edge of the first lumbar transverse process.

An insensitive skin weal is first produced, using a short and comparatively fine needle (20 gauge or 0.9 mm external, 3 cm long) and injecting about 3 ml of solution. This serves to counteract spasm of the longissimus dorsi muscle during subsequent insertion of the long needle. After an appropriate pause, an 18 gauge needle, 8 cm long, is inserted directly downwards until its point strikes the transverse process or the intertransverse ligament. After penetration of the ligament 5–10 ml of solution is injected. During withdrawal of the needle a further 5 ml is infiltrated along its track. During the final withdrawal of the needle, the skin is pressed downwards to prevent separation of the connective tissue and the aspiration of air through the needle.

Dissections carried out at the Cambridge Veterinary School (Fig. 12.8) indicated that a more certain location of the nerves might be obtained by always directing the needle towards the cranial border of the transverse process of the vertebra behind the nerve to be blocked. For example, to block the first lumbar nerve it appeared that the needle should be directed to strike the cranial border of the process of the second lumbar vertebra about 5 cm from the midline.

Moreover, it was noted that at such sites the cranial borders of the transverse processes were usually in the same cross-sectional plane of the body as the most prominent parts of their lateral borders. It seemed, therefore, that palpation of the most prominent part of the lateral border of the process would be of value in locating the site for the insertion of the needle. From these observations a technique was developed which has proved to be satisfactory even in the hands of inexperienced students.

In this technique, to block the thirteenth thoracic and the first, second and third lumbar nerves, skin weals were raised in line with the most obvious parts of the transverse processes of the second, third and fourth lumbar vertebrae, about 5 cm from the midline of the body. Location of the transverse process of the first lumbar vertebra is usually difficult so that in most cases the site for infiltration around the thirteenth thoracic nerve is found by simple measurement. The distance between the skin weals over the second and third lumbar transverse process is measured and another skin weal is produced at a distance equal to this, cranial to the anterior weal to mark the site where the needle is to be introduced to strike the cranial border of the first lumbar transverse process. A stout needle (7 cm long, 3 mm bore) is inserted through each skin weal and the underlying longissimus dorsi muscle infiltrated with 2–3 ml of 1% lignocaine hydrochloride injected through these needles as they are advanced to a depth of about 4 cm from the skin surface. The needles used for the injections around the nerves (10 cm long, 2 mm bore) have 'short-bevel' points so that penetration of the tough intertransverse ligaments can be appreciated as the needle is advanced. These needles are introduced through the holes made in the skin by the stout needles used for infiltration of the longissimus dorsi muscle, and advanced to strike the cranial border of the vertebral process. Each needle is then redirected forwards over the edge of the process and advanced until it is felt to penetrate the intertransverse ligament. Injection of 15 ml of 2% lignocaine hydrochloride with 1:400 000 adrenaline is made immediately below the ligament and a further 5 ml of this solution is injected as the needle is withdrawn to just above the ligament. It is important to ensure that the needles shall be vertical when contact is first made with the cranial border of the processes for, if they are not, redirection over the edge of the processes may cause their points to come to lie well away from the course of the nerves. Successful infiltration of the nerves is indicated first by the development of a belt of hyperaemia which causes an appreciable rise in the skin temperature. Full analgesia develops in about 10 minutes and persists for about 90 minutes. When a unilateral block is fully developed it produces a curvature of the spine, the convexity of which is towards the analgesic side.

A method of producing lumbar paravertebral block which utilizes a lateral approach to the nerves has been described by Magda [22]. The skin is clipped and disinfected at the ends of the first, second, third and fourth lumbar transverse processes and about 10 ml of local analgesic solution is injected beneath each transverse process towards the midline. The needle is withdrawn a short distance and redirected first cranially and then caudally, more analgesic solution being injected along each line of insertion. A total of about 20 ml of solution is used for each site and the last portion of each 20 ml is injected slightly dorsal and caudal to the transverse process to block the dorsolateral branches of the nerves. Cakala [23] considers this technique to be easier, safer and more satisfactory than that of Farquharson. R. Gianturco (personal communication) has described a method of blocking the thirteenth thoracic nerve, in which accurate location of the transverse process of the first lumbar vertebra is not required. He blocks the nerve just before it divides (Fig. 12.8), about 0.5 cm behind the caudal border of the last rib.

It is inevitable that failure or at least partial failure will sometimes attend attempts to inject local analgesic solution in the immediate vicinity of a series of nerve trunks situated at a depth of 5–7 cm from the surface of the body, however careful the technique of injection and no matter which method of approach is adopted. Among the factors which reduce the precision of the method are: the nerves traverse the intransverse spaces obliquely; in some animals the nerve roots are double, emerging from double foramina; it is difficult to ensure that the site of injection is the same as that assessed from the body surface; penetration of the muscular mass of the back tends to cause spasmodic contraction of the muscles with consequent modification of the needle track. Precise location of the sites for injection is also more difficult in the new large breeds of cattle.

Pudic (internal pudendal) block

Exposure of the glans penis for examination is a frequent requirement of veterinary practice, particularly in cases of inability fully to protrude the organ, for the treatment of injuries and infections and for the removal of neoplasms. While epidural block is a reliable means of provoking exposure of the penis in the bull, it must be acknowledged that the method also has disadvantages, particularly in the heavier individuals. The chief of these is that the volume of the analgesic solution required to cause complete exposure may result in severe interference with the motor power in the hind-limbs, and in order to prevent injury to the limbs and pelvis it becomes necessary to keep the animal cast and restrained for several hours. But prolonged recumbency in a heavy bull, often associated with struggling, may result in injury elsewhere.

Larson developed the method of bilateral pudic nerve block to bring about exposure of the bull's penis without causing locomotor impairment [24]. Since the publication of Larson's article the method has also been used in the cow in the treatment of prolapsed uterus and to prevent straining in inflamed conditions of the vagina.

The pudic nerve is made up of fibres arising from the ventral branches of the third and fourth sacral nerves. It passes ventrally and caudally on the medial surface of the sacrosciatic ligament where it is in association with the middle haemorrhoidal nerve, to cross the lesser sacrosciatic foramen where it is accompanied by the internal pudic vessels; they then pass along the floor of the pelvis to the ischial arch supplying motor fibres to the urethra and the erector and retractor muscles of the penis and, the middle haemorrhoidal nerve, sensory fibres to the skin on either side of the midline from the anus to the scrotum. Between the sacrosciatic ligament and the rectum in the region of surgical approach to the nerve lies the sheet-like coccygeal muscle. The pudic nerve lies between the ligament and the muscle, while the accompanying middle haemorrhoidal nerve lies deep to the muscle, that is between it and the rectal wall. The lesser sacrosciatic foramen is closed by a sheet of fascia which is an extension of the fascia of the coccygeal muscle. Habel [25] pointed out that in addition to the pudic and middle haemorrhedial nerves some fibres which enter into the dorsal nerve of the penis are obtained from a branch of the sciatic nerve which, leaving the parent nerve on the outer aspect of the sacrosciatic ligament, passes into the lesser sacrosciatic foramen and anastomoses with the ventral branch of the pudic nerve where that lies immediately above the internal pudic vessels close to the ventral border of the foramen.

The pudic nerve is located per rectum, the hand being introduced as far as the wrist and the fingers directed laterally and ventrally to detect the lesser sacrosciatic foramen. Its outline is not clearly identifiable, but its position is recognized by the softness and depressability of the pelvic wall at this point. Moreover, the internal pudic artery which can readily be detected running along the lateroventral aspect of the pelvic cavity passes out of the pelvis at the cranial part of the foramen. Care should be taken not to introduce the hand too far, for on entering the rectum the foramen lies immediately ventrolateral to the fingers. The nerve can readily be felt, the size of a straw, lying on the sacrosciatic ligament immediately cranial and dorsal to the foramen. The pulsation of the artery which lies about a finger's breadth below the nerve can also be felt.

The site of insertion of the needle is at the point of deepest depression of the ischiorectal fossa immediately medial to the ligament and it is directed in a cranial and slightly ventral direction. During the whole procedure a hand is kept in the rectum. When the needle has penetrated to a depth of 5–7 cm, it will be felt through the rectal wall and its point is directed to the position of the nerve a little cranial to the foramen. Here some 20–25 ml of 2% lignocaine hydrochloride (or its equivalent) is injected. A further 10–15 ml is injected a little caudal and dorsal to this point in order to block also the middle haemorrhedial nerve which may carry some sympathetic fibres to the penis. Habel, in view of the fact that the results following Larson's technique are not always as good as might be expected, suggests from his anatomical experience that a third injection should be made after redirecting the needle a little ventrally just inside the lesser sacrosciatic foramen where the ventral branch of the pudic nerve can be palpated distal to the anastomosis previously referred to. The onset of adequate exposure and desensitization for treatment is delayed for a period varying from 30–45 minutes after injection.

The method was used in the Liverpool University School by Professor J. G. Wright who found that location of the pudic nerve was relatively easy in adult bulls but less so in yearlings. Location of the point of the needle through the rectal wall was not always easy, and it was thought that there might be a danger, should the animal move suddenly during the procedure, of penetration of the rectum. The duration of the effect was prolonged; in several cases the penis could still be exposed with ease after 6 hours while in a young bull there was still some relaxation of the retractor muscles after 24 hours.

In so far as Habel's criticism of Larson's method is concerned it is probable, having regard to the considerable volume of solution in the method, that its dispersion is so widespread that the nerve anastomosis to which he refers is in many instances effectively blocked.

The technique of pudic block for provoking exposure of the penis in the bull is more exacting, more cumbersome and probably less certain than that of epidural injection. Nevertheless it overcomes that serious objection of epidural analgesia, namely prolonged recumbency.

A lateral approach to pudendal nerve block has been described [26]. In this technique one injection is made over the pudendal nerve just as it passes medial to the dorsocranial quadrant of the lesser sciatic foramen, and a second injection is performed between the posterior haemorrhedial and pudendal nerves. This latter injection necessitates penetration of the sacrosciatic ligament. The site of insertion of the needle is determined by using the cranial tuberosity of the tuber ischii as a fixed point and the length of the sacrotuberous ligament as a radius. The distance is used to establish the site on a line drawn parallel to the midline, anterior to the fixed point. After clipping, cleaning and disinfecting, the site is marked by the subcutaneous injection of 2 ml of 2% lignocaine hydrochloride. This injection makes subsequent manipulations less painful and renders the subject more amenable to handling. Either hand is then introduced into the rectum and the lesser sciatic foramen located. A 12 cm long, stout needle (1.8 mm bore) is inserted at the skin site and directed towards the middle finger held in the foramen until the point can be felt to lie alongside the nerve. About 10 ml of local analgesic solution is injected at this site. The needle is withdrawn 4–5 cm and redirected caudally and dorsally so that it penetrates the sacrosciatic ligament at a point about 2.5 cm above and behind the first site of injection. Five millilitres of solution is injected at this point, the needle is withdrawn and the sites massaged to spread the solution in the tissues. Similar injections are carried out on the other side of the animal.

Local analgesia for castration of the bull

For castration the site of the proposed incision in the scrotum may be desensitized by the subcutaneous infiltration of local analgesic solution but this does not, of course, block the nerve fibres which run in the spermatic cord. These fibres may be blocked by the direct injection of 5–10 ml of local analgesic into each cord at the neck of the scrotum, or by injecting 5–25 ml (depending on the size of the animal) into the substance of each testicle. In this latter method the drug is said to pass out from the testicle along the lymph vessels and to block, after diffusion, the nerve fibres present in the cord [27]. The bulk of the drug is carried on in the lymph stream to enter the blood stream and for this reason excessive dosage must be avoided or intoxication will occur.

For the closed or bloodless (Burdizzo) castration the skin of the neck of the scrotum must be infiltrated by subcutaneous injection and the spermatic cord itself is also infiltrated at the same site. About 10–20 ml of 2% lignocaine hydrochloride solution is used on each side.

Caudal analgesia

In the ox the spinal cord ends in the region of the last lumbar vertebra but the meningeal sac is continued as far as the junction of the third and fourth sacral segments. The diameter of the neural canal as it passes through the sacrum is approximately 1.8 cm in the caudal part and 2 cm in the cranial. In the lumbar regions the dimensions of the canal are much greater, its width at the last segment being 4 cm. This helps to explain why paralysis of the spinal nerves as far forward as the first sacral is effected with comparatively small quantities of local analgesic solution (20 ml), whereas paralysis of the anterior lumbar nerves necessitates the injection of much larger quantities (100 ml or more).

Caudal block is performed through the space between the arches of the first and second coccygeal vertebra — i.e. beyond the termination of the spinal cord and its meninges. This site is selected in preference to the sacrococcygeal space because it is larger and thus more easily penetrated, and, in fat animals particularly, is more easily detected. Location of the site for the introduction of the needle is not difficult and the operator may be guided by one or more of the following ways:

1. The tail is gripped about 15 cm from its base and raised 'pump-handle' fashion. The first obvious articulation behind the sacrum in the first intercoccygeal.
2. Standing on one side of the animal and observing the line of the croup, the prominence of the sacrum is seen. Casting the eye back towards the tail, the next prominence to be observed is the spine of the first coccygeal bone. The site is the depression immediately behind it.

3. The caudal prominence of the tuberosity of the ischium is palpated and the point selected 10–11 cm in front of it. A line drawn directly over the back from this point passes, in a medium-sized animal, through the depression between the first and second coccygeal spines.

The dimensions of the opening in the dorsal wall of the neural canal are approximately 2 cm transversely and 2.5 cm craniocaudally. The depth of the canal is about 0.5 cm. The canal is occupied by six caudal nerves, together with a vein on each side. The aperture between the two vertebral arches is closed by the interarcual ligament and the space between the vertebral spines occupied by connective tissue. Surmounting the spines is a variable amount of subcutaneous fat covered by skin. The distance from the surface of the skin to the floor of the canal varies from 2 to 4 cm. The floor comprises, about the centre of the space, the intervertebral cartilaginous disc, and, in front of and behind this, the upper surface of the vertebral centrum.

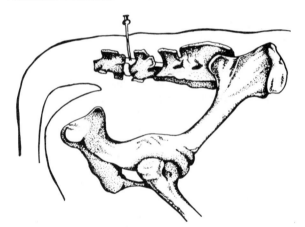

Fig. 12.9 Caudal epidural injection made into the first intercoccygeal space.

An insensitive skin weal is made with the object of preventing movement during insertion of the injection needle and thus ensuring that the latter is introduced in the correct position and direction. For insertion of the epidural needle the tail is allowed to hang naturally. The point of the needle is applied to the centre of the depression between the first and second coccygeal spines, taking care that it is exactly in the midline. If the dermis is tough and considerable pressure is necessary to pierce it, the thumb and forefinger of the left hand are used to grip the needle immediately beneath its adaptor in order to steady it while pressure is applied to the adaptor with the fingers of the right hand. The needle is thrust ventrally and cranially at an angle of 15° with the vertical, until its point impinges on the floor of the

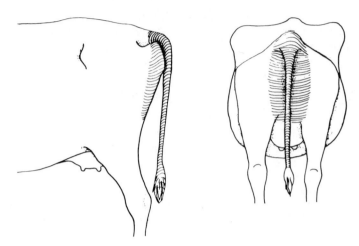

Fig. 12.10 Area of skin desensitization after the caudal injection of 10 ml of 2% lignocaine solution in a 4 year old shorthorn cow of average size.

canal. Often contact with a caudal nerve causes the animal to move suddenly, and the operator should be prepared for this.

Provided that the needle has been inserted in the proper position and direction, there is no doubt that it has entered the epidural space. Sometimes, however, the point of the needle has traversed the space and penetrated the intervertebral disc. This is detected, on attaching the syringe and attempting to inject the solution, by the great resistance offered to the plunger. Should this error occur, the needle should be slightly withdrawn and the syringe reapplied. When the point of the needle lies in the neural canal there is, for all practical purposes, no resistance, and the injection can be made quite easily. Sometimes blood escapes from the needle due to rupture of a vein. In this event the analgesic solution can still be injected without harm, or, if it is thought preferable, the needle can be withdrawn, cleansed of blood clot and reinserted. The rate of injection should be comparatively slow, a volume of 15 ml being given over 10–15 seconds; 2% lignocaine hydrochloride is now almost universally used but the duration of the block can, if needed, be increased by using 0.5% bupivacaine.

Production of a caudal block means that motor control of the hind-limbs is uninfluenced. When 2% solutions of lignocaine hydrochloride are used the total dose lies between 5 and 10 ml, depending on the size of the animal. Provided that the concentration used has been sufficient to paralyse completely the sensory fibres, skin analgesia of the following area will develop: the tail and croup as far as the midsacral region; the anus, vulva and perineum; the posterior aspect of the thighs. Paralysis of the motor fibres will cause the anal sphincter to relax and the posterior part of the rectum to balloon. Defaecation will be

suspended. Stretching of the vulva will provoke no response and the vagina will dilate. In parturition cases 'straining' ceases, but uterine contractions will be uninfluenced.

Obstetrical indications include: to overcome straining for the manipulative correction of malpresentations and the performance of the more simple embryotomy operations; operative treatment of parturient injuries; reduction of the prolapsed uterus.

General indications include: surgical operations on the tail (5–10 ml sufficient); suture of tears of the perineum and vulva, horn gores, etc.; Gotze's operation for reconstruction of the perineum; examination of the vagina and external uterine cervical os in fractious animals; retraction of the uterine cervix; Albrechtson's uterine irrigation treatment; ovariectomy.

The onset of muscular paralysis of the tail occurs in from 1 to 1½ minutes, and affords reliable evidence that the injection has been correctly made. When lignocaine is used analgesia attains its maximum extent in the course of 5–10 minutes, and persists for about an hour, after which there is progressive recovery. The block has completely disappeared by the end of the second hour.

The introduction of epidural analgesia was immediately followed by its use as a means of causing relaxation and exposure of the penis in the bull. At first, relatively large volumes of solution were used to ensure complete relaxation of the organ, but these doses caused marked motor disturbance of the hind-limbs and it was necessary that the animal be cast and restrained for several hours to ensure it did not sustain injury. It is probable that these quantities were used because it was not realized that there was a greater delay in the onset of relaxation of the penis than in sensory and motor paralysis of the tail. An initial minimal dose should be given and the needle left in position; if extrusion does not occur after the elapse of an appropriate interval additional small doses should be given until it does, for in this way exposure of the penis can be obtained with the animal still standing. Edgson and Scarnell [28] employed this method for the treatment of the penis of bulls infected with *Vibrio fetus*. In the Liverpool Veterinary School a 3% lignocaine solution with 1:50 000 adrenaline has been used for surgical operations on the penis. It was possible to provoke complete relaxation and desensitization with the animal still able to maintain the standing position although there was some locomotor incoordination. It would seem that the dose capable of causing complete relaxation of the penis is very close to that which will cause a degree of incoordination which necessitates casting and restraint. As yet there is no accurate method of determining dosage in relation to weight or other measurements and it is probable there will be cases in which too much or too little has been given. Penile relaxation attains its maximum some 25 minutes after injection; return of tone commences in 2 hours and is complete in $4\frac{1}{2}$ hours.

For this particular purpose epidural analgesia has, nowadays, been replaced to a large extent by pudic nerve block, sympathetic blockade or by the use of tranquillizers such as the α_2-adrenoceptor agonists or acepromazine.

Epidural analgesia

Epidural analgesia may be induced through a needle introduced as for the production of a caudal block. The degree of motor interference in the hind-limbs will vary from a partial paralysis affecting primarily the flexors and the stifle-joint, and the flexors and extensors of the hocks and digital joints, to complete paralysis. In partial cases, attempts to move may be associated with spasmodic flexing and extending of the hocks, and arrangements should be made either to support the animal in the standing position or restrain it by hobbles in recumbency. Plenty of bedding should be available to prevent the animal bruising itself when it goes down. In cases where complete hind-limb paralysis is induced, the animal should be kept on its breast with the hind-limbs placed beneath it for a period of 10–15 minutes to ensure the onset of bilateral analgesia. When unilateral analgesia only is required, the animal should be restrained on its side, with the appropriate side downwards, until the full development of analgesia, after which it is turned over. Loss of sensation spreads progressively forwards according to the dose, over the croup, between the hind-limbs to the inguinal

regions, prepuce and scrotum, the hind-limbs, mammary glands, and finally flanks and abdominal wall to the region of the umbilicus. The duration of paralysis is longer. The animal will be unable to rise for 2 hours or so, and incoordination may persist for 3–4 hours or even longer. When epidural analgesia is attained, as is the case when the method is used for the operation of digital amputation, it is imperative that the limbs shall be kept in hobbles, with the animal in breast recumbency, until it is certain that full motor function of the hind-limbs has returned, for otherwise attempts to rise may result in severe injury. The tail serves as a good guide. When power has returned to it, it may be taken that the animal can rise and stand.

Epidural block may be used for: difficult manipulative reposition; extensive embryotomy; amputation of the prolapsed uterus; caesarean section; examination of and operation on the penis; cutting operations about the prepuce and inguinal regions; castration; operative interferences on the udder; operations on the hind-limb such as amputation of the digit.

For difficult obstetrical interferences and amputation of the uterus doses of 100–150 ml of 2% lignocaine with 1:200 000 adrenaline may be used.

Benesch [29] states that its application, when properly performed, is entirely free of danger. Wright (personal communication) observed no ill effects other than a temporary lameness in a cow which fell awkwardly. Cuille and Chelle [30] noted that sometimes the tail is carried in a twisted manner, but with normal mobility, for 5–6 days following injection, after which it becomes normal again, and they ascribe this to injury of the coccygeal nerves during injection. Brook [31] recorded a case in which permanent paralysis of the tail followed epidural injection for the delivery of a dead and oedematous fetus. The animal was unable to elevate the tail even during defaecation and urination, with the result that excoriation of the tail and perineum developed. There was some lateral mobility. A hard, diffuse and painful enlargement developed in the region of the first coccygeal spine. It is probable that infection of the neural canal with the subsequent inflammatory changes was the cause. Fortunately the accident is rare, but every effort must be made to avoid it, for it detracts greatly from the animal's value. The greatest care must be taken that the analgesic solution is not a source of infection. It may be assumed with confidence that when prepared by a manufacturing house of repute, the solution is sterile when received, but the danger is that it will become contaminated during use. It is preferable when using comparatively small volumes to employ ampoules. There is a grave risk that asepsis will break when dealing with a dead or putrid fetus, particularly if a vaginal examination has been made prior to the induction of analgesia, or if a second injection is required after operation has commenced.

When inducing epidural analgesia, the possible development of hypotension must be borne in mind. Although Wright (personal communication) recorded no signs of hypotension when injecting volumes of 100–150 ml at the caudal site for amputation of digits, he noted the condition in bulls after doses of 150–200 ml of 2% solution. Symptoms are those of collapse, with a racing heart and small pulse, and rapid and shallow respirations.

Hypotension may be combated by the intravenous or intramuscular injection of vasopressors such as metaraminol or methoxamine. Metaraminol tartrate is a sympathomimetic amine which has a dual action in that it increases both the force of myocardial contraction and peripheral resistance. It has no central excitatory effect; side-effects such as tremor and tachycardia are not seen. Unlike adrenaline, metaraminol has no effect on blood sugar. It is best given to cattle by intravenous injection in doses up to 20 mg, after which the maximum effect takes 1–3 minutes to develop and lasts for about 25–30 minutes.

Methoxamine hydrochloride is another sympathomimetic amine but its main action is one of peripheral vasoconstriction. It does not affect the force of myocardial contraction and is devoid of stimulatory action on the central nervous system. When given to adult cattle by intravenous injection in doses of 30–60 mg it acts almost immediately and its action lasts for about an hour. Alternatively, it may be given in doses of up to 60 mg by intramuscular injection.

Lumbar epidural analgesia

Injection of local analgesic solutions in the caudal region affords a method of inducing epidural analgesia, but it is not always easy to produce satisfactory cranial spread when this site of injection is used. Consequently, some workers make the injection at the lumbosacral foramen. However, needles introduced through the lumbosacral foramen may enter the subarachnoid space and once this has been entered it is no longer safe to proceed with the induction of an epidural block until the puncture in the dura has become sealed. The patency of the hole in the dura persists for several hours and if an immediate spinal block is considered to be essential, a deliberate, controlled subarachnoid block must be performed. It is because subarachnoid block can be adequately managed only in relatively small animals, in which full use can be made of gravity to control the extent of neural blockade, that injection at the lumbosacral foramen is normally only employed in sheep, small pigs and dogs.

Injection into the epidural space in the lumbar region has been employed to produce analgesia of a number of body segments in cattle. By careful control of the dose of local analgesic injected it is possible to produce a belt of analgesia around the animal's trunk without interfering with the control of the hind-limbs. This type of spinal block may be referred to as 'lumbar segmental epidural analgesia'. Although not an easy technique to perform it is one which warrants inclusion in any discussion of lumbar epidural analgesia.

The desensitization of the flank in cattle by the epidural injection of local analgesic solution into the vertebral canal in the cranial lumbar region was first described in 1948 by Bucholz working in the Giessen School. Later the Russian writers Magda *et al.* [32] described their technique and Arthur in the London Veterinary School introduced the method to British veterinarians [33]. By a single injection, analgesia of the whole of the flanks may be attained with the animal still able to maintain the standing position and operations such as caesarean section and rumenotomy performed. Bucholz injected 10–15 ml of 2% Tutocaine solution, Magda and his colleagues 10 ml of a 4% procaine hydrochloride solution, while Arthur has employed 3% lignocaine hydrochloride and 5% procaine hydrochloride, varying the volume injected according to the size of the animal; a yearling heifer received 6 ml and an adult cow 10 ml. St Clair and Hardenbrook [34] in the USA who were investigating the method at about the same time as Arthur have since recorded very similar findings. Usually 10 ml of 2% lignocaine gave satisfactory results.

Arthur's technique is as follows: with the animal standing, the site for insertion of the needle is just to the right of the lumbar spinous processes on a line 1.5 cm behind the cranial edge of the second lumbar transverse process. An initial skin weal is produced using a fine needle and a longitudinal skin incision some 2–3 cm long is made to facilitate penetration by the spinal needle. The spinal needle (14 gauge, 12 cm long) is directed ventrally and medially at an angle of 10–13° with the vertical for a distance of 7.5 cm at which point the needle has entered the neural canal. By adopting the preliminary skin incision the spinal needle can be moved with relative ease and the operator is able to appreciate the differences in resistance offered by the muscle and the interarcual ligament, respectively. Even when small quantities of local anaesthetic are injected along the track of the needle, penetration of the interarcual ligament is apparently painful and thus the animal should be effectively restrained by the head. It should be noted that the intervertebral space through which the needle must pass to enter the epidural space is actually an interosseous canal formed by the bases of the spinous processes cranially and caudally and by the intervertebral articular processes laterally. In an

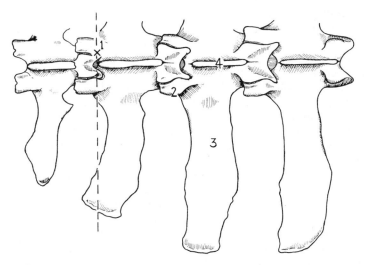

Fig. 12.11 First four lumbar vertebrae viewed from above: 1, point of insertion of spinal needle through skin; 2, articular processes; 3, transverse processes; 4, spinous processes.

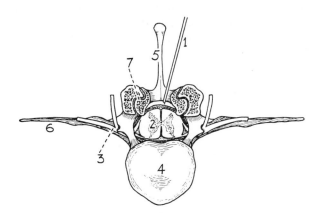

Fig. 12.12 Transverse section through the joints between the articular processes of the first and second lumbar vertebrae. The body of the first lumbar segment is viewed from its caudal aspect. 1, Needle in position; 2, spinal cord surrounded by meninges; 3, left first lumbar nerve; 4, body of first lumbar vertebra; 5, spinous process; 6, transverse process; 7, sectioned interlocking articular processes.

adult Jersey cow this canal measures 1 cm deep, 0.8 cm long and 0.5 cm wide (these dimensions will be considerably greater in the average Friesian or Ayrshire cow), and unless the needle is properly inclined its point will abut on the lateral wall of this canal rather than enter the neural canal (Fig. 12.11). Immediately the needle is felt to penetrate the interarcual ligament, the stilette is withdrawn and if air is heard to enter the needle it is certain evidence that the epidural space has been entered. Alternatively, in the absence of inspiration of air, and if no fluid flows from the needle, a trial injection is made. If the needle is in the epidural space scarcely any pressure

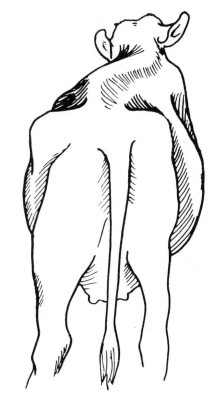

Fig. 12.13 Unilateral analgesia with either paravertebral block or lumbar epidural block produces spinal curvature towards the affected side.

on the plunger is needed. If, on withdrawing the stilette, cerebrospinal fluid flows from the needle, the latter should be quickly but gently withdrawn until the flow ceases and then injection made. (Arthur recorded three cases of accidental puncture of the subarachnoid space but no ill effect resulted presumably because of the relatively small volume of solution injected.)

Lumbar segmental epidural injection results in a broad belt of analgesia encircling the abdomen and involving the whole depth of the wall including the parietal peritoneum. Analgesia develops some 10 minutes after injection and persists for about 3 hours.

Further observations recorded by Arthur include a case of a small Guernsey cow in which the injection of 10 ml caused a partial paralysis of the left cranial crural and obturator nerves in addition, which resulted in 'dropping' of the stifle with abduction of the limb and a tendency to fall on to the left side. In several cases only unilateral analgesia developed, usually of the left side but occasionally of the right. This unilateral action may be due to an insufficient volume of local anaesthetic solution as was indicated by a cow in which 7 ml provoked unilateral analgesia only but an additional 3 ml, without altering the position of the needle, caused a complete belt of analgesia. A feature of unilateral block is a pronounced bending of the spine with the convexity of the curve on the desensitized side. Two interesting side-effects on the sympathetic nervous system were noted. The first was the passage of urine within a few minutes on the onset of analgesia, due presumably to paralysis of the sympathetic fibres controlling the trigonum, and the second was an increase in skin temperature behind the site of injection of some 15°C. No clinical evidence of hypotension due to paralysis of the splanchnic nerves was observed. Arthur's conclusion is that preliminary trials of the method have confirmed its value for operations about the flank and udder performed with the animals standing.

More recently, the technique has been investigated by Skarda and Muir [35, 36] who failed to reach the epidural space at L1–L2 in seven out of 25 cows. They found that the cardiovascular response to unilateral segmental epidural block (T13–L1 and L1–L3) was associated with a reduction in mean systemic arterial blood pressure and an increase in cardiac output. The increase in cardiac output was believed to be due to an increase in heart rate in response to the decreased vascular resistance. These changes appeared to be of no clinical significance and it was concluded that the sympathetic blockade caused by segmental epidural injection was well tolerated by non-sedated healthy cows.

GENERAL ANAESTHESIA

Because it is only safe when the trachea is intubated with a cuffed tube and the inspired gases are enriched with oxygen, general anaesthesia is seldom used when surgery has to be carried out on the farm. However, under hospital conditions where expert anaesthetists are available, general anaesthesia is often more convenient, more certain and less time consuming than methods of local analgesia.

Endotracheal intubation

In adult cattle the larynx cannot be seen without the use of the Rowson laryngoscope and 'blind' intubation through the mouth is successful only on rare occasions unless manipulation of the tube is very gentle indeed. However, when the Rowson laryngoscope is not available, a tube may be introduced into the trachea with certainty if the procedure known as 'intubation by palpation' is adopted.

For this, a wedge-shaped gag is insinuated between the molar teeth of the anaesthetized animal and a hand is passed through the mouth to identify the epiglottis and arytenoid cartilages (Fig. 12.14). The fingertips are placed on the arytenoid cartilages and the lubricated tube is passed between the dorsum of the tongue and arm. The tube is directed through the glottis by the exploring hand which is then withdrawn

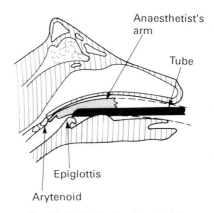

Fig. 12.14 Intubation by palpation.

from the mouth as the tube is pushed on into the trachea.

A 25.0 mm tube is suitable for cattle of about 450 kg body weight. It is sometimes impossible to accommodate a tube of this size and the forearm in the mouth cavity. Under these circumstances a stomach tube is directed into the trachea, the arm withdrawn and the endotracheal tube threaded down over the stomach tube and when it is correctly placed the stomach tube is removed.

The use of the Rowson laryngoscope (Longworth

Scientific Instrument Co. Ltd) makes intubation a relatively simple matter. The head and neck of the anaesthetized animal are positioned so that the head is in full extension and a wedge-shaped mouth gag is introduced between the molar teeth. The blade of the laryngoscope is inserted into the pharynx with the open side of the C-section blade against the hard palate, until contact is made with the epiglottis. The handle is then moved to the left or right so as to rotate the blade, when one of the two distal tips will lift the epiglottis, exposing to view the vocal cords and the interior of the larynx. No attempt is made to lift the jaw of the animal during this procedure. A large endotracheal tube cannot be passed down the blade of the instrument so a rubber-covered, fairly stout wire guide is introduced down the blade and into the trachea. The laryngoscope is withdrawn as soon as the guide is in position and the endotracheal tube is passed around the guide wire. The guide must be about three times as long as the endotracheal tube to avoid the possibility of its being lost into the trachea during this manoeuvre, and it is, of course, withdrawn from the lumen of the tube once this has been introduced. One problem is that the tube may catch on the epiglottis unless it is rotated at the appropriate moment.

The lubricant applied to any endotracheal tube used in ruminant animals should never contain a local analgesic drug for if it does the mucous membrane of the trachea and larynx may remain desensitized for some time after the tube is withdrawn. The protective cough reflex will then be absent and foreign material may be inhaled into the bronchial tree.

In calves, endotracheal intubation is best performed with the aid of a more conventional laryngoscope. The anaesthetized animal is placed on its back with its head and neck in full extension. An assistant draws the tongue well out of the mouth and fixes the upper jaw by pulling on the ends of a tape placed just behind the dental pad. The laryngoscope is then introduced so that the tip of the blade is behind the base of the tongue and in front of the epiglottis. The laryngoscope blade is lifted to expose the larynx and vocal cords and the tube passed into the trachea under direct vision. It is important to note that the larynx is brought into view by a lifting movement and not by employing the laryngoscope blade as a lever using the incisor teeth as a fulcrum.

Endotracheal tubes may also be passed through the mouth and 'threaded' through the larynx which is gripped between the anaesthetist's finger and thumb. Using this method it is sometimes necessary to stiffen the tube by passing down it a piece of straight brass rod of suitable length which is withdrawn as soon as the tube is in the trachea. It is difficult to pass tubes by this method unless the calf is quite deeply anaes-

thetized, but the method is useful if a laryngoscope is not available. Most newborn calves will accommodate tubes of 12 mm internal bore, and 16 mm tubes are adequate for animals of 3–4 months of age.

Intravenous agents

Pentobarbitone sodium

Satisfactory anaesthesia can be induced in small bovine animals by the slow intravenous injection of pentobarbitone sodium. The injection should occupy at least 4 minutes. Induction is quiet and the dose taken to induce light anaesthesia varies from 1 to 1.45 g/50 kg body weight. Surgical anaesthesia persists for about 30 minutes and is followed by a lightening narcosis. The animal will not be able to regain its feet in less than 3 hours. For the very young calf — animals up to 1 month old — pentobarbitone is unsuitable. Narcosis is prolonged for 2 days or even longer, and there is a grave danger that during this period the animal will succumb from oedema of the lungs, or that it may subsequently develop pneumonia.

Thiopentone sodium

Thiopentone sodium has come to be used in adult cattle either alone to provide full anaesthesia for operations of short duration or to induce anaesthesia which is then maintained by inhalation agents. It enables anaesthesia to be induced in the standing animal so that casting tackle is unnecessary and only one assistant is required to hold the animal while the injection is being made.

Premedication is seldom indicated but if essential it must be remembered that its use may delay recovery from anaesthesia. Thiopentone sodium is injected rapidly into the jugular vein in a dose of 11 mg/kg estimated body weight; if xylazine premedication has been used a dose of 5–6 mg/kg is usually adequate. (The 5 g pack of the drug is particularly convenient.) The dose should be dissolved in a maximum of 50 ml of water for larger volumes cannot be injected rapidly enough to produce unconsciousness when this minimal dose is employed. The animal sinks quietly to the ground within 20–30 seconds of injection and there is a brief period of apnoea. Apnoea seldom lasts for more than 15–20 seconds and artificial respiration is not required. Surgical anaesthesia of about 3–4 minutes' duration is followed by recovery which is usually complete within 45 minutes. Recovery is invariably quiet and free from excitement. The animal can be propped up, and will maintain a position of sternal recumbency, about 12–15 minutes after the injection of the drug. The period of surgical anaesthesia, although brief, is adequate for operations of very short duration or the performance of endotracheal intubation, and can be prolonged by the administration of inhalation agents such as halothane.

Apart from the usual risks of general anaesthesia in ruminant animals the method is safe. The margin of safety is wide and serious overdosage is impossible unless there is a gross error in the estimation of body weight. Underdosage, on the other hand, is not infrequent and when subanaesthetic doses are given the animal remains standing. Subanaesthetic doses do not cause excitement. Another reason for failure to induce anaesthesia is slow injection of the drug; it is essential that the injection should be completed within 8 seconds. When subanaesthetic doses are given, or the injection is made too slowly, a second injection of the drug may be made without delay and apart from some delay in recovery no harmful effects occur. Perivascular injection will also account for failure to induce anaesthesia and should this mishap occur the site of injection must be infiltrated with 0.5–1.0 litre of saline. Severe tissue reaction will not occur if the irritant thiopentone is promptly diluted with saline in this manner; but it is unwise to persist with attempts to induce anaesthesia by further injections of thiopentone once a perivascular injection has been made.

Thiopentone should not be administered by this rapid injection technique to shocked animals or to animals suffering from non-compensated cardiovascular disease. Young calves up to 14 days old are not good subjects for thiopentone anaesthesia as in these animals recovery may be very prolonged and the use of even very small doses for induction of anaesthesia is probably unwise.

Methohexitone sodium

Because recovery after methohexitone sodium is so much more rapid than it is after thiopentone sodium, it might appear to be the better of the two compounds for use in ruminants. However, preliminary trials at the Cambridge School have shown that, in cattle, the action of methohexitone sodium is rather unpredictable. The reason for this is unknown and, at the moment, the rapid intravenous injection of a computed dose cannot be recommended. Given to cows by slow intravenous injection, assessing the effects produced as injection proceeds, the compound has so far proved to be quite satisfactory. Slow injection is usually associated with the occurrence of muscle tremors during induction but these seem to be of no importance. Methohexitone sodium appears to produce better conditions for endotracheal intubation than are produced by thiopentone sodium. The jaw is more relaxed and the laryngeal closure and cough mechanisms appear to be less active. Adult cows have

been given up to 2.5 g of methohexitone sodium by intravenous injection for induction, anaesthesia has been uneventful, and recovery has been smooth and extremely rapid but occasionally accompanied by a return of muscle tremors seen during induction of anaesthesia.

Tavernor [37] suggested the use of methohexitone in young calves and commented that a dose of 1 mg/kg by rapid intravenous injection is sufficient to enable endotracheal intubation to be carried out Robertshaw [38] has reported the satisfactory use of methohexitone in castrated Ayrshire calves whose ages ranged from 1.25 to 10 months.

Ketamine

When used with xylazine, ketamine can provide excellent anaesthesia in cattle. Induction is quiet, good muscle relaxation is produced and recovery is smooth and uncomplicated. Xylazine is given either by intramuscular injection (0.2 mg/kg) or intravenously (0.1 mg/kg) to produce deep sedation, often with recumbency. Ketamine is then given intravenously in doses of 2 mg/kg and the animal goes quietly to sleep. Endotracheal intubation can be performed soon after the xylazine injection and before the ketamine is given. Whenever possible this should be done, for ketamine appears to be associated with excessive salivation, but whether this is the result of excessive production or simply failure to swallow the normal production is uncertain. It is possible to prolong anaesthesia with a drip infusion containing 2 mg/ml of ketamine and recovery is usually complete within 45 minutes of stopping this infusion. It is usually necessary to run this drip infusion at a rate of 10 ml/min [39] for the maintenance of anaesthesia. In view of the apparently satisfactory nature of this technique, it is surprising that there appear to be only two brief reports of it in the literature [40, 41]. Equivalent doses of detomidine may be used instead of xylazine.

Waterman [42] recorded the very successful use of xylazine/ketamine mixtures in calves between the ages of 1 week and 1 year. She stated that xylazine and ketamine were miscible in the same syringe and that there appeared to be no disadvantages in giving them simultaneously by intramuscular injection (0.2 mg/kg of xylazine with 10 mg/kg ketamine), to provide anaesthesia of about 35 minutes duration followed by complete recovery in a further 80–90 minutes.

Guaiphenesin

Approximately 80–100 mg/kg of 5% guaiphenesin on its own is needed to produce recumbency in cattle.

More commonly, and always if pain-producing procedures are to follow, a combination of guaiphenesin and thiopentone is used (50 g guaiphenesin to 2 g thiopentone sodium). This mixture is run slowly into a vein to produce the desired effect; the prior administration of xylazine greatly diminishes the necessary quantity. Its administration results in a decrease in tidal volume and arterial blood pressure and an increase in respiratory and heart rates. A similar technique involves the use of 1 g of ketamine mixed with 50 g of guaiphenesin infused intravenously to effect.

Inhalation agents

Halothane

Because of its great potency and because it does not appear to have any toxicity, halothane is a most useful inhalation anaesthetic for cattle. It will produce very satisfactory anaesthesia and it is usually administered by low-flow methods with carbon dioxide absorption. Using these methods, between 30 and 40 ml of the liquid must be vaporized to induce anaesthesia in a cow weighing 450 kg and for the maintenance of anaesthesia for 1 hour a further 30 ml is required. After the induction of anaesthesia with thiopentone sodium in a cow of similar weight anaesthesia can be maintained for 1 hour by the use of 25–30 ml of the liquid agent. However, when anaesthesia is induced by a drug such as thiopentone sodium much of the flexibility of halothane anaesthesia is lost and recovery from anaesthesia is, to some extent, delayed.

In cattle, as in horses, halothane is best vaporized from a special vaporizer unit and the inexperienced anaesthetist may find the maintenance of smooth anaesthesia is not easy. The loss of flexibility which occurs when thiopentone is used to induce anaesthesia does to some extent overcome any tendency towards swinging anaesthesia.

If prolonged anaesthesia is contemplated no time should be lost in puncturing the rumen through the left body wall with a trocar and cannula. The trocar is withdrawn and the cannula left in the rumen. It is better to perform this operation early on in the anaesthetic rather than be forced to carry it out as an emergency measure later on for the relief of established tympany.

Once the administration of the anaesthetic is terminated, recovery is rapid. Most animals can support themselves on the brisket within 10 minutes from the termination of anaesthesia. The animal should be propped up in sternal recumbency as soon as possible to allow eructation to occur. The endotracheal tube is left in the trachea with the cuff still inflated and manipulated at intervals until its manipulation causes the animal to cough. As soon as coughing is provoked by this manoeuvre the tube is withdrawn without prior deflation of the cuff.

Enflurane and isoflurane

There is very little information about the use of enflurane and isoflurane in cattle. They may be used in a manner similar to that employed for halothane, but recovery is more rapid because of their lower solubilities (p. 104). There is a clinical impression that isoflurane anaesthesia is associated with more respiratory depression than is halothane.

Methoxyflurane

When used in the appropriate apparatus, methoxyflurane will anaesthetize cattle, but because of its high solubility and low volatility which can lead to slow induction and recovery, it cannot be recommended for bovine anaesthesia.

Ether

It is generally agreed that it is almost impossible to anaesthetize adult cattle by ether when this agent is given by open or semi-open methods. Nevertheless, satisfactory anaesthesia has been maintained in narcotized adult cattle using a closed or low-flow system. Narcosis was usually induced by the intravenous injection of a thiobarbiturate and after endotracheal intubation ether was administered from a to-and-fro or circle-type system with soda lime for absorption of carbon dioxide. Recovery after ether anaesthesia is quiet and reasonably rapid.

Ether can be used to anaesthetize small calves but its inhalation in the concentrations necessary for the induction of anaesthesia usually produces a profuse outpouring of salivary and bronchial secretion and for this reason even in young animals anaesthesia should be induced with another agent. The best agent to use for this purpose is debatable but thiopentone sodium given as a 2.5% solution by slow intravenous injection in quantities just sufficient to produce loss of consciousness has given good results.

Cyclopropane

Cyclopropane was used as an anaesthetic agent for cattle of all ages and although it was an expensive gas the cost per anaesthetic was small.

Cyclopropane anaesthesia is easily controlled and recovery is rapid but because mixtures of cyclopropane and air or oxygen are explosive it has been replaced by newer agents such as halothane, enflurane or isoflurane.

Chloroform

It is extremely doubtful if the use of chloroform in cattle can be justified today.

Nitrous oxide

Usually, nitrous oxide/oxygen mixtures are only used to maintain anaesthesia following induction with an intravenous agent such as a barbiturate.

Anaesthesia is induced, the animal intubated with a cuffed endotracheal tube and the nitrous oxide/oxygen mixture administered by a low-flow method with carbon dioxide absorption. Maintenance of satisfactory anaesthesia with nitrous oxide/oxygen alone is impossible and the judicious introduction of small quantities of halothane, enflurane or isoflurane into the anaesthetic circuit is necessary. Provided that only minimal quantities of the intravenous drug and supplementary agents have been used, recovery is smooth and extremely rapid. When anaesthesia has been induced with nitrous oxide the animal usually regains its feet within 10 minutes of the termination of the anaesthetic.

Although the use of 50% nitrous oxide with oxygen will reduce the MAC of halothane by about 27% [43] its ability to diffuse into gas-filled spaces within the body means that ruminal distension is not uncommon. Many anaesthetists will not use nitrous oxide in ruminants because of this.

Signs of unconsciousness

In cattle the signs referable to depth of unconsciousness vary depending on the agents employed. The position of the eye, coupled with the presence and briskness of the eyelash reflex, usually provides useful information. During the transition from light levels of unconsciousness under the inhalation agents, barbiturates and the combinations of guaiphenesin with them, the eyeball usually rotates ventrally and the briskness of the eyelash reflex decreases. The eyelash reflex is abolished and the eyeball moves to a central position as deeper levels of unconsciousness are reached.

Ketamine produces tension in the extraocular muscles so that under its influence the eyeball maintains a central position and the eyelash reflex remains strong.

During general anaesthesia the respiratory rate in adult cattle is commonly between 20 and 40 breaths per minute, being higher when the animal is in a supine position. Hypoventilation is usual and to maintain a normal P_aCO_2 it is necessary to ventilate the lungs with tidal volumes of 5–6 litres at rates of 10–12 breaths/min. Heart rates in properly anaesthetized adult cattle are usually between 60 and 70 beats/min, but if ketamine is used to induce anaesthesia after xylazine premedication the rate may be between 50 and 60 beats/min. Arterial systolic blood pressures are very variable and pressures between 130 and 280 mmHg have been recorded with diastolic pressures between 70 and 200 mmHg.

NEUROMUSCULAR BLOCK

Neuromuscular blocking agents are seldom used in routine, clinical, bovine anaesthesia because facilities for performing IPPV and monitoring the degree of block must be available if they are to be used with safety. Pancuronium (0.1 mg/kg) has been used in experimental animals and produces relaxation of some 30–40 minutes duration. As in horses, but in contrast to other species of animal, the facial muscles are more resistant to neuromuscular block than are the limb muscles. Monitoring of block should, therefore, be carried out by stimulation of nerves to limb muscles (see p. 125).

REFERENCES

1. Schatzman, U., Held, J. P. and Rohr, W. (1979) *Proceedings of the Association of Veterinary Anaesthetists of Great Britain and Ireland* **8**, 108.
2. Symonds, H. W. (1976) *Veterinary Record* **99**, 234.
3. Symonds, H. W. and Mallinson, C. B. (1978) *Veterinary Record* **102**, 27.
4. Eichner, R. D., Prior, R. L. and Kvasnika, W. G. (1979) *American Journal of Veterinary Research* **40**, 127.
5. Alitalo, I. (1986) *Acta Veterinaria Scandinavia*, Suppl. 82, p. 193.
6. Jedruch, J. and Gajewski, Z. (1986) *Acta Veterinaria Scandinavia*, Suppl. 82, p. 189.
7. Kitzman, J. V., Booth, N. H., Hatch, R. C. and Wallner, B. (1982) *American Journal of Veterinary Research* **43**, 2165.
8. Ruckebusch, Y. and Toutain, P. L. (1984) *Veterinary Medica Review* **1**, 3.
9. Doherty, T. J., Ballinger, J. A., McDonell, W. N., Pascoe, P. J. and Valliant, A. E. (1987) *Canadian Journal of Veterinary Research* **51**, 244.
10. Toosey, M. B. (1959) *Veterinary Record* **71**, 24.
11. Browne, T. G. (1938) *Veterinary Record* **50**, 1336.
12. Peterson, D. R. (1951) *Journal of the American Veterinary Medical Association* **118**, 145.
13. Taylor, J. A. (1960) *Veterinary Record* **72**, 1212.
14. Pincemin, Y. (1933) *Record Medicin Veterinaire* **109**, 341.
15. Collin, C. W. (1963) *Veterinary Record* **85**, 833.

16. Brown, C. W. (1956) Quoted by Arthur, G. H. (1960) *Veterinary Record* **82**, 1215.
17. Keown, G. G. (1956) *Canadian Journal of Comparative Medical Science* **20**, 12.
18. Raker, C. W. (1956) *Journal of the American Veterinary Medical Association* **128**, 238.
19. Bogan, J. A. and Weaver, A. D. (1978) *American Journal of Veterinary Research* **39**, 1672.
20. Parkinson, P. I., Margolin, L. and Dickinson, D. S. P. (1970) *British Medical Journal* **ii**, 29.
21. Farquharson, J. (1940) *Journal of the American Veterinary Medical Association* **97**, 54.
22. Magda, I. I. (1949) *Soviet Veterinariya* **16**, 96.
23. Cakala, S. (1961) *Cornell Veterinarian* **51**, 64.
24. Larson, L. S. (1953) *Journal of the American Veterinary Medical Association* **123**, 18.
25. Habel, R. E. (1953) *Journal of the American Veterinary Medical Association* **128**, 16.
26. McFarlane, L. S. (1963) *Journal of the South African Veterinary Medical Association* **34**, 73.
27. Rieger, H. (1954) *Berlin Munchen Tierarztliche Wochenschrift* **67**, 107.
28. Edgson, F. A. and Scarnell, J. (1955) *Veterinary Record* **67**, 469.
29. Benesch, F. (1938) *Proceedings of the XIIIth International Veterinary Congress*, Zurich.
30. Cuille, J. and Chelle, P. (1931) *Review General Medicine Veterinaire* **40**, 393.
31. Brook, G. B. (1935) *Veterinary Record* **15**, 601, 605, 606.
32. Magda, I. I., Shalduga, N. E. and Voskovoinikov, M. (1952) *Veterinariya* **29**, 47.
33. Arthur, G. H. (1956) *Veterinary Record* **68**, 254.
34. St Clair, L. E. and Hardenbrook, J. H. (1956) *Journal of the American Veterinary Medical Association* **129**, 405.
35. Skarda, R. T. and Muir, W. W. (1979a) *American Journal of Veterinary Research* **40**, 52.
36. Skarda, R. T. and Muir, W. W. (1979b) *American Journal of Veterinary Research* **40**, 645.
37. Tavernor, W. D. (1964) *Veterinary Record* **74**, 595.
38. Robertshaw, D. (1964) *Veterinary Record* **76**, 357.
39. Taylor, P., Hopkins, L., Young, M. and McFadyean, I. R. (1972) *Veterinary Record* **90**, 35.
40. Fuentes, V O. and Tellez, E. (1974) *Veterinary Record* **94**, 482.
41. Fuentes, V. O. and Tellez, E. (1976) *Veterinary Record* **99**, 338.
42. Waterman, A. E. (1981) *Veterinary Record* **109**, 464.
43. Steffey, E. P. and Howland, D. (1979) *American Journal of Veterinary Research* **40**, 372.

CHAPTER 13

ANAESTHESIA OF THE SHEEP, GOAT AND OTHER HERBIVORES

Domestic sheep and goats are placid animals of manageable size and most clinical surgical procedures can be performed under some type of local analgesia with only the minimum of physical restraint or narcotic sedation. However, provided precautions are taken to avoid the development of ruminal tympany, they are also good subjects for general anaesthesia, and many anaesthetists consider that this is always more convenient and less time consuming than local analgesia. Nearly all major surgery is best performed under inhalation anaesthesia but the intravenous agents have a place as induction agents and for surgery of very short duration.

SEDATION OF THE SHEEP AND GOAT

In general, sheep and goats do not need sedation; the presence of an attendant to control the head is all that is required to keep the animal from moving about during surgery. Occasionally, however, goats and some of the wilder breeds of sheep (e.g. Welsh mountain or Soay) do need more than this and today there are numerous drugs which may be employed.

Chloral hydrate

Although in the past chloral hydrate has been used as a sedative and, indeed, as an anaesthetic in sheep and goats [1–3], much better agents are available today.

α_2-Adrenoceptor agonists and antagonists

Most sheep can be sedated by the intramuscular injection of xylazine (0.2 mg/kg); some goats appear much more sensitive to this drug and doses of 0.05 mg/kg may result in profound sedation for 12 or more hours. Because results following intramuscular injection are unpredictable, in both sheep and goats it is probably best to administer the drug by very slow intravenous injection, assessing the degree of sedation as injection is made over some minutes. When given in this way doses of 0.1–0.15 mg/kg are usually required to sedate sheep, while 0.01 mg/kg are sufficient for most goats. In sheep, xylazine administration has occasionally been associated with the development of pulmonary oedema.

The intrathecal spinal injection of xylazine has been shown to result in analgesia and doses of 50 µg appear equivalent to an intravenous dose of 50 µg/kg but the duration of action is much shorter when the drug is given intravenously (45 minutes versus 120 minutes after intrathecal injection) [4].

Medetomidine, in intravenous doses of 10–20 µg/kg, produces very deep sedation in sheep, similar to that seen after the use of 0.2 mg/kg of xylazine.

Although little information is available, there is no reason why the α_2-adrenoceptor antagonists should not be used to counteract the effects of the α_2-adrenoceptor agonists in sheep and goats. In sheep, atipamezole given intravenously in doses of 25 or 50 µg/kg awakens animals sedated with 0.3 mg/kg of xylazine, but some animals given the lower dose relapse into a sedated state.

Benzodiazepines

Diazepam can be given by mouth in doses of about 15 mg/kg and wild sheep or aggressive male goats may be sedated by mixing this in a small meal of oats and bran, or a small quantity of concentrates. For procedures such as radiography or foot-trimmings, large rams or male goats may be given 2 mg/kg of diazepam by intramuscular injection, but these intramuscular injections appear to cause pain.

Midazolam may be given intravenously and a dose of 4 mg/kg produces, after about 3–5 minutes, very satisfactory sedation for most non-painful procedures.

Further increments of 1–2 mg/kg may be given intravenously to produce recumbency which lasts about 30 minutes, but it is difficult to produce full anaesthesia with this agent. A total dose of 1 mg of the antagonist, flumazenil, produces very rapid awakening when given by intravenous injection but relapse to deep sedation may follow [5].

Phenothiazine derivatives

Acepromazine (or, on the Continent of Europe, the half as potent compound propiopromazine) is the only phenothiazine tranquillizer likely to be used today for sedating sheep or goats. Acepromazine is usually used in sheep by intramuscular injection in doses of 0.05 mg/kg but the smaller breeds such as the Soay may need up to 0.1 mg/kg for effective sedation. Most goats can be satisfactorily sedated by the intramuscular injection of 0.1 mg/kg. As in all ruminants, the phenothiazines relax the gastro-oesophageal junction and increase the risk of regurgitation of ruminal contents.

LOCAL ANALGESIA OF THE SHEEP AND GOAT

Nerve blocking for dishorning

The sites for producing nerve blocks for the dishorning of goats were well described by Vitums [6].

Anatomical considerations

The nerve supply to the horns is provided by the cornual branches of the lacrimal and infratrochlear nerves. The cornual branch of the lacrimal nerve emerges from the orbit behind the root of the supraorbital process. The nerve, covered by a thin frontalis muscle, divides into several branches, two of which course towards the caudolateral aspect of the base of the horn and supply mainly the lateral and caudal parts of it. The main trunk of the infratrochlear nerve emerges from the orbit dorsomedially and divides into two branches, the dorsal or cornual branch, and the medial or frontal branch. The cornual branch soon divides, one division running towards the dorsal aspect of the base of the horn and ramifying in its dorsal and dorsomedial parts. The other division courses toward the medial aspect of the base of the horn and gives off branches to the medial and caudomedial parts of it. Both divisions are covered in part by the orbicularis and in part by the frontalis muscles.

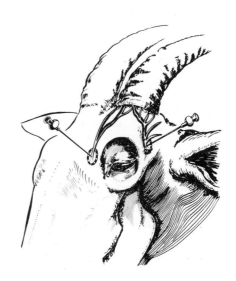

Fig. 13.1 Nerve blocks for dishorning of goats. The cornual branches of both the lacrimal and infratrochlear nerves must be blocked. Care must be taken in young kids to ensure that attempts to block both these nerves do not lead to the injection of toxic quantities of local analgesic solution.

Technique

The site for producing block of the cornual branch of the lacrimal nerve is caudal to the root of the supraorbital process (Fig. 13.1). The needle should be inserted as close as possible to the caudal ridge of the root of the supraorbital process to a depth of 1.0–1.5 cm.

The site for blocking the cornual branch of the infratrochlear nerve is at the dorsomedial margin of the orbit (Fig. 13.1). In some animals the nerve is palpable by applying slight pressure and moving the skin over this area. The needle should be inserted as close as possible to the margin of the orbit to a depth of about 0.5 cm. In adult animals, about 2–3 ml of local analgesic solution should be injected at each site.

These nerves may be blocked for the disbudding of kids, but kids are very small animals and it is all too easy to administer a toxic dose of local analgesic. The authors agree with Taylor [7] that light general anaesthesia with halothane/oxygen is much safer for disbudding of these very young animals provided the oxygen mixture is switched off before any cautery is used.

Paravertebral block

In sheep and goats lumbar paravertebral block is carried out using techniques similar to those employed in cattle. In most animals palpation of the transverse processes of the lumbar vertebra presents no difficulty, and because the nerves lie nearer to the skin surface the injections can be made with greater precision than in cattle. For operations carried out through the flank the thirteenth thoracic and the first three lumbar nerves are blocked. For each of these nerves 5 ml of 1% lignocaine hydrochloride with 1:100 000 adrenaline is injected ventral to the inter-transverse ligament and a further 2 ml is injected dorsal to the ligament. An increase in the skin temperature due to hyperaemia can be detected very soon after injection and full analgesia is present about 5 minutes later. Analgesia persists for about 60 minutes.

Pudendal block

A technique for producing pudendal nerve block in sheep has been described by McFarlane [8]. The site for the introduction of the needle is determined by using the cranial tuberosity of the tuber ischii as a fixed point and the length of the sacrotuberous ligament as a radius. This distance is used to establish the site on a parallel to the midline, cranial to the fixed point. After clipping and skin disinfection a finger is introduced into the rectum and the slit-like lesser ischiatic notch is located on one side (usually about finger depth from the anus). The needle is inserted at the corresponding site and 7 ml of local analgesic solution (e.g. 2% lignocaine hydrochloride with 1:100 000 adrenaline) is injected at the notch. After massage through the rectal wall to distribute the solution, the other side is injected keeping the same finger in the rectum. Complete analgesia and, in the ram, exposure of the penis follow within about 5 minutes of injection of the second side.

Local analgesia for castration

In the UK the Protection of Animals (Anaesthetics) Act, 1964 specifies that castration of male sheep over 3 months of age and of male goats over 2 months of age must be carried out under anaesthesia. Although general anaesthesia of short duration can be given for this operation, in practice it is likely that some form of local analgesia will be employed. Intratesticular injection would appear to be the most convenient procedure for use on the farm, although all of the methods described for the bull (p. 248) are applicable.

Dosage for intratesticular injection depends on the size and age of the animal concerned and from 2–10 ml of local analgesic solution (1% lignocaine hydrochloride) is injected into each testicle. The needle is plunged perpendicularly through the tensed scrotal skin into the testicle and the bulk of the dose is injected into its substance. The line of the skin incision is infiltrated with the remainder of the dose after the point of the needle has been withdrawn to a subcutaneous position.

Caudal block

For intravaginal obstetrical procedures caudal epidural analgesia may be induced by the injection of 3–4 ml of local analgesic solution into the canal through the sacrococcygeal space. This is a valuable technique and if careful aseptic precautions are observed no complications are encountered.

For the symptomatic relief of painful conditions of the vagina and rectum which provoke severe and continuous straining the technique of continuous caudal block can be extremely useful. A fine nylon catheter is introduced into the canal through a Tuohy needle (Fig. 13.2) at the sacrococcygeal space and advanced cranially for 6–8 cm. The needle is then withdrawn leaving the catheter *in situ*. Local analgesic solution (3–4 ml) is injected through the catheter whenever the animal shows signs of sensation returning to the pelvic organs. If all injections are made with aseptic precautions and the free end of the catheter is maintained in a sterile condition — capped and bound up in a sterile gauze swab, for example — between injections, analgesia can be safely maintained for many hours by this technique.

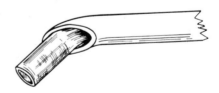

Fig. 13.2 Catheter emerging from tip of Tuohy needle.

The injection of 0.75–1 ml of 1% lignocaine hydrochloride, or its equivalent, at the sacrococcygeal space provides excellent analgesia for the docking of lambs' tails but it must be remembered that analgesia takes about 5 minutes to develop after the injection is made.

Epidural and subarachnoid block

Both epidural and subarachnoid spinal nerve blocks provide excellent conditions for intra-abdominal, pelvic or hind-limb surgery. In sheep restraint of the head and fore-limbs is simple and if the animal is made comfortable upon the operating table it will not interfere with the surgeon's work by struggling. Provided that careful technique and the most scrupulous asepsis are employed there is very little risk to the animal. The vast majority of the complications which have been described as occurring after spinal nerve blocks can be traced to faulty or clumsy technique or to the introduction of infection into the epidural or subarachnoid space.

Although the needle may be introduced between any two lumbar vertebrae there is less risk of puncturing the meninges if it is introduced through the lumbosacral space. The site for lumbosacral injection is located as follows: The cranial border of the ilium on each side is located by palpation. A line joining these crosses the dorsal spinous process of the last lumbar vertebra. The needle is introduced immediately caudal to this.

Procedure

A large area around the site of injection is clipped and the skin thoroughly cleaned and disinfected. The sheep is then restrained in lateral decubitus with the lumbosacral spine in full flexion. The restraint must be good, for the animal usually attempts to move as the needle penetrates the ligamentum flavum and movement at this juncture may result in accidental puncture of the dura mater.

Some workers [9] recommend that sheep be restrained in the prone position with their hind-limbs over one edge of the table for the insertion of the needle but this is much less comfortable for the animal, interferes with breathing and makes it more difficult to prevent movement as the needle is introduced through the ligamentum flavum.

With full aseptic precautions, the site of the introduction of the epidural needle is infiltrated with 2 or 3 ml of local analgesic solution using a very fine needle. A large-bore needle is introduced through the insensitive zone made by this injection and then withdrawn to leave a clearly defined skin puncture. The epidural needle (6 cm long, 16 gauge with a fitted stilette) is inserted through the skin puncture and directed towards the lumbosacral space (Fig. 13.3). When the needle point is judged to have entered the tough ligamentum flavum the stilette is removed and a 20 ml syringe containing about 5 ml of air is attached to the needle. The needle is advanced cautiously with one hand while the thumb of the other

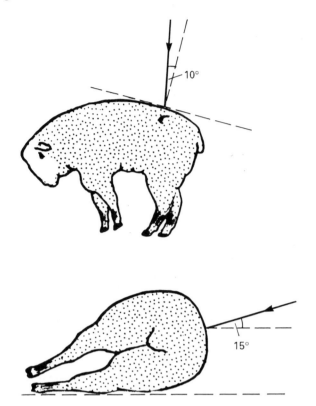

Fig. 13.3 Direction of insertion of needle for lumbar epidural injection in sheep in lateral recumbency.

hand maintains a continuous pressure on the plunger of the syringe. The sudden loss of resistance to injection of the air when the needle emerges from the ligamentum flavum is immediately apparent by movement of the syringe piston. The loss of resistance indicates that the epidural space has been entered and the injection of air tends to force the dura away from the advancing needle point. Next, an attempt is made to aspirate cerebrospinal fluid into the syringe. If fluid is drawn into the syringe or drips from the needle when the syringe is detached it must be assumed that the dura has been punctured and in these circumstances either a subarachnoid injection is made (see p. 264) or the whole procedure should be abandoned, for experience has shown that it is not safe merely to withdraw the needle slightly and proceed with the epidural injection. If all is well and the dura has not been punctured a syringe containing the local analgesic solution is attached to the needle and the injection made. If predominantly unilateral analgesia is required the sheep is maintained in lateral recumbency (the side to be desensitized being undermost) but if bilateral analgesia is desired the animal is turned on to its back as soon as the needle is removed. In either case it is an advantage to apply a 10° head-down tilt to the animal's body by raising the end of the table. The animal is maintained in position until analgesia is complete and the time taken for this will depend on the analgesic drug employed.

The drug used is usually 1.5% lignocaine hydrochloride with the addition of adrenaline from an ampoule to give a final concentration of 1:100 000 adrenaline. This gives excellent analgesia of about 2 hours' duration. The volume of lignocaine solution injected is, of course, dependent upon the size of the sheep and ranges from 8–15 ml.

The injection of this quantity of 1.5% lignocaine solution usually causes a slight fall in blood pressure due to paralysis of the splanchnic nerves. Occasionally (in about 5% of cases) the fall in blood pressure may be severe and the animal will show signs of distress due to hypotension. In these circumstances 5–10 mg of methoxamine hydrochloride should be given immediately by intravenous injection. It is always a wise precaution to insert a catheter into a vein before any spinal nerve block is performed so that difficulties of venepuncture do not delay the intravenous administration of the vasopressor drug. Hypotension can usually be minimized by the intravenous infusion of 0.5–1 litre of Hartmann's solution prior to the administration of the block but this is seldom practical in veterinary clinical practice. Systolic arterial blood pressure is easily monitored by using a sphygmomanometer with the cuff cranial to the hock and a Doppler-shift pulse detector sited over the metatarsal artery.

Motor nerve fibres are not blocked by a 1.5% solution of lignocaine hydrochloride or equivalent solutions of other drugs so an animal can still move its hind-legs during an operation. However, because the afferent sensory fibres are blocked the reflex arc is not intact and the sheep is unable to stand for 4–6 hours from the time of injection. The phrenic nerves and the motor nerves to the intercostal muscles are also unaffected and respiration is not embarrassed even if the solution permeates high up into the cervical region.

The sheep should be allowed to lie quietly while recovering from the effects of the epidural block. The animal can maintain itself in sternal recumbency and any attempt to hasten it to rise may cause it to become excited. Damage to hip joints or pelvic bones by forceful uncoordinated movements may occur if the animal is frightened or excited during the recovery period.

Continuous epidural block may be produced by repeated injections given through a fine nylon catheter introduced with a Tuohy needle (Fig. 13.2). 'Top-up' injections should generally be limited to half the initial dose used.

It is probable that there are no indications for the deliberate induction of a subarachnoid or 'true spinal' nerve block in sheep for on all occasions when it might be used an epidural block is to be preferred. Subarachnoid block is, therefore, only likely to be induced when the dura is accidently punctured during an attempt to perform an epidural injection.

The specific gravity of the fluid injected into the subarachnoid space, coupled with the posture of the animal, has a most important bearing on the spread of analgesia. It has been found that cinchocaine as Heavy Nupercaine (i.e. 1:200 Nupercaine in 6% glucose) is a satisfactory agent for use in sheep (although specially prepared solutions of lignocaine and bupivacaine may be used). This solution is hyperbaric and sinks to the most dependent part of the meningeal sac. Its spread within the subarachnoid space is shown in Fig. 13.4 and it is important to note that the natural curvature of the spine plays an important part in the distribution of the solution when this is injected in the lumbar region and allowed to spread under the influence of gravity. Diffusion of the drug in the cerebrospinal fluid usually plays only a small part in the spread of analgesia.

If the dura is accidentally punctured and it is decided to carry on and perform a subarachnoid block then 1.5–2 ml of Heavy Nupercaine are injected through the needle and the needle withdrawn. For a unilateral block the sheep is maintained in lateral decubitus so that the nerve roots on the

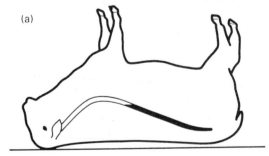
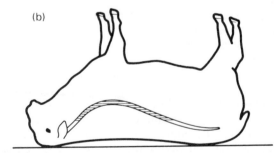

Fig. 13.4 Spread of solution in subarachnoid space when injected in the lumbar region. (a) Hyperbaric solution, i.e. specific gravity of solution is greater than that of the cerebrospinal fluid. (b) Hypobaric solution, i.e. specific gravity less than that of cerebrospinal fluid.

underside of the animal become impregnated with the drug, while for a bilateral block the sheep is placed on its back as soon as possible after the needle has been removed. Spread of analgesia towards the head or tail is obtained by tilting the table so that the sheep's body is either head down or head up. The extent of analgesia is tested from time to time by pinching the skin with a pair of forceps or towel clips and when the desired area of analgesia is attained the table top is returned to the horizontal position. Analgesia persists for about 3 hours and the sheep is able to stand after a further 2–3 hours have elapsed. Subarachnoid block appears to cause a more pro-

found fall in blood pressure than is encountered with an epidural block.

After a dural puncture, whether or not this has been followed by a spinal block, most sheep exhibit signs which may well indicate that they are suffering from a headache. They grind their teeth, avoid bright lights and press their heads against walls or cold water buckets. Headache is a well-recognized sequel to spinal puncture in man. The intrathecal injection of 50 μg of xylazine immediately after the local analgesic solution may prolong the period of post-operative analgesia but as yet there are no reports of its efficacy.

ANAESTHETIC TECHNIQUES IN THE SHEEP AND GOAT

Intravenous injection

Venepuncture in sheep and goats presents few difficulties and the site chosen depends mainly on the assistance available and the personal preference of the anaesthetist.

The marginal and central ear veins are easily visible after the hair has been clipped and the skin soaked with a skin-preparation solution. A 0.63 mm (23 gauge) butterfly needle or a catheter (23 gauge, 2.5 cm long) may be introduced into the vein and secured to the ear pinna with adhesive strapping. Once this is in position the animal may be allowed to settle down for several minutes before anaesthesia is induced by injection through it and the animal is unaware that this is being made. Ear-punch marks may render this route impossible but when it can be used it is very convenient for most anaesthetic purposes.

The cephalic vein in the fore-leg and the recurrent tarsal vein in the hind-leg are also convenient vessels. They are usually quite obvious after the hair or wool over them has been clipped. A butterfly needle (0.8 mm, i.e. 21 gauge) or a catheter (19 gauge, 5 cm long) introduced into the cephalic vein may be secured in position by taping it to the leg with adhesive strapping but it is not easy to secure these in the recurrent tarsal vein. If the recurrent tarsal vein has to be used for repeated injections a plastic cannula (19 gauge, 5 cm long) should be used for these are much easier to tape in position or to secure to the leg by a skin stitch. Sheep's veins have fragile walls so it is relatively easy to transfix the vein with a needle; plastic catheters are much less likely to give rise to this problem.

Goats have relatively long, thin necks with obvious jugular veins so that jugular venepuncture presents no problems and this may be carried out as described for horses (p. 210). Sheep, on the other hand, have

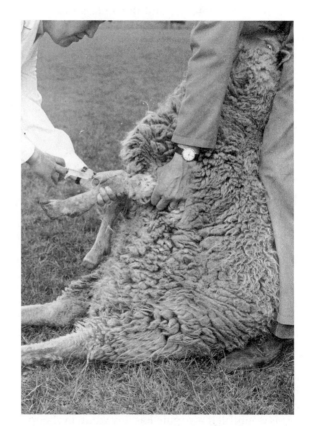

13.5 Restraint of sheep for injection into the cephalic vein. For jugular venepuncture the sheep is similarly restrained in the sitting position but it is not easy to place the needle correctly in the vein with the sheep in this position and hence the injection of irritant substances into the jugular vein of the sitting sheep is to be avoided.

relatively short, thick necks and the jugular furrow is often obscured by fat so that the vein is not obvious. The taking of blood samples from the sheep's jugular vein is a simple matter when the animal is held in the sitting position with the head turned away from the person taking the sample, but the accurate intravenous injection of agents is not so easy. Most anaesthetists prefer to use another vein for the injection of tissue irritants such as thiopentone for this reason.

Endotracheal intubation

In sheep and goats endotracheal intubation is best performed under direct vision with the aid of a laryngoscope. The anaesthetized animal is placed on its back with its head and neck in full extension. An assistant draws the tongue well out of the mouth, holding it in a gauze sponge for better grip, and fixes the upper jaw by pulling gently downwards on the ends of a tape placed just behind the dental pad. The anaesthetist uses a gauze sponge on a sponge-holding forceps to clear the mouth of saliva and any regurgitated ruminal contents, and introduces the laryngoscope so that the tip of its blade is behind the base of the tongue and in front of the epiglottis. The laryngoscope blade is then lifted horizontally to expose the larynx and vocal cords and the tube passed into the trachea under direct vision. It is important that the larynx is brought into view by a lifting movement and not by employing the laryngoscope blade as a lever using the dental pad as a fulcrum.

Endotracheal tubes may also be passed through the mouth and 'threaded' through the larynx which is gripped between the anaesthetist's finger and thumb. When using this method it is sometimes necessary to stiffen the tube by passing down a piece of thick copper wire of suitable length which is withdrawn as soon as the tube is in the trachea. It is difficult to pass tubes of really adequate size by this technique but it is useful if a laryngoscope is not available.

Tubes lubricated with an analgesic jelly may also be passed through the nostril. The inferior nasal meatus is relatively large in sheep and goats and although tubes passed via the nostril must be smaller than those introduced through the mouth reasonably adequately sized ones can be used. If the tube passed up the nostril cannot be introduced blindly through the larynx a laryngoscope is used to expose the tip of the tube in the pharynx and the vocal cords. The tip of the tube is grasped with Magill's intubation forceps and assisted into the laryngeal opening as it is advanced through the nostril.

For large sheep (such as Dorset horn) a 16 mm tube can be passed through the mouth and a 12 mm tube through the nostril. For intubation of adult goats by the oral route 11 and 12 mm tubes are usually adequate.

PREPARATION FOR ANAESTHESIA OF THE SHEEP AND GOAT

Most clinical surgery performed on sheep is carried out at short notice — e.g. caesarean section for dystocia — and there is no time to prepare the animal for anaesthesia. Experience of such situations suggests that there may be little need to withhold food and water before anaesthesia for non-emergency surgery since sheep do not regurgitate copiously at the time of induction of general anaesthesia and any ruminal tympany may be dealt with by passing a stomach tube or by needle paracentesis of the rumen. In goats, planned surgery (e.g. for the repair of fractures) is more common and for this preanaesthetic preparation is possible but, again, experience has shown there is no good reason for denying access to food and water right up to the time of operation.

It is doubtful if atropine has any value in sheep and

goats. The doses necessary to prevent salivation completely (0.2–0.8 mg/kg) produce undesirable tachycardia and ocular effects, while smaller doses merely make the saliva more viscid and hence more difficult to drain from the oropharynx. On the rare occasion when bradycardia develops during general anaesthesia an anticholinergic (e.g. atropine, 0.6–1.2 mg) may be given intravenously.

Sedative premedication is seldom necessary before general anaesthesia and, if given, can delay recovery. It may, however, be useful in counteracting some of the undesirable side-effects of the anaesthetic agents. Probably the best sedative premedication is diazepam given intravenously in doses of 1 mg/kg, or 2 mg/kg intramuscularly; it is particularly effective in both sheep and goats in countering the unwanted actions of ketamine.

GENERAL ANAESTHESIA OF THE SHEEP AND GOAT

Sheep and goats should not be maintained for any longer than is essential in the supine position during general anaesthesia. In this position the weight of the ruminal and intestinal contents compresses the aorta and posterior vena cava, leading to circulatory embarrassment (supine hypotensive syndrome) and

restricts the free movement of the diaphragm, giving rise to respiratory acidosis with decreased tidal volume and alveolar collapse. Whenever possible surgery shoudld be carried out with the animal in lateral decubitus, or in the prone position with the pelvis supported in such a way as to allow free movement of the abdominal wall during breathing. A jointed operating table which is tilted so that the hind-quarters of the laterally recumbent or prone animal are about 15 cm below the level of the withers, to allow the abdominal viscera to fall away from the diaphragm, and the head is inclined downwards to allow saliva and any regurgitated ruminal contents to drain from the mouth, is highly desirable if much surgery is to be performed on sheep and goats.

A cuffed endotracheal tube should always be passed as soon as possible after the induction of anaesthesia to prevent the inhalation of saliva and regurgitated ruminal contents, and for all but the shortest anaesthetics a stomach tube should be intro-duced into the rumen to prevent the development of ruminal tympany. If the rumen still becomes dis-tended with gas in spite of the presence of the stomach tube no time should be lost in performing paracentesis through the left flank with a 14 gauge needle.

Unconscious sheep and goats will continue to produce saliva and because this will not be swallowed and reabsorbed, progressive acidosis develops. These animals may lose up to 500 ml of saliva per hour and during long operations this loss should be replaced by the injection of sodium bicarbonate solution at a rate of 1 mmol/(kg h).

Intravenous anaesthesia of the sheep and goat

What little clinical surgery has to be performed on sheep and goats is probably best carried out under inhalation anaesthesia and the role of the intravenous drugs should only be that of inducing anaesthesia in particularly vigorous animals. Nevertheless, in cer-tain situations, especially when only relatively minor surgery is contemplated, intravenous anaesthesia can be useful.

Pentobarbitone sodium

Many years ago Phillipson and Barnett [10] reported the use of pentobarbitone sodium in sheep. They found that in lambs up to 2 months old a dose of 29 mg/kg by slow intravenous injection gave anaes-thesia of sufficient depth and duration for abdominal surgery. With adult sheep they found great variation in response to the drug. In all cases the duration of anaesthesia was shorter than in lambs — about 15 minutes only. In adult sheep they found that the dose for induction varied from 28 to 33 mg/kg. (Workers in the USA have also observed the greater susceptibility of castrated animals to pentobarbitone sodium.)

Pentobarbitone sodium appears to be a satisfactory anaesthetic for minor operations of short duration in sheep but, in contrast to its effects in other species of animal, detoxication is rapid; the duration of anaes-thesia from a single injection is short and thus it is not satisfactory for prolonged intra-abdominal surgery. Today, most workers prefer to use pentobarbitone simply as an induction agent and to maintain anaes-thesia with an inhalation anaesthetic administered through the endotracheal tube.

Hill [11] and Lukens [12] were probably the first to report the use of pentobarbitone sodium in goats. A more recent record is that of Linzell [13] who reported that the full anaesthetic dose for the goat is about 30 mg/kg for an adult animal and the animal is on its feet in 20–60 minutes from the time of injection. To maintain anaesthesia, further doses of 6–36 mg/(kg h) (according to the depth of anaesthesia required) must be administered.

It is important to note that commercially available solutions of pentobarbitone sodium often contain propylene glycol and this causes haemolysis and haematuria in both goats and sheep [13, 14]. Pento-barbitone solutions for use in these animals should be made up from powder, using 10% ethyl alcohol in saline as a solvent.

Thiopentone sodium

An initial dose of about 10 mg/kg of thiopentone in a 2.5% solution given by intravenous injection pro-duces induction of anaesthesia and, often, 30–50 seconds of apnoea. During the period of apnoea, muscle relaxation is profound enough for the jaw to be opened widely and endotracheal intubation to be performed. Recovery from thiopentone is consider-ably quicker than from pentobarbitone and is usually quiet and uneventful. Defaecation always occurs during anaesthesia and regurgitation of ruminal con-tents is not uncommon. Today, thiopentone sodium is extensively used to induce anaesthesia which is to be maintained by endotracheal inhalation methods.

Methohexitone sodium

In both sheep and goats the intravenous injection of 4 mg/kg of a 2.5% solution of methohexitone sodium produces anaesthesia of 5–7 minutes' duration. Re-covery to the standing position is complete within 10–14 minutes of the injection but the recovery is usually associated with violent jerking or convulsive move-ments and excitement if the animal is disturbed by noise during this period. Anaesthesia may be pro-longed by the injection of 50–75 mg/min of the drug [15].

Recovery excitement may be prevented by pre-medication with diazepam or xylazine. After such premedication the dose of methohexitone required for induction of anaesthesia is about 2 mg/kg and the whole course of anaesthesia is smoother.

Methohexitone has been used as an induction agent before inhalation anaesthesia in very small lambs of 1–2 weeks of age with reasonably satisfactory results, but it is probable that in lambs of this age induction with the inhalation anaesthetic is safer.

Ketamine

Clinically, ketamine appears to be an extremely safe drug for sheep and goats but experimental evidence to support this observation is difficult to obtain because these animals are so nervous or excitable that control values for the various physiological functions which need to be studied are almost impossible to determine. The drug is used on its own or with other agents to increase skeletal muscle relaxation and to suppress its excitatory effects.

When used on its own, ketamine produces in both sheep and goats a peculiar state in which there appears to be profound analgesia yet the animal seems aware of its surroundings and the ability to eructate, cough and swallow is maintained. Intravenous injection of the drug causes an initial fall in arterial blood pressure, the extent of which is dose dependent. The hypotension is short lived and at surgically useful dose levels is usually followed by a mild hypertensive phase. It also causes an initial brief period of respiratory depression but because of the difficulty in establishing control values it is impossible to say whether this is associated with any significant alteration in blood gas tensions.

Taylor *et al.* [16] considered that 2 mg/kg produced ideal anaesthesia for intrauterine surgery in sheep, and Thurman *et al.* [17] also found ketamine alone to be a satisfactory agent for these animals. Clinical experience at the Cambridge Veterinary School has not confirmed these reports. Intravenous doses of up to 20 mg/kg have been found to be necessary for caesarean section and after this the shepherd has commented that the lambs delivered behaved 'peculiarly' for some hours. Intramuscular doses of 20 mg/kg appear to be effective for the sedation of sheep and it is claimed that they do not affect physiological variables [18].

It seems that more generally satisfactory results are obtained when ketamine is used in combination with other agents and numerous techniques and combinations are currently in vogue.

In many sheep reasonably satisfactory anaesthesia may be produced by the simultaneous intravenous injection of 4 mg/kg of ketamine and 0.05 mg/kg of xylazine or 2 mg/kg diazepam. In some animals, however, really adequate surgical anaesthesia is only obtained when, in addition, nitrous oxide/oxygen mixtures are administered. Mixtures of medetomidine and ketamine (25 µg/kg plus 1 mg/kg ketamine) will produce reasonable anaesthesia when given by intramuscular injection and anaesthesia can be prolonged by the administration of half doses of this mixture as necessary.

In goats, Kumar *et al.* [19] considered intramuscular xylazine/ketamine to be both safe and useful. In 20 animals quoted, anaesthesia was induced with 0.22 mg/kg xylazine and 11 mg/kg ketamine after premedication with 0.4 mg/kg of atropine. Intravenous injection of a mixture of 2 mg/kg diazepam with 4 mg/kg of ketamine also seems satisfactory.

It must be noted that xylazine, diazepam and ketamine are all expensive agents and their use in sheep and goats may be difficult to justify when other much less expensive and equally satisfactory agents (e.g. thiopentone, Saffan, halothane) are available.

Saffan

In both sheep and goats anaesthesia may be induced in healthy animals by the intravenous injection of 2.2 mg/kg Saffan [20]. Waterman [21] also found these doses satisfactory for induction of anaesthesia and endotracheal intubation when intubation could be performed within 2 minutes of the injection but she preferred a slightly higher dose of 3 mg/kg as it gave more time for moving the sheep and positioning it on the operating table for intubation. In old or debilitated animals, however, doses of 2 mg/kg may produce profound anaesthesia with marked relaxation of the jaw muscles and suppression of protective pharyngeal and laryngeal reflexes.

Heart rate, arterial blood pressure, cardiac output and respiratory rate are extremely labile in sheep and it is difficult to obtain control values but in general the intravenous injection of 2.2 mg/kg of Saffan produces a short-lived decrease in heart rate and arterial pressure with some slowing of respiration and myocardial depression. Apnoea is not produced and the animal's mucous membranes remain pink throughout the period of anaesthesia when the animal is breathing room air. These doses of 2.2 mg/kg can be expected to provide about 10 minutes of surgical anaesthesia with recovery to the standing position about 20 minutes after injection.

The effects of Saffan on the heart rate, blood pressure and respiratory rate are dose dependent. Higher doses of 4.4 mg/kg produce about 15 minutes of anaesthesia with complete recovery after a further 30 minutes. They usually produce an immediate decrease in heart rate and blood pressure with temporary apnoea.

Circulatory depression appears to result from a direct action of the steroids on the myocardium (C.

M. Stowe, personal communication), and cannot be attributed to the vehicle Cremophor EL.

Salivation occurs during anaesthesia and some animals regurgitate so, as is usual in ruminants, endotracheal intubation with a cuffed tube is essential to prevent aspiration. The absence of marked respiratory depression means that in healthy animals oxygen supplementation of the inspired air is usually unnecessary, although it may be in anaemic animals or in those with abdominal distension. Muscle relaxation is good and lambs delivered from ewes anaesthetized with Saffan show few signs of respiratory or circulatory depression. Recovery from anaesthesia may be associated with an increased sensitivity to noise and physical stimulation; there may be some muscle twitching and limb paddling but this is seldom seen if the animal is left undisturbed.

Saffan may be given to maintain anaesthesia for longer periods either by intermittent injection or intravenous infusion. After induction with 2.2 mg/kg, continuous infusion of 0.23 mg/(kg min) [20] to 0.24 mg/(kg min) [21] is sufficient to maintain anaesthesia. Recovery is remarkably rapid and most sheep will stand up well within 30 minutes of termination of the infusion.

When facilities for inhalation anaesthesia are not available, Saffan seems to be the best agent for the induction and maintenance of anaesthesia in sheep. Experience in goats is more limited, but these animals appear to behave in a very similar manner [22] and there is no reason to suppose Saffan to be any less useful in them.

Inhalation anaesthesia of the sheep and goat

All the factors which complicate inhalation anaesthesia in cattle are also encountered in sheep and goats. The anaesthetist must be prepared to deal with copious salivation, the regurgitation of rumen contents and, when anaesthesia is prolonged, the occurrence of ruminal tympany.

Nitrous oxide

In sheep and goats nitrous oxide is often used to maintain anaesthesia which has been induced with an intravenous agent. Anaesthesia is induced, the animal intubated with a cuffed endotracheal tube and a mixture of nitrous oxide and oxygen administered. Either a non-rebreathing system or a semi-closed system with carbon dioxide absorption may be used. Nitrous oxide is run into the circuit at the rate of 4 l/min and oxygen at a rate of 2 l/min, and quite commonly the mixture is supplemented by the addition of minimal quantities of halothane, ether, meth-

oxyflurane, enflurane or isoflurane. Nitrous oxide will always diffuse into the rumen and gut so that tympany, serious enough to interfere with breathing, may develop.

Ether

Although sheep and goats can be forcibly restrained and compelled to breathe the pungent vapour of ether, its inhalation by the conscious animal produces profuse salivation. Furthermore, induction of anaesthesia with ether is a slow process which is most unpleasant for the animal. For these reasons ether is usually only used as an agent for the maintenance of anaesthesia following induction with an intravenous drug. It is either volatilized with oxygen and administered by endotracheal low-flow methods, or used to supplement nitrous oxide/oxygen mixtures given by non-rebreathing techniques.

Halothane

Because of its potency halothane is an excellent anaesthetic for sheep and goats of all ages. It is usually vaporized with oxygen or a nitrous oxide/oxygen mixture and administered by non-rebreathing or low-flow techniques.

Anaesthesia is induced almost to the point of respiratory failure with a mixture containing 3–4% of halothane vapour delivered through a close-fitting face-mask. This usually takes from 3 to 4 minutes. The mask is removed from the face and endotracheal intubation is performed rapidly as anaesthesia lightens. Anaesthesia is maintained with an inspired mixture containing 1–1.5% of halothane vapour and inexperienced anaesthetists find it easier to maintain smooth anaesthesia when a non-rebreathing or low-flow system, rather than a completely closed system, is used.

During halothane anaesthesia arterial blood pressure is decreased in a dose-dependent manner and adjusting the inspired halothane concentration to maintain a constant blood pressure is often used as a means of ensuring a constant level of central nervous depression. At surgical levels of anaesthesia the spontaneous respiratory rate is usually between 15 and 18 breaths/min but shallow, rapid breathing is not uncommon and its cause is not always obvious.

Recovery from anaesthesia is rapid even after prolonged administration. Induction of anaesthesia with an intravenous agent makes endotracheal intubation less of a hurried procedure, but prolongs the recovery period.

Methoxyflurane

In sheep and goats methoxyflurane is usually used to supplement nitrous oxide/oxygen mixtures delivered through non-rebreathing systems. It has no obvious advantage over halothane.

Other fluorinated agents

Enflurane, isoflurane and sevoflurane have apparently not been used to anaesthetize sheep or goats for clinical surgery. They are more expensive and are unlikely to offer any major advantages over halothane in these animals.

The recovery period

After general anaesthesia the endotracheal tube should be left in place until the animal has regained the swallowing and cough reflexes. As in all ruminants, sheep and goats should be propped up in the prone position, supported on either side by bales, so that eructation can take place during the recovery period. They should be kept under observation to ensure that tympany does not develop due to them slipping into lateral recumbency. Hypothermia is unlikely to occur unless the environment is exceptionally cold.

The relief of postoperative pain demands the same care in sheep and goats as in all other animals. Because they do not become violent when in pain it is often assumed that they are comfortable when in fact pain may be acute. The different, much more normal behaviour seen after the administration of a suitable analgesic is often remarkable. Up to 10 mg of morphine or 250 mg of pethidine by intramuscular injection is usually adequate for up to 4 hours in spite of experimental evidence of a much shorter period of effectiveness.

OTHER HERBIVORES

Anaesthesia of species of animal which are of economic importance is still evolving in developing countries as drugs and anaesthetic apparatus become available. In an era where tremendous advancement has been made in veterinary anaesthesia there is still a place in these countries for relatively simple and inexpensive techniques. The main concern is with buffaloes, camels and elephants but the importance of the llama is increasing. Satisfactory techniques of sedation and anaesthesia for use in these animals are emerging but clearly there is scope for improvement. Research in anaesthesia is hampered by restrictions on the import of drugs, the prohibitive price of anaesthetic apparatus and the non-availability of trained personnel [23].

Camels (*Camelus dromedarius*)

Local and regional analgesia

Nerve blocks of the hind-limb in camels were reported by Dudi *et al.* [24]. These workers described the topographical anatomy and technique of nerve blocks of the peroneal, tibial and plantar nerves with 2% lignocaine. However, it is probable that intravenous regional analgesia for foot operations as reported by Purohit *et al.* [25], being easier to perform, will always be preferred for desensitization of the digit. Intravenous regional analgesia may be produced by the injection of 60 ml of 2% lignocaine (without adrenaline) distal to a tourniquet applied half-way down the limb without prior exsanguination.

Epidural block may be produced by the injection of 2% lignocaine or its equivalent at the sacrococcygeal or first intercoccygeal space. A 5 cm long, 19 gauge needle is inserted at an angle of about 45° with the horizontal in an animal restrained in the sitting position. For caudal block 12–15 ml of solution is adequate; 50 ml will produce sensory block caudally from the umbilicus.

Chloral hydrate

The use of chloral hydrate to produce anaesthesia in camels was described many years ago [26, 27] and this drug is still extensively used to sedate or even anaesthetize camels in developing countries [28]. Intravenous administration of 100 mg/kg as a 10% solution produces a marked tachycardia, sustained arterial hypotension, respiratory acidosis and mild hypoxaemia but no changes in the electrocardiogram [28]. Muscle relaxation is not marked.

The use of a combination of chloral hydrate and magnesium sulphate results in less tachycardia and greater muscle relaxation with less respiratory depression than the use of chloral hydrate alone [29].

Guaiphenesin and thiopentone

Guaiphenesin (100–110 mg/kg) intravenously produces ataxia and intravenous thiopentone (4.5 mg/kg) may then be used to produce anaesthesia [29] which can be maintained with halothane/oxygen administered by mask or through an endotracheal tube using a low-flow absorption method.

α_2-adrenoceptor agonists

Xylazine given intramuscularly at a dosage rate of 0.4 mg/kg produces obvious sedation after about 9 minutes, followed quite quickly by recumbency. Recovery to the standing position occurs some 3 hours after injection. Arterial hypotension is not associated with elevated central venous pressure or bradycardia, but marked hyperglycaemia occurs [30]. It is presumed that vagal stimulation is responsible for first-degree atrioventricular block, sinoatrial block, sinus arrhythmia and wandering pacemaker in the sinoatrial node. This dose of xylazine is claimed to provide adequate sedation and analgesia with sufficient muscle relaxation for minor surgery of short duration.

Intravenous xylazine 0.5 mg/kg produces a state bordering on full anaesthesia which lasts for approximately 30 minutes; the animals usually sit up after about 45 minutes and stand about 15 minutes later. The xylazine antagonist, tolazoline, given intravenously in doses of 0.4 mg/kg 15 minutes after the administration of the xylazine, enables the animals to stand 15 minutes later [31].

Detomidine in doses of 50 μg/kg by intramuscular injection usually produces recumbency within 10 minutes. As sedation develops the neck muscles relax and the head droops. Ataxia is followed by voluntary sternal recumbency. Preliminary studies indicate that analgesia can be expected to be present for the next 1½ hours. The heart rate, respiratory rate and rectal temperature show little change from preinjection levels during the period of sedation. Recovery is quiet and the animals stand about 3 hours from the time of injection. Although there are no reports of their use it is likely that the α_2-adrenoceptor antagonists can be given to hasten recovery from detomidine sedation.

Ketamine

Ketamine (1–2 mg/kg intravenously) may be used after xylazine (0.4–0.5 mg/kg intramuscularly) to produce anaesthesia of approximately 30 minutes' duration with good muscle relaxation. Full recovery takes about 3 hours from the time of the ketamine injection. Because intravenous ketamine injection may be followed by a rather long period of apnoea many workers prefer to give this drug intramuscularly. The doses of both xylazine and ketamine may be reduced in tame, working camels and in the very young.

Inhalation anaesthesia

Inhalation anaesthesia is best administered through an endotracheal tube but intubation in male animals can be difficult due to the 'goola' pouches. Interference from the pouches can be minimized by ensuring free respiration through the nostrils during the intubation process; the tube is not likely to enter the pouch opening for this faces caudally and not cranially. It is advisable to induce complete relaxation of the jaw muscles with an intravenous or intramuscular agent so that the mouth can be opened widely. In the adult the technique of intubation is similar to that used in cattle (p. 254) but the male animal has prominent canine teeth and in both sexes the cheek teeth are usually very sharp. The use of a good mouth gag to protect the anaesthetist's arm is almost essential. Small, young animals are best intubated using a laryngoscope and difficulties arise when the animal has grown too large for this and the mouth cavity is too small to admit a palpating hand. Blind intubation is possible if the head and neck are extended and the tube is stiffened with a maleable stilette but can be more difficult than in cattle.

Halothane is the least expensive of the inhalation agents used today and is usually given after induction of unconsciousness with an intravenous or intramuscular agent. Respiratory depression is marked and it is a common practice to fast camels for 48 hours prior to general anaesthesia to minimize the weight of the forestomach and prevent tympany from developing. Respiratory function is best maintained when the animal is in sternal recumbency and this position should always be adopted for the recovery period.

It is generally agreed that regurgitation of stomach contents occurs more readily in camels than in cattle. In camels the oesophagus enters directly into the forestomach unlike in cattle where the oesophageal opening is at the junction of the rumen and the reticulum. It is not known whether this difference accounts for the higher incidence of regurgitation in anaesthetized camels.

Buffaloes (*Bubalus bubalis*)

Most anaesthetic techniques for the buffalo have been adapted from those used in cattle but there are marked differences in the way in which they respond to some agents.

α_2-adrenoceptor agonists

The effects of xylazine on buffalo calves have been reported [32–34]. Intravenous doses of 0.22–0.44 mg/kg produce dose-related duration of sedation from 65 to 130 minutes. Intramuscular doses of 0.44 mg/kg produce inability to stand for some 150 minutes while intramuscular administration of 0.22 mg/kg of xylazine produces excellent sedation, analgesia and moderate muscle relaxation with an onset time of 10–15 minutes and a duration of approximately 45–60 minutes.

Preliminary trials of detomidine indicate that 20 µg/kg by intramuscular injection produces deep sedation of about 30 minutes' duration. This dose may be associated with recumbency, but there is no evidence of cutaneous analgesia and the swallowing reflex is not abolished in the sedated animal. Intramuscular doses of 40 µg/kg cause the animal to lie down and saliva runs from the mouth but it is not clear whether this indicates increased production of saliva or inability to swallow the normal quantities; recovery is usually complete in 50–70 minutes. Micturition is usual as sedation develops and vocalization is not uncommon. Under deep detomidine sedation the P_aCO_2 is usually about 43 mmHg (5.7 kPa) and the P_aO_2 about 75 mmHg (10 kPa).

There appear to be no reports of α_2-adrenoceptor antagonists being used to hasten the awakening of buffaloes given xylazine or detomidine, but there is no obvious reason why they should not be given for this purpose.

Chloral hydrate

Administered intravenously at doses of between 0.13 and 0.18 g/kg, chloral hydrate was found to be superior to the barbiturates by Gadzhiev [35]. The drug has also been administered mixed with magnesium sulphate and a barbiturate [36] in the proportions of 30 g chloral hydrate, 15 g magnesium sulphate and 2.5 g thiopentone per litre. Some 2 ml/kg of this mixture produce anaesthesia of 15–25 minutes' duration.

Guaiphenesin

The intravenous infusion of 165 mg/kg of guaiphenesin to buffalo calves has been found to produce unacceptable levels of arterial hypotension and respiratory depression [36]. Smaller doses may be free from these disadvantages.

Ketamine

The use of ketamine on its own and with chlorpromazine hydrochloride in buffalo calves on blood glucose, serum glutamic pyruvic transaminase, serum glutamic oxaloacetic transaminase and lactic dehydrogenase was investigated by Pathak *et al.* [37].

In buffalo calves up to 1.5 years old, 2 mg/kg of ketamine by intravenous injection produces an anaesthetic effect of 3–5 minutes' duration. This is characterized by rigidity of the limb muscles but analgesia seems profound. Intramuscular injection of 2 mg/kg of chlorpromazine 15 minutes prior to the intravenous injection of this dose of ketamine is reported to double the duration of analgesia and abolish the muscle rigidity [38].

The combination of xylazine (0.22 mg/kg intramuscularly) with ketamine (2 mg/kg intravenously) has been reported [39]. It produces satisfactory general anaesthesia of 30–45 minutes' duration with good muscle relaxation. Recovery to the standing position is seen some 80 minutes after the ketamine injection. Slight ataxia persists for a further 10–15 minutes.

Inhalation anaesthetics

Buffaloes may be intubated and anaesthesia maintained as for cattle.

Llama

In the developed countries interest in llamas as companion or pack animals is increasing. As yet there is little information available regarding their anaesthetic management but this is currently being investigated in many centres so that more knowledge should soon be available. One such investigation was that of Gavier *et al.* [40] who studied the use of xylazine, ketamine and halothane with spontaneous breathing and with mechanically controlled ventilation of the lungs. The intravenous administration of 0.25 mg/kg of xylazine followed 5 minutes later with ketamine (2.5 mg/kg intravenously) produced satisfactory conditions for endotracheal intubation. The adult llama was intubated with a 12 mm bore tube, 45 cm long, and anaesthesia maintained with halothane in oxygen. Hypercapnia and respiratory acidosis were seen during spontaneous respiration. During both spontaneous breathing and controlled lung ventilation marked cardiovascular depression developed during maintenance of anaesthesia with halothane. Thus, it appears that the problems of general anaesthesia may be very similar to those encountered in horses.

Elephant

Only the Indian or Asiatic elephant can be regarded as a domestic animal. Trained elephants are usually relatively quiet and intravenous injection into an ear vein presents no great difficulty but animals that are not so tame may need to be dosed by dart-gun.

Xylazine (0.08–0.15 mg/kg) given by intravenous or intramuscular injection may be used to sedate elephants. They become somnolent but usually remain standing and recovery from a single dose takes about 3 hours.

Etorphine at a dose of 2 µg/kg will yield satisfactory sedation for the performance of venepuncture and the administration of drugs such as thiopentone to produce the desired depth of anaesthesia. Endotracheal intubation presents no difficulty for the mouth can usually be opened widely. Maintenance of anaesthesia is usually with halothane/oxygen and, at the end, the administration of diprenorphine at twice the etorphine dose hastens recovery. Some anaesthetists prefer the use of Immobilon (2.45 mg etorphine plus 10 mg/ml acepromazine per ml) to plain etorphine, claiming the mixture to be more effective than etorphine on its own.

The most detailed account of anaesthesia in elephants is that of A. Webb (personal communication). At the University of Florida School, Webb sedated juvenile elephants (between 3 and 5 years old) weighing between 300 and 650 kg for transport with a xylazin/ketamine cocktail (0.1 and 0.6 mg/kg respectively by intramuscular injection). He then induced anaesthesia with intramuscular etorphine (2 µg/kg) which took about 20 minutes to produce recumbency and unconsciousness. Oral intubation with a cuffed endotracheal tube was performed by manual palpation, checking to exclude the presence of food residues in the mouth. Bivona, thick-walled, endotracheal tubes of 18 mm internal diameter i.d. were used for elephants up to 250 kg bodyweight, 22 mm i.d. for those up to 300 kg, 26 mm i.d. for up to 450 kg, and 30 mm i.d. tubes were used for any larger animals. Anaesthesia was maintained with halothane in oxygen, the initial vaporizer setting with a fresh gas flow rate of 3–5 l/min (i.e. a 'low-flow'

setting) to a large animal circle absorber system being less than 1%, rising to 1–2% after the first 40–60 minutes. With spontaneous breathing blood gas values were in the region of 80–150 mmHg (10.7–20 kPa) for the P_aO_2 and 50–60 mmHg (6.7–8 kPa) for the P_aCO_2, with typical respiratory rates of 6–12 breaths/min. If the P_aCO_2 climbed to around 60 mmHg (8 kPa) IPPV was performed using an equine ventilator set to deliver between 5 and 10 ml/kg. Heart rates were between 40–60 beats/min and the systolic blood pressure was well maintained at over 100 mmHg. Of 20 elephants, two developed episodes of ventricular arrhythmias and one showed second-degree heart block. Monitoring was via an ECG (lead 2 with the electrodes set for a base–apex system) and arterial blood pressure by intra-arterial pressure recording from an auricular artery or by using a Doppler-shift flow detector distal to a pressure cuff on the tail. At the end of anaesthesia the halothane was turned off and when good jaw muscle tone was present diprenorphine was given at twice the dose of etorphine used for the induction of anaesthesia. Extubation was carried out as soon as the animals rose to sternal recumbency. Because of hot weather conditions all the animals were given balanced electrolyte solutions at the rate of 10–20 ml/kg/h from the time of induction of anaesthesia until just before extubation. In his series of cases Webb encountered one animal which seemed to collapse when given the diprenorphine and ventilatory support was needed.

REFERENCES

1. De Koch, G. and Quinlan, J. (1926) *11th and 12th Reports*, Part I. Department of Agriculture Union of South Africa, p. 361.
2. Bessalaar, H. J. and Quin, J. I. (1935) *Onderstepoort Journal of Veterinary Science* 5, 501.
3. Dukes, H. H. and Sampson, J. (1937) *Cornell Veterinarian* 27, 139.
4. Waterman, A. E., Livingstone, A., Bouchenafa, O. and Dash, A. (1988) *Advances in Veterinary Anaesthesia, Brisbane*, p. 94.
5. Klein, L., Tomasic, M. and Nann, L. (1988) *Advances in Veterinary Anaesthesia, Brisbane*, p. 70.
6. Vitums, A. (1954) *Journal of the American Veterinary Medical Association* 125, 294.
7. Taylor, P. M. (1980) *Goat Veterinary Society Journal* 1, 4.
8. McFarlane, L. S. (1963) *Journal of the South African Veterinary Medical Association* 34, 73.
9. Grono, L. R. (1966) *Australian Veterinary Journal* 42, 58.
10. Phillipson, A. T. and Barnett, S. F. (1939) *Veterinary Record* 51, 869.
11. Hill, R. T., Turner, C. W., Uren, A. E. and Gomez, E. T. (1935) *Research Bulletin Montana Agriculture Experimental Station*, No. 230.
12. Lukens, F. D. W. (1937) *American Journal of Physiology* 122, 729.
13. Linzell, J. L. (1964) *Small Animal Anaesthesia*. Oxford: Pergamon Press.
14. Potter, G. B. (1958) *British Journal of Pharmacology* 13, 385.
15. Robertshaw, D. (1966) *Veterinary Record* 78, 433.
16. Taylor, P., Hopkins, L., Young, M. and McFadyean, I. R. (1972) *Veterinary Record* 90, 35.
17. Thurman, J. C., Kumar, A. and Link, R. P. (1973) *Journal of the American Veterinary Medical Association* 162, 293.
18. Britton, B. J., Wood, W. G. and Irving, M. N. (1974) *Laboratory Animals* 8, 41.
19. Kumar, A., Thurman, J. C. and Hardenbrook, H. J. (1976) *Veterinary Medicine/Small Animal Clinician* 71, 1707.
20. Hall, L. W. (1972) *Postgraduate Medical Journal* 48 (Suppl. 2), 55.
21. Waterman, A. E. (1981) *Research in Veterinary Science* 30, 144.
22. Foex, P. and Prys-Roberts, C. (1972) *Postgraduate Medical Journal* 48 (Suppl. 2), 24.
23. Tyagi, R. P. S. (1988) *Advances in Veterinary Anaesthesia, Brisbane*, p. 21.
24. Dudi, P. R., Chouhan, D. S., Choudhary, R. J., Deora, K. S. and Gahlot, T. K. (1984) *Indian Veterinary Journal* 61, 848.
25. Purohit, N. R., Chouhan, D. S., Chaudhary, R. J. and Deora, K. S. (1985) *Indian Journal of Veterinary Sciences* 55, 435.

26. Singh, R., Rathore, S. S. and Kohli, R. N. (1962) *Indian Veterinary Journal* **39**, 614.
27. Said, A. H. (1964) *Veterinary Record* **76**, 550.
28. Sharma, S. K., Jit Singh, Peshin, P. K. and Singh, A. P. (1983) *Zentralblatt für Veterinarmedizin* **30**, 674.
29. Sharma, S. K., Jit Singh, Singh, A. P. and Peshin, P. K. (1984) *Research in Veterinary Science* **36**, 12.
30. Peshin, P. K., Nigam, J. M., Singh, S. C. and Robinson, B. A. (1980) *Journal of the American Veterinary Medical Association* **177**, 875.
31. Bonarth, K. H., Nouth, S. R., Evans, J., Amelang, D., Axt, U. and Bonarth, I. (1988) *Advances in Veterinary Anaesthesia, Brisbane*, p. 227.
32. Peshin, P. K. and Kumar, A. (1983) *Indian Journal of Animal Health* **22**, 139.
33. Peshin, P. K. and Kumar, A. (1983) *Indian Veterinary Journal* **60**, 981.
34. Peshin, P. K., Kumar, A. and Singh, H. (1978) *Pantnagar Journal of Research* **3**, 245.
35. Gadzhiev, M. A. (1955) *Trud. Mosk. Vet. Akad.*, p. 236.
36. Johari, M. P. and Sharma, S. P. (1962) *Indian Journal of Veterinary Science* **32**, 235.
37. Singh, J., Sobti, V. K., Kohli, R. N., Kumar, V. R. and Khanna, A. K. (1981) *Zentralblatt für Veterinarmedizin* **28**, 60.
38. Pathak, S. C., Nigam, J. M., Peshin, P. K. and Singh, A. P. (1982) *Indian Journal of Animal Science* **52**, 319.
39. Singh, A. P. Jit Singh, Peshin, P. K., Gahlawat, J. S., Prem Singh and Nigam, J. M. (1985) *Zentralblatt für Veterinarmedizin* **32**, 54.
40. Gavier, D., Kittleson, M. D., Fowler, M. E., Johnson, L. E., Hall, G. and Nearenberg, D. (1988) *American Journal of Veterinary Research* **49**, 2047.

CHAPTER 14

ANAESTHESIA OF THE PIG

On the farm, surgery may be carried out on pigs using either local analgesia or general anaesthesia. Where local analgesia is used, the pig is usually first heavily sedated or even lightly anaesthetized to prevent the loud squealing noises which these animals make when restrained. When general anaesthesia is employed under farm conditions, simple methods giving short-term anaesthesia suffice, as surgery is usually limited in complexity. However, the pig is often used as an experimental animal in research projects involving long and complicated surgery and in such circumstances sophisticated anaesthetic techniques, possibly even including cardiopulmonary bypass, may be required.

Pigs range in size from small newborn piglets to adult boars weighing 350 kg, and methods of restraint and for the administration of anaesthesia must be varied accordingly. Whilst small pigs are easily re-

strained, large sows and boars may prove both difficult and dangerous. Large pigs are usually restrained by a rope or wire snare around the upper jaw, behind the canine teeth (Fig. 14.1). In most cases the pig will try to escape by pulling back against this rope or snare and thus immobilizes itself, but this method does not work if the animal moves forward to attack (as a sow attempting to defend her litter may do). Smaller pigs are usually restrained on their sides by grasping the undermost legs and leaning on the body. Pigs are easily trained and, at a research establishment, the problems of restraint are greatly reduced by regular handling, as often as possible. In a large intensive farming unit, however, there is a lack of individual handling and some animals may be extremely difficult to control.

In general, pigs are good subjects for general anaesthesia. Although they resent restraint, as is

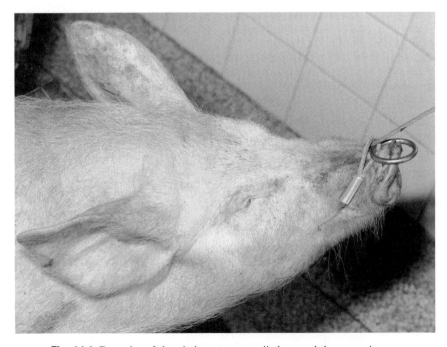

Fig. 14.1 Restraint of the pig by a snare applied around the upper jaw.

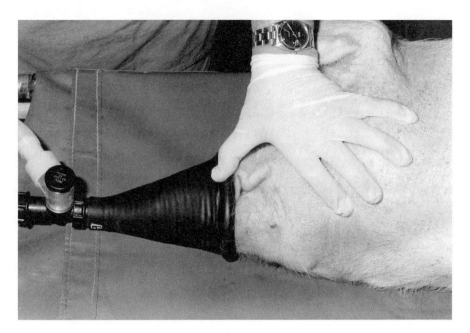

Fig. 14.2 Maintaining a clear airway by pushing forward on the vertical ramus of the mandible with the tongue drawn forward out of the mouth. For ease of photography, in this illustration the mask is held firmly on the face by the thumb, but the position of the hand is usually reversed, the thumb being used to push on the mandible and the fingers to hold the mask on the face.

shown by the struggling and loud squeals which they produce, this does not seem to result in adrenaline release with the attendant dangers during subsequent anaesthesia. Recovery from anaesthesia is usually calm. As they have little body hair, pigs are liable to develop hypothermia when sedated or anaesthetized, but this lack of hair does enable the anaesthetist to assess the state of peripheral circulation by monitoring the skin colour. Pigs tend to be fat and adipose tissue forms a depot for anaesthetics. The fatty nature of the tissue also makes accurate intramuscular injection more difficult in these animals. The shape of the pig's head, together with the fat in the pharyngeal region coupled with the small larynx and trachea, makes respiratory obstruction likely in both sedated and anaesthetized animals. The airway is best maintained by applying pressure behind the vertical ramus of the mandible and thus pushing the jaw forward, while the tongue is drawn out between the incisor teeth (Fig. 14.2). Salivation, even if not excessive, can contribute to airway obstruction in these animals so anticholinergic premedication should be used before general anaesthesia.

PORCINE MALIGNANT HYPERTHERMIA

Although in the vast majority of pigs general anaesthesia presents few problems other than those associated with the maintenance of a clear airway, some strains and breeds suffer from a biochemical myopathy which manifests itself during general anaesthesia with some anaesthetic and ancillary agents. Hall *et al.* [1] first reported its occurrence in Landrace-cross pigs following the use of suxamethonium during halothane anaesthesia, but it was later found that it could occur without the administration of suxamethonium. Breeding experiments with this strain of pigs showed the abnormality to be inherited as an autosomal dominant with variable penetrance, occasional litters being found without susceptible animals. In some litters, however, piglets died before testing with a non-lethal test procedure which had been devised [2], so this finding must be treated with some reserve. It is also possible that two genes might have been involved but, unfortunately, due to withdrawal of funding, opportunity for investigation of this possibility was not followed up.

The abnormal response of these pigs to anaesthetic and other drugs was characterized by the development of generalized muscle rigidity, a severe and sustained rise in body temperature, hyperkalaemia and metabolic acidosis. Since this first report of the porcine syndrome there have been numerous other reports of similar abnormal responses to anaesthetic agents, both in humans and animals and it is generally agreed that the syndrome has certain resemblances to the 'stress reaction' seen in Pietrain and Poland–China pigs. There are, however, some striking differences between the syndrome as manifested in the various breeds and strains. For example, in South Africa, Harrison [3] was able to use thiopentone/nitrous oxide anaesthesia to set up experimental preparations in their strain of Landrace-cross animals before inducing the syndrome by the administration of halothane and suxamethonium. Hall *et al.* [2] were unable to trigger the reaction in their Landrace-cross pigs after they had received thiopentone. The South African workers also found that halothane would initiate the typical syndrome in the presence of neuromuscular block produced by tubocurarine but while this relaxant did not abolish it did modify the response in the British strain of pigs. In Poland–China and Pietrain pigs, dyspnoea, hyperthermia and immediate rigor mortis can be induced by environmental stress associated with exercise, transportation, and high ambient temperatures (according to Nelson, quoted by Ellis [4]). Landrace pigs develop the syndrome only when anaesthetized and, as far as is known, exercise, transportation, and exposure to high ambient temperatures never produce anything resembling the condition.

In 1970, Kalow [5] suggested that malignant hyperthermia in man could be a syndrome resulting from more than one defect, and the same may be true for the porcine syndrome. It seems likely that it is the resistance or susceptibility to triggering factors which differs, and that the final metabolic derangement which leads to death is common to all. Experience to date is that while the pig is proving a valuable experimental animal for the study of this condition, great caution is necessary in transposing results from one breed or strain of pigs to another breed or strain, to another species of animal, or to man.

Early clinical findings suggested that the primary abnormality is to be found in the voluntary muscle of the affected animals and attempts have been made to find a biochemical 'marker' which could support this suggestion and which might serve to identify experimental animals (and more particularly human beings) at risk. Raised serum creatine phosphokinase (CPK) levels have been reported in a number of myopathies both in humans and in experimental animals [6, 7] and there have been reports of raised serum CPK levels in relatives of human patients who have reacted abnormally to halothane or suxamethonium [8, 9]. The serum levels of this enzyme were studied in Landrace-cross pigs [10] and it was found that raised CPK levels in unanaesthetized animals had a fair predictive value for the development of abnormal muscle contracture following induction with halo-

thane and the use of suxamethonium. Of 34 closely related animals studied, 25 had serum CPK levels in excess of 250 units/l and 20 of these were abnormal reactors. Clearly the finding in an animal of a serum CPK level of less than 250 units/l does not rule out the possibility of an abnormal reaction, but the chances of this happening are much lower.

A non-lethal test procedure for identifying potential reactors was described by Hall *et al.* [2], halothane administration, close intra-arterial injection of suxamethonium and intravenous injection of this relaxant being used to detect susceptible animals. The animals were anaesthetized with a halothane/oxygen mixture delivered through a face-mask and some developed muscular rigidity during induction. In these the administration of halothane was stopped and the animal was immediately immersed up to its neck in a bath of cold water. This measure prevented a fatal rise in body temperature, and the muscle rigidity passed off after 15–25 minutes' immersion. Recovery of consciousness was delayed for 1–2 hours. In animals which did not become rigid during induction 2–5 mg of suxamethonium chloride (depending on the size of the animal) was injected as a 1% solution in normal saline into one femoral artery. In normal pigs this produced fasciculation followed by complete flaccidity in the muscle deriving its blood supply from that artery. The muscular flaccidity was easily recognized by comparing the ease of flexion of the joints of the hind-legs. After obtaining a negative response to these tests normality was confirmed by the lack of abnormal response to an intravenous injection of 10–25 mg of suxamethonium to the anaesthetized animal. In animals classified as reactors the fasciculation following the intra-arterial injection was unusually severe and was succeeded by rigidity of the involved muscles. Occasionally, bulging of the affected muscles was observed, but in every case muscle rigidity was easily recognized by comparison of the ease with which the joints of the hind-limbs could be flexed and extended. The rigidity passed off within 1–2 minutes and the animals were allowed to regain consciousness without being challenged with an intravenous dose of suxamethonium.

It must be emphasized that the clinical veterinary anaesthetist is very unlikely to encounter cases of porcine malignant hyperthermia except in the Poland–China and Pietrain breeds, but it may occur in Large White and Landrace pigs (particularly in view of the modern practice of breeding from boars known to carry the trait) so he or she should be aware that the condition exists and be able to recognize it should it be encountered. In a typical case, where a susceptible pig is given a triggering agent, its muscles develop contracture making the animal very stiff or even rigid ('stiff pig disease'). Often, the first sign the anaesthetist notices is a spreading apart of the digits. Next, the body temperature starts to rise and the skin often shows blotchy reddening. If no attempt is made to treat the condition, the body temperature continues to rise (rectal temperatures of over 42°C have been recorded); eventually respiration ceases and death ensues. Presumably death is due to cellular hypoxia, for at temperatures over 42°C oxygen utilization exceeds oxygen supply [11].

Although various treatments have been described, there is no specific therapy for malignant hyperther-mia and, at present, immediate cooling coupled with the administration of sodium bicarbonate provides the best chance of success. Dantrolene sodium, a skeletal muscle relaxant, given orally before the induction of anaesthesia, may prevent the onset of the syndrome in susceptible pigs [12] and in doses of between 2 and 10 mg/kg it has proved of some use in the treatment of the established condition [13, 14]. Induction of anaesthesia with Saffan also affords a measure of protection against the development of the syndrome in some strains of susceptible animals [2].

SEDATION

The pig's reaction to restraint (struggling accompanied by ear-splitting squeals) is unpleasant for all concerned and, therefore, sedation is widely used to facilitate all handling and minor procedures, as well as for restraint prior to local or general anaesthesia.

In the pig, α_2-adrenoceptor agonists may help in smoothing reactions to ketamine but, for reasons as yet unknown, they are generally ineffective as sedatives.

Azaperone

This butyrophenone drug is inexpensive and extremely safe and effective in pigs so that other sedatives are now seldom used in these animals. It is marketed both to the veterinary profession for clinical use and directly to farmers who use it to control fighting when mixing litters in intensive units [15].

Azaperone must be given by deep intramuscular injection, the neck muscles behind the ear usually proving to be the most convenient and best site. Subcutaneous injection is ineffective and intravenous injection results in a phase of violent excitement. The doses used depend on the effects sought and range from 1–8 mg/kg, but it is recommended that a dose of 1 mg/kg is not exceeded for adult boars as higher doses cause protrusion of the penis with the risk of subsequent damage to that organ. Following an intramuscular injection of 1–8 mg/kg of azaperone, the pig should be left undisturbed for 20 minutes, as interference before this time may provoke an excitement reaction. Excitement may occur during this induction phase even in the absence of stimulation, but it is usually mild and rarely of clinical significance. After the induction period of some 20 minutes, the pig is deeply sedated and handling for the administration of other drugs or minor procedures is greatly facilitated.

Azaperone causes vasodilatation resulting in a small fall in arterial blood pressure, and some slight respiratory stimulation [16]. The vasodilatation of cutaneous vessels makes the sedated pig particularly likely to develop hypothermia in a cold environment so warm surroundings are essential, but the dilated ear veins are easy to enter for the intravenous injection of drugs.

Droperidol

The butyrophenone compound, droperidol, has been used in pigs by Mitchell [17] and doses of 0.1–0.4 mg/kg give similar sedation to that produced by azaperone. Mitchell also studied the effects of butyrophenone/analgesic drug mixtures for sedation but found that fentanyl with droperidol produced better sedation than droperidol alone [17].

More recently at the Cambridge Veterinary School it has been found that a combination of droperidol (0.5 mg/kg) with midazolam (0.3 mg/kg) given separately or, where appropriate, from the same syringe, into the gluteal or biceps femoris muscles, produces ideal sedation for radiography, lancing of abscesses, etc. (P. G. G. Jackson, personal communication).

Dependable sedation of approximately 15 minutes follows some 10 minutes from the time of injection, but it is important to leave the pig undisturbed whilst the effects are developing. As with ketamine, sudden awakening without prior warning may occur.

Acepromazine

Pigs are easily restrained for intravenous injection if acepromazine (0.03–0.1 mg/kg) is given by intramuscular injection before venepuncture is attempted. Under the influence of acepromazine they do not squeal when handled and are much less likely to dislodge the venepuncture needle by head shaking. Acepromazine may itself be given intravenously but may cause thrombosis of the vein unless very dilute solutions are used. When given by intravenous injection the drug should be allowed 10–20 minutes to produce its full effects. Intravenous injection may be

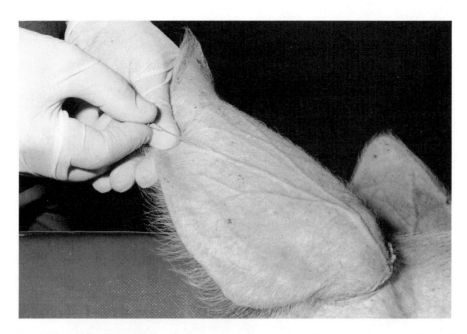

Fig. 14.3 Distension of the ear veins by the application of an elastic band around the base of the ear.

followed by hyperpnoea which lasts for about 15 minutes, but the reason for this is unknown.

Dissociative agents

Tavernor [18, 19] described the use of phencyclidine in pigs and this drug was used very successfully as a sedative for pigs for some years until the hallucinatory effects produced in man led to a ban on the use of the drug in food animals. Phencyclidine has been withdrawn from the market and the dissociative agent in current use, ketamine, is generally used as an anaesthetic rather than as a sedative.

PREPARATION FOR GENERAL ANAESTHESIA

In pigs, 6–8 hours' fasting and 2 hours' deprivation of water is usually adequate to ensure that the stomach is empty. Vomiting at induction is rare in pigs (although it used to be seen regularly during recovery from cyclopropane anaesthesia) but a full stomach exerts pressure on the diaphragm and reduces respiratory efficiency. The majority of surgery carried out in pigs, whether clinical or experimental, is elective and fluid deficits are seldom present before anaesthesia. An intravenous infusion may be needed, however, before anaesthesia for the correction of a strangulated hernia. Details of existing drug therapy such as antibiotic food additives, or anthelmintics, should be noted — especially if muscle relaxants whose action they may lengthen are to be used in the anaesthetic technique.

PREMEDICATION

During general anaesthesia salivation, even if not excessive, may cause respiratory obstruction. Atropine, intramuscularly or intravenously, in doses of 0.3–2.4 mg, or glycopyrrolate (0.2–2.0 mg), depending on the size of the pig, will usually control this salivation.

The degree of sedation required depends on the anaesthetic technique which is to follow. Some anaesthetists prefer to dispense with sedation at this stage, while others use it to facilitate the administration of the anaesthetic and to reduce the squealing which would otherwise occur at induction. Only rarely is there any need for analgesics to be included in the premedication but if required they may be employed in slightly larger doses than are used in dogs. It is probable that azaperone is the most widely used

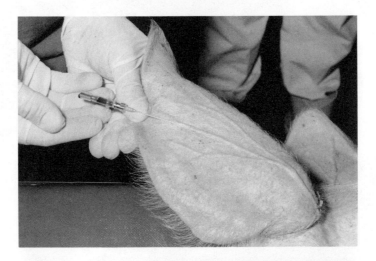

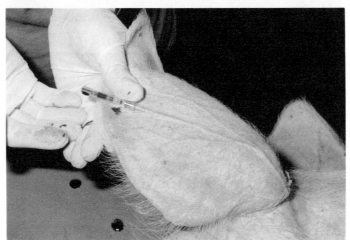

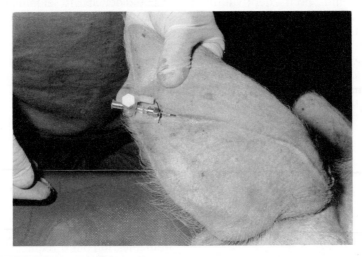

Fig. 14.4 Stages in the introduction of a catheter into the ear vein of a pig.
The stitch securing the catheter does not penetrate the ear cartilage.

premedicant drug for porcine anaesthesia. As already mentioned, it is given by intramuscular injection in doses of 1–8 mg/ kg according to the degree of sedation required.

INTRAVENOUS TECHNIQUE

Intravenous injections are best made into one of the auricular veins on the external aspect of the ear-flap. Small pigs are restrained on their side on a table. One assistant leans on the neck and trunk, at the same time gripping the legs, whilst the second assistant holds the uppermost ear at the base of the conchal cartilage and applies pressure to the vein as near to the base of the ear as possible. If a second assistant is not available, a rubber band is applied around the base of the ear-flap. In large pigs, a noose is applied around the upper jaw behind the tusks as previously described (see Fig. 14.1). As in small pigs, the ear veins are distended by the application of pressure as near to the base of the ear-flap as possible.

Once the ear-flap has been cleaned, the veins are usually easily visible (Fig. 14.3), but if necessary they can be made more obvious by gentle slapping and brisk rubbing of the ear-flap with an alcohol-soaked gauze swab. Venepuncture is then caried out using a needle about 2.5 cm long and, depending on the calibre of the vessel, 21–23 gauge (0.8–0.65 mm). In large pigs blood can be aspirated into an attached syringe once the needle has been inserted into the vein but in small pigs the amount of blood in the vein between the points of pressure and insertion of the needle may be so small that it is impossible to withdraw any into the syringe. In such cases injection must be attempted and if the needle is not in the lumen of the vein a subcutaneous bleb will develop. When it is certain that the needle is in the vein the pressure is released (if a rubber band has been applied to the base of the ear-flap the band must be cut with scissors) and the injection made. It will be noticed that the solution injected washes the blood out of the vein and this affords further evidence that the needle is correctly placed in the lumen of the vessel.

Introduction of a catheter into an ear vein is not difficult (Fig. 14.4) but these veins are not very suitable for the administration of large quantities of fluid. Fortunately such treatment is seldom needed, but if it is necessary it is usually best to implant surgically a catheter into the jugular vein of the anaesthetized pig, as the subcutaneous fat makes percutaneous puncture of this vein difficult. Some workers prefer to catheterize the anterior vena cava by a blind technique. Small pigs are restrained on their backs in a V-shaped trough with the neck fully extended and the head hanging down. The fore-legs are drawn back and a 5–7.5 cm long, 16 s.w.g. (1.65 mm) needle is pushed through the skin in the depression which can be palpated just lateral to the anterior point of the sternum and formed by the angle between the first rib and trachea. The needle is directed towards an imaginary point midway between the scapulae and advanced until blood can be freely aspirated when a syringe is attached to it. A fine plastic catheter is then threaded through the needle into the anterior vena cava and after its position has been verified by the aspiration of blood through it, or by radiography, the needle is completely withdrawn and the catheter secured in position with a skin suture. In large animals the procedure is carried out with the animal standing and hanging back on a nose snare. It is always important to ensure that the head does not deviate from the midline and that the neck is well extended (Fig. 14.5).

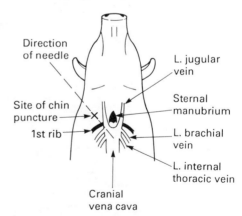

Fig. 14.5 Site for the introduction of a needle to penetrate the anterior vena cava. The needle tip is advanced towards an imaginary point midway between the scapulae.

INTRAPERITONEAL INJECTION

This method of administration of anaesthetic drugs is sometimes employed by the less skilled veterinarian, but it is far from ideal. Response is variable, and accidental injection into the liver, kidney or gut lumen may occur. The injection of irritant solutions may lead to the subsequent formation of intraperitoneal

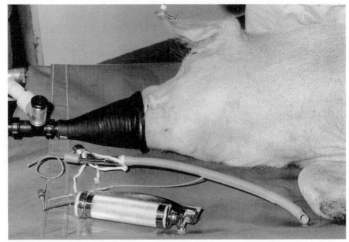

(a)

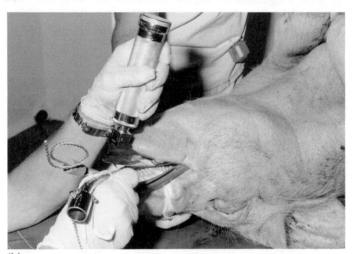

(b)

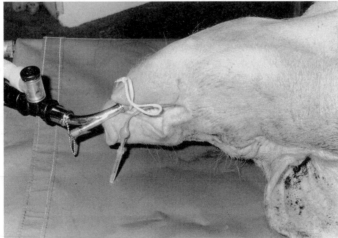

(c)

adhesions. However, if for any reason intravenous injection is impossible, this route of administration may have to be used. Preferably, pigs should be starved for 24 hours to reduce the gut volume before the injection is made. The animal is then restrained on its back, or by its hind-legs, and an area of skin in the region of the umbilicus is clipped and cleaned. A needle is inserted 2–5 cm from the midline at the level of the umbilicus and the injection made. A complete absence of resistance to pressure on the plunger of the syringe indicates that the solution is being injected into the peritoneal cavity or, possibly into the lumen of the gut.

ENDOTRACHEAL INTUBATION

Endotracheal intubation in the pig is not easy. The shape and size of the head and mouth make the use of a laryngoscope difficult. The rima glottis is extremely small, and the larynx is set at an angle to the trachea, causing difficulty in passing the tube beyond the cricoid ring. Laryngeal spasm is easily provoked so that intubation must be carried out under deep general anaesthesia or with the aid of a relaxant.

The sizes of endotracheal tubes suitable for pigs are unexpectedly small when compared with those used in dogs of similar body weight. A 6 mm tube may be the largest which can be passed in a pig weighing about 25 kg; a 9 mm tube is suitable for a 50 kg animal, and large boars and sows may accommodate tubes of 14–16 mm diameter. Introduction of the tube may be made easier by the use of a metal stilette. The ideal stilette is a copper rod with one end carefully rounded or covered to prevent damage to the mucosa of the larynx or trachea. The rod is placed inside the endotracheal tube, and a moveable side-arm adjusted to ensure that the tip does not protrude beyond the end of the tube (Fig. 14.6). Whenever an endotracheal tube is reinforced in this way care must be taken not to use force in its introduction, as damage to the laryngeal mucosa with subsequent oedema and, after extubation, respiratory obstruction, can easily occur. Laryngoscopes designed for use in man, as used in dogs, are suitable for use in small pigs, but in large ones the Rowson laryngoscope may be needed to expose the larynx to view.

The anaesthetized pig is placed on its back with the neck and head fully extended. An assistant pulls on the tongue and fixes the upper jaw while the laryngoscope is introduced and the larynx brought into view (Fig. 14.7). Under direct vision the tube is passed between the vocal cords and kept dorsal to the middle ventricle of the larynx. If its progress is arrested at the cricoid ring, the stilette must be partially withdrawn and the head flexed slightly on the neck. The tube may then be advanced into the trachea.

Fig. 14.6 Endotracheal intubation in the pig: (a) apparatus needed (note the malleable wire stilette inside the tube but not protruding its bevelled end); (b) use of the laryngoscope to lift the lower jaw and displace the base of the tongue to one side; (c) tube tied in position with tape around lower jaw and cuff inflated.

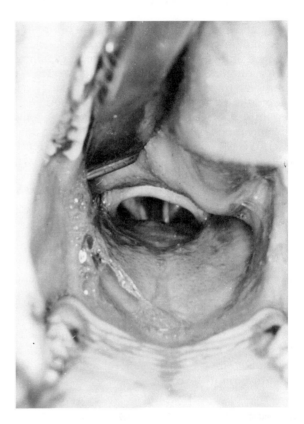

Fig. 14.7 View of the pig's larynx when the laryngoscope is used correctly in the supine animal. As can be seen, the laryngoscope blade is used to elevate the base of the tongue and does not come into contact with the epiglottis. The epiglottis is often so soft and flexible that unless due care is taken it folds back into the glottic opening as the tube is passed.

Endotracheal intubation in the pig is greatly facilitated by the use of muscle relaxants, such as suxamethonium, which relax the jaw muscles and prevent the larynx from going into a spasm. The anaesthetized pig is given oxygen to breathe through a face-mask and the relaxant is administered intravenously. The pig is intubated as soon as the jaw muscles relax and IPPV is carried out until spontaneous respiration is resumed. If suxamethonium is the relaxant used, spontaneous respiration will begin within 1–2 minutes from the time of its injection. Should an attempt at intubation fail, small pigs may easily be ventilated by squeezing the reservoir bag of the anaesthetic system while a face-mask is applied (Fig. 14.2), but this is more difficult in adult sows and boars, so it is recommended that relaxants are only used in these larger animals by anaesthetists who are experienced at endotracheal intubation in this species of animal and are capable of ventilating large individuals through a face-mask.

GENERAL ANAESTHESIA

Although the pig is a good subject for general anaesthesia the anaesthetist may find problems in maintaining spontaneous breathing and a clear airway.

When dealing with fat pigs, cessation of breathing is a common complication of deep anaesthesia. A striking feature of this apparent respiratory failure is that it is different from that seen in other species, for expulsion of the air from the lungs by pressure on the abdomen is immediately followed by a spontaneous deep inspiration of the type seen when there is some mechanical obstruction to respiration during anaesthesia. It is possible that in the fat pig mere extension of the head is enough to cause pressure on the larynx sufficient to arrest breathing. The animal's head should be placed at the natural angle and artificial respiration applied. This is performed by applying pressure to the abdomen about every 4 seconds and unless spontaneous breathing returns within 1–2 minutes, endotracheal intubation to facilitate IPPV should be considered. IPPV may also be carried out through a closely applied face-mask without endotracheal intubation but, if it is, care must be taken to avoid inflation of the stomach.

The prudent anaesthetist avoids trouble by avoiding the need to produce deep anaesthesia — if necessary by the simultaneous use of techniques of local analgesia when light general anaesthesia does not suffice on its own.

Intravenous anaesthesia

The intravenous injection of suitable agents into an already sedated animal is an excellent way of inducing general anaesthesia in pigs. Under farm conditions it may be necessary to maintain anaesthesia by the use of intravenous drugs but if suitable apparatus is available anaesthesia can be continued, even on the farm, with inhalation agents. Numerous agents are available for induction of anaesthesia by the intravenous route and many of them can be used to maintain anaesthesia in situations where this is necessary. In pigs, some of these agents may also be administered by intraperitoneal injection.

Metomidate

This hypnotic drug, usually used in combination with azaperone, is a safe agent for the production of basal narcosis in pigs both under field conditions and prior to the use of more sophisticated methods for the maintenance of anaesthesia in the operating theatre. Ideally, metomidate is given intravenously at a dose rate of 3.3 mg/kg about 20 minutes after the intramuscular injection of 2 mg/kg of azaperone. Often the pig moves as the metomidate is injected and this may be a response to pain for the intravenous injection of the related drug, etomidate, is known to cause pain in man. Following the intravenous injection of the metomidate the pig becomes recumbent and remains so for some 10–20 minutes. Respiration is well maintained and further doses of metomidate can be given as required to prolong the time of recumbency. Analgesia is very limited with this combination of drugs and painful stimuli sometimes result in dramatic, even if short-lived, awakening, so it is advisable to utilize some form of analgesia to enable surgery to be carried out. The combination of azaperone and metomidate is compatible with all inhalation and neuromuscular blocking agents used in anaesthesia so that they may be used subsequently as needed.

It is possible to give azaperone intramuscularly or intraperitoneally and metomidate intraperitoneally at the same time. Narcosis follows about 20 minutes after injection but P. Lees and M. J. Meredith (personal communication) have found that intraperitoneal injection results in peritonitis and the formation of adhesions.

Thiopentone sodium

Anaesthesia can be induced in pigs by the intravenous injection of minimal (5–10 mg/kg) quantities of a 2.5% solution of thiopentone. As in all other species of animal, larger doses or incremental doses are cumulative and can result in delay in recovery.

In the literature many different dose rates and concentrations of thiopentone have been recommended for use in pigs. Muhrer [20] recorded an extensive experience of thiopentone sodium as an intravenous anaesthetic in pigs. He used a 5% solution (1 g in 20 ml) injected into the ear vein, half the computed dose being injected rapidly and the remainder more slowly over the next 2–3 minutes. He found that the dose required to produce his desired degree of anaesthesia varied considerably, for quite apart from weight factors pigs showed marked differences in their susceptibility to the drug. In his experience, induction doses generally gave 5–10 minutes' anaesthesia with a total recovery period of 30–60 minutes.

S. Jennings (personal communication) recommended doses of up to 29 mg/kg for small pigs and 24 mg/kg for larger ones, again administered in two stages to unsedated animals.

Experience at the Cambridge Veterinary School has been that the quantity of thiopentone taken to induce medium surgical anaesthesia and the duration of the anaesthetic period are chiefly governed by the speed at which the injection is made. When rapid injection techniques are practised in healthy pigs, the quantity used will be surprisingly small, and the recovery period short. Surgical anaesthesia can be induced in sows weighing about 100 kg by the injection of no more than 500 mg of the drug. Moreover, it has been observed that the use of a 2.5% solution decreases the total dose required for any operation. Induction of anaesthesia with thiopentone sodium is greatly facilitated by the use of azaperone premedication. Provided that the pig is left undisturbed for 20 minutes after the injection of the azaperone, controlled injection into an ear vein is easy and complete anaesthesia can be obtained with surprisingly small quantities of a 2.5% solution of thiopentone. It seems that the butyrophenone antagonizes the respiratory effect of the thiopentone, but this clinical impression still awaits controlled investigation.

As with all barbiturate anaesthetics, respiration may fail with the onset of anaesthesia. When rapid injection techniques are used this period of apnoea is short and should not necessitate the use of artificial respiration. Apnoea of more than a few seconds' duration must, of course, be treated by artificial respiration and, provided this is applied efficiently, spontaneous breathing soon returns. Recovery after a very great overdose of thiopentone may be expected if efficient artificial ventilation of the lungs is performed until the concentration of thiopentone in the brain has diminished.

Methohexitone sodium

It would seem that provided the anaesthetist is aware of the basic principles underlying the use of intravenous anaesthetic agents, and has some knowledge of the special characteristics of methohexitone (such as its tendency to produce muscle tremors during induction), it can be used quite safely in pigs [21]. Anaesthesia can be produced in unsedated animals by the intravenous injection of 5–6 mg/kg as a 2.5% solution and recovery is complete 10–15 minutes after the injection of a single induction dose [22].

Premedication with azaperone reduces the dose of methohexitone required, and enables small incremental doses to be used to prolong anaesthesia without delay in recovery.

Pentobarbitone sodium

This drug still has a place for surgery carried out on the farm. The most satisfactory method of administration of pentobarbitone sodium in pigs is slow intravenous injection into the ear vein, continuing until the desired depression of the central nervous system is obtained. However, intraperitoneal injection using a computed dose or intratesticular injection may be adopted.

For healthy, unsedated male and female pigs up to 50 kg live weight, the average intravenous dose necessary to induce medium depth anaesthesia is about 30 mg/kg. In small pigs there is a considerable margin of safety, but in larger ones great variations in susceptibility may occur. Castrated animals appear to be slightly more susceptible than entires. Provided that the injection is made slowly and the onset of muscle relaxation is observed, the method is safe. Induction is not associated with narcotic excitement; in fact, in the case of a squealing animal, the progressive reduction, and finally cessation of squealing, is a good guide to the progress of narcosis. Depths of anaesthesia may be difficult to assess in pigs. The presence of complete relaxation of the abdominal muscles and the absence of response to pricking of the skin is evidence that anaesthesia has been attained. Its duration will be sufficient for the performance of rapid operations such as castration. For very large subjects the dose per kilogram must be reduced and marked variations in susceptibility will be encountered.

The duration of surgical plane will depend upon the initial depth of anaesthesia induced. As a rule it is shorter than in the dog. With light levels of unconsciousness — a brisk corneal reflex and a reflex response to skin pricking — it is of 10–15 minutes only; when there is a sluggish corneal reflex and loss of reflex response to pricking — 20–25 minutes. Anaesthesia is followed by a period of progressively lightening narcosis which persists for 3–8 hours. The period of recovery is not accompanied by narcotic excitement and the animal usually passes into a state of sleep.

In small, unsedated subjects in which intravenous injection may be found to be difficult, the intraperitoneal route may be adopted although, in general, it is not to be recommended. It becomes necessary to compute an anaesthetic dose. For animals up to 20 kg this is put at 30 mg/kg; for those between 20 and 30 kg, at 24 mg/kg. Variations in response are inevitable with such a method. In some cases narcosis only will be obtained and it will be necessary to augment it by inhalation or local injection, while in others anaesthesia may become alarmingly deep and even fatal. Provided a careful watch is kept on respirations, and artificial respiration applied should they cease, fatalities should, however, be of rare occurrence. In fat subjects there is a possibility that, despite the length of the needle employed, the injection will be made into retroperitoneal fat. In this case absorption will be so slow it is improbable that even light narcosis will develop. When employing this route of administration, the action of the drug will attain its maximum depth in a period of 20–30 minutes after injection. The duration of the period of anaesthesia and of narcosis tends to be rather longer than with the intravenous method.

Intratesticular injection.   A strong solution of pentobarbitone sodium, such as one commercially available for euthanasia of small animals (300 mg/ml) may be administered by intratesticular injection prior to castration [23]. A dose rate of about 45 mg/kg is employed, a very large boar being given 20 ml of solution in each testicle, and adequate anaesthesia for castration develops within 10 minutes of injection. Removal of the testicles removes any excess drug, so that to prevent overdosage this must be carried out as soon as the boar becomes anaesthetized. Care must be taken in the disposal of the testicles after their removal since they still contain enough barbiturate to produce fatal poisoning of any animal which might eat them.

Saffan

Since its first reported use in pigs [24] Saffan has proved to be a useful induction agent. When no premedication is used, intravenous doses of 6 mg/kg produce surgical anaesthesia of 10–15 minutes duration followed by smooth recovery. In larger pigs intravenous doses of 6 mg/kg constitute too large a volume for convenience and it is usual to employ premedication to reduce the dose needed. Following sedation with 4 mg/kg of azaperone intramuscularly, the intravenous injection of 2 mg/kg of Saffan produces good surgical anaesthesia with adequate muscle relaxation and minimal respiratory depression. Further increments of Saffan can be given to prolong anaesthesia.

Ketamine

Pigs are said to be rapidly immobilized by the intramuscular injection of 20 mg/kg of ketamine [25, 26] which produces adequate analgesia for the performance of minor operations. Wakening is often

disconcertingly abrupt and many pigs seem to remain sensitive to noise throughout the period of anaesthesia. Much better results are obtained by the intravenous injection of 2–5 mg/kg of ketamine after pretreatment with 1 mg/kg of xylazine, although this latter drug seems to produce no obvious sedation in pigs. Reasonably satisfactory results are also obtained when 10–18 mg/kg of ketamine are given intramuscularly after the intravenous injection of 1–2 mg/kg of diazepam. It must be remembered that ketamine, xylazine and diazepam are all rather expensive for use in farm animals.

Inhalation anaesthesia

Under field conditions, simple methods of administration may be used to administer volatile agents to pigs. For example, chloroform masks designed for use in horses have been used, equally well, for large pigs. Such methods use large quantities of the volatile anaesthetic agent. Where anaesthetic apparatus is available, the patient breathing circuit employed depends mainly on the size of the pig. Breathing circuits designed for use in man, and which are used for dogs, may be used for all but the largest of boars and sows where the systems designed for equine anaesthesia are more appropriate.

Endotracheal intubation is essential if IPPV is to be used but otherwise volatile agents may be administered via a face-mask. Large Hall-pattern facemaks are adequate for small pigs but masks suitable for large pigs are not commercially available. Fortunately, conical or snout-shaped masks are fairly easy to design and construct and although they may not fit really tightly around the pig's snout a gas-tight seal can be obtained by wrapping wet towels around the edge of the mask. The pig breathes through the nose, so whatever mask is used it is essential to ensure that it does not block the flow of gas into the nostrils. Luckily, the anterior position of the external nares in pigs makes their obstruction by the mask much less likely than in animals such as horses and cattle where the nares are situated more laterally. If a suitable snout mask for a large pig is not available the anaesthetic may be administered through a Hall's mask placed just over the nostrils, although it is obviously impossible to make this a gas-tight fit and a considerable quantity of anaesthetic escapes to the atmosphere. Whenever the pig is not intubated the tendency towards respiratory obstruction must be overcome by pushing the mandible forward as previously described (Fig. 14.2).

Induction of anaesthesia with inhalation agents is usually free from excitement but, except in small pigs, it is usually more convenient to induce anaesthesia with a parenterally administered agent and to use the inhalation just for the maintenance of anaesthesia. Under farm conditions, when methods of administration lead to a considerable wastage of anaesthetic, the older, less expensive agents are usually employed, but when more sophisticated apparatus is available any inhalation agent may be used.

Trichloroethylene

Trichloroethylene — once quite widely used in porcine anaesthesia — is no longer available.

Ether

Inhalation of ether by the conscious pig produces copious salivation and bronchial secretion, even after atropine premedication, so it cannot be regarded as a satisfactory induction agent for this species of animal. Given by semi-closed or low-flow methods following suitable premedication and induction with intravenous agents, it can produce good anaesthesia with marked muscle relaxation.

Halothane

Because of its potency and relative absence of toxicity, halothane is an excellent anaesthetic for pigs of all ages. Induction of anaesthesia is rapid and provided the animal can be effectively restrained there is seldom any need to use an intravenous drug for this purpose before halothane is given. Squealing ceases after as few as 4–5 breaths of halothane vapour have been taken and inhalation of the vapour does not provoke salivation or breath holding. Recovery from anaesthesia is equally smooth and rapid.

Unfortunately, the cost of halothane and the need to transport bulky anaesthetic apparatus limits its use on farms but, where low-flow or semi-closed methods can be used, halothane may be considered to be the agent of choice for porcine anaesthesia. Its association with the condition of malignant hyperthermia must, however, be remembered and the pig should be observed very closely during the induction period so that the earliest possible warning sign that this condition is developing may be recognized in time for effective cooling to be instituted. The main disadvantages in pigs, as in all species, are those of cardiovascular depression leading to hypotension, respiratory depression, and the comparative lack of ability to suppress motor response to surgical stimulation.

Methoxyflurane

Induction with methoxyflurane is too slow for convenience, but it may be used to supplement nitrous oxide/oxygen mixtures.

Enflurane and isoflurane

These agents produce a rapid induction and satisfactory anaesthesia in pigs, but are far too expensive to be used except in low-flow systems of administration. Their effects are very similar to those of halothane and it remains to be seen whether they will ever have a place in porcine anaesthesia.

The haemodynamic effects of isoflurane compared with halothane in newborn piglets have been reported by Schieber *et al.* [27].

Nitrous oxide

It is impossible to induce anaesthesia in pigs with nitrous oxide but as long as sufficient oxygen is provided it may be supplemented with a volatile anaesthetic agent. In particular, the sequence of premedication, induction with thiopentone sodium, endotracheal intubation under a relaxant, and the maintenance of anaesthesia by endotracheal nonrebreathing administration of nitrous oxide with an intravenous or inhalational supplement has proved to be a very satisfactory method for lengthy experimental surgical procedures in pigs of all ages. By this system very light anaesthesia can be maintained and relaxation is produced as required by the administration of muscle relaxants. Recovery from anaesthesia is rapid.

USE OF MUSCLE RELAXANTS

Neuromuscular blocking agents are used in pigs to facilitate endotracheal intubation and for thoracic, abdominal or experimental surgical procedures. As in all species of animal, two things are essential if these drugs are to be administered:

1. The pig must be anaesthetized and, therefore, unconscious

2. The means to apply IPPV must be available

Techniques involving muscle relaxants are not designed for use in the field, and can only be properly applied by a skilled, experienced anaesthetist. All those intending to use these drugs in porcine anaesthesia should be fully familiar with the pharmacology (Chapter 7) and with the methods of IPPV (Chapter 8).

Suxamethonium

Suxamethonium is used in pigs to facilitate endo-tracheal intubation. Atropine premedication is essential to counter the autonomic stimulant effect of the initial depolarizing process. Following induction of anaesthesia, doses of 2 mg/kg suxamethonium produce complete paralysis of about 2 minutes' duration, i.e. long enough to allow unhurried, atraumatic intubation. It is, of course, necessary to perform IPPV until full spontaneous breathing is resumed.

Non-depolarizing relaxants

All the non-depolarizing relaxants used in man may be employed in the anaesthetized pig to facilitate

Table 14.1 Relaxant drugs which have been used in pigs

Name	Dose (mg/kg)	Approximate duration of action (min)
Suxamethonium	2	2–3
d-Tubocurarine	0.3	25–35
Gallamine	4	15–20
Alcuronium	0.1	30–40
Pancuronium	0.12	25–30
Vecuronium	0.1	15–20
Atracurium	0.5	20–60

surgical or experimental procedures. The choice of relaxant depends on the duration of action needed, on the route of elimination of the drug, and on the cardiovascular effects it produces. The drugs which have been used in pigs are listed in Table 14.1.

The technique most commonly employed is as follows. The pig is premedicated with atropine and, usually, azaperone. Anaesthesia is induced with a suitable intravenous agent such as thiopentone or metomidate, the pig is intubated (generally with the aid of suxamethonium) and anaesthesia is maintained with nitrous oxide and oxygen supplemented with agents such as fentanyl or morphine given intravenously, or volatile inhalation agents such as halothane administered at an inspired concentration of $1.2 \times MAC$ (i.e. about 1.2%). Following the administration of the chosen relaxant, IPPV is carried out using a ventilator or by manual squeezing of the anaesthetic reservoir bag. Ventilators designed for use in adult human beings are adequate for the majority of pigs, but large boars and sows may have to be ventilated with one of the ventilators designed for use in large animals. At the end of the procedure, atropine (0.6–2.4 mg) is administered to counter the muscarinic effects of neostigmine which is given in doses of up to 0.1 mg/kg to restore spontaneous breathing.

LOCAL ANALGESIA

Caudal blocks are not employed in pigs and epidural analgesia is usually used simply for economic reasons.

Epidural block

In the pig the spinal cord ends at the junction of the fifth and sixth lumbar vertebrae and the spinal meninges continue, around the phylum terminale, as far as the middle of the sacrum. At the lumbosacral space the sac is comparatively small, and it is improbable that a needle introduced at this point will penetrate into the subarachnoid space. The lumbosacral aperture is large. Its dimensions in the adult are approximately 1.5 cm craniocaudally and 3 cm transversely. The depth of the canal is about 1 cm.

The site for insertion of the needle is located as follows. The cranial border of the ilium on each side is found with the fingers. A line joining them crosses the spinous process of the last lumbar segment. The needle is inserted in the midline immediately behind this spine and directed downwards and backwards at an angle of 20° with the vertical. The depth to which the needle must penetrate in pigs of 30–70 kg will vary from 5–9 cm. The landmarks described are readily detected in animals of smaller size but they

may be entirely masked by the overlying tissues in larger ones. In these, a point 15 cm cranial to the base of the tail serves as a fairly accurate guide. Provided the needle is introduced in approximately the correct position and direction, the size of the lumbosacral space makes its detection comparatively easy. Eighteen gauge needles are used; for pigs between 30 and 50 kg one 8 cm long and, for animals of 70 kg and above, one 12 cm long.

Before inserting the epidural needle an insensitive skin weal should be produced. The animal is restrained either on its breast or side. For small pigs the latter is preferable, as sudden movement can be better controlled. In large sows and boars the injection is made in the standing animal. Owing to difficulties with restraint, it is generally necessary to make the injection comparatively rapidly. Penetration of the canal is often associated with sudden movement, for which attendants must be prepared. In pigs weighing from 10–20 kg the interarcuate ligament is at a depth of about 2–3.5 cm from the skin surface while in adult sows and boars it may be at a depth of up to 15 cm.

Epidural analgesia has been used for the castration of pigs of 40–50 kg, injecting 10 ml of 2% lignocaine solution with adrenaline. Complete desensitization of the scrotum, testes and spermatic cord was present in 10 minutes, and there was a partial motor paralysis of the hind-limbs. Recovery was complete at the end of the second hour. Although a similar volume dose was recommended by Frank [28] for procaine solutions it is difficult to know up to what weight this computation should be employed, for in adults fat often represents a considerable proportion of body weight; 100 kg is suggested as the upper limit, with a maximum dose of 20 ml.

When 2% lignocaine solution without adrenaline is used analgesia lasts for up to 90 minutes after full development of the block [29].

Other indications are obstetrical manipulations, return of the prolapsed rectum and amputation of the prolapsed uterus.

Analgesia for castration

Local analgesia is quite suitable for the castration of male pigs up to about 5 months of age but general anaesthesia is probably more satisfactory for older animals.

Intratesticular injection is probably the most practical method of local analgesia. A needle of suitable size is thrust perpendicularly through the tensed scrotal skin and advanced until its point lies in the middle of the testicle. Between 3 and 15 ml, depending on the size of the animal, of 2% lignocaine hydrochloride solution are injected into the testicle and a further 2–5 ml are injected subcutaneously beneath the scrotal skin as the needle is withdrawn. Both sides are treated in the same manner. Operation may commence about 5 minutes after completion of the injections.

POSTOPERATIVE CARE

It is absolutely essential that pigs should be kept in a warm environment until they are completely mobile after sedation or general anaesthesia because due to their lack of body hair they are prone to develop hypothermia if left in cold surroundings. Close observation during the recovery period is necessary so that immediate measures may be taken to relieve any respiratory obstruction which may occur. Postoperative pain relief is essential, particularly following extensive experimental surgical procedures. Narcotic analgesics may be given as necessary, in doses similar to those used in dogs and among those most commonly employed are morphine (0.1 mg/kg up to a maximum of 20 mg) and pethidine (2 mg/kg up to a maximum of 1.0 g in large boars and sows).

REFERENCES

1. Hall, L. W., Woolf, N., Bradley, J. W. P. and Jolly, D. W. (1966) *British Medical Journal* **ii**, 1305.
2. Hall, L. W., Trim, C. M. and Woolf, N. (1972) *British Medical Journal* **ii**, 145.
3. Harrison, G. G. (1969) *British Journal of Anaesthesia* **41**, 844.
4. Ellis, F. R. (1971) *Anaesthesia* **26**, 540.
5. Kalow, W. (1970) *Proceedings of the Royal Society of Medicine* **63**, 178.
6. Eppenberger, M., Nixon, C. W., Baker, J. R. and Homburger, F. (1964) *Proceedings of the Society of Experimental Biology and Medicine* **117**, 465.
7. Wilson, K. M., Evans, K. A. and Carter, C. O. (1965) *British Medical Journal* **i**, 750.
8. Denborough, M. A., Ebeling, P., King, J. O. and Zapf, P. (1970) *Lancet* **i**, 1138.
9. Isaacs, H. and Barlow, M. B. (1970) *British Medical Journal* **i**, 275.
10. Woolf, N., Hall, L. W., Thorne, C., Down, M. and Walker, R. G. (1970) *British Medical Journal* **iii**, 386.
11. Pettigrew, R. T., Galt, J. M and Udgate, C. M. (1974) *British Medical Journal* **4**, 679.
12. Harrison, G. G. (1977) *British Medical Journal* **4**, 315.
13. Gronert, G. A., Milde, J. H. and Theye, R. A. (1976) *Anesthesiology* **44**, 488.
14. Alitalo, I. and Schulman, A. (1983) *Nordisk Veterinarmedicin* **35**, 239.
15. Symoens, J. and Van den Brande, M. (1969) *Veterinary Record* **85**, 64.
16. Clarke, K. W. (1969) *Veterinary Record* **85**, 649.
17. Mitchell, B. (1966) *Veterinary Record* **79**, 651.
18. Tavernor, W. D. (1963) *Veterinary Record* **75**, 1377.
19. Tavernor, W. D. (1964) *Small Animal Anaesthesia*. Oxford: Pergamon Press.
20. Muhrer, M. E. (1950) *Journal of the American Veterinary Medical Association* **117**, 293.
21. Emberton, G. A. (1966) *Veterinary Record* **78**, 541.
22. Noakes, D. E. (1966) *Veterinary Record* **78**, 669.
23. Henry, D. P. (1968) *Australian Veterinary Journal* **44**, 418.
24. Hall, L. W. (1972) *Postgraduate Medical Journal*, June Suppl., p. 55.
25. Roberts, F. W. (1971) *Anaesthesia* **26**, 445.
26. Thurman, J. C., Nelson, D. R. and Christie, C. J. (1972) *Journal of the American Veterinary Medical Association* **160**, 1325.
27. Schieber, R. A., Namnoum, A., Sugden, A., Shiu, G. V., Orr, R. A. and Cook, D. R. (1986) *Anesthesia and Analgesia* **65**, 633.
28. Frank, E. R. (1931) *Veterinary Record* **11**, 867.
29. Hopcroft, S. C. (1965) *British Journal of Anaesthesia* **37**, 982.

CHAPTER 15

ANAESTHESIA OF THE DOG

A well-administered general anaesthetic to a dog which is fit and healthy is a very safe procedure and there should be little risk to the life of the animal. Unfortunately there is evidence that this is not always so. Although the mortality rate in veterinary school clinics does appear to be very low a recent survey of anaesthesia in UK general veterinary practices, carried out by the Association of Veterinary Anaesthetists of Great Britain and Ireland, revealed a rate of one death per 870 fit healthy dogs anaesthetized. Moreover, morbidity due to anaesthesia, which is often overlooked, is also not uncommon.

Apart from any direct toxic effects of the agents administered, most damage during anaesthesia occurs as a result of hypoxia, either through respiratory depression or lack of oxygen in the blood or, more commonly, through failure of the blood to reach the tissues. The tissues most sensitive to a short period of hypoxia include the heart, brain, liver and kidneys. In man, severe hypoxic brain damage will be obvious postoperatively, but less serious damage may well be unnoticed by the hospital staff as the patient recovers and returns home. Decreased intelligence, which may even mimic senility will, however, be very obvious to friends and relatives. It is very difficult to measure the intelligence of animals, but following the use of anaesthetic techniques known to carry the risk of hypoxia, owners have been heard to comment that their dog or bitch has 'never been the same since the anaesthetic'. A much more dramatic and obvious cause of postanaesthetic morbidity in dogs is renal failure. Many elderly dogs suffer from some degree of chronic interstitial nephritis and in such animals even mild renal hypoxia may prove fatal within a relatively short time. These dogs are also completely dependent on an unrestricted fluid intake to maintain renal function at an adequate level, and may require intravenous fluids, particularly if recovery is long.

The wide range of size and breeds of dogs makes it impossible to rely solely on one technique of anaesthesia, or to utilize only one patient breathing circuit. Different sizes and different breeds of dogs may be more or less sensitive to drugs and the environment. On average, as expressed in terms of milligrams per kilogram, larger dogs need considerably smaller doses of anaesthetic drugs, while smaller dogs are more liable to suffer from hyperthermia and hypothermia. Many breed differences are important — for example, some families of the boxer breed are very sensitive to the effects of the phenothiazines — and respiratory obstruction may complicate recovery from anaesthesia in brachycephalic breeds. Greyhounds and similar breeds have relatively large hearts which may become hypoxic if coronary perfusion falls in a hypotensive episode.

Drugs which cause central nervous stimulation, such as ketamine, should be used with care because dogs have a very low threshold to their convulsive effects. The particular sensitivity to histamine means that Saffan and other preparations which contain Cremophor EL are contraindicated in all Canidae.

ANALGESIA

Opioid analgesics

Opioid analgesics selected for use in dogs to provide analgesia before, during and after surgery are those usually of medium potency and duration of action, such as morphine, pethidine, methadone and papaveretum, but buprenorphine and butorphanol appear to be an acceptable alternative to these and are not 'controlled' drugs. It must be remembered that all are potent respiratory depressants, particularly when combined with barbiturates, so that subsequent anaesthesia should be administered with this in mind. Potent short-acting analgesics such as fentanyl may be used during surgery to obtain an increased analgesic effect and this and similar drugs are components of 'neuroleptanalgesic' mixtures. For postoperative

Table 15.1 Opiate analgesics used in the dog

	Dose (mg/kg)	Approximate duration of effect	Route of administration	Main uses
Morphine	0.1–0.2	4 hours	i.m.	Premedication and postoperative
Pethidine	1–2	2–4 hours	i.m.	Premedication and postoperative
Methadone	0.1	4 hours	i.m. or i.v.	Premedication and postoperative
Fentanyl	0.001–0.007	20–30 minutes	i.v.	During surgery and postoperative
Buprenorphine	0.006	6–8 hours	i.m. or i.v.	Postoperative

analgesia any of these drugs may be used but its long duration of action may make buprenorphine particularly useful at this time provided its bell-shaped dose response curve is remembered. Suitable dose rates and the durations of the action in dogs are given in Table 15.1 and for premedication the lower dose rates should be selected unless preoperative pain is severe.

Morphine frequently causes ambulatory dogs to vomit and defaecate. This side-effect also occurs following the use of other narcotic analgesics (except pethidine) but it is much less likely to occur if the animal is in pain when the drug is administered. When given intravenously to dogs pethidine causes a severe but usually short-lived hypotension which is thought to be due to histamine release. It is, therefore, best given by other routes. The other drugs of this group may be given by the intravenous or intramuscular routes depending on the need for rapidity of action, but intramuscular injection is to be preferred for both premedication and postoperative analgesia because it tends to produce a more level, prolonged effect.

Pentazocine and butorphanol have the advantage of being subject to less stringent statutory controls, and both have the added advantage that they may be given by the oral route (although much higher doses are needed). Butorphanol has proved a useful analgesic in experimental trials and is said to be a satisfactory premedicant [1] but in clinical use it has sometimes proved disappointing. To avoid dysphoric reactions with pentazocine it is important not to overdose. There is no question that the best analgesia is provided by the pure μ agonists (p. 65).

Non-steroidal anti-inflammatory drugs (NSAIDs)

Flunixin meglumine, a potent analgesic with anti-inflammatory, antipyretic and antiendotoxic properties is indicated for the alleviation of inflammation and acute pain in musculoskeletal disorders and as an adjuvant in the treatment of endotoxic or septic shock. In dogs it is important not to exceed a maximum of three doses because the drug can have serious gastrointestinal effects. The recommended dose is 1 mg/kg by slow intravenous or subcutaneous (not intramuscular) injection every 12 hours and this can produce dramatic pain relief following surgery involving the musculoskeletal system.

SEDATION

Many nervous, 'highly strung' dogs do not tolerate minor procedures such as clipping, grooming or bathing without vigorous protest, and handling at these times is greatly facilitated by the use of suitable sedation. The genuinely vicious animal is, fortunately, not often encountered but when it is, it may need to be heavily sedated for the safety of the veterinarian, nursing staff and, not infrequently, the owner during even a simple physical examination. Heavy sedation is usually necessary to preserve an aseptic routine when operations are performed under epidural or other nerve block. Owners often seek advice about the prevention of travel sickness and although in some cases specific antiemetics may be necessary, for many dogs a simple sedative given in good time before the journey commences is all that is required to solve the problem.

Phenothiazine derivatives

In the UK acepromazine (p. 52) is the phenothiazine derivative most commonly used for the sedation of dogs. For small animal use it is supplied as a yellow, 2% solution for injection, and as 10 and 25 mg tablets for oral administration. The response to acepromazine is by no means uniform, depending as it does on the animal's temperament, physical condition and breed. In general, the giant breeds (e.g. Newfoundland) are exceptionally sensitive to the drug and will become recumbent and reluctant to move following doses of about 0.03 mg/kg. Although unable to get up, they can usually be roused easily and pulse and respiration are well maintained. The sight-hound breeds such as the greyhound are also fairly sensitive to its sedative effects — which may be complicated by profound hypotension. Small breeds, in particular the terrier breeds, are much more resistant and may not show signs of sedation following even large doses.

Dogs of the boxer breed are renowned for their liability to 'faint' following even small doses of phenothiazine derivatives (e.g. 0.02 mg/kg acepromazine by intramuscular injection). This response may occur quite suddenly, with no prior sedation; the animal becomes unconscious and there is severe hypotension with bradycardia. Because this response is similar to a vasovagal reaction which might be blocked by atropine or glycopyrrolate, the authors suggest that not only should minimal doses (0.02 mg/kg) be employed in this breed, but also that they should always be combined with anticholinergics even if being given for purposes other than premedication before anaesthesia.

The actions of acepromazine are potentiated by hypovolaemia, by uraemia, and even by old age. The hypotensive effects of the drug can become particularly serious in the presence of hypovolaemia, and if this condition is suspected it is advisable to establish ready access to a vein before administering acepromazine, as percutaneous venepuncture can become very difficult once hypotension has developed. Hypotension is best treated by the rapid intravenous infusion of fluid and, possibly, once the circulating blood volume has been restored, by vasopressor drugs (e.g. methoxamine in doses up to 5 mg by intravenous injection).

The action of acepromazine is primarily of an anxiolytic nature. In nervous animals its sedative effects are often marked, but in the fortunately rarely encountered genuinely vicious animal it is usually ineffective. Because of the nature of the dose–response curve, increasing the dose in these vicious animals will not increase sedation, although ataxia and a reduced speed of response may make them slightly easier to handle.

Doses of 0.03–0.05 mg/kg, preferably by intramuscular injection, are usually quite adequate for the production of sedation and are certainly adequate when the drug is used for premedication. These are lower doses than those recommended on the product data sheets, but increasing the dose rarely increases the sedative effect of the drug and merely prolongs its action. Acepromazine and atropine solutions may be mixed in the same syringe, and if time is short the intravenous route may be employed (at 0.03 mg/kg), but the drug may still take up to 20 minutes to produce its full effects. Acepromazine is said by some to be poorly absorbed from subcutaneous sites but has, in fact, been used satisfactorily by this route in dogs. Oral administration is much less reliable and doses of 1–3 mg/kg are needed at least 1 hour prior to induction of anaesthesia.

Where prolonged or particularly deep sedation is needed the higher dose rates recommended in the product data sheets may be used. In the authors' experience side-effects do not occur any more frequently at this higher dosage than at the lower doses used for premedication but the duration of the side-effects and, therefore, the need for resuscitation, is increased. The duration of action of the drug is almost completely dependent on the dose and while low doses given to healthy animals may need to be repeated after 4 hours, higher doses may still be exerting some effect 24 hours later.

Other phenothiazine derivatives which are used include propionyl promazine, promazine, promethazine, trimeprazine and chlorpromazine. The side-effects produced by them and the provisions of use are similar to those of acepromazine but methotrimeprazine, which is used as part of the neuroleptanalgesic mixture Small Animal Immobilon, is said to have the added advantage of possessing analgesic properties.

α_2-Adrenoceptor agonists

Xylazine

Xylazine was the first α_2-adrenoceptor agonist to be widely used in veterinary medicine. Given by intramuscular injection in doses of 1–3 mg/kg it will produce good sedation and even hypnosis in dogs. As the drug is classified as a sedative/hypnotic, as might be expected, increasing the dose leads to greater sedation as well as increased duration of action. Although high doses will apparently produce unconsciousness (absence of response to external stimuli) this is associated with very severe cardiovascular effects and prolonged recovery, so that high doses cannot be recommended. The major side-effect of xylazine in dogs is vomiting or severe retching as sedation develops. Although on occasion this vomiting is useful for emptying the stomach of a dog which has been fed, it appears to be distressing to the dog as well as being unpleasant for the staff who have to clear up the vomited material.

In dogs, xylazine often causes a rise in arterial blood pressure which is followed by hypotension with severe bradycardia and dose-related respiratory depression. Although atropine may be given to prevent bradycardia its effect is variable, sometimes being apparently ineffective while in other cases its administration results in tachycardia accompanied by severe arterial hypertension.

Even if sedation is not marked, the doses of induction agents which are needed after xylazine premedication are greatly reduced, and any agent which is given subsequently must be used with great care. Xylazine slows the circulation, so there is a long delay between the intravenous injection of an anaesthetic drug and its effects becoming apparent; unless due allowance is made for this, intravenous anaesthetic agents will be over-dosed.

Medetomidine

Medetomidine is a recently introduced α_2-adrenoceptor agonist (see p. 62) for use in dogs and cats. It is a very potent, selective drug which produces a dose-dependent decrease in the release and turnover of noradrenaline in the central nervous system which is manifested as sedation, analgesia and bradycardia. In the periphery, medetomidine causes vasoconstriction by activation of postsynaptic receptors in the vascular smooth muscle. Thus, as with xylazine, there is an initial increase in arterial pressure due to an increase in systemic vascular resistance. However, when used by the intramuscular route at doses which produce moderately deep sedation (40 µg/kg) the rise is minimal and arterial blood pressure rapidly falls to slightly below the normal resting level [2]. Following medetomidine administration dogs often breathe in an irregular manner, periods of up to 45 seconds of apnoea being followed by several rapid breaths. Although the mucous membranes sometimes appear cyanotic, P_aO_2 is only slightly depressed.

In comparative trials of equisedative doses of xylazine and medetomidine both the type of sedation achieved and the side-effects of bradycardia, respiratory depression and cyanosis were similar, although medetomidine had a longer duration of action. Vomiting occurs in about 20% of dogs receiving medetomidine, but is more frequent and prolonged after xylazine [3]. Both xylazine and medetomidine decrease gut motility and increase blood sugar levels and these effects must be recognized if these drugs are used in dogs undergoing investigational procedures.

Medetomidine has a very steep dose–response curve and doses should, theoretically, be calculated on a body surface area basis rather than on body-weight. In practice this means that smaller dogs require relatively higher doses than large dogs. Over the rising phase of this dose–response curve sedation and analgesia are dose dependent. Thus, in medium-sized dogs 5 µg/kg given intramuscularly produces only slight sedation — the animals can stand and walk (albeit with some ataxia) and are generally amenable to restraint for clipping or intravenous injection — whilst at intramuscular doses of 40 µg/kg deep sedation, bordering on hypnosis is achieved. Although higher doses may be needed in small or difficult animals, once the maximum sedative dose is reached higher doses simply increase the duration of effect.

Although appearing deeply sedated vicious dogs may still be aggressive and must be handled with care.

Medetomidine can be given intramuscularly or intravenously and it is also rapidly absorbed through mucous membranes. Following intravenous injection the dog becomes sedated within 5 minutes but maximal effects may take longer to appear. In medium-sized quiet dogs, maximal sedation is often achieved with intravenous doses of 20 µg/kg. After intramuscular injection maximal sedation and peak blood concentration is reached within 15–20 minutes. The volume of distribution is between 2.8 and 3.5 l/kg and its half-life of elimination (in urine and faeces) from 1 to 1.6 hours (data from Farmos Group Ltd).

The drug is also effective when squirted from a syringe into the oral cavity of vicious dogs in doses of 30–80 µg/kg, but in quiet dogs it may be administered carefully under the tongue and doses of 5–10 µg/kg are very effective by this sublingual route which avoids a first-pass through the liver.

In the UK the data sheet for medetomidine recommends that impervious gloves be worn when handling the drug.

As for all α_2-adrenoceptor agonists, the use of medetomidine for premedication greatly reduces the doses of subsequent anaesthetic required in a dose–effect manner. Its sedative and hypnotic effects have been shown to be synergistic with those of opioids such as fentanyl and butorphanol [2, 4] and with those of all the anaesthetic agents studied. These effects are discussed later (p. 294).

α_2-Adrenoceptor antagonists

In recent years the use of antagonists to terminate prolonged sedation induced by the α_2-adrenoceptor agonists has become more common (p. 63). Yohimbine, at intravenous doses of 0.1 mg/kg, will antagonize the sedation produced by xylazine [5]: higher doses will cause convulsions. Yohimbine for injection is not available in the UK. Atipamezole is a new, specific α_2-adrenoceptor antagonist and in dogs arousal occurs within minutes of its intramuscular injection at five times the dose of medetomidine, the respiratory rate also returning to normal. Although this dose of atipamezole increases the heart rate this does not return to presedation levels. For this, a dose of 10 times the original medetomidine dose must be given or the sedation allowed to wane before the antidote is administered. After large doses of atipamezole dogs have been described as 'over alert' but convulsions have not been encountered. Although atipamezole is marketed specifically for use as an antidote to medetomidine, in the authors' experience intramuscular doses of 200 µg/kg are equally effective in reversing the sedation induced by 3 mg/kg of xylazine in the dog.

Antagonists are useful in limiting the duration of sedation and in counteracting accidental overdosage. They may be particularly valuable in limiting the hypothermia that occurs in small animals under prolonged sedation. However, it must be remembered that they antagonize not only the sedation but also the analgesia induced by the α_2-adrenoceptor agonists, so that in some circumstances reversal of sedation may not be advisable.

Skin contact with solutions of atipamezole should be avoided and impervious gloves worn when administering it.

Sedative/opioid combinations

In general, to produce simple sedation, one of the phenothiazines is combined with an opioid, each drug being used at the dose usually used for premedication. Combelen/Polamivet, consisting of methadone, propionyl promazine and an atropine-like compound, is a commercially available mixture widely used on the Continent of Europe. Another such mixture is that of Omnopon–Scopolamine with acepromazine, and the authors find that 20 mg of Omnopon (papaveretum) and 0.4 mg Scopolomine (hyoscine) combined with 3 mg of acepromazine is a very good premedication for really vicious German shepherd dogs. Other combinations recommended include acepromazine (0.07 mg/kg) with buprenorphine (9 µg/kg) or pethidine (3.3 mg/kg) given by intramuscular injection [6] and xylazine or medetomidine may be used as the sedative instead of acepromazine. Intramuscular medetomidine (40 µg/kg) with butorphanol (0.05 mg/kg) produces deeper sedation than that achieved with medetomidine alone [4] and xylazine has been widely used in combination with methadone. For deeper levels of sedation, and light levels of anaesthesia, the more powerful opiates such as fentanyl or etorphine are used. The best method is undoubtedly to administer the analgesic intravenously to the already sedated dog. Fentanyl is the ideal agent for this because of its short duration of action and if respiratory depression occurs it is short lived because of the limited duration of action of this drug. If respiratory support is needed it should be by IPPV with oxygen rather than resort to antagonist drugs which also antagonize the analgesia.

With the various premixed combinations of drugs which are marketed for sedation in dogs it is impossible to obtain the same degree of control and balance between the components than can be achieved if the drugs are given separately. These formulations are designed to produce optimal effects in about 60% of animals and hence in a large proportion of cases they will be less than satisfactory.

Hypnorm consists of fentanyl with fluanisone. Intramuscular injection produces deep sedation and analgesia of about 20 minutes' duration, which is suitable for minor surgical procedures. Dogs remain sensitive to sound and may react violently to noises, making the preparation unsuitable for use for radiography where the click of the exposure control may make the animal move just as the radiograph is being taken. Supplementary anaesthesia is needed for major surgery and if possible this should take the form of inhalation anaesthesia as intravenous drugs, especially the barbiturates, may produce profound respiratory depression.

The effects of the fentanyl component of Hypnorm may be antagonized by opioid antagonists but the duration of action of the preparation is such that this is seldom necessary.

Innovar-Vet is a combination of fentanyl (0.4 mg/ml) with droperidol (20 mg/ml) which has been used extensively in dogs in North America but it has not been available in the UK.

Small Animal Immobilon contains the powerful and very long-acting opioid etorphine in combination with methotrimeprazine. Given at the manufacturer's recommended doses to the dog by the intravenous, intramuscular or subcutaneous routes, it produces a profound and prolonged state of unconsciousness and analgesia. Intramuscular and subcutaneous injections are painful. Respiratory depression can be severe and the dog may appear cyanotic. Very little work has been published on the cardiovascular effects of Immobilon in dogs but clinical impression suggests that a proportion of animals suffer from severe hypotension, as the mucous membranes become almost white while the pulse becomes almost imperceptible. Convulsions following the use of Immobilon have been reported to the Association of Veterinary Anaesthetists Committee concerned with deaths and adverse reactions of drugs used in anaesthesia.

At the end of surgery, the etorphine component of the mixture may be antagonized by the injection of diprenorphine (p. 72) but the patient remains sedated from the effects of methotrimeprazine. It must be remembered that once the antagonist has been given, attempts to provide analgesia with pure agonist opioids will be unsuccessful. Following reversal of the effects dogs tend to return to a state of deep sedation, or even unconsciousness, several hours after the antagonist has been given.

Although reported mortality is low, morbidity may be high. Owners have reported that dogs 'appear to be different' and instances of postsedation renal failure have occurred after the use of Immobilon. Such morbidity could well be a result of hypoxia and/or hypotension during the period of sedation.

Benzodiazepines

Diazepam is not often used in dogs as it produces no obvious sedation. However, following its use for premedication the dose of induction agents is reduced and diazepam is, perhaps, particularly useful for suppressing the excitatory phenomena which may be seen when methohexitone is used for induction of anaesthesia. It may be used intravenously in doses of 0.25 mg/kg, or intramuscularly at doses of 0.5–1 mg/kg, where the phenothiazine tranquillizers are contraindicated and *obvious* sedation is not required. Intramuscular injection of all the available preparations of diazepam appears to be painful and even intravenous injection of preparations other than 'Diazemuls' is often resented. There is a clinical impression that better sedation results when diazepam is given by mouth so it may be that products formed in the first-pass through the liver are important in producing the sedative effects in dogs.

Midazolam is a potent, short-acting, water-soluble benzodiazepine. It is about twice as potent as diazepam and is very useful for potentiating the effects of other centrally active drugs. Midazolam is not painful on intravenous injection and does not cause thrombophlebitis. Its half-life in dogs has not been accurately defined but appears to be about 60–90 minutes. Attempts to use midazolam in dogs to induce anaesthesia have produced disappointing results, mainly because of considerable variation between individual dogs and currently it can only be recommended for intravenous use in doses of 0.2–0.5 mg/kg for its anxiolytic effects.

Temazepam does not form active metabolites and has a relatively short duration of action. It may be given to dogs in a soft gelatine capsule in doses of approximately 0.25 mg/kg. Although not as flexible as intravenous sedation it may have a place when an orally administered sedative is indicated.

Antagonists which are currently being developed may increase the usefulness of the benzodiazepines. It is possible that one of them, Flumazenil (Ro 15–1788), will fulfil an antagonist role to benzodiazepines as naloxone does with the opioids but, as yet, there is little information on its effects in dogs. The only report to date is that of Erhardt *et al.* [7] on the use of this drug with naloxone to antagonize the effects of a respiratory depressant mixture of fentanyl/climazolam (a benzodiazepine not generally available). Recovery following the injection of the antagonists was quiet and had no pathophysiological sequelae.

PREPARATION FOR ANAESTHESIA

The significance of many of the conditions which may be discovered from the case history and preanaesthetic examination have been discussed in Chapter 1 but there are some aspects of the preanaesthetic preparation of dogs which warrant further consideration.

Previous drug therapy can alter the response of the dog to anaesthesia and operation so that it is essential that details of any such therapy should be sought from the case history. A full discussion of all possible drug interactions is beyond the scope of this book and reference should be made to textbooks on pharmacology, but interactions which are encountered fairly commonly in canine anaesthesia are described below.

Dogs which have been treated with corticosteroid drugs at any time in the 2 months preceding anaesthesia may have a reduced ability to respond to stress. Steroid cover should be given during the surgical period, and if major surgery has been performed this cover should be continued for 3 days. Hydrocortisone hemisuccinate may be given by intramuscular injection in doses of 100–300 mg at the time of premedication and, if necessary, continued at 6-hourly intervals. Other steroids which may be used for this purpose include prednisone and predisolone (three to five times as potent as cortisone), and betamethasone or dexamethasone (35 times as potent) given in divided doses intramuscularly.

Long-term barbiturate therapy for epilepsy may lead to enzyme induction and a decrease in duration of action of similar drugs given for anaesthesia. However, the remaining effects of the long-acting barbiturates will be additive to those of the anaesthetic drugs. In practice, it is difficult to judge which of these two effects will predominate, and intravenous drugs of the barbiturate type should be administered with particular care.

Many antibiotics, in particular those of the streptomycin group, the polymixins and tetracyclines exert an influence at the neuromuscular junction which enhances the effects of competitive muscle relaxants. Chloramphenicol has been reported to increase the length of action of barbiturate drugs but this rarely presents a clinical problem. Organophosphorus compounds used as insecticides reduce available pseudo-cholinesterases and, therefore, prolong the action of suxamethonium.

Anaesthesia in dogs which are digitalized requires skill and caution. Excessive bradycardia during anaesthesia is a danger in digitalized patients and other drugs such as suxamethonium can cause serious ventricular arrhythmias. Many dogs which have been given digitalis no longer need it, and in these cases the drug should be withdrawn some weeks prior to anaesthesia. Where digitalis is essential for the proper maintenance of cardiac function, then careful stabilization is needed to ensure that an overdose is not being given, and treatment should be maintained over the surgical period.

Starvation for about 12 hours usually ensures a dog will have an empty stomach but gastric emptying is delayed in the parturient bitch and in dogs which have been involved in accidents or fights. If the stomach is not empty before anaesthesia dogs often vomit during the induction or recovery periods and inhalation of this vomit may be fatal. Dogs appear to have very weak protective laryngeal reflexes and have been known to inhale vomit even after they have regained

their feet following anaesthesia. Water need not be withheld until premedication is given or until about 2 hours prior to anaesthesia and, indeed, further deprivation can cause renal failure in dogs which have compensated chronic kidney disease.

When a dog is obviously fluid depleted, or when blood loss during surgery is likely to be unavoidably great, an intravenous infusion should be set up before anaesthesia is induced. Percutaneous venepuncture may prove to be almost impossible if left until circulatory failure is established. Ideally, fluid deficits should be replaced before anaesthesia but if this is impracticable, then at least an adequate circulatory volume should be ensured by infusion of blood, plasma or plasma substitute.

PREMEDICATION

Premedication in the dog usually involves the administration of anticholinergic, sedative and analgesic drugs, the combination chosen depending on the circumstances and the anaesthetic technique which is to follow.

Anticholinergic drugs

In dogs, the use of anticholinergic agents is only essential if irritant volatile anaesthetics are to be given, or if techniques involving the administration of neuromuscular blocking agents are to be employed because dogs are not particularly sensitive to vagal reflexes so that their prevention is less necessary than in some other species of animal. In breeds such as the St Bernard which tend to produce excessive quantities of saliva, the use of drying agents is often less helpful than expected as it rapidly makes the saliva thick and viscid rendering it more likely to cause obstruction of the airway. However, the reduction of vagal tone produced by the anticholinergics is useful in counteracting the tendency towards bradycardia when agents such as halothane are used, but their use to counteract the effects of the α_2-adrenoceptor agonists remains controversial. The only contraindications to their use are pre-existing tachycardia, and certain ocular conditions where the dilatation of the pupil which they produce may be undesirable.

Atropine sulphate is the anticholinergic drug frequently used in dogs, and may be given by the intramuscular, subcutaneous or intravenous routes. Dose rates commonly range from 0.02–0.1 mg/kg (about 0.25 mg to a puppy and up to 1.8 mg for a large dog when the 0.6 mg/ml solution is used). The dose rate is not critical as atropine is very rapidly removed from the bloodstream of a dog, and over-

dose is very rare. When it does occur, it results in convulsions which, if the dose is high enough, may be followed by coma and death.

Other anticholinergic drugs are sometimes used as part of neuroleptanalgesic mixtures. Hyoscine is combined with papaveretum in Omnopon–Scopolamine (p. 75) and diphenylpiperidinoethylacetamide in Combelen/Polamivet and when such mixtures are used atropine is not required. Glycopyrrolate has also been used in dogs at a dose rate of 0.01 mg/kg. It appears to have no clear advantages in this species of animal over atropine except that it does not readily cross the blood–brain barrier and is less likely to produce central nervous stimulation.

Sedative and analgesic premedication

Premedication with sedative and opioid drugs contributes to a smooth induction of anaesthesia by reducing stress and allowing easy handling of the dog. It also reduces the dose of subsequent anaesthetics and helps to provide a calm and pain-free recovery from anaesthesia. Thus, it becomes an integral part of the anaesthetic procedure. It is, therefore, particularly important to allow sufficient time to elapse for the maximal effects of premedication to develop before anaesthesia is induced, as failure to do this may result in overdosage of induction agents. The influence of high doses of premedicant drugs on subsequent induction doses of anaesthetics can be dramatic (Table 15.2) and the decision to use high or low doses is influenced by the personal preferences of the anaesthetist.

Any of the analgesic and sedative drugs already discussed may be used for premedication but those most commonly employed for this purpose in dogs

Table 15.2 Examples of the effects of premedication on the subsequent dose of induction agent

Premedicant drug and dose	Induction agent and dose
No premedication	Thiopentone 10 mg/kg
Acepromazine 0.03–0.05 mg/kg i.m.	Thiopentone 7–8 mg/kg
Medetomidine 5 μg/kg i.m.	Thiopentone 7–8 mg/kg
Medetomidine 10 μg/kg i.m.	Thiopentone 6–7 mg/kg
Alfentanil 5 μg/kg i.v.	Thiopentone 3–5 mg/kg
No premedication	Propofol 6–7 mg/kg
Acepromazine 0.03–0.05 mg/kg i.m.	Propofol 4 mg/kg
Medetomidine 40 μg/kg i.m.	Propofol 1–1.5 mg/kg
Alfentanil 5 μg/kg i.v.	Propofol 3–4 mg/kg
Alfentanil 10 μg/kg	Propofol 1–2 mg/kg

The examples in this table refer to the situation in fit, healthy dogs. Sick animals may require considerably less while individual dogs may require more or less of the induction agent following premedication.

are the opioids, the phenothiazines and the α_2-adrenoceptor agonists.

The use of opioids may increase preoperative sedation and contribute to intraoperative and postoperative analgesia. Generally, opioids with a fairly long action are chosen (e.g. morphine 0.1–0.3 mg/kg, or pethidine 1–4 mg/kg, or butorphanol 0.2 mg/kg, all by intramuscular injection) and recently buprenorphine (0.006 mg/kg intramuscularly) has become particularly popular because of its prolonged length of action. When opioids of this level of potency are used at the doses suggested for premedication they have a minimal effect on the dose of anaesthetic subsequently required. However, at higher doses the reduction in dose of induction agent needed may be marked. This is particularly true when potent opioids such as fentanyl, alfentanil or etorphine are employed. Dogs given the mixtures of Hypnorm®, Innovar-Vet® or Immobilon® are usually considered to be anaesthetized rather than sedated and should these mixtures be followed by other anaesthetic agents only very small doses will be needed. Fentanyl is usually used to provide intraoperative analgesia, but recently alfentanil, given intravenously immediately prior to injection of an intravenous induction agent has been found to be useful in reducing the dose of that agent and so speeding recovery from its effects.

Acepromazine in intravenous or intramuscular doses of 0.03–0.05 mg/kg calms most animals effectively for venepuncture and reduces the induction dose of thiopentone or propofol by about one-third. Higher doses do not reduce the induction dose further but considerably lengthen the anaesthetic recovery period. For vicious dogs acepromazine may be combined with an opioid such as buprenorphine (0.006 mg/kg); this increases effective sedation without appreciably reducing the induction doses still further. Acepromazine is long acting so it contributes to postoperative sedation and has the added advantage that it seems to reduce myocardial irritability. However, its hypotensive action means that it is contraindicated in hypovolaemic animals.

Xylazine and medetomidine may produce profound sedation and greatly decrease the dose of anaesthetics used subsequently. Unfortunately, it is not always easy to predict the dose of subsequent anaesthetic that will be required as although in general there is a decrease in anaesthetic dose with increased dose of sedative there is considerable variation from animal to animal. The situation is complicated by the fact that the fall in cardiac output induced by these sedative drugs greatly increases the vein/brain circulation time so that there may be a considerable delay (1 minute or more) between injection of an intravenous drug and its full effect being obvious. The slow circulation also delays the uptake of volatile inhalation agents, again leading to danger of overdosage if this is not appreciated. Many anaesthetists therefore prefer to use these sedatives at low doses (e.g. medetomidine at 5–10 μg/kg intramuscularly) for premedication but, if higher doses have been given, for example to a vicious dog, then all subsequent agents should be given slowly, allowing adequate time to assess fully their effects. Xylazine and medetomidine are perhaps particularly useful in preventing the convulsant effects of ketamine, but as they cause marked cardiovascular changes (p. 59) their use in dogs suffering from cardiovascular or pulmonary diseases, or those with body fluid deficits, is inadvisable.

INTRAVENOUS ANAESTHESIA

In dogs, as in other animals, intravenous agents may be used either to induce anaesthesia which is then maintained by inhalation methods, or as sole anaesthetic agents. Despite their dangers and disadvantages when used as sole anaesthetic agents, this use is increasing because of fears over the effects of pollution of the atmosphere by volatile inhalation anaesthetics.

The use of intravenous drugs as sole anaesthetics does not mean that anaesthetic machines are unnecessary. All the measures normally taken to maintain proper respiratory function during anaesthesia must still be employed. The intravenous agents commonly produce respiratory depression and endotracheal intubation, the administration of oxygen, and even IPPV,

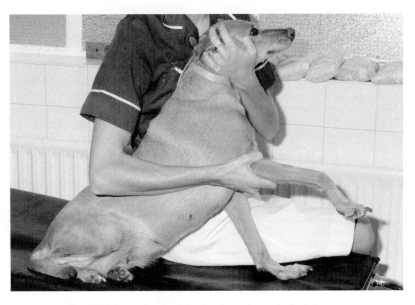

Fig. 15.1 Restraint for injection into the cephalic vein.

may be necessary if hypoxaemia and hypercapnia are to be avoided.

Some intravenous agents may also be given by subcutaneous or intramuscular injection but these routes of administration always suffer from the disadvantages of variable absorption leading to a sometimes stormy induction, and the difficulty of gauging the dose.

Intravenous technique

Intravenous injections in dogs are most commonly made into the cephalic vein, but other convenient sites include the recurrent tarsal vein, the femoral vein, the jugular vein and, in anaesthetized subjects, the sublingual veins. Whichever site is used, the conscious dog should be handled quietly and forcible restraint reserved for those occasions when it is essential. Muzzles should only be applied to dogs showing an inclination to bite. The quick removal of the muzzle which is entangled in the facial hair is not always easy and any delay in its removal from dogs which vomit during the induction of anaesthesia can lead to inhalation of the vomited material.

Haematoma formation after venepuncture should be prevented by the application of pressure to the site for an adequate period — usually about a minute. Haematoma are not only painful for the patient; they may prevent the subsequent use of the particular vein for venepuncture for several days. Where a vein has been entered during an unsuccessful attempt at venepuncture, the pressure which was keeping the vein distended should be released and firm pressure applied to the site to stop bleeding before another attempt is made.

If the vein on the right fore-leg is to be punctured an assistant stands on the left side of the animal, passes his or her left arm around the animal's neck and raises its head (Fig. 15.1). The assistant's right hand grips the animal's right fore-leg so that the middle, third and fourth fingers are immediately behind the olecranon and the thumb is round the front side of the limb. The limb is extended by pushing on the olecranon and the vein is raised by applying pressure with the thumb. Venepuncture must, of course, be carried out with the usual aseptic precautions, so the hair over the vein is clipped and the skin is disinfected.

It is an advantage to use a syringe which has an eccentrically placed nozzle for this allows the syringe to rest securely on the fore-arm with the needle more or less flush to the vein. In this way the angle of entrance, that is, the angle between the needle and the vein, is small and consequently there is much less risk of the needle being pushed right through the vein.

Suitable needle sizes depend to some extent on the size of the dog and the quantity and viscosity of the fluid to be injected. For most purposes a needle 2.5 cm long and 23 gauge (0.6 mm bore) is quite satisfactory. The points of the needle should not be cut too acutely, the so-called 'short bevel' or 'dental cut' being preferred.

Two methods of stabilizing the vein prior to needle puncture are employed. In one, the skin over the vein is kept taut by the thumb and fore-finger of the

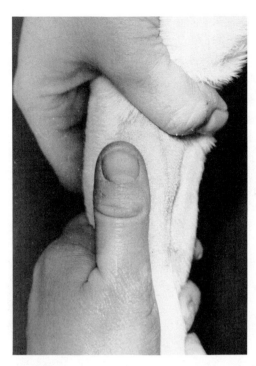

Fig. 15.2 Stabilization of the cephalic vein against the thumb.

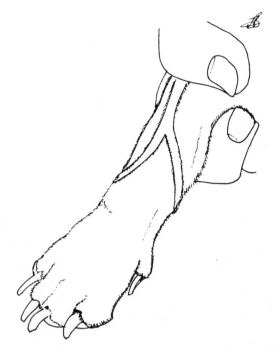

Fig. 15.3 In short-legged dogs such as Dachshunds with very mobile skins the easiest point for venepuncture is at the junction of the veins from the medial and lateral aspects of the carpus where they form the cephalic vein.

anaesthetist's left hand which grasps the animal's fore-arm immediately below the site of puncture. In this position it is easy for the anaesthetist to grip the syringe between the left thumb and fore-finger once the vein has been entered. The skin should be pierced immediately over the vein to avoid the branches of the radial nerve which run on either side of the vein in the region of the limb.

In the second method, the anaesthetist's left thumb is placed just alongside the vein, and the skin is not tensed (Fig. 15.2). The vein is stabilized between the needle and the thumb as the needle is advanced through the skin into the vein. With this method there is a greater tendency to make contact between the needle point and the branch of the radial nerve running alongside the vein.

In Dachshunds and dogs with similar short, bent fore-limbs venepuncture is best attempted in the angle where the veins join to form the cephalic vein just cranial to the carpus (Fig. 15.3).

All air should be expressed from the syringe before venepuncture is attempted and there must be sufficient space left in the syringe to allow slight withdrawal of the piston in order to test whether the needle is within the lumen of the vessel. Blood should enter the syringe when this is done, and no injection must be made if blood does not appear in the syringe. Failure to draw blood usually means that either the vein has not been entered, or that the needle has

become occluded. Failure to aspirate blood into the syringe is also encountered if the vein is already thrombosed, or if peripheral perfusion is very poor as it may be after the use of α_2-adrenoceptor agonists.

The recurrent tarsal vein may be used for intravenous injection at the point where it passes cranially and dorsally on the lateral aspect of the leg just cranial to the tarsus. Either hind-leg may be used with the animal restrained on its side, but two assistants may be required. One places an arm under the animal's neck and grips both fore-legs, and with the other arm exerts pressure on the neck and head. The other assistant holds the limb to be used for the injection in a state of full extension and raises the vein as shown in Fig. 15.4. The recurrent tarsal vein is usually more prominent than the cephalic vein but it is more mobile and therefore more difficult to puncture. When the needle has been introduced well into the vein the syringe is fixed to the leg by pressing on the needle hub with the thumb while the fingers encircle the limb.

The femoral vein in the middle part of the medial aspect of the thigh may also be used. It is rendered obvious by pressure applied to the inguinal region and is usually more prominent in the cranial part of the thigh. Care should be taken to ensure that injections are not made into the femoral artery which lies directly beneath the vein.

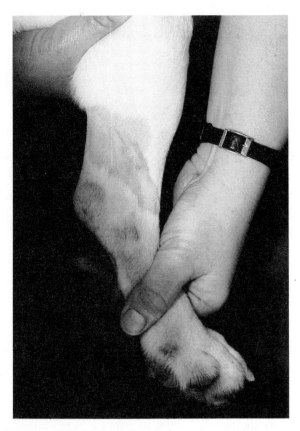

Fig. 15.4 Method of extending the limb and raising the recurrent tarsal vein.

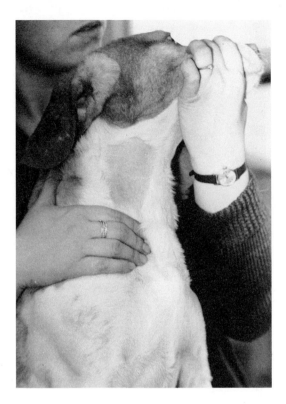

Fig. 15.5 Jugular venepuncture in the conscious, sitting dog.

Venepuncture of the jugular vein in the dog is a very simply procedure. It can be carried out with the dog standing or sitting with the head raised (Fig. 15.5) and the technique is very similar to that used in horses (p. 211). In smaller or ill patients it is easier when the animal is restrained on its side and the vein is raised by occlusion near the sternal inlet. A small foam pad or sandbag placed under the neck of the dog makes the position of the vein more obvious. This vein is particularly useful when fluids are to be infused and because of the mobility of the skin a 5.25 inch (13 cm) long catheter (Angiocath, Deseret) or a longer one should be introduced and sutured in place when long-term intravenous fluid therapy is anticipated.

The sublingual veins may be used for intravenous injections in anaesthetized dogs. The tongue is pulled over the anaesthetist's finger so that its ventral surface is exposed and injection is made into one of the easily visible veins. It is usually impossible to aspirate blood through the needle introduced into one of these veins, but extravascular injection causes very obvious swelling when only small amounts (less than 0.1 ml) of solution has been injected. It is important to use the smallest available needle (25 gauge or smaller) for even when such needles are used the vein will bleed very freely after their withdrawal, and pressure has to be applied to the site for several minutes if very painful sublingual haematomata are to be avoided.

Intravenous agents

Thiopentone sodium

Solutions of thiopentone have a high pH and the drug can only be given by the intravenous route. It should always be used in dogs as a 2.5% or weaker solution for more concentrated solutions are unnecessary and dangerous. Use of a 5% solution increases the total quantity of the drug required, causes thrombosis of the vein and, if any is injected perivascularly, produces a serious slough of the overlying tissues and skin. The thrombosis caused by the concentrated solutions of thiopentone occurs over several days following the injections so it is seldom noticed unless there is a need for further venepuncture in this period. Sloughing of the skin may give rise to litigation for the recovery of damages and the injection of any quantity of even a 2.5% solution into the tissues outside the vein is an indication for the immediate injection of at least 10–20 ml of saline into the area.

The dose of thiopentone depends on the condition of the dog, its state of hydration, and on previous medication. For these reasons it is often stated to be 'sufficient and no more' but as a rough guide the anaesthetist should expect to have to use up to 10 mg/kg in any individual case which is presented for induction. In the fit but lightly premedicated dog, two-thirds of this, i.e. about 7 mg/kg, given rapidly as a bolus of a 2.5% solution, should produce a rapid induction of anaesthesia adequate to permit a smooth transition to inhalation anaesthesia with or without endotracheal intubation. Large dogs require relatively less than smaller animals but if the drug is given slowly, or to an inadequately premedicated dog, then the total dose of 10 mg/kg which should have been drawn up into the syringe, may be required. In the sick or heavily premedicated dog considerably lower doses may be sufficient. Induction with these quantities produces little serious circulatory depression and although there may be a period of apnoea it is brief.

Potent opioids also reduce the dose of thiopentone needed to induce anaesthesia — for example, it may be greatly reduced by the administration of alfentanil. The alfentanil is given intravenously in a dose of 5 µg/kg over a 30 second period immediately before the injection of the thiopentone. The use of a dilute solution of alfentanil helps in the slow administration which is necessary to prevent the occurrence of apnoea when thiopentone is injected. Alfentanil may produce bradycardia and, therefore, many anaesthetists mix it with a small dose of atropine (e.g. 0.3 mg) or glycopyrrolate, for although this may be unwise on strictly pharmacological grounds, in practice it is both safe and effective. The initial dose of thiopentone required after alfentanil is about 3 mg/kg and if this is insufficient to allow endotracheal intubation, increments of 10–25 mg are given to effect. Recovery is fast due to the small dose of thiopentone needed.

In dogs, thiopentone is very slowly metabolized and attempts to prolong anaesthesia with multiple or higher doses which saturate the body fat result in very prolonged anaesthesia followed by 'hangover' for 24 or more hours. In thin dogs such as greyhounds (which may also be deficient in the liver enzymes necessary for detoxication of thiopentone), this level is reached very rapidly indeed, and little more than the minimum induction dose may be given with safety [8–10]. Thiopentone differs from some other intravenous agents in that high doses cause severe respiratory depression so that prolonged anaesthesia cannot be produced by an initial high dose, but must be maintained by incremental doses. Where thiopentone is used as a sole anaesthetic, recovery may be violent and noisy. Sedative premedication can prevent this, so should always be employed, but if it is omitted, a sedative or analgesic should be given intravenously at the end of anaesthesia.

The maximum total dose of thiopentone for a fit dog is about 25 mg/kg — and this would represent a gross overdose in a thin or sick patient. Full consciousness may not be regained for 24 hours after a dose of this magnitude. Because of its lack of analgesic properties, attempts to use thiopentone for painful procedures, even short ones such as the removal of a barley-grass awn from the external ear canal, tend to result in overdosage. It must be emphasized that thiopentone should be regarded as more as a hypnotic rather than an anaesthetic agent, and it is better to ignore slight limb movements or respiratory irregularities caused by surgical stimulation than to administer larger quantities of thiopentone in an attempt to abolish them. With experience, the correct, *small* dose for the operation or examination procedure may be given in an initial very rapid injection, but if this does not produce satisfactory conditions, there is no alternative but to inject further small doses or to use some other technique to produce the desired depression of the central nervous system. Because the dose used will depend so much on the anaesthetist's appreciation of the depth of anaesthesia, in learning to use the drug the anaesthetist will have to rely upon observation of almost all of the reflex signs in order to assess depth but, with increasing experience, concentration on the breathing and the response to surgical stimulation will suffice. The experienced anaesthetist aims to produce, at all times, the minimum of respiratory depression while only just abolishing, or perhaps on occasion only modifying, the response to stimulation. This is accomplished by very careful, sometimes subconscious, attention to detail.

Doses of up to 5 mg/kg of thiopentone may be given by very rapid intravenous injection to unpremedicated dogs before the application of a facemask for the completion of induction with an inhalation agent. No attempt is made to give sufficient thiopentone to allow endotracheal intubation to be performed, and the sole object is to produce just sufficient depression to overcome struggling when the dog is introduced to the inhalation agent. (Too much thiopentone depresses the respiration and interferes with the uptake of the inhalation agent.) This is probably the best way to use thiopentone for outpatients, for if an agent such as halothane is employed as the main anaesthetic agent, recovery of consciousness should be complete within very few minutes of the termination of anaesthesia. Because of the rapid recovery, this is a good method to employ in brachycephalic breeds of dogs, although in these the anaesthetist must be prepared to give slightly greater quantities of thiopentone so that endotracheal intubation may be carried out under its influence should respiratory obstruction develop as soon as consciousness is lost.

As with all anaesthetics, the best results are only obtained by an anaesthetist who is thoroughly familiar with thiopentone and who is able to exercise a little artistry in its administration. To illustrate this point it may be noted that anaesthetists beginning their training find it necessary to administer far larger doses than are used in comparable cases by experienced anaesthetists, yet it is often extremely difficult to understand why this should be so. Possibly the manner in which the animal is handled, the difficulty encountered in atraumatic venepuncture, and the lack of familiarity with the signs of thiopentone anaesthesia, all contribute to the necessity for a larger dose of the drug.

In the absence of surgical stimulation the first indication that thiopentone anaesthesia is passing off is that stiffening of the jaws and curling of the tongue occur when the mouth is opened. There may be licking of the nose and from this point recovery is rapid. In 5 minutes or so the animal will be attempting to raise its head and in a further 10 minutes it will be able to maintain the prone position. The dog is obviously quite conscious and aware of its environment about half an hour after induction where no other anaesthetic agent has been given to prolong anaesthesia. Limb coordination, especially the hind, is delayed, and the dog may stagger in a rather drunken manner for about an hour. There is no postanaesthetic malaise or vomiting.

Thiamylal sodium

The properties of thiamylal sodium are very similar to those of thiopentone sodium but it is slightly more potent, a 2% solution being equivalent to 2.5% thiopentone. It is claimed that this drug is less cumulative than thiopentone and gives rise to fewer signs of excitement during induction and recovery, but this has never been substantiated by controlled trials.

Thiamylal is widely used in North America, but in the UK it is so much more expensive than thiopentone that its use has been very limited. When used in equivalent concentrations there is little obvious difference between the two drugs.

Methohexitone sodium

Although recovery from a single 'slug' dose of methohexitone is due mainly to redistribution to the body fat, the drug is rapidly eliminated from the body by metabolism and excretion so that dogs recover from even large doses quite quickly. In general it is advisable to use a sedative premedication to smoothe induction and recovery, because without such sedation both periods may be violent. Intravenous doses of 4–6 mg/kg in a 1 or 2% solution injected at a rate of approximately 10 ml/s are suitable for the induction of anaesthesia in dogs premedicated with acepromazine, and further small increments given as required may be used to prolong anaesthesia. Because of its rapid elimination from the body, recovery after prolonged methohexitone anaesthesia usually occurs within half an hour of the last dose being given. Overdose produces severe respiratory depression, and even anaesthetic doses produce more respiratory depression than equipotent doses of thiopentone. Depression of cardiac output with low anaesthetic doses is also greater than after equipotent doses of thiopentone [11].

Because recovery is so rapid and complete, methohexitone is most useful for outpatient anaesthesia, although it must be recognized that the need for sedative premedication or the administration of sedatives at the end of anaesthesia does produce some prolongation of recovery. It is also useful as an induction agent in thin dogs, young dogs and for caesarean section. If given as an infusion it can be used as the sole agent for anaesthesia provided the inspired air is enriched with oxygen. However, its pharmacokinetics are such that cumulation does occur in doses in excess of 10–12 mg/kg, which therefore limits its use by infusion.

As with thiopentone the dose of methohexitone can be reduced by the prior intravenous injection of 5 µg/kg of alfentanil. Provided this is given slowly over more than 30 seconds the subsequent injection of 2–3 mg/kg methohexitone does not result in significant apnoea. The incidence of myoclonia, movement and hiccups is greatly reduced and, consequently, induction of anaesthesia is much smoother. This procedure is useful in dogs such as greyhounds to minimize the dose of barbiturate used but if they are stimulated in the recovery period violent narcotic excitement can result.

Today, the indications for the use of methohexitone in dogs are few. It has largely been replaced by propofol.

Pentobarbitone sodium

Pentobarbitone was formerly widely used in canine anaesthesia and there can be no doubt that at the time of its introduction in the early 1930s it caused a revolution in small animal practice. By the end of 1938 the slow intravenous injection of pentobarbitone had been used to produce anaesthesia in more than 2000 operation cases in the Beaumont Hospital of the Royal Veterinary College, London, by J. G.

Wright and his colleagues, and in over 800 consecutive ones without a death attributable to the anaesthetic. These results were so much better than any that had been achieved by earlier methods that pentobarbitone soon became the standard agent for producing anaesthesia of about an hour's duration.

Although pentobarbitone is not often used now for clinical canine surgery it still has a place in situations where facilities for the administration of inhalation anaesthetics are not available. It is still widely employed in experimental laboratories and the veterinary anaesthetist must be prepared to advise and instruct laboratory workers in its use. Another use for pentobarbitone is in the treatment of poisoning with substances which produce convulsions (e.g. strychnine).

After weighing the animal the approximate dose is estimated on a basis of about 30 mg/kg body weight. This dose, together with a little more of the drug, is drawn up into a syringe. In fit animals, about two-thirds of the computed probable dose is injected rapidly as soon as venepuncture has been performed, in order to ensure that the dog passes quickly through the excitement phase of induction of anaesthesia. The remainder of the dose is administered over 3–4 minutes, pausing after the injection of each increment and assessing its effect. When complete relaxation of the head and neck is obtained, the assistant releases the fore-limbs and if a muzzle has been used it is removed. Opening the mouth provokes movement of the tongue and jaws varying from a complete yawn to a slight curling of the tip of the tongue. A little more of the anaesthetic is injected and after an appropriate wait the jaws are again opened. The aim is to reach the point at which the jaws are completely relaxed and the tongue, when drawn out, hangs limply.

When this is attained, a light level of unconsciousness can be assumed. The corneal reflex is present, the pupil reacts to light and the pedal reflex is brisk. Respirations are regular and deep. This is the degree of anaesthesia to be induced for superficial operations. If an intra-abdominal interference is to be made, it may be decided to deepen from this point during peritoneal manipulations by an inhalation agent. At any rate, it may be taken that this depth of anaesthesia is perfectly safe. If it is decided to induce deeper unconsciousness with pentobarbitone, the so-called 'pedal reflex' is then used as the index of depth. If the web between the digits is pinched firmly with the finger and thumbnails, it will be found that the pedal reflex comprises a definite upward and backward jerking of the limb. Often the response continues for several seconds after the stimulus has ceased. Administration is slowly continued until the reflex is just lost and then the depth of unconsciousness is adequate for the performance of intra-abdominal procedures.

Propofol

Propofol, as the free-flowing oil-in-water emulsion which does not give rise to histamine liberation, is now commonly used in dogs [12–15]. It is compatible with all the adjuvant drugs used in canine anaesthesia.

The dose for induction of anaesthesia in unpremedicated dogs is 6 mg/kg and premedication with 0.02–0.04 mg/kg of acepromazine reduces this to about 4 mg/kg. Females are more susceptible than males, the induction dose in unpremedicated females being 5.23 mg/kg (SD 1.58, $n = 68$) and in males 5.74 mg/kg (SD 1.53, $n = 39$) [14]. After induction, propofol may be given in incremental doses as needed to maintain anaesthesia and in unpremedicated dogs the requirements approximate to 0.8 mg/(kg min) [14]. In dogs premedicated with acepromazine (0.05 mg/kg) and atropine (0.02 mg/kg) propofol continuously infused at a rate of 0.4 mg/(kg min) produces acceptable operating conditions but although apparently quite safe, maintenance of anaesthesia is associated with some complications such as muscle rigidity, limb tremors and hiccough [16] in a proportion of animals. Induction and recovery are usually quite trouble free but retching and vomiting have been encountered in the recovery period in 16% of dogs after continuous infusion of the agent. Dogs left unstimulated in the recovery period appear to sleep — arousal during this stage can result in immediate awakening with an ability to walk without ataxia. Dogs given one dose of propofol recover completely in about 18 minutes from the time of its injection and those given intermittent injections recover in about 22 minutes from the time of injection of the final increment. Acepromazine premedication (0.02–0.04 mg/kg) slightly, but not statistically, prolongs recovery [14].

The effect on respiratory rate is variable but dogs which are panting before the induction of anaesthesia are likely to continue to do so throughout anaesthesia. Propofol undoubtedly produces dose-dependent respiratory depression. A most alarming feature is that a small number of dogs become cyanosed for some minutes after the injection of propofol although normal breathing movements are present during the cyanotic episode. To date there are no reports of blood gas values during this time, but the fact that air is moving in and out of the lungs and the cyanosis does not disappear when oxygen is administered seems to indicate that there may be opening up of pulmonary shunts in these animals. Propofol produces no consistent effects on pulse rate or arterial blood pressure. The dose-dependent arterial hypotension reported in man does not appear to be a feature of propofol anaesthesia in dogs.

At the moment it seems that propofol should be confined to the role of an induction agent or single-dose anaesthetic for although Hall and Chambers [16] concluded that the continuous infusion of propofol to maintain anaesthesia in healthy dogs was safe, it appeared to be less satisfactory than the use of thiopentone–halothane/nitrous oxide–oxygen.

Undoubtedly, the most striking feature of propofol anaesthesia is the rapid, excitement-free, complete recovery. This is invaluable when a dog has to be returned to the owner's care with the minimum of delay.

Because propofol is expensive attempts have been made to reduce the quantity required to induce anaesthesia. Chambers [17] reported that the use of alfentanil (10 µg/kg intravenously mixed with 0.3 mg atropine) immediately before the intravenous injection of propofol reduced the dose of propofol needed to induce unconsciousness to about 2 mg/kg. However, apnoea of more than 3 minutes' duration occurred in 11% of his dogs and 6% showed twitching or paddling, usually of the fore-legs. Later trials (Hall, unpublished observations) demonstrated that a dose of 5 µg/kg of alfentanil (again mixed with 0.3 mg of atropine) given over 30 seconds resulted in less apnoea without significantly increasing the subsequent dose of propofol needed. Recovery time from injection to full awakening (no ataxia) is of the order of 7 minutes — a very fast recovery. The elimination of both alfentanil and propofol in dogs can be described by a three-compartment model. Both have very short distribution half-lives, 3.6 and 7.4 minutes respectively, and short metabolic half-lives of 24 and 53 minutes (J. B. Glen, personal communication). Awakening from a bolus dose probably occurs rapidly by redistribution. Further studies to determine the optimum dose of alfentanil before propofol are needed.

Ketamine

The dose of ketamine which produces anaesthesia in dogs is very near to that which causes convulsions, and ketamine cannot be recommended as a sole agent for canine anaesthesia. In North America it has been used in dogs in combination with various sedative agents to induce deep sedation or light general anaesthesia. Atropine premedication has been used to prevent excessive salivation which otherwise occurs, and if deep general anaesthesia has been needed these mixtures have been supplemented with inhalation anaesthetics. A very wide range of sedatives has been used, including xylazine, acepromazine, promazine and diazepam, in many different doses. Commonly, ketamine has been used in doses of about 5.5 mg/kg together with, for example, 2 mg/kg xylazine [18] or 2.75 mg/kg promazine [19]. Such mixtures give about 30 minutes of anaesthesia with the dog

regaining its feet approximately 2 hours from the time of injection. Both intramuscular and intravenous injections have been used, but even these comparatively low doses of ketamine produce convulsions in some patients. In the trial carried out by Stephenson and coworkers [18] convulsions occurred in four out of 17 dogs. It is said that although ketamine does not often cause respiratory depression, it does occasionally produce respiratory arrest, so that the patient should be kept under constant observation from the time of injection until complete recovery has occurred.

Metomidate

Little has been published in the English language about the use of metomidate in dogs although it has been quite widely used in this species of animal on the Continent of Europe. Its effect is hypnotic rather than anaesthetic; additional analgesia is needed before surgery is possible and heavy sedative or analgesic premedication is essential to prevent the occurrence of twitching and spontaneous muscle movements during anaesthesia.

Etomidate

Erhardt [20] reported the use of etomidate and alfentanil mixed in a ratio of 1 mg to 0.015 mg for anaesthesia in dogs. He recorded its successful use for short-term anaesthesia and commented that recovery was rapid. The drug has not, however, achieved popularity in canine anaesthesia and, in the Cambridge Veterinary School, etomidate anaesthesia without the simultaneous use of alfentanil has been associated with pain on injection and emergence excitement.

Steroids

Saffan, the only steroid anaesthetic currently on the market, is specifically contraindicated by the manufacturers for use in dogs, as it is solubilized in Cremophor EL — a compound which may cause massive release of histamine in all Canidae. Although it has been claimed that following heavy premedication with potent antihistamines Saffan can be used quite safely in dogs [21, 22], reports to the Association of Veterinary Anaesthetists of Great Britain and Ireland indicate that even after this premedication Saffan administration is still followed by anaphylaxis. It is the authors' view that to administer an anaesthetic which is known to have dangerous side-effects and to counteract these with other drugs which are not without their own disadvantages is simply not justifiable when simple and safe alternatives exist.

Minaxalone, a water-soluble steroid anaesthetic,

has undergone clinical trials in both man [23] and dogs [24] but following chronic toxicity studies it was withdrawn by the manufacturers and is unlikely to be reintroduced.

INHALATION ANAESTHESIA

A wide variety of inhalation agents has, in the past, been used in canine anaesthesia but today the presence of electrical apparatus potentially capable of igniting flammable or explosive gas mixtures discourages the use of any but non-flammable, non-explosive agents in the hospital environment. The choice of agent or agents in any particular case is largely governed by the anaesthetist's knowledge of the limitations of each agent and, of course, by the apparatus, assistance and other drugs available at the time. The properties of the gaseous and volatile agents commonly employed in dogs which influence their choice are summarized from a practical point of view in Table 15.3.

Table 15.3 Properties of inhalation agents commonly used in dogs

Agent	Rapidity of action	Analgesic activity	Other properties
Nitrous oxide	++++	Good	Inadequate on its own
Enflurane	+++	Poor	Spontaneous movements
Halothane	++	Poor	Hypotension, respiratory depression
Isoflurane	+++	Poor	Hypotension, respiratory depression
Methoxyflurane	+	Good	Supplement to nitrous oxide

Anaesthetic ether, now only obtainable with difficulty, is slow acting but produces good analgesia. Its main disadvantage is its flammable and explosive nature in air and oxygen.

The inhalation agents may be used in dogs both to induce or maintain anaesthesia, or, more commonly, to maintain anaesthesia which has been induced with an intravenous agent. With intravenous agents induction of anaesthesia is rapid, pleasant and safe for the animal; contraindications to their use are very few. However, it is not too difficult to obtain a smooth, quiet induction of anaesthesia with the inhalation agents in cases where it is really necessary. The dog should be placed on a table at a convenient height and gently restrained by an assistant. Oxygen, together with up to 66% of nitrous oxide if available (to make use of the second-gas effect — Chapter 6, p. 110), should be fed from the anaesthetic machine to a non-rebreathing system such as the Magill which is connected to a malleable face-mask. The mask is put near, but not on, the dog's muzzle.

The volatile agent is introduced gradually into the gas mixture, its concentration being increased slightly after every three or four breaths of the animal. Once the maximum desired concentration has been achieved the mask is slowly and carefully brought closer to the dog's muzzle until finally it is closely applied to the face. Attempts to introduce high concentrations of a volatile agent too early in the procedure usually result in the patient struggling, breath holding and becoming excited. With care, induction of anaesthesia can be rapidly obtained with halothane, isoflurane and enflurane.

Once anaesthesia has been induced the breathing system may be changed to a rebreathing circuit if so desired. During induction, however, a non-rebreathing system is essential. If a low-flow system is used with minimal gas flows, the uptake of anaesthetic by the animal results in dilution of the anaesthetic in the reservoir bag, and delays the onset of anaesthesia. This dilution factor is equally important when first administering volatile agents following intravenous induction of anaesthesia. Another factor to be considered is that if a rebreathing circuit is used, the nitrogen exhaled by the dog may accumulate in the circuit and thus reduce the inspired oxygen concentration.

If the only apparatus which is available is an absorber system, then it must be used with a high gas flow rate and an open relief valve, while the rebreathing bag must be emptied at frequent intervals. The larger the dog, the longer the time dilution occurs and the greater the period before the flow rate may be reduced. In circuits such as the Stephens machine, where the vaporizer is incorporated in the breathing circuit (see p. 165), so that more anaesthetic is vaporized with every breath, dilution of the volatile agent at induction does not occur. However, nitrogen accumulation in the system occurs so that frequent emptying of the rebreathing bag is still needed.

The different types of breathing systems which are available are described in Chapter 9 and the choice of system in any particular case will depend on the size of the dog. For small dogs the resistance and deadspace of the apparatus must be sufficiently low. The non-rebreathing systems commonly used in dogs include the Ayre's T-piece, the Magill circuit, and the coaxial circuits such as the Bain or Lack systems (p. 159). These systems have the great advantage that the concentrations of gases which are breathed by the patient are those delivered from the anaesthetic machine, so that a stable level of anaesthesia is very easy to maintain. This is particularly useful when monitoring the depth of anaesthesia becomes difficult because of the location of the surgical site. These circuits also have a low dead-space and a low resistance, but their use causes the dog to lose heat from the inspiration of cold, dry gases. This cooling effect may be an advantage or disadvantage depending on the ambient temperature. Their main disadvantage is that a relatively high total gas flow rate is needed to prevent rebreathing and consequently running costs are greater than with closed systems. Pollution of the air in the room can be simply overcome by the use of ducting from the expiratory valve or open end of the reservoir tube (p. 393).

An Ayre's T-piece is the circuit of choice for all dogs of less than 5 kg of body weight because of its exceptionally low dead-space and resistance to breathing. To prevent rebreathing it is generally agreed that the fresh gas flow to the system should be twice the minute volume of respiration. The Magill or Lack circuits (p. 159) may be used for all larger dogs and although theoretically a supply of fresh gas equal to the minute volume of alveolar ventilation should be sufficient to prevent rebreathing, in practice most anaesthetists allow a flow equal to the total ventilation per minute. Clearly, one problem which arises in the use of non-rebreathing systems is estimation of the minute volume of the patient so that the appropriate fresh gas flow rate can be set. Minute volume depends on the size of the dog and on the depth of anaesthesia and Fig. 15.6, which shows the relationship between body weight and respiratory variables in dogs, may be used as a guide to the fresh gas flow rates required.

Inhalation anaesthesia is also administered to dogs from both to-and-fro and circle absorber circuits. Their main advantage over non-rebreathing systems are that they are economical in use because they conserve anaesthetic agents, and without any special measures being necessary, reduce pollution of the room air to a minimum. Heat is generated by the action of the exhaled carbon dioxide on the soda lime of the absorber, water vapour is conserved in the circuit and the animal consequently breathes warm, moist gases. Because there is no heat loss with breathing, high ambient temperatures may give rise to heat stroke, however. The resistance afforded to breathing generally limits the use of these circuits to larger dogs unless, as is common in North America, they have been specifically designed for human paediatric or small animal use. The to-and-fro system, incorporating a perspex soda lime canister capable of holding 0.5 kg of soda lime, is the absorber circuit still most commonly used in the UK. Many years ago it was relatively inexpensive to purchase when compared with a circle system, and it was often improvised.

The resistance to breathing limits its use to dogs weighing more than 10 kg, while the effect of steadily increasing dead-space makes it inefficient for all sizes of animal. The presence of the soda lime canister so close to the dog's head is physically awkward, and the inhalation of soda lime dust can make the dog cough in the postoperative period. Today, the to-and-fro system of absorption has no place in canine anaesthesia since inexpensive, much more satisfactory circle systems are freely available from several commercial sources.

In circle absorber systems the dead-space is within the Y-junction connected to the face-mask or endotracheal tube and can, therefore, be made very small. The soda lime is placed some distance from the patient, and is utilized efficiently as all the expired gases pass right through the canister. The resistance to breathing depends on the diameter and length of the tubing, the resistance afforded by the unidirectional valves, and the shape and size of the soda lime canister. Many different circle absorber systems are commercially available but in the UK most are designed for use in adult human beings and have such a high resistance to breathing as to limit their use in dogs to those weighing 25 kg or more. Circle systems incorporating in-circuit vaporizers are also marketed for veterinary use. The advantages and disadvantages associated with the use of in-circuit vaporizers have been discussed in Chapter 9.

Although it is perfectly possible to administer anaesthetics from any of these various systems quite satisfactorily through an airtight face-mask, for all but the very briefest of procedures on dogs, endotracheal methods of administration are to be preferred.

Low-flow administration of inhalation anaesthetics

A low-flow system can be defined as one in which there is substantial rebreathing of previously expired gas which has passed through a carbon dioxide absorber (usually in a circle system). The fresh gas inflow to the system is greater than the mere consumption of anaesthetic and oxygen by the animal for when these are equal the arrangement becomes a closed system with no spill-over to the atmosphere. For all practical purposes, in dogs a low-flow system is one in which the fresh gas inflow to the circuit is between 0.5 and 2 l/min.

Until comparatively recently low-flow systems were used only by enthusiasts and the lack of interest by others was probably due to the fact that if the fresh gas inflow is low there may be a considerable difference between the concentrations of gases and vapours set on the anaesthetic machine and the inspired concentration available to the animal. Many veterinarians

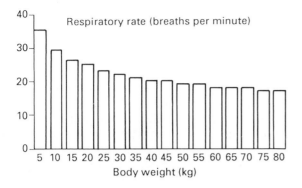

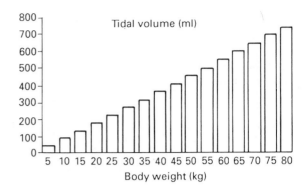

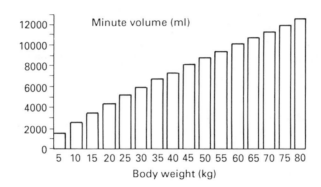

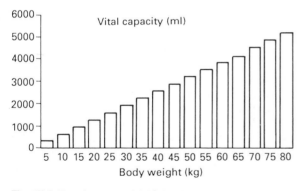

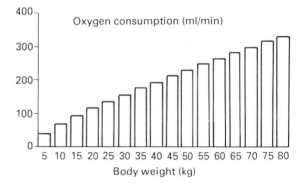

Fig. 15.6 Respiratory variables for the conscious dog. Calculated from the allometric equations in *Scaling* by K. Schmidt-Nielsen (1984, Cambridge University Press, Cambridge).

may have concluded, in their uncertainty about these differences, that there is a danger of unexpectedly high or low concentrations of any volatile agent being inhaled by the animal or, worse still, or accidental hypoxia.

As in horses (p. 226) the simplest way to use a low-flow system is to restrict the method to only one gas as the carrier gas — oxygen — and a volatile anaesthetic such as halothane. At the outset the anaesthetic system should be full of air and the animal should have been breathing air. Thus, the animal/system will contain a considerable amount of nitrogen at a concentration of around 80%. This is undesirable and the nitrogen should be eliminated by a fresh gas flow of oxygen sufficient to allow significant spillage through the exhaust valve, although it is not possible to eliminate nitrogen from the system entirely. For practical purposes a concentration of 3–5% nitrogen is acceptable and to produce this a fresh gas flow of above 3 l/min is necessary for the first 10–15 minutes of anaesthesia. Given this high initial gas flow rate a vaporizer such as a 'Fluotec' placed outside the breathing circuit but in the fresh gas supply line will behave in exactly the same way as it does when used in a circuit in which there is no or virtually no rebreathing, i.e. the concentration set on the vaporizer will be more or less the same as the concentration inspired by the animal. At the end of 10–15 minutes, provided the reservoir bag is filling well *and the vaporizer setting has been adjusted in accordance with the clinical needs of the animal*, the fresh gas flow can be reduced to about 2 l/min, for while the inspired concentration of the volatile agent may become slightly less than set on the vaporizer, the difference for all practical purposes is too small to be significant.

Later on in the course of the anaesthetic the fresh gas flow may be reduced still further (e.g. to 1 l/min) provided that the reservoir bag continues to fill well at the end of expiration and is not totally collapsed at the end of inspiration. There will now be an important difference between the likely inspired concentration of the volatile agent and the vaporizer setting. The reason for this is simply that the mass of volatile agent delivered to the circuit at this low flow rate is insufficient in the first few hours of the anaesthetic period to make up the net losses from the breathing system to the animal's tissues. A reliable approximation is that the inspired concentration of the volatile agent will be one-half to one-third of that set on the vaporizer. In the case of isoflurane, which is rather less soluble in the tissues than halothane, closer to one-half the vaporizer set concentration will be available as the inspired concentration for the animal. This 'rule of thumb' has been found to be reliable but in any particular case the inspired concentration to be aimed at is that which is *judged to be appropriate to the clinical need of the animal* and this will vary from animal to animal and, in the same animal, between different phases of the surgical procedure.

The conditions which make the fresh gas/inspired gas concentration differences when the fresh gas flow is low also dictate that an alteration in the inspired concentration in response to a change in vaporizer setting will be slower in becoming effective than is the case with high-flow systems. This disadvantage may be overcome in one of two ways — the vaporizer can be set to its highest setting if anaesthesia becomes inadequate or, alternatively, the fresh gas flow can be increased and the vaporizer setting adjusted as if a non-rebreathing system were in use. To achieve a rapid reduction in inspired concentration it is necessary to increase the fresh gas flow rate while turning the vaporizer off.

When nitrous oxide/oxygen mixtures are used as the carrier gas problems arise from the different rates at which nitrous oxide and oxygen will be consumed from the breathing system. The uptake of gases by the animal obeys the so-called square root of time law — i.e. the amount taken up is proportional to the square root of the elapsed time. At the start of an anaesthetic nitrous oxide consumption by the tissues is much greater than that of oxygen, but after a variable period of time it becomes less than that of oxygen, so that the great fear is that under these circumstances a state could be reached in a low-flow system in which nitrous oxide accumulation within the system would occur with a serious reduction in the oxygen concentration, leading to severe or fatal hypoxia. While there is no doubt that such a situation could arise during low-flow anaesthesia it is reassuring to note that:

1. If the fresh gas inflow is 2 l/min or more, the difference between the proportions of oxygen to nitrous oxide in the fresh gas supply and the inspiratory limb of the circuit are likely to be so small as to be negligible.
2. For the vast majority of animals whose metabolic rate is normal it is quite safe to use a fresh gas flow comprising equal proportions of nitrous oxide and oxygen (e.g. 'Entonox') at flow rates above 1 l/min. To use smaller flows of fresh gases is probably unwise unless the oxygen concentration is increased or the concentration of oxygen in the inspired limb of the circuit is actually monitored.

Circle systems which incorporate the vaporizer inside the breathing circuit (e.g. the Stephens machine) are more difficult to use and *very close observation of the dog is needed to obtain the correct setting of the vaporizer control*. Particular care needs to be taken to ensure that the first breaths an animal takes from the circuit are not deep ones of the saturated vapour accumulated in the previously unused vaporizer; it is always wise to flush the circuit with oxygen before connecting the animal to it.

Endotracheal intubation

Endotracheal intubation of dogs is easily performed. The level of anaesthesia required is that which is just adequate to allow the dog's mouth to be held open without risk of the anaesthetist being bitten, for the dogs' larynx does not go into spasm when it is stimulated during light levels of anaesthesia. The anaesthetized dog is placed in lateral recumbency

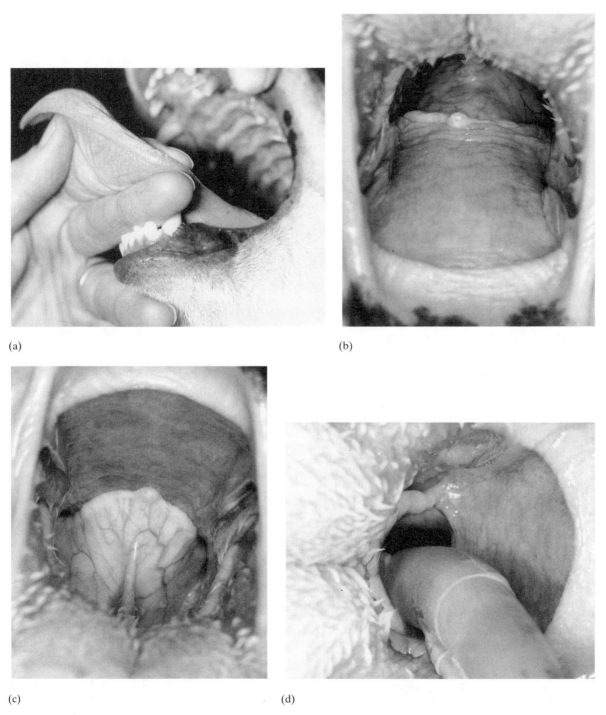

(a)

(b)

(c)

(d)

Fig. 15.7 Endotracheal intubation as seen by a right handed anaesthetist. (a) The nurse assistant holds only the upper lips and the anaesthetist draws the tongue out of the mouth, protecting its undersurface by placing a finger over the dog's incisor teeth. (b) Only the tip of the epiglottis is visible below the soft palate. (c) The soft palate has been lifted by the tip of the tube to allow the tip of the epiglottis to come forward. (d) The tube has been passed behind the epiglottis, through the vocal cords and on towards the sternum.

with its mouth held open in such a way that neither the assistant nor the anaesthetist will get bitten should the depth of anaesthesia not have been judged correctly. The assistant holds only the upper lips and the anaesthetist's finger is placed between the dog's lower incisor teeth and its tongue to prevent injury to the underside of the tongue as this is drawn forward out of the mouth (Fig. 15.7A). The epiglottis is clearly visible when the tongue is held in this position but its tip is usually positioned behind the soft palate (Fig. 15.7B). The lubricated tube is introduced into the mouth and its tip used to deflect the soft palate upwards and backwards so as to bring the entire epiglottis into view (Fig. 15.7C). The tube is then used to depress the epiglottis anteriorly on to the base of the tongue and to keep it there whilst the tube itself is advanced in front of the arytenoid cartilages into the trachea (Fig. 15.7D). Should any difficulty be encountered, a laryngoscope may be used as described on p. 282 to allow vocal cords to be seen or, alternatively, a finger may be inserted into the pharynx and used to direct the tube into the glottis.

Care should always be taken to avoid injury to the larynx and forceps should never be applied to the epiglottis, or to the fold of mucous membrane between the epiglottis and the tongue, in order to expose the laryngeal opening. Trauma to the larynx or to the tissues around it may give rise to oedema which can, when the tube is removed, cause complete obstruction of the airway and necessitate the performance of an emergency tracheostomy.

Standard cuffed Magill endotracheal tubes are suitable for use in all but small dogs, the tube sizes up to 11 mm internal diameter are those designed for use in man. However, man has a very small trachea in comparison with that of dogs, so that the larger tubes required for medium and big dogs are produced only for veterinary use. In very small dogs it is preferable to use uncuffed tubes because the added dimensions of the cuff-inflating tube increase the overall diameter and thus decrease the bore of the tube which can be accommodated by the trachea. When these uncuffed, or plain, tubes are used a pharyngeal pack of ribbon gauze will prevent inhalation of foreign material into the trachea.

The diameter of the largest tube which can be introduced into the trachea is related to both the size and breed of the dog. For example, a 16 mm tube can usually be passed into the trachea of an adult German shepherd whilst, in an Airedale of similar size, a 12 mm tube may be the largest which can be used. For their size, bulldogs and bull terriers have exceptionally small-diameter tracheas and it is often preferable to use uncuffed tubes in these breeds.

All new Magill tubes should be cut to the correct length so that endobronchial intubation is impossible

and dead-space is reduced to a minimum. To anchor the tube in position once it has been introduced a tie should be placed tightly around the tube where it goes over the endotracheal tube connector; this tie is secured either to the jaw where the canine teeth will prevent movement (Fig. 15.8) or around the back of the head in the case of brachycephalic dogs. It is very dangerous to place the tie half way along the tube where it cannot be tied tightly, for looseness will allow the tube to move in the mouth and possibly to slip out of the trachea during surgery.

Agents employed

Nitrous oxide

It is generally agreed that dogs cannot be anaesthetized with unsupplemented mixtures of nitrous oxide and oxygen and thus in canine anaesthesia the gas is used only where it can be given with other agents. It is used in a non-rebreathing or low-flow system either:

1. As a vehicle for the vaporization and delivery of volatile anaesthetic agents. The proportion of oxygen in the mixture — provided it is at least 30% — is unimportant because the maintenance of anaesthesia does not depend on the potency of nitrous oxide.

or:

2. In conjunction with thiopentone, pethidine and other analgesic supplements such as fentanyl, and with muscle relaxants, for maintaining a light plane of anaesthesia. In these circumstances the proportion of oxygen in the nitrous oxide/oxygen mixture delivered to the animal becomes of great importance and two factors must be considered.

To make the most of the advantages offered by nitrous oxide it must not be diluted with nitrogen or oxygen, and the oxygen concentration in the respired mixture must only be sufficient to satisfy the animal's metabolic requirements. The animal must be saturated with nitrous oxide; this can only occur after nitrogen has been eliminated from the body and the time needed for this to occur depends upon five factors:

1. The degree of ventilation of the lungs
2. The solubility of nitrous oxide in the blood, brain and tissues
3. The flow of gases delivered to the animal
4. The percentage of nitrous oxide in the respired mixture
5. The tension of nitrogen in the respired mixture

Another factor which must be considered in low-flow systems is that although the percentage of oxygen in the mixture leaving the anaesthetic

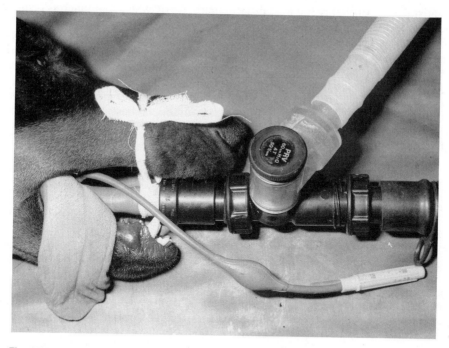

Fig. 15.8 Endotracheal tube secured in place by a tie placed tightly around the connector and then tied around the upper jaw behind the canine teeth. Note that the tube has been shortened so that the expiratory valve is at the nostrils ensuring minimum dead-space. The inflating tube for the cuff has been doubled over and sealed by a disposable needle-case; this does not damage the tube and is more convenient than other methods.

machine may appear to be adequate, the actual concentration inhaled by the animal may fall below the minimum required. This is because even when the animal is fully saturated with nitrous oxide it still requires oxygen for its metabolic processes. This point may be illustrated by considering a hypothetical example of an animal which is fully saturated with nitrous oxide breathing into a closed system. If this animal consumes oxygen at the rate of 200 ml/min and oxygen and nitrous oxide are both fed into the circuit at the rate of 250 ml/min then the oxygen content of the gases actually respired will be

$$\frac{250 - 200}{250 + (250 - 200)} \times 100$$

or approximately 16.6% although the flowmeter readings indicate that mixture containing 50% oxygen is being supplied to the animal. The smaller the total gas flow of the machine, the larger must be the proportion of oxygen in the mixture.

It is important that the mixtures of nitrous oxide and oxygen should not be diluted with air. In dogs such dilution is usually prevented by delivering the mixture through a cuffed endotracheal tube.

Satisfactory results may be obtained when nitrous oxide/oxygen mixtures are used to maintain anaesthesia which has been induced by the intravenous injection of thiopentone sodium following well-chosen premedication. In many cases, however, the degree of surgical stimulation produced by the operative procedure is sufficiently marked as to make the animal restless when nitrous oxide and oxygen alone are employed. This restlessness often proves to be an embarrassment both to the surgeon and the anaesthetist. In these circumstances the anaesthetist is often tempted to introduce a degree of hypoxia into the administration of the anaesthetic, but this temptation should always be resisted. Better methods are available which produce smooth anaesthesia without sacrificing the benefits of nitrous oxide.

The simplest and safest method of obtaining smooth anaesthesia is to supplement the basal nitrous oxide/oxygen mixture with a volatile agent or an intravenous drug. When a volatile agent is chosen a low concentration is introduced and the concentration is steadily increased until the desired depth of unconsciousness is reached.

The technique of induction with thiopentone sodium given after rather heavy premedication of acepromazine with a narcotic analgesic, followed by nitrous oxide/oxygen (allowing at least 30% oxygen in the respired mixture) supplemented by the intravenous injection of small doses of an analgesic as required is very satisfactory. Probably the best intra-venous supplements for spontaneously breathing dogs are alfentanil (2–5 µg/kg) and fentanyl (0.5 to 1 µg/kg). A muscle relaxant may be used with this technique if abdominal section is to be performed or a thorax opened. Recovery is rapid and there seems to be the minimum of postanaesthetic nausea and hang-over for if their surgical condition allows it most dogs will eat a normal meal soon after regaining consciousness. The safety of α_2-adrenoceptor agonist premedication for this technique has not been established.

Chloroform

It is generally agreed that because of its toxic effects on the liver and kidneys, coupled with its ability to sensitize the heart to adrenaline-induced arrhythmias, chloroform is not a safe anaesthetic for dogs. Only on an occasion where there is no possible alternative, such as may occur unexpectedly in the field, should chloroform now be used as an anaesthetic agent for dogs.

Halothane

Because of its potency and because it is well tolerated by the respiratory tract halothane is often used alone as an anaesthetic agent for dogs. The animal is restrained and anaesthesia induced using a face-mask, the halothane being vaporized and delivered to the animal by a stream of oxygen or nitrous oxide/oxygen mixture. In small dogs (up to 10 kg) induction of anaesthesia is rapid and the duration of the period of narcotic excitement is brief. In larger dogs induc-tion and the narcotic excitement stage are more prolonged and it is usually advisable to give a minimal sleep dose of an intravenous agent before halothane is used.

Halothane is potent and anaesthesia is often diffi-cult to control, for small alterations in the con-centration of the vapour being respired result in quite gross alterations in the depth of anaesthesia. No attempt should be made to produce profound muscle relaxation by increasing the depth of halothane anaesthesia for this results in a severe fall in blood pressure and marked respiratory depression. The respiratory depression is often manifested by fast shallow breathing and the inexperienced anaesthetist may mistake this as sign of too light anaesthesia. Because of the respiratory depressant properties of the drug only minimal premedication and the smallest possible quantity of thiopentone should be given prior to the use of halothane.

Halothane lends itself to supplementation of the intravenous agent/nitrous oxide/oxygen sequence, particularly when spontaneous respiration is desirable, since very small concentrations produce a good result without marked side-effects. When deeper anaesthesia or more marked muscle relaxation is required it is probably better to use a muscle relaxant rather than increase the inspired concentration of halothane.

Like any other potent volatile anaesthetic agent, halothane is best administered from a calibrated vaporizer (see p. 157) so that the concentration delivered to the animal is known. In any case it is important that the anaesthetist should be fully acquainted with the actual concentrations delivered by any vaporizer which is used.

Enflurane

In dogs, enflurane, like halothane, produces a dose-dependent depression of both respiratory and cardio-vascular function. Side-effects such as muscle twitch-ing during clinical anaesthesia were not encountered by Cribb *et al.* [25], although these have been reported as occurring in experimental situations and by some other clinicians. The ability to produce rapid changes in the depth of anaesthesia and the rapid recovery suggest that this agent may be useful in dogs undergoing surgery as day-patients. However, enflurane is a poor analgesic and dogs need pain relief very early in the postoperative period to prevent restlessness or excitement and a rather stormy recovery from anaesthesia. It is possible that the inclusion of an analgesic in the premedication would avoid the problem, but this might delay recovery and thus negate the major advantage offered by the use of this anaesthetic agent.

Isoflurane

The high volatility and low blood solubility of iso-flurane suggest that it might be better than enflurane for day-patient surgery in dogs. Its high cost tends to limit its use in canine anaesthesia and when it is used low-flow methods of administration are usually employed. Up to 4% isoflurane vapour may be needed to induce anaesthesia but inspired concentra-tions of 1.5–2% are adequate for anaesthetic main-tenance. The authors' opinion is that for dogs it offers no significant advantage over halothane although there are theoretical considerations for preferring it in certain situations — for example, it has properties which make it particularly suitable for use in dogs suffering from cardiac disease.

Methoxyflurane

Methoxyflurane is a useful inhalational supplement. It is both non-explosive and non-flammable and by its use reasonably good muscle relaxation can be obtained. It is extremely difficult to administer an overdose of methoxyflurane when administration is through a non-rebreathing system. In practice, it is best vaporized in a calibrated vaporizer and since the maximum concentration of the vapour which can be obtained from a vaporizer is less than about 4% (see p. 109), this agent is of little use in the induction of unconsciousness.

Although it can be administered with oxygen alone, this mixture may not provide satisfactory operating conditions in large dogs and it is probable that methoxyflurane is best used as a supplement to nitrous oxide/oxygen mixtures. Moreover, because of the relatively prolonged recovery period after its use, it is best restricted to anaesthesia for major surgery where rapid recovery to full consciousness is not essential and where the apparent postoperative analgesia provided by it is an advantage.

Currently, it appears that methoxyflurane will be withdrawn by the manufacturers in the near future, presumably due to the relatively small demand for it.

NEUROMUSCULAR BLOCKING AGENTS

The use of neuromuscular blocking agents as part of the anaesthetic procedure is a technique which has much to offer in canine surgery for the profound relaxation produced enables the surgeon to work more efficiently. Relaxants enable the anaesthetist to take full control of respiration during a thoracotomy. Laparotomies, particularly those involving dissection deep within the abdomen, are more easily performed, and dislocated joints are more easily reduced. The profound relaxation which can be produced is also helpful for laminectomies and lumbar disc fenestrations, especially in large dogs where the surgeon has to retract deep and powerful muscles to expose the surgical target. The use of neuromuscular blocking agents and their general pharmacology has been considered in Chapter 7 but some points of particular relevance to canine anaesthesia are summarized in Table 15.4.

Table 15.4 Neuromuscular blocking agents in dogs. Approximate doses and effects

	Dose (mg/kg)	Effective length of action (minutes)	Remarks
Depolarizing			
Suxamethonium	0.3–0.4	20	Initial muscle fasciculation. No reversal
Non-depolarizing			
Atracurium	0.5	15–80	Can be given by infusion
Alcuronium	0.06–0.1	30–40	Residual effects can last some hours
Gallamine	1.0	15–20	Tachycardia
Pancuronium	0.06–0.1	20–40	Further 1 or 2 doses if required. Some tachycardia
Vecuronium	0.06–0.1	15–20	'Pure' neuromuscular blocker

Neuromuscular blocking agents paralyse the patient and thus by abolishing respiration and preventing somatic response to impulses in afferent nerves, they suppress many of the signs used to assess the depth of unconsciousness. When these agents are used, therefore, facilities for IPPV must be available and the anaesthetist must be capable of judging the depth of anaesthesia in the absence of many of the reflex responses normally used. In dogs, the following signs are useful in judging the depth of unconsciousness when the animal is paralysed:

1. *Pulse.* If anaesthesia becomes too light the pulse rate may increase, or the animal may show signs of vasovagal syncope with pallor of the mucous membranes and bradycardia.
2. *Pupil.* Paralysis of the ocular muscles means that the eye is central and the pupil is easily visible. The pupil dilates if anaesthesia becomes too light, is constricted at surgical levels, and dilates again as anaesthesia becomes too deep. Atropine premedication has no significant effect on these signs.
3. *Lacrimation and salivation.* Overflow of tears, or visible production of saliva both indicate that anaesthesia is becoming too light.
4. *Tongue.* Despite the use of neuromuscular blocking agents, in dogs the tongue will be observed to twitch if anaesthesia becomes too light. This twitching is readily detected if the anaesthetist is monitoring the sublingual artery.

If any of these signs are observed it must be taken that the level of unconsciousness should be deepened by one of the methods discussed on p. 311.

Agents used

The agents currently used to produce neuromuscular block in canine anaesthesia are listed in Table 15.4 but the doses shown in this table must be regarded as only a guide to the initial dose to be administered to

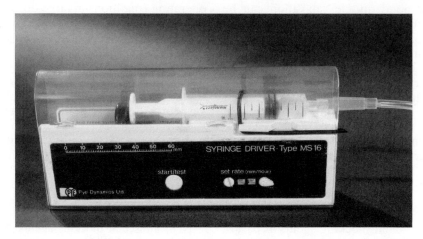

Fig. 15.9 Grazenby Dynamics MS16 Syringe Driver used to infuse atracurium in dogs according to the method of Jones and Brearley [22].

any particular animal. It is quite impossible to be dogmatic about the dose likely to be needed because the actual one used will depend on the physical build of the dog, the normality of its myoneural junction, the anaesthetic agents in use, and the requirements of the operation.

Atracurium is not particularly short acting in dogs; total neuromuscular block requires a dose of 0.5 mg/kg and the duration of this block varies from 15 to 80 minutes. Maintenance of the block requires about 0.6 mg/kg/h of atracurium. Jones and Brearley [26] described an interesting infusion technique. Following an initial bolus dose of 0.5 mg/kg the train-of-four response is monitored from the facial nerve. After a variable time when at least two of the twitches have returned, the atracurium infusion is begun. This infusion is delivered from a Grazenby Dynamics MS16 Syringe Driver (Fig. 15.9) at a drive setting equal to the weight of the animal in kilograms, and the infusion solution is made by diluting a 2.5 ml ampoule of atracurium (25 mg) with an equal volume of saline in a 5 ml syringe so that the infusion rate becomes equal to 0.5 mg/(kg h) of atracurium. After cessation of the infusion towards the end of the operation, at least two of the train-of-four twitches normally return within 10–15 minutes and reversal of the block is then carried out with atropine and neostigmine.

Initially, it was believed that atracurium did not cause histamine release in dogs but more recently evidence of this has been observed in some individuals. Cases of apnoea have been reported within the first half-hour after apparent adequate reversal of atracurium block [27, 28]; it is not certain whether the apnoea was due to recurarization but the dogs appeared to respond to additional antagonist.

There seem to be no reports of histamine release

following the use of gallamine, pancuronium or vecuronium and thus these non-depolarizing neuromuscular blockers are probably the agents of choice for dogs.

Vecuronium appears to be the 'purest' neuromuscular blocker and a dose of 0.1 mg/kg produces complete block with abolition of all the twitches of the train-of-four. Recovery is apparent after about 20 minutes.

Unless precautions are taken to prevent it, the body temperature of dogs is particularly liable to fall during long operations and it must be remembered that changes in muscle temperature affect the duration of action of the relaxant drugs. The action of suxamethonium is markedly prolonged by hypothermia which, at least clinically, appears also to make antagonism of the block due to competitive agents more difficult and uncertain.

Termination of neuromuscular block

Suxamethonium-induced block requires no antagonist; doses of 0.3 mg/kg give about 20 minutes of profound relaxation in most dogs and its action usually terminates in a rapid and complete manner. Assuming the anaesthetic depth to be that of surgical anaesthesia, the dog's eyes, which have been central, start to rotate downwards and spontaneous respiration returns. With the possible exception of dogs that have been given atracurium, once spontaneous breathing becomes adequate it can be safely assumed that neuromuscular block will not become re-established unless a further dose of relaxant is given.

Neostigmine is probably the most widely used anticholinesterase antagonist of non-depolarizing neuromuscular block in dogs. The action of these neuromuscular blockers can only be antagonized when it starts to wane (p. 128). When full paralysing doses are given it is usually impossible to restore spontaneous breathing until a period of 10–15 minutes (vecuronium) or 25–40 minutes (pancuronium, alcuronium) has elapsed from the time of administration. When twitch height is being monitored it will be found that it is best to wait until all four twitches in the train-of-four are visible. In the absence of this monitoring, decreasing chest compliance, attempts at spontaneous breathing or response to stimuli afforded by movement of the endotracheal tube in the trachea should be observed before attempts are made to restore normal neuromuscular transmission.

An anticholinergic should always be given to counteract the muscarinic effects of neostigmine and a common practice is to mix atropine in a syringe with neostigmine (1.2 mg atropine to 2.5 mg of neostigmine). This practice is safe because the anticholinergics exert their effects before the onset of neostigmine activity. A commercially available preparation (Robinul, A. H. Robins) mixes neostigmine (2.5 mg) with glycopyrrolate (0.5 mg). Neostigmine in one of these mixtures is given intravenously in increments of 0.5 mg until full muscle power is restored. Some anaesthetists consider it is

better practice to administer the anticholinergic drug intravenously about 60–90 seconds before injecting neostigmine, rather than mixing them. The total dose of neostigmine needed should not exceed 0.1 mg/kg and its muscarinic actions must always be blocked by atropine or glycopyrrolate whichever procedure is adopted.

With non-depolarizing neuromuscular blockers a degree of residual block remains even after the restoration of apparently adequate breathing. In the dog, this is shown by the eyes remaining central with an absence of palpebral reflexes whatever the depth of anaesthesia. Palatine and laryngeal muscles may also remain weak following incomplete antagonism of the neuromuscular block so that the dog may develop respiratory obstruction once the endotracheal tube is removed. It is, therefore, most important not to allow any residual block to remain at the end of anaesthesia and the residual effects even of the relatively short-acting agent vecuronium should be antagonized with neostigmine.

Even if given with full doses of anticholinergic agents neostigmine may cause serious cardiac arrhythmias if there has been gross underventilation during anaesthesia or if carbon dioxide has been allowed to accumulate at the end of operation with a view to stimulating breathing.

ARTIFICIAL VENTILATION OF THE LUNGS

In dogs, IPPV may be required as an emergency measure when respiratory depression or arrest has occurred, when the thoracic cavity has been opened, and when neuromuscular blocking agents are employed. It can be carried out either by manual compression of the rebreathing bag, or by using one of the many ventilators commercially available (Chapter 8).

In small dogs the Ayre's T-piece is usually used. Ventilation may be carried out by the anaesthetist obstructing the outflow of gases from the reservoir tube so that the fresh gas inflow inflates the lungs, but this may result in an undesirable pattern of lung inflation with a long inspiratory period. With the Jackson–Rees modification of the T-piece circuit which incorporates the open-ended bag at the distal end of the expiratory limb, the anaesthetist allows the bag to inflate by partially blocking the open end, inflates the lungs by squeezing the bag and allows expiration to occur by releasing its open end. By this means the inspiratory period can be kept short and the mean intrathoracic pressure reduced.

The Magill circuit is unsuitable for IPPV as manual squeezing of the reservoir bag simply empties gases

through the inspiratory valve. If the expiratory valve is partially closed, it is possible to inflate the lungs but total rebreathing may occur as it is fresh gas which is spilled out of the expiratory valve when the bag is squeezed. In an emergency the lungs may be inflated using a Magill circuit with a very high gas flow rate but it cannot be used for long-term IPPV because of the rebreathing entailed. The circle rebreathing system allows very effective IPPV to be carried out by manual squeezing of the reservoir bag but any vaporizer incorporated in the breathing circuit must be switched off, as the flow rates generated through it by squeezing of the reservoir bag could result in lethally high concentrations of volatile anaesthetics being delivered to the dog.

The majority of mechanical ventilators which are available from commercial sources were designed for use in man, and may be used for all but the smallest of dogs. Some compress the bag of rebreathing systems and others simply divide the flow of fresh gas from the anaesthetic machine to provide the tidal volume. Ventilators designed for human paediatric use may be used on small dogs but the majority of these are probably better ventilated by manual methods.

NEONATAL ANAESTHESIA

Occasionally it is necessary to anaesthetize very young or newborn puppies. Premedication should consist of only a very small dose of an anticholinergic agent, and as such very young animals lack the enzymes necessary for the elimination of many parenterally administered drugs and the fat needed for their redistribution, it is best to induce and maintain anaesthesia with inhalation anaesthetics. Endotracheal intubation is usually unnecessary, and indeed many consider it to be actually contra-indicated, for it may induce sufficient laryngeal oedema and swelling to cause respiratory obstruction when the tube is removed. Hypothermia is easily

induced and must be prevented by active warming during both surgery and the anaesthetic recovery period. Particular attention must also be paid to the replacement of fluid deficits and the maintenance of fluid balance.

In general, any inhalation anaesthetic delivered through a face-mask to the puppy provides anaesthesia adequate for the majority of surgical procedures which have to be performed on puppies of this age group, and is followed by a rapid recovery. Major procedures requiring other anaesthetic techniques should, whenever possible, be deferred until the pup is at least 8 weeks old.

LOCAL ANALGESIA

In the dog, the simplicity and safety of modern general anaesthesia means that local analgesia is rarely employed except for very minor procedures. However, certain techniques of local analgesia can still prove useful where poor facilities or the condition of the patient preclude the use of general anaesthesia.

Intravenous regional analgesia

This method provides a very safe and simple way of obtaining analgesia of the distal part of the limb and proves useful for operations such as the wiring of dislocated toes and toe amputations in tractable dogs such as greyhounds, or in sedated dogs.

The animal is restrained on its side and its systolic blood pressure measured (see p. 18). The appropriate limb is held as high as possible above heart level for 2–3 minutes to partially exsanguinate it while a sphygmomanometer cuff is being applied. The cuff is placed around the fore-arm cranial to the carpus, or around the tibial region cranial to the hock, and is quickly inflated to just above the systolic blood pressure. An intravenous injection of 2–3 ml of 1% lignocaine is made through a very fine needle into any superficial vein which can be identified distal to the occluding cuff. The lignocaine should not include adrenaline which may impair its diffusion. Some animals show signs of slight discomfort as the injection is made, but the onset of analgesia up to the level of the cuff is rapid. Analgesia lasts as long as the pressure within the cuff is maintained above the animal's systolic pressure. Sensation returns to the foot within a few minutes after deflation of the cuff tourniquet.

In a series of 20 greyhounds, good results were achieved in 17 cases, while in three, although the operation could be performed satisfactorily, the

animal appeared to experience slight discomfort. The tourniquet was in place for 25–55 minutes and even during the longest of these operations there was no waning of analgesia. No harmful results were observed to follow the release of the lignocaine into the general circulation, but it must be noted that none of the dogs were allowed to stand up for 2–3 minutes after removal of the tourniquet.

The major difficulty in the application of this technique in canine surgery is the identification of a suitable superficial vein distal to the occluding cuff. In greyhounds and other thin-skinned dogs this presents no problems, but in thick-skinned dogs it may be necessary to introduce an indwelling needle or catheter before partial exsanguination of the limb.

The main reasons for failure with this technique are the use of a tourniquet which does not occlude the arterial blood supply to the region, or not allowing the necessary 5 minutes for analgesia to develop after injection of the local analgesic.

Brachial plexus block

A technique for the production of brachial block has been described by Nutt [29] for attaining regional analgesia of the fore-limb.

With the dog standing on all four legs, the tri-angular area bounded by the anterior border of the supraspinatus muscle, the chest wall and the dorsal border of the brachiocephalicus muscle, is clipped and prepared for injection. The animal's head is held away from the side to be injected and the depression in the centre of the clipped area is palpated and the first rib located. A 7.5 cm needle of 1.6 mm bore is inserted into the centre of the depression and guided caudally lateral to the chest wall and medial to the subscapularis muscle until its point is judged to be level with the spine of the scapula. After aspiration to confirm that the point of the needle does not lie within a blood vessel, 1–3 ml of lignocaine hydrochloride, according to the size of the dog, is injected through the needle. Onset of analgesia should be observed in most cases within 10 minutes of injection. There is a gradual loss of motor power, followed by complete relaxation and loss of sensation below and including the elbow joint as the block develops. It is possible that paraesthesia occurs soon after injection, for some animals chew at the leg.

Certain complications may occur consequent upon this procedure: a major blood vessel may be punctured by the needle and a large haematoma develop as a result of this; the local analgesic solution may be injected intravascularly; the brachial plexus may be damaged, causing neuritis or permanent paralysis; the needle may enter the thorax and admit the entry of air into the pleural cavity; infection may be introduced into the axilla. However, if due care is exercised the technique may be regarded as a relatively safe procedure, of particular value where general anaesthesia is contraindicated owing to the state of the patient when presented for surgery.

Nutt reports that fat dogs are difficult subjects on which to perform this block and says that some failures may be anticipated in these animals. However, it must be noted that he used very small volumes of a concentrated solution of lignocaine hydrochloride (3%). Tufvesson [30] records the use of 5–10 ml of 2–3% procaine hydrochloride solution for this block. If this volume of solution can be injected into a dog's axilla, it would appear that Nutt might have obtained more certain results by the injection of 10–15 ml of a 1% lignocaine hydrochloride solution containing 1:200 000 adrenaline to delay absorption and diminish the risk of toxic reactions.

Infiltration of the digital nerves

The digital nerves are approached lateral and medial to the first phalanx of the digit to be rendered analgesic. A fine needle is introduced subcutaneously on each side of the digit (Fig. 15.10) and 2 ml of local analgesic solution is injected on each aspect.

Auriculopalpebral nerve block

The nerve runs caudal to the mandibular joint at the base of the ear and, after giving off the cranial auricular branch, proceeds as the temporal branch along the dorsal border of the zygomatic arch towards the orbit. Before reaching the orbit the nerve divides into two branches, which pass medially and laterally to supply the orbicularis muscle.

The needle is introduced through the skin and

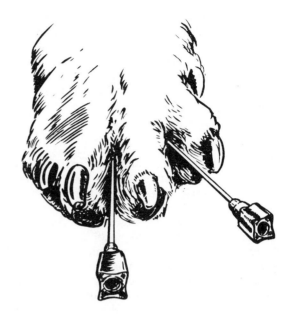

Fig. 15.10 Injection of the digital nerves.

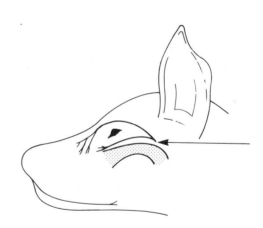

Fig. 15.11 Auriculopalpebral nerve block. The nerve is blocked just where the zygomatic ridge dips medially.

fascia over the midpoint of the caudal third of the zygomatic arch (just where the arch can be felt to dip sharply medially) and 1 ml of solution is injected (Fig. 15.11).

The blocking of this branch of the facial nerve does not produce any analgesia. By paralysing the orbicularis muscle it facilitates examination of, and operations on, the eyeball. It is of particular value in preventing squeezing of the eyeball after intraocular operations.

Caudal block

In the dog, caudal nerve block may be given between the sacrum and the first coccygeal vertebra or between the first and second coccygeal vertebra. The same principles are followed as in the larger animals. The procedure is technically easy and the dose administered should not exceed 1 ml of 2% lignocaine hydrochloride solution. This block is useful for docking the tail in adult dogs and for other surgical operations upon the tail.

Epidural block

In the dog, with practice, lumbar epidural analgesia can be a safe and simple method of obtaining analgesia and muscle relaxation of the abdominal, perineal, caudal, and hind-limb regions. It is contraindicated in dogs suffering from skin sepsis in the lumbar region or blood-clotting problems.

The technique consists of the injection of local analgesic solution into the epidural space at the lumbosacral junction, so that the solution spreads both caudally and cranially. The anatomical considerations involved in this technique have been discussed in detail in Chapter 10 which should be read carefully before attempting to carry out the technique.

In the dog the spinal cord ends at the junction of the sixth and seventh lumbar vertebrae, and the meninges continue to the middle of the sacrum. Brook [31], who studied the sacral meningeal cul-de-sac in the dog, pointed out that its dimensions at the lumbosacral space are so small that it may be taken that injection here is always extradural. The greater splanchnic nerve arises from the twelfth thoracic ganglion and a fall in blood pressure may occur if the anaesthetic solution extends cranial to the first lumbar segment. To reduce this danger Brook advised that the animal be restrained on its back during the onset of analgesia so that the ventral spinal nerve roots which contain the vasomotor fibres are less profoundly affected than the dorsal roots containing the sensory fibres.

To locate the site the illiac prominences on either side are identified. An imaginary line joining them crosses the dorsal spinous process of the last lumbar segment. The site for insertion of the needle is in the midline immediately caudal to this process. The interarcual ligament lies at a depth of 2–4 cm from the skin and the approximate dimensions of the space in a 14 kg dog are: craniocaudally, 0.4 cm; laterally, 0.7 cm.

Lignocaine hydrochloride 2% with 1:200 000 adrenaline is commonly used for epidural block but bupivacaine 0.75% will produce longer periods of analgesia. Lignocaine produces analgesia in about 5–10 minutes while after bupivacaine the onset time may be from 15 to 30 minutes. Lignocaine block usually lasts 1.5–2 hours which is quite adequate for most surgery but bupivacaine will produce analgesia of 5–6 hours so that this drug is to be preferred if postoperative analgesia is required.

For the injection the dog is probably best restrained firmly on its right side with its back adjacent to the edge of the table. (Some anaesthetists make the injection with the dog in the standing position or restrained on its breast. Sudden forceful movement, however, cannot effectively be prevented when the animal's limbs are beneath it.) An insensitive skin weal is made just caudal to the last lumbar spine by the injection of a little of the local analgesic solution, using a short, fine needle. For the epidural injection a 21 gauge needle 3–5 cm long is employed. Its point should be cut at an angle of 45°. It is introduced directly in the midline, immediately caudal to the last lumbar dorsal spine, and pressed slightly caudally (assuming the animal to be in the normal position), taking care that its direction does not deviate to one side (Fig. 15.12). Penetration of the interarcual ligament imparts a distinct 'popping' sensation to the finger. Should bone rather than ligament be encountered, it indicates that the direction of the needle has been wrong and that its point has struck an articular process or the roof of the first sacral segment. If this occurs the needle is slightly withdrawn and a search made for the space by redirecting it a little caudally, cranially or laterally.

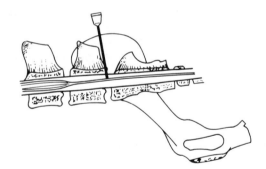

Fig. 15.12 Epidural analgesia. The site and direction for insertion of the needle.

That the canal has been entered is indicated by the complete absence of resistance to the injection. In the majority of animals no difficulty will be experienced in locating the space, but in very fat dogs it may be impossible to palpate either the illiac tuberosities or the last lumbar spine and, in these, failure may attend efforts to induce epidural analgesia. Again, with highly nervous animals, movement during injection may cause failure. The injection must be made slowly, over some 10–15 seconds, otherwise vomiting and possible convulsions may occur. The local analgesic solution should be warmed by placing ampoules in hot water before use.

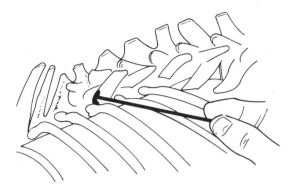

Fig. 15.13 Block of the eleventh thoracic nerve. The needle is advanced along the cranial border of the twelfth rib towards the body of the eleventh thoracic vertebra.

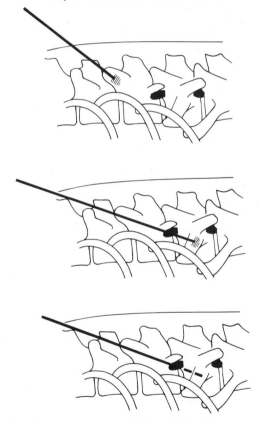

Fig. 15.14 Block of the thirteenth thoracic nerve. The needle is introduced to strike the caudal articular process of the twelfth thoracic vertebra and then directed to contact the transverse process of the first lumbar vertebra. It is then withdrawn slightly and the injection made.

There is a rather remote possibility that the meningeal cul-de-sac will be penetrated, in which case cerebrospinal fluid will escape from the needle. If this occurs it is probably best to withdraw the needle and abandon the attempt to produce epidural analgesia.

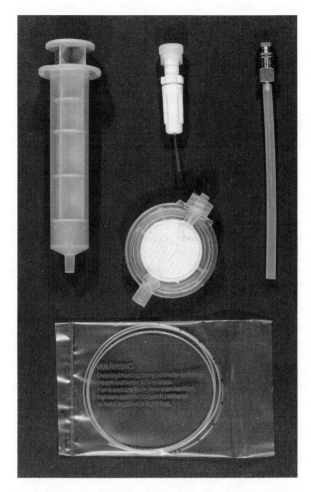

Fig. 15.15 Epidural 'Minipack' set (Portex Ltd) which is ideal for the introduction of a catheter into a dog's epidural space. The set contains a 10 ml syringe, 19 G Tuohy needle graduated 10–45 mm × 5 mm, open-ended catheter marked at 20–100 mm × 10 mm from tip, loss-of-resistance device, flat filter and Luer Lock connector.

A catheter can be introduced easily some 2–3 cm into the epidural space through a correctly placed Tuohy needle.

In the dog interference with motor power of the hind-limbs is of no consequence. To produce analgesia up to the first lumbar segment a dose of approximately 1 ml per 4.5 kg body weight is required and for cranial laparotomies where analgesia is needed to the fourth or fifth thoracic segment this dose is usually increased to about 1 ml per 3.5 kg.

The complication most likely to occur is hypotension and this is perhaps best minimized by the infusion of about 20 ml/kg of Hartmann's solution as the block develops. Certainly, a catheter should be placed in a vein before epidural block is induced so that vasopressors can be injected without delay should hypotension develop. Arterial blood pressure should be monitored by non-invasive means in every case. The dose of methoxamine, by intravenous or intramuscular injection, is up to 5 mg.

It must be borne in mind that the neural canal at the lumbosacral space is almost completely occupied by the nerves comprising the cauda equinum and it is by no means impossible that some permanent injury may result from epidural injection. Again, the greatest care must be taken that all apparatus and local analgesic solution are sterile, otherwise the canal may become a focus of sepsis.

Place of epidural analgesia in dogs

Among the advantages over general anaesthesia are: the absence of respiratory worries when dealing with the brachycephalic breeds; the completeness of muscle relaxation; the absence of straining when traction is applied to the peritoneum; the absence of depression of the fetuses in caesarean section.

Disadvantages include the need for more planning in the organization of operating lists; waiting for the block to develop, so delaying busy surgical schedules; the possibility of some dogs moving during surgery even with profound sedation given to control the head end of the animal, and occasional failure to produce a satisfactory block.

Paravertebral nerve block

Paravertebral block of the last three thoracic and first four lumbar nerves affords a useful, safe method of producing relaxation of the abdominal muscles. Used in conjunction with light general anaesthesia it produces excellent operating conditions for the surgeon working within the abdomen. The technique for blocking these nerves has been described by Micheletto [32] and this technique has been slightly modified by several workers.

To block the eleventh thoracic nerve the twelfth rib is used as a landmark. This rib is traced upwards to the point where it disappears under the lateral border of the longissimus dorsi muscle. A skin weal is made over this point and through the weal a needle (about 7 cm long, 1 mm bore) is introduced to strike the anterior border of the rib. The needle is advanced carefully, keeping its point in contact with the anterior border of the rib, until its progress is arrested by the eleventh thoracic vertebra (Fig. 15.13). An injection of 2 ml of 1% lignocaine hydrochloride solution with 1:200 000 adrenaline is made at this point. The twelfth thoracic nerve is blocked in a similar manner, the thirteenth rib being used as the landmark.

To block the thirteenth thoracic nerve a skin weal is raised at the posterior border of the dorsal spine of the twelfth thoracic vertebra, and a needle is introduced through this and directed slightly caudally and laterally to strike the caudal articular process of the vertebra. The needle is then withdrawn slightly and advanced again over this process until it meets the transverse process of the first lumbar vertebra. After withdrawing the needle point about 1 cm, 2 ml of local analgesic solution is injected. The lumbar nerves are treated in a similar manner, the landmarks sought being the caudal articular processes of the vertebrae immediately cranial to the nerves to be blocked (Fig. 15.14).

For laparotomy, it is necessary to block seven nerves on each side of the body and, clearly, this is a time-consuming procedure. However, when combined with light general anaesthesia, it is a technique which is very useful under conditions of general practice, since it produces operating conditions equal to those obtained by the use of muscle relaxants; yet it does not necessitate the IPPV of the lungs which must be employed when relaxants are used.

POSTOPERATIVE CARE

In most dogs which have been intubated the endotracheal tube should be removed early in the recovery period. The habit of leaving the tube in place until the dog regains full control of its larynx is to be deplored as it appears to be responsible for laryngeal oedema, postoperative coughing and a very sore throat which may make the animal reluctant to take food. Exceptions to this general rule are made where there is a particularly high risk of respiratory obstruction occurring in the recovery period either due to the surgery which has been performed, or to the anatomy of the brachycephalic breeds. Whether or not the endotracheal tube has been left in place, the dog must be carefully watched until it has regained its protective reflexes, and should remain under continuous observation until it is fully conscious. Laryngeal spasm and oedema sufficient to cause respiratory obstruction is fortunately rare in the dog, but occasionally (usually in elderly dogs with a history of chronic cough) laryngeal paralysis and collapse is encountered. The arytenoid cartilages appear to collapse into the laryngeal orifice and emergency tracheostomy may be necessary to relieve obstruction from this cause. Dogs with chronic respiratory insufficiency may require the administration of oxygen in the recovery period. Initially this may be given through a face-mask, but later on a nasal catheter delivering oxygen into the pharynx is usually better tolerated by the animal. Oxygen tents, oxygen cages or human baby incubators are sometimes useful for prolonged administration of oxygen in the postoperative period but when inside one of these the patient is not readily available for routine nursing attention.

Dogs need to be kept warm and comfortable after anaesthesia. A slow return to consciousness may be due to a disease condition, to failure to eliminate anaesthetic drugs, or to the development of cerebral oedema following hypoxaemia or hypotension during anaesthesia, but it is probably most commonly due to hypothermia. Hypothermia is better prevented than treated, as energetic, rapid rewarming of the patient results in cutaneous vasodilatation which can be responsible for serious hypotension in animals which have a depleted blood volume after surgery. The rectal temperature, as measured by a mercury-in-glass clinical thermometer, is often extremely low in the postoperative period, but ballooning of the rectum may make this measurement unreliable; pharyngeal temperature or oesophageal temperature measured by a thermistor probe thermometer is a much better guide to the condition of the dog. Heat loss during anaesthesia may be prevented by maintaining the ambient temperature between 29 and 30°C, but this can be unpleasant for the surgical team so it is more usual to adopt a lower environmental temperature and place the dog on the thermostatically controlled heating pad or water blanket. If hot water bottles are used care must be taken to avoid burning the unconscious animal. Dogs often shiver during recovery from anaesthesia, particularly when halothane has been used, and although shivering increases oxygen consumption considerably it does have the effect of raising the body temperature. It is usually in dogs which fail to shiver that hypothermia becomes a serious problem.

Excitement in the recovery period is always undesirable and the animal may even thrash about to the extent of causing itself injury, although fortunately this is uncommon. Excitement or restlessness is more common after barbiturate anaesthesia than after the use of inhalation agents and can often be prevented from occurring by adequate suitable premedication. When it does occur, however, diagnosis of its cause may not be easy. Sometimes it seems to be due to nothing more than the peculiar temperament of the animal which manifests itself when the residual effects of the anaesthetic drugs suppress the inhibitory influences which operate in the fully conscious state to make the animal socially acceptable. For this diagnosis to be made correctly, all other possible causes must be excluded. If the restlessness is due to pain, it should be relieved by analgesics but it is necessary to eliminate other causes before administering these potentially harmful drugs. When

an intravenous infusion has been given during anaesthesia and the animal has not been catheterized, distension of the bladder can cause very great discomfort and it should also be remembered that many dogs will not urinate in a kennel. Evidence of bladder distension should always be sought whenever a dog is restless in the postoperative period and the condition should always be relieved by emptying the bladder, if necessary by catheterization. The administration of analgesics to these animals may make distension of the bladder more tolerable, and may even promote urinary retention when the animal is fully conscious and is taken out for exercise. Another cause for postanaesthetic discomfort in dogs is lying on a cold, unyielding surface. Noisy, brightly lit surroundings can also be responsible for restlessness. Unless all these various causes are appreciated it may be difficult to understand why recovery may be anything but smooth in a dog which has been given a full dose of analgesic.

Postoperative pain relief is a subject which has been rather neglected in canine surgery. In man, almost all surgery is associated with pain in the postoperative period, and there is no reason to suppose that dogs are not affected in the same way. It is easy to see why the situation with regard to postoperative pain in dogs is unsatisfactory. Postoperative pain does not directly cause death, it is short lived and the animal cannot communicate its feelings to its attendants other than by biting or struggling to avoid exacerbation of its pain. For these reasons postoperative pain relief has been given little serious attention. Even when its presence is recognized, pain is often treated inadequately for fear of causing respiratory or circulatory depression with the pain-relieving drugs. Surgical pain is usually severe for only the first 1 or 2 days; in this period it can usually only be relieved effectively by the narcotic analgesics, but after this non-steroidal anti-inflammatory drugs often provide adequate analgesia. Morphine may not be the best of the powerful analgesics available for use in dogs, but with the possible exception of papaveretum ('Omnopon', Roche), other drugs do not seem to be greatly superior. Early trials of the partial antagonist buprenorphine suggested it to be a valuable drug in the dogs as its prolonged action (8–12 hours) made it particularly satisfactory for postoperative use (P. M. Taylor, personal communication). Subsequent experience with it has proved somewhat disappointing. Because of the shape of its dose–response curve and the normal variation in response between individuals it seems to be very difficult to estimate the dose needed in any one dog. The drug also seems to produce psychic disturbances and dogs will vocalize when unlikely to be suffering postoperative pain. This vocalization may be taken as an indication for the further administration of buprenorphine which may then do no more than to decrease any analgesia it was providing.

It is generally agreed that it is better to prevent the development of severe pain by giving a powerful analgesic early on, rather than waiting until the dog seems to be in agony. The drugs and doses required depend on the condition of the dog, the remaining depressant effect of anaesthesia, and the surgery which has been performed. The practice of giving the first dose of an analgesic such as morphine or methadone by slow intravenous injection before the dog leaves the operating theatre has much to commend it for it allows the effect of the drug to be monitored. A slow intravenous injection of analgesic gives more rapid relief of pain than does an intramuscular or subcutaneous injection but it may only be possible to give the first dose by this route.

An alternative method for long-term pain relief following operations is to inject 1.0 mg of morphine in 3 ml of aqueous solution (with no preservative in the solution) per 10 kg of body weight into the epidural space at the lumbosacral junction. It is uncertain how long the pain relief lasts but some dogs have been apparently pain free for up to 24 hours.

If a combination of 0.1 mg of morphine and 0.7–1.0 ml of 0.5% bupivacaine per 10 cm of vertex–coccyx length is injected into the epidural space at the lumbosacral junction, nerve block up to the level of the last rib can be expected and this gradually converts to postoperative analgesia of some 24 hours duration without affecting motor activity in the hindlimbs or cardiopulmonary function [33].

It is essential that dogs which have undergone major surgery and require intensive care postoperatively are kept sedated and pain free, so that nursing procedures can be carried out as necessary. These animals may be receiving intravenous fluids, on chest drainage or pulmonary ventilators, or have urinary catheters or vascular catheters for monitoring purposes. Most dogs, as long as they are made comfortable and have effective pain relief, will tolerate these procedures, especially if they are also given what is aptly referred to as 'tender loving care', but occasionally they become restless and difficult for the nurses to restrain. Doses of diazepam given by intravenous infusion have proved very helpful in these situations [34]. Initially, doses as high as 1 mg/kg/h may be needed to settle the dog but much less diazepam is required as time goes on.

A dog's fluid intake should be restored as soon as possible following surgery. Oral intake is best, and if there are no surgical contraindications, the dog may be allowed access to small amounts of water as soon as it is fully conscious. Should it be impossible to provide an adequate intake by mouth, fluids must be given intravenously. This is particularly important in elderly dogs where fluid deprivation may lead to renal failure.

Again, if there are no surgical contraindications, small quantities of food may be offered as soon as the dog is fully conscious. A full stomach appears to be an excellent sedative and most dogs will settle down and sleep quietly once they have had a meal. Post-operative vomiting can be a problem, both immediately on recovery and during the next few hours, but it is usually related to the surgical condition, to preoperative feeding unknown to the anaesthetist, or to specific drugs used in the anaesthetic technique. As long as the quantities allowed are not too large, it is rare for a dog to vomit postoperatively once it has eaten voluntarily.

REFERENCES

1. Short, C. E. (1987) *Principles and Practice of Veterinary Anesthesia*, p. 45. Baltimore: Williams and Wilkins.
2. England, G. C. W. and Clarke, K. W. (1989) *Acta Veterinaria Scandinavica*, Suppl. 4, p. 179.
3. Clarke, K. W. and England, G. C. W. (1989) *Journal of Small Animal Practice* 30, 343.
4. Clarke, K. W. and England, G. C. W. (1988) *Advances in Anaesthesia, Proceedings of the 3rd International Congress of Veterinary Anaesthesia*, Brisbane, p. 104.
5. Hatch, R. C., Kitzman, J. V., Zahnar, J. M. and Clark, J. D. (1985) *American Journal of Veterinary Research* 46, 371.
6. Taylor, P. M. and Herrtage, M. E. (1986) *Journal of Small Animal Practice* 27, 325.
7. Erhardt, W., Stephen, M., Schatzmann, U., Westermayr, R., Schindele, M., Murisier, N. and Blumel, G. (1987) *Journal of the Association of Veterinary Anaesthetists of Great Britain and Ireland* 14, 99.
8. Bogan, J. (1970) *Journal of the Association of Veterinary Anaesthetists of Great Britain and Ireland* 1, 18.
9. Robinson, E. P., Sams, R. A, and Muir, W. W. (1986) *American Journal of Veterinary Research* 47, 2105.
10. Sams, R. A., Muir, W. W. and Deltra, R. L. (1985) *American Journal of Veterinary Research* 46, 1677.
11. Clarke, K. W. and Hall, L. W. (1975) *World Veterinary Congress*. Thessiloniki 2, 1688.
12. Hall, L. W. (1984) *Journal of the Association of Veterinary Anaesthetists of Great Britain and Ireland* 11, 115.
13. Watkins, S. B., Hall, L. W. and Kellagher, R. E. B. (1985) *Proceedings of the 2nd International Congress of Veterinary Anesthesia*, Sacramento, p. 177.
14. Watkins, S. B., Hall, L. W. and Clarke, K. W. (1987) *Veterinary Record* 120, 326.
15. Morgan, D. W. T. and Legge, K. (1989) *Veterinary Record* 124, 31.
16. Hall, L. W. and Chambers, J. P. (1989) *Journal of Small Animal Practice* 28, 623.
17. Chambers, J. P. (1989) *Journal of the Association of Veterinary Anaesthetists of Great Britain and Ireland* 16, 14.
18. Stephenson, J. C., Blevins, D. I. and Christie, G. J. (1978) *Veterinary Medicine/Small Animal Clinician* 3, 303.

19. Schulman, J. (1981) *Canine Practice* **8**, 53.
20. Erhardt, W. (1984) *Journal of the Association of Veterinary Anaesthetists of Great Britain and Ireland* **12**, 196.
21. Corbett, H. R. (1977) *Australian Veterinary Practice* **7**, 184.
22. Bomzon, L. (1981) *Journal of Small Animal Practice* **22**, 769.
23. Dundee, J. W. (1981) *Anaesthesia* **36**, 579.
24. Clarke, K. W. and Hall, L. W. (1984) *Journal of the Association of Veterinary Anaesthetists of Great Britain and Ireland* **12**, 83.
25. Cribb, P. H., Hird, J. F. R. and Hall, L. W. (1977) *Veterinary Record* **101**, 50.
26. Jones, R. S. and Brearley, J. C. (1987) *Journal of Small Animal Practice* **28**, 197.
27. Jones, R. S. and Clutton, R. E. (1984) *Journal of Small Animal Practice* **25**, 473.
28. Hall, L. W., Kellagher, R. E. B. and Watkins, S. B. (1985) *British Journal of Anaesthesia* **57**, 1046.
29. Nutt, P. (1962) *Veterinary Record* **74**, 874.
30. Tufvesson, G. (1951) *Nordiske Veterinaermedicin* **3**, 183.
31. Brook, G. B. (1935) *Veterinary Record* **15**, 549, 576, 597, 659.
32. Micheletto, B. (1954) *Annali Facultie Medicine Veterinaire*, vol. 4.
33. Bonarth, K. H. and Saleh, A. S. (1985) *Proceedings of the 2nd International Congress of Veterinary Anaesthesia*, Sacremento.
34. Hall, L. W. (1976) *Journal of Small Animal Practice* **17**, 661.

CHAPTER 16

ANAESTHESIA OF THE CAT

Despite the cat's reputation for having nine lives, anaesthetic fatalities are not unknown in apparently fit, healthy animals. Indeed, in veterinary general practice in the UK a recent survey by the Association of Veterinary Anaesthetists indicated a death rate of one in 550 for fit, healthy cats [1].

Cats object to being restrained so that even friendly cats may prove difficult to inject intravenously, and unhandled cats may be impossible to anaesthetize using this route of administration. For this reason it may be necessary to use parenteral drugs by other routes, or to induce anaesthesia using inhalation agents. Cats are small in size and this means that the margin of error is small; anaesthetic overdoses can easily be administered and, for inhalation anaesthesia, special apparatus is necessary if asphyxia is to be avoided. Respiratory obstruction can occur due to the small diameter of the cat's trachea and the tendency for laryngeal spasm to develop. Endotracheal intubation may not reduce this danger, as trauma to the larynx during this procedure may result in ob-struction from mucosal oedema postoperatively. Adrenaline release during a stormy induction or recovery can cause ventricular fibrillation and this is especially likely to happen if the heart is suffering from the insults of hypoxia or hypercapnia due to partial respiratory obstruction, or to the use of inappropriate anaesthetic apparatus. In the cat, vagal reflexes are very active during light anaesthesia, they are triggered by surgery of the head and neck, particularly of the eyes, nose and larynx, and give rise to laryngeal spasm or, occasionally, to cardiac arrest.

The cat must not be regarded, as it so often is in veterinary medicine, as a small dog; its temperamental and physiological make-up is very different. Provided that this is recognized, suitable premedication, a quiet induction of anaesthesia, careful monitoring, the maintenance of a clear airway, adequate oxygenation and the efficient removal of carbon dioxide, and appropriate attention to fluid and electrolyte balance, should ensure a very low mortality rate.

ANALGESIA

Cats have often been denied adequate analgesia on the mistaken grounds that the use of opioids causes maniacal excitement in Felidae. Certainly, the use of high doses can do so and violent excitement may be seen after intravenous injection of these drugs, as this method of administration may expose the brain to a (temporary) overdose. Thus, the intravenous administration of potent opioids such as fentanyl or alfentanil to conscious cats cannot be recommended. However, in the correct doses, opioids will not induce excitement even in fit, healthy animals [2] and if the cat is in pain when the drug is given high doses are tolerated without problems. Any of the opioids of moderate potency which have been recommended for use in other species of animal, given at the lowest dose rates used in dogs, may be used to provide pre- or postoperative analgesia in cats. It is probable that pethidine, given by the intramuscular route at total doses of 10–20 mg to average-sized animals has been the opioid most widely used, but cats in severe pain may safely be given intramuscular morphine at doses of 0.1–0.15 mg/kg. Of the partial agonist drugs, butorphanol given intramuscularly at doses 0.05–0.1 mg/kg has been recommended by Short [3] and buprenorphine (0.006 mg/kg) given intramuscularly at the end of surgery provides excellent postoperative analgesia although at the expense of considerably delayed recovery from anaesthesia.

The non-steroidal anti-inflammatory drug phenylbutazone is quite toxic to cats, even in moderate doses, but aspirin may be given in small doses by mouth. When indicated, 10–20 mg/kg of aspirin should be given in divided doses over a period of 24 hours. This dose given for 1 or 2 days is generally both safe and effective and allows for the fact that the rate of hepatic drug metabolism is slow due to a deficiency of bilirubin-glucuronoside glucuronosyltransferase. Long-term aspirin administration can lead to aplastic anaemia or thrombocytopenia.

SEDATION

Phenothiazine derivatives

Acepromazine may be given at the dose rate of 0.03–0.05 mg/kg and by the routes already described for dogs (p. 291), but in cats the sedation produced is very variable and is seldom adequate to assist in control of the animal. However, premedication with phenothiazine derivatives results in a smoother recovery from anaesthesia and reduces excitement side-effects induced by certain anaesthetics. Promethazine, a potent antihistamine, is sometimes used before Saffan anaesthesia to reduce the risk of allergic-type reactions.

α₂-Adrenoceptor agonists

Xylazine (Rompun) has been widely used, but it may produce variable results. Its action is that of a sedative/hypnotic so that increasing the dose increases the depth and duration of the sedation produced, and doses of 1–3 mg/kg by the intramuscular route are used to give mild to fairly profound sedation. Subcutaneous injection may be used but gives less reliable results. Vomiting and retching occur as the drug starts to exert its effect and are most commonly seen after the lower dose rates are employed [4]. Cardiovascular effects are dose dependent and the authors have found that although there may be an initial period of hypertension, doses of more than 3 mg/kg result in cardiac depression and hypotension. Dunkle *et al.* [5], using echocardiography, found xylazine to have a marked depressive effect on cardiac performance and showed that glycopyrrolate may not completely alleviate the bradycardia due to this α₂-adrenoceptor agonist. Very high doses of xylazine have been used to anaesthetize cats but they are associated with respiratory depression, cardiovascular depression and a very protracted recovery. They represent overdosage and such misuse cannot be condoned.

When xylazine is used for premedication, its effects summate with those of all other central nervous depressant drugs, so that doses of all parenterally administered anaesthetics have to be greatly reduced. This additive effect seems to depend on the dose of xylazine given rather than on the effect which it has produced, so that great care is necessary in even apparently lightly sedated cats. Following xylazine premedication doses of barbiturate drugs are at least halved, and doses of Saffan have to be reduced even more than this. Xylazine has often been used with

ketamine and the use of these two drugs will be discussed later on p. 333.

The more recently introduced drug medetomidine may well replace xylazine. An intramuscular dose of 80 μg/kg appears to give sedation similar in type and depth to that produced by 3 mg/kg of intramuscular xylazine. Maximal effect is obtained within 10–15 minutes. Duration of effect is dose related, but after an 80 μg/kg dose the clinically useful effect lasts for approximately 1 hour and recovery appears to be complete in about 2.5–3 hours. Side-effects are as expected for an α₂-adrenoceptor agonist, there being marked bradycardia and transient arterial hypertension followed by hypotension; depression of respiratory rate, pallor of mucous membranes and vomiting early on as sedation develops. Prolonged sedation with high doses of medetomidine may cause hypothermia.

Should there be any worries about the condition of an animal sedated with these drugs bradycardia may be treated with atropine or glycopyrrolate, although this may not be altogether beneficial [5]. The sedative effects of medetomidine may be antagonized with atipamezole. However, there are some arguments as to the ideal dose to employ and doses of one to four times the original dose of medetomidine have been recommended. Higher doses, or doses given at a time when sedation is already waning, have led to some cats being over-alert. The over-alert state did not progress to obvious excitement and, when left quiet in a cage, the animals resumed normal behaviour over the course of the next hour. As there are times when it may be desirable for a cat to remain very slightly sedated (e.g. for the journey home) the decision as to the most suitable dose of atipamezole for any individual case should be adjusted according to the time lapsed since the administration of medetomidine and the degree of reversal required. It should be noted that in the authors' experience, under-reversal using lower doses of atipamezole still leaves the cat liable to hypothermia.

Benzodiazepines

Diazepam and other drugs of the benzodiazepine group produce no obvious sedation when given to domestic cats. They are sometimes used in premedication for their muscle-relaxing properties and this use is associated with an increased duration of action of other drugs used in anaesthesia. Diazepam is given in doses of up to 0.5 mg/kg by intramuscular injection; its injection appears to give rise to pain no matter what preparation is used.

SEDATIVE/OPIOID COMBINATIONS

Neuroleptanalgesic techniques employ large doses of opiate analgesics to which the cat may respond with violent excitement. They are, therefore, contra-indicated for use in cats or, indeed, in all other Felidae.

Low doses of opioids such as pethidine (1–2 mg/kg) may be used together with acepromazine but the improvement in sedation over that provided by acepromazine is usually minimal.

PREANAESTHETIC PREPARATION

Preanaesthetic examination should be carried out in a manner similar to that described in Chapter 1, and any pathological conditions found, together with any pre-existing drug therapy, taken into account during the subsequent anaesthetic. In clinical practice it is common to find that cats have been exposed to organophosphorus insecticides from flea collars or sprays and this may increase the length of action of suxamethonium given for intubation. Corticosteroids are frequently used in cats to control allergies to external parasites and corticosteroid cover should be given over the anaesthetic and operating periods if

the cat has received such therapy in the 2 months preceding anaesthesia.

About 12 hours of fasting will usually ensure that the cat has an empty stomach and water need only be withheld for 2 hours prior to anaesthesia, or the water bowl removed at the time premedication is given. If surgery is to be carried out on the day of admission, enquiry should be made as to whether the cat was closely confined throughout the previous night for a roaming, hunting cat may have filled its stomach by eating its prey.

ANAESTHETIC TECHNIQUES

Intravenous injection

The minimum of forcible restraint should be used to enable intravenous injection to be carried out. Cats object strongly to restraint and respond to its imposition by trying to escape from it, thus inviting more forcible measures which only too often result in scratched and bitten assistants and a very frightened, excited cat. Such stormy conditions during the induction of anaesthesia can lead to the cat dying from ventricular fibrillation.

In the conscious cat, intravenous injections are best made into the cephalic vein. The animal is placed in a sitting position on a table of convenient height and for injection into the right cephalic vein the assistant stands to the cat's left side, raising and supporting its head between the thumb and fingers of the left hand. In this position the assistant can usually help to keep the cat calm by tickling it below the ears (Fig. 16.1). The assistant's right hand is placed so that the middle, third and fourth fingers are behind the olecranon, and the thumb is around the front of the right fore-limb. The limb is extended by pushing on the olecranon and the vein is raised by applying gentle pressure with the thumb. The limb must not be held in a vice-like grip because this cuts off the arterial blood supply and distresses the cat. Venepuncture is carried out as described on p. 299 for the dog. Most friendly household cats will allow venepuncture to be carried

out easily as long as the needle is sharp (and modern disposable ones are) and no thrust is made with the needle. The needle must be introduced steadily and gently through the skin and into the lumen of the vein without stabbing. Should it become obvious that more restraint is needed, the assistant can provide this rapidly by holding the cat between his or her body and right arm while preventing movement from the hind limbs by pressing the cat firmly on to the surface of the table. The cat's head can easily be controlled when held firmly in the left hand as described. If it is clear that greater restraint than this is needed, it is probably preferable to abandon attempts at intravenous injection until an appropriate premedication has had time to take effect, or to induce anaesthesia by other means. A short needle with a fine bore is suitable for injections into the cephalic vein and, in general, a 25 gauge needle (0.5 mm external diameter), 15 mm long is ideal.

Although in theory any of the methods of venepuncture described for use in dogs may be applied in cats, the problems of restraint make them difficult to use in conscious animals. In moribund or anaesthetized animals, the jugular vein can be used. The cat is placed in lateral recumbency with its neck over a small pad or sandbag, its fore-limbs are stretched backwards towards its tail, and the uppermost jugular vein occluded in the jugular groove near to the sternal inlet by the assistant's thumb. Venepuncture is then

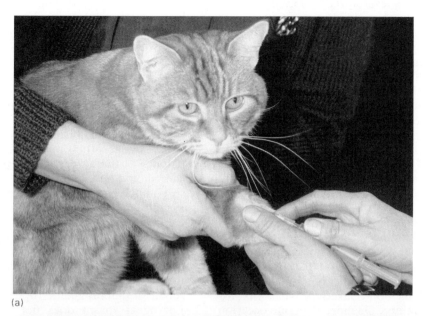

(a)

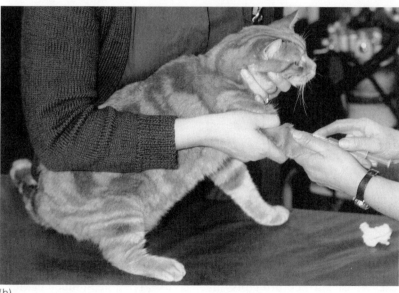

(b)

Fig. 16.1 Injection into the cephalic vein. (a) In the majority of cats if only minimal restraint is used, as here, the animal does not become frightened or otherwise upset by the procedure. (b) Less calm animals can often be calmed by 'ear tickling' as the procedure is being carried out.

carried out as described for the dog (p. 300). The jugular vein route is a particularly useful one for the administration of intravenous fluid therapy and when relatively large blood samples are required for diagnostic or other purposes the jugular vein is the only practicable source.

Endotracheal intubation

In cats, laryngeal spasm is easily provoked, and after induction of anaesthesia atraumatic intubation can only be carried out by adopting one of the following methods:

1. The laryngeal mucous membrane of the anaesthetized cat can be desensitized by spraying it with a solution of a local analgesic drug, such as 4% lignocaine hydrochloride. The larynx usually goes into a spasm when the spray is applied and attempts of intubation should be delayed for about 30 seconds until it is seen to relax again. Following intubation by this method it must be remembered that the larynx will be insensitive, and the normal protective reflexes absent, until the effects of the local analgesic have worn off. Spraying the larynx has been shown to produce tissue oedema [6] and the amount of local analgesic used is critical for Heavner has shown that lignocaine is capable of causing neurogenically mediated ventricular arrhythmias [7].

   In cases where quick intubation is essential this technique is not suitable since spraying the larynx with local analgesic solution does not produce immediate desensitization and paralysis of the vocal cords. Attempts should not be made to force a tube through the non-relaxed, active larynx, for this can cause injury. On more than one occasion attempts to force a tube through a larynx showing spasm have resulted in penetration of the pharyngeal wall and passage of the tube down the neck between the oesophagus and trachea.

2. The anaesthetized cat may be paralysed by the administration of a relaxant drug after inhaling pure oxygen from a face-mask for 30–60 seconds to prevent hypoxia during the subsequent intubation procedure. Paralysis is usually produced rapidly by the intravenous injection of 3–5 mg of suxamethonium (for an adult cat), and oxygen administration is continued during the fasciculations caused by the initial depolarizing action of this agent. When relaxation is complete the cat is intubated through completely flaccid vocal cords. Artificial ventilation of the lungs is continued through the endotracheal tube until spontaneous respiration returns some 5 minutes later. Should intubation prove difficult the cat is prevented from becoming hypoxic whilst further attempts are made by manual ventilation of the lungs using a face-mask. The mask is applied and the lungs inflated several times with pure oxygen whenever (but preferably before) the mucous membranes take on a dusky, cyanotic appearance and a further attempt is made to intubate as soon as the colour is restored to a normal pink by the lung inflation.

   Manual ventilation of the lungs through a face-mask is not difficult. Cats' faces are reasonably uniform in shape and it is easy to get a gas-tight seal between a properly designed mask and the face. The lower jaw must be pushed forward to ensure the airway is clear and only gentle pressure applied to the bag to ventilate the lungs or gas will be forced down the oesophagus into the stomach. It is possible to ventilate almost all unconscious cats with pure oxygen at any time and the well-oxygenated cat can be intubated under the influence of a muscle relaxant such as suxamethonium without need for haste.

   Ventilation of the lungs through a face-mask is only impossible in cats with upper respiratory obstruction (usually an abscess or tumour) and in these a tracheostomy may be the only way in which patency of the airway can be assured. Particular care should be taken to exert only minimal pressure on the bag in cats with ruptured diaphragms, for in them it is very easy to inflate the stomach.

   Obviously, this technique of introducing an endotracheal tube should be practised when intubation of the cat is not strictly needed so that it can be performed competently and quickly when this is essential — e.g. in cats anaesthetized for repair of diaphragmatic ruptures.

3. Laryngeal spasm does not occur during deep anaesthesia. This is not recommended as a routine procedure but where emergency intubation is required following an accidental overdose of anaesthetic, it is never necessary to employ either of the methods described above to secure relaxation of the jaw muscles and vocal cords.

Attempts to carry out forceful intubation by any technique through tightly apposed vocal cords, even if initially successful, will result in damage to the mucous membrane with oedema and the danger of obstruction after extubation. The cat's larynx may also go into a spasm after extubation, so endotracheal tubes should, if there are no surgical contraindications, be removed without any previous deliberate lightening of anaesthesia.

Intubation is performed under direct vision as soon as the jaw muscles are relaxed by general anaesthesia or the effects of the relaxant, and intubation is, of course, possible at much lighter levels of anaesthesia when relaxants are used. Although the expert should be able to intubate regardless of the position of the cat, the technique is best learned if one standard position is employed until the technique is mastered. The head and neck of the supine cat are extended by placing a small sandbag under the neck, or by an assistant supporting the head with a hand placed beneath the neck, and the tongue is pulled out of the mouth, taking care not to injure it on the teeth. A standard laryngoscope with an infant-sized blade is introduced and the tip of the blade placed so that it is over the dorsum of the tongue and resting just in front of the epiglottis. The laryngoscope blade is then lifted

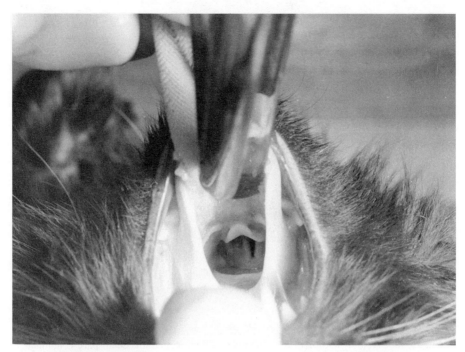

Fig. 16.2 Exposure of the larynx by lifting of the laryngoscope blade.

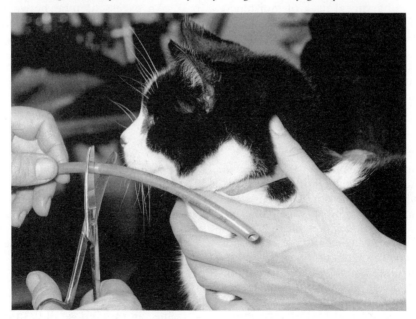

Fig. 16.3 New endotracheal tubes must be cut to the correct length before use. This is from the nostrils to the point of the shoulder.

to expose the glottic opening and giving a good view of the vocal cords (Fig. 16.2). The endotracheal tube may then be passed between the cords without any difficulty. If a laryngoscope is not available, a lighted tongue depressor such as the 'Twinlight' can be used in much the same way but these tongue depressors are not so easy to control and it may be found easier to expose the larynx if the cat is lying on its side as described for the dog (p. 309).

A 5 or 5.5 mm uncuffed endotracheal tube is suitable for most adult cats. A tight seal, such as may be needed to prevent inhalation of foreign materials,

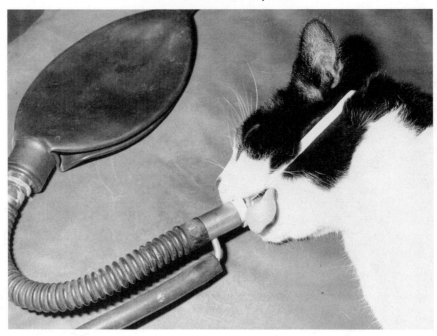

Fig. 16.4 A correctly intubated cat with no excess length of tube protruding from the mouth and the tube securely anchored in position with a tape. Apparatus dead-space is minimal.

can be ensured by a pharyngeal pack of moistened ribbon gauze. Endotracheal tubes should be long enough to pass well beyond the larynx but not so long that they will enter the main bronchus. The correct length may be assessed as being from the nostrils to the point of the shoulder of the cat, and all new tubes should be cut to this measurement before use (Fig. 16.3). An excess of tube between the mouth and breathing circuit should not be tolerated because this, in small animals, adds significantly to the respiratory dead-space. A tape tied tightly around the tube over the endotracheal connector can be secured behind the cat's ears to anchor the tube in position once it has been introduced (Fig. 16.4).

PREMEDICATION

Anticholinergic drugs should generally be included in the premedication given to cats, both to prevent saliva and bronchial secretions from obstructing the small-diameter airway, and to block vagal reflexes. The only contraindications to their use are the general ones of pre-existing tachycardia or glaucoma and they should be given whenever it is proposed to use suxamethonium for endotracheal intubation. Analgesics should be given whenever it is necessary to relieve pain. The use of sedatives is governed by the temperament of the cat and by the anaesthetic technique to follow. Phenothiazines do little to calm a wild cat, but are useful in quieter animals to counteract excitement caused by some drugs and to improve the quality of recovery. Xylazine and medetomidine markedly reduce the dose of all other drugs used for anaesthesia and should be used with very great care. In the survey of anaesthetic problems carried out recently by the Association of Veterinary Anaesthetists of Great Britain and Ireland, xylazine was associated with a particularly high number of fatalities (one per 117 cats given the drug), that were primarily due to overdosage with agents given later to produce anaesthesia. However, xylazine and medetomidine appear to be particularly useful in reducing the side-effects of ketamine (p. 333), as indeed are the benzodiazepines.

Anticholinergic agents

Atropine, at a total dose of 0.3 mg for an adult cat, may be given by the intramuscular or subcutaneous route. Atropine interferes with vision and cats which have received this drug should be handled particularly carefully to avoid inducing panic reactions.

Glycopyrrolate, in doses of about 0.01 mg/kg by intramuscular injection, or at half this dose by the intravenous route, is probably a better anticholinergic for cats. It does not cause as marked an increase in heart rate nor does it readily cross the blood–brain barrier.

PARENTERALLY ADMINISTERED ANAESTHETICS

Intravenous injection is relatively easy in dogs but in cats problems of restraint may make intravenous injections more difficult or even impossible, so that agents which can be given by other routes tend to have a greater role to play in feline than in canine anaesthesia. The disadvantages of such administration — slow induction, variable absorption, variable results, often prolonged recovery, and inability to dose to effect — must be weighed against the temperament of the cat and the likelihood of being able to carry out a controlled intravenous injection.

Thiopentone sodium

Thiopentone may only be given intravenously and in cats it should be used as a 1.25% or even more dilute solution. It may be used for induction of anaesthesia at doses of up to 10 mg/kg, as described for the dog (p. 301), and if the cat has not been given a sedative premedication it is probable that the full dose will be required. As in dogs, very small doses will be needed after premedication with the α_2-adrenoceptor agonists. If thiopentone is to be used as the sole agent, incremental doses up to a total dose of 20 mg/kg may be used but, at these high doses, saturation of the fat depots may mean that recovery will take several hours and effects may still be observed the next day. If recovery is prolonged, the cat must be kept warm, for development of hypothermia will delay recovery still more.

Methohexitone sodium

Methohexitone may be given only by intravenous injection, and is used at a concentration of 0.5% for feline anaesthesia. Although it can be used for induction of anaesthesia at a dose of about 5 mg/kg, and given in incremental doses to maintain anaesthesia, in cats its tendency for causing excitement means that recovery is often far from uneventful. The use of sedative premedication helps to reduce the incidence of excitatory phenomena but, in general, methohexitone is only employed in cats when very rapid recovery is essential (e.g. after caesarean section).

Pentobarbitone sodium

Until about 20 years ago pentobarbitone was widely used in general practice and experimental laboratories as an anaesthetic for cats. Doses of 25 mg/kg by intravenous injection, half given fast to avoid induction excitement and the rest given slowly over 2–3 minutes to effect, give about 2 hours of surgical anaesthesia. Recovery from such doses is very prolonged, the cat not becoming fully conscious until the next day. Despite the long-acting nature of the drug and the respiratory depression it causes, pentobarbitone anaesthesia has, over the years, been successfully and safely administered to many hundreds of thousands of cats. Most deaths following pentobarbitone anaesthesia probably result from hypothermia and it is essential that the cat is kept warm in the recovery period.

Pentobarbitone can also be given by intraperitoneal injection but the results are variable, depending on its absorption from the peritoneal cavity. Induction of anaesthesia is slow and cats frequently show a stage of marked excitement so that if released at this stage they may literally run around the walls of the room. Some veterinarians have administered pentobarbitone to cats by intrapleural injection and although absorption from this cavity is better than from the peritoneum, injection is very painful and the potential complications are such that the intrapleural route is quite unacceptable [8–11].

Saffan

Since its introduction into clinical feline anaesthesia [12] this steroid mixture has become an extremely popular agent, especially in general practice.

The two steroids in Saffan are dissolved with Cremophor EL to give a total steroid concentration of 12 mg/ml and in veterinary practice it has become customary to express doses in terms of milligrams of this total steroid content. (In medical practice doses of the identical preparation 'Althesin' were usually given in ml/kg or μg/kg.) The solution is non-irritant and is given to cats intravenously or intramuscularly. In the unsedated cat, doses of 3 mg/kg by intravenous injection produced unconsciousness for a few minutes, whilst doses of 9 mg/kg give 10–15 minutes of anaesthesia with very little increase in the initial depth of unconsciousness or respiratory depression. The increased duration of action with initial dose increase reaches a plateau at about 18 mg/kg and giving higher doses is pointless and may be dangerous [13]. If it is necessary to prolong anaesthesia further, increments of Saffan may be given later on, or an inhalation agent employed. Saffan is rapidly metabolized in the liver so that the incremental dose regimen does not result in undue delay in recovery and cats are usually completely conscious 2 hours after the last dose has been given. The rapid breakdown of the steroids, coupled with the minimal cardiovascular effects, is undoubtedly responsible for the wide safety margin as far as dose is concerned.

Intravenous induction of Saffan anaesthesia is usually smooth and rapid, but occasionally it is complicated by retching, vomiting and laryngeal spasm. Although in the majority of healthy, unpremedicated cats the dose of Saffan needed to produce some 15 minutes of anaesthesia (9 mg/kg) may be given intravenously as a single injection, in a few it may be an overdose. It certainly causes a significant depression of cardiac output, stroke volume and systemic vascular resistance [14]. The authors much prefer to give an initial intravenous injection of 2–3 mg/kg and administer the rest of the dose after gauging the response to the initial injection. Where sedative premedication is employed the dose of Saffan may have to be reduced and if xylazine is employed as a sedative a reduction of more than 50% may be necessary. The use of other intravenous anaesthetic agents with Saffan may result in severe respiratory and cardiovascular depression and the manufacturers state that Saffan should not at any time be combined with any other intravenous anaesthetic. There is little respiratory depression during Saffan anaesthesia, although the intravenous injection of high doses (more than 12 mg/kg) may give rise to some depression and a period of apnoea [14]. Hypothermia may occur but is rarely clinically significant unless the operation involves wide opening of the body cavities, or the cat is fluid depleted. Recovery from Saffan anaesthesia is often rather restless and if the animal is stimulated in some way recovery may be violent, the cat becoming rigid, twitching, convulsing and even showing opisthotonus. The smoothness of recovery can usually be greatly improved by ensuring that the animal is pain free and left undisturbed in a quiet, warm, comfortable, roomy cage. Acepromazine premedication is also claimed by many to improve the quality of recovery from Saffan anaesthesia.

When Saffan is used as an induction agent before inhalation anaesthesia it is often necessary to increase the concentration of any volatile agent to above what might be expected in order to suppress the twitching associated with recovery from Saffan. Laryngeal spasm may be provoked by head and neck surgery under light Saffan anaesthesia (reports to the Association of Veterinary Anaesthetists of Great Britain and Ireland) and for this type of surgery cats must be premedicated with atropine and intubated.

Saffan may also be given by intramuscular injection and doses of 18 mg/kg are followed in about 10 minutes by anaesthesia which lasts some 10–20 minutes. These large doses represent a rather large volume (4.5 ml for a 3 kg cat) but the injection appears painless and cats do not resent administration. Lower doses can be used for minor procedures such as dematting the coat. As the anaesthetic is eliminated so rapidly from the body, it is ineffective if it is given either subcutaneously or into the fascial planes between the muscles, so to ensure its proper effect it should be given deep into the vastus group of muscles. Intramuscular administration is never as reliable as intravenous injection and it is, therefore, generally employed either where deep sedation rather than anaesthesia is needed or where it is possible to supplement by an intravenous injection once the cat is unconscious.

Hyperaemia and swollen paws, ears and noses are common following the administration of Saffan and there are reports of laryngeal and pulmonary oedema. Other side-effects include sneezing, retching, vomiting and laryngeal spasm, but provided a clear airway is maintained and respiration and cardiac function are not depressed, Saffan is undoubtedly a safe induction and maintenance agent for use in general practice. Evans estimated the mortality rate to be less than 1:10 000 [13] but it seems more likely that the true mortality rate for Saffan in cats is nearly 10 times greater than this at about one in 900 [1].

Propofol

Propofol has now been used quite extensively in cats as an intravenous anaesthetic. The dose needed to induce anaesthesia is 6–7 mg/kg in both unpremedicated animals and in animals premedicated with acepromazine (0.03 mg/kg). The dose following medetomidine premedication has yet to be established but is likely to be very low. Induction is smooth and blood pressure and heart rate are well maintained but there is some significant respiratory depression. Maintenance of anaesthesia with propofol requires about 0.5 mg/(kg min). Recovery is generally smooth but retching, sneezing or pawing of the face may occur in about 15% of cases.

The cats' liver does not metabolize phenols as rapidly as does the dogs' liver so that in cats rapid recovery is not a marked feature of propofol anaesthesia as it is in dogs. Also, some cats have disturbed recoveries, pawing at their noses in a manner reminiscent of that seen after the use of Saffan. Acepromazine premedication appears to improve the quality of recovery. Propofol seems less likely than Saffan to produce anaphylactoid reactions in cats but these reactions with Saffan are, in the vast majority of animals relatively mild, so this is not a reason to prefer the use of propofol. It is doubtful whether propofol offers any major advantage over the other intravenous agents to the feline anaesthetist.

Ketamine

Ketamine is a dissociative agent which is widely used in cats. Although not well received when first introduced into the UK it has become more popular as its peculiar characteristics have gradually been recognized.

The fact that ketamine can be administered by intramuscular or subcutaneous injection makes it a very useful agent for the induction of anaesthesia in cats which are difficult or impossible to handle. The volume of solution which has to be injected is small and the injection can be made by a dart projectile fired from a blowpipe. If it is possible to give it from a syringe, the small volume can be injected very rapidly. It should be noted, however, that intramuscular or subcutaneous injection of ketamine appears to be painful, in that it is very often violently resented by the animal, and that for all but the most minor of procedures it is necessary to supplement its action with an inhalation agent, as the marked muscle tone limits the surgery possible. When given by intravenous injection there is a delay of 1–2 minutes before its effects become apparent but this is the best route for administration. Application to the mucous membrane of the mouth (squirting from a syringe) can be an effective route of administration in cats which are difficult to handle.

Other concentrations are available for medical use but ketamine is marketed for veterinary purposes in an aqueous solution containing 100 mg/ml.

When used alone, the duration of action of ketamine depends on the dose of the drug which is given. Glen [15] found that the cat became recumbent 3–5 minutes following intramuscular injection of either 10 or 20 mg/kg. Sternal recumbency was regained 30 minutes after the lower dose and 50 minutes following the higher one, but it was considerably longer before the cat was able to stand and behave normally. Higher doses were seldom more reliable and resulted in very long recovery. Glen concluded that while the drug might be satisfactory as an anaesthetic for minor procedures, it should be considered as being more of an agent for the induction of anaesthesia to be maintained by inhalation methods. The manufacturers recommend intramuscular doses of 11–33 mg/kg, depending on the depth and duration of anaesthesia required. Very small kittens of less than 4 weeks of age appear to need still higher doses of up to 35 mg/kg. Doses up to the lower end of this range are used when the drug is given by intravenous injection.

Under ketamine cats exhibit marked muscle tone, their eyes remain open and spontaneous movement quite unrelated to any stimulation may occur. Such movements may lead the anaesthetist who is unaccustomed to the effects of the drug to assume that anaesthesia is lightening, but this is not the case and further doses given in an attempt to suppress them result in overdosage. Laryngeal and pharyngeal reflexes are often said to be retained, but the anaesthetist should not count on this protection and should take all the normal precautions to ensure that the airway remains clear. Salivation is often profuse, so atropine or glycopyrrolate premedication is advisable. Although ketamine is claimed to cause minimal respiratory depression, relative or absolute overdoses can cause apnoea [1]. Non-fatal adverse reactions relate to cats given the drug by the intramuscular route for a short procedure and apnoea occurring once the cat has been returned to its cage; it is probable that deaths reported at a similar time resulted from apnoea. Therefore, it is essential that cats should be kept under continuous observation from the time ketamine is administered until it is obvious that recovery is complete. Ketamine produces some slight stimulation of the circulatory system and cardiovascular problems are seldom encountered in cats under its influence.

During recovery from ketamine some cats show marked emergence phenomena which are extremely difficult to describe. The cat becomes hypersensitive to stimuli and shows marked tonicity of the skeletal muscles. The pupils are widely dilated but the animal appears unable to see. These signs are most marked in wild or feral cats or in cats recovering in noisy or uncomfortable surroundings. In man, such emergence phenomena are associated with unpleasant dreaming or hallucinations, but it is obviously impossible to know whether this is also true for cats.

A wide range of sedative agents have been used for premedication, or in combination with ketamine, in order to reduce the side-effects, in particular those of emergence phenomena and increased muscle tone. Where the use of such premedication allows a reduction in the dose of ketamine, speed of recovery may be enhanced. Acepromazine (0.1 mg/kg by intramuscular injection) although widely used is not totally effective in reducing the unwanted side-effects and has little influence on the dose of ketamine subsequently required. Intramuscular diazepam in doses of 1 mg/kg has also often proved disappointing. However, midazolam (0.2 mg/kg) mixed in the syringe with ketamine (10 mg/kg) and administered intramuscularly [16] provides deep sedation suitable for radiotherapy; useful sedation lasts about 30 minutes (some cats become cyanosed when breathing air) and recovery is usually complete within 2–3 hours. Undoubtedly, to date, xylazine has been the most commonly used sedative for cats receiving ketamine. Xylazine is extremely effective in preventing emergence excitement and increased muscle tone and it permits reduction in the ketamine dose, but its use is also associated with the side-effects of bradycardia (unless anticholinergics have been used for premedication) and vomiting. In the UK, combined doses recommended were 1 mg/kg of xylazine with 22 mg/kg of ketamine by intramuscular injection [17] but this combination leads to deep anaesthesia with fairly prolonged recovery and, as discussed above, has been associated with cases of apnoea and death. In many other countries, the dose of ketamine following 1 mg/kg of xylazine has been reduced to 10 or even 5 mg/kg, the latter dose ensuring a considerably faster recovery. A reduction in xylazine to 0.5 mg/kg with a larger dose (20–25 mg/kg) of ketamine has been used by Arnbjerg [18] with only three deaths in over 7000 cats. None of these cats received an anticholinergic. Thus, his method must be regarded as safe but the prolonged recovery period (of 3–5 hours) may present problems in busy practice conditions.

More recently, medetomidine (80 µg/kg) has been combined with ketamine (5 mg/kg) by intramuscular injection for operations such as ovarohysterectomy. Because of the length of action of medetomidine, recovery is prolonged [19]. Atipamezole may be given to speed recovery but should not be given until the effects of ketamine have waned — probably about 1 hour after a dose of 5 mg/kg.

Zolazepam/tiletamine

Zolazepam is a member of the benzodiazepine group of drugs (p. 55), while tiletamine is a drug of the phencyclidine family (p. 92). Their combination in equal proportions has been used intravenously and intramuscularly to produce deep sedation or even anaesthesia in cats and dogs. Intravenous doses of 15 mg/kg of the mixture produce unconsciousness in one injection site/brain circulation time and after intramuscular injection full effects are seen in 2–5 minutes. Anticholinergic premedication should be given to limit excess salivation which is a feature of the anaesthetic state. Anaesthesia or sedation may be prolonged by the injection of one-third to one-half of the initial dose. After one dose the duration of surgical anaesthesia is of the order of 20–60 minutes and recovery is prolonged, frequently taking 6 or more hours or even longer. If more than the one initial dose has been administered recovery can be very prolonged.

INHALATION ANAESTHESIA

Inhalation agents may be used in cats to induce and maintain anasthesia but because of the small size of the animals it is relatively easy to administer an overdose of the volatile anaesthetics. The fit, un-sedated cat strongly resents attempts to induce anaesthesia with volatile agents given through a face-mask and it is seldom possible to avoid struggling or fighting with the animal at some time during the induction process. For this reason many anaesthetists prefer to induce anaesthesia by placing the cat in a rectangular glass or clear plastic chamber such as a battery jar and piping the anaesthetic gases and vapours into the chamber. The cat usually accepts this procedure quite calmly provided it can see out of the container and the transparent walls enable the behaviour of the animal to be observed. It must be removed from the chamber as soon as it loses consciousness and collapses in a state of light anaesthesia.

To induce anaesthesia using a face-mask in a restrained cat, the animal is usually placed in lateral recumbency with all four legs held by an assistant while the anaesthetist controls the head with one hand and uses the other to apply the face-mask.

Cats seldom object to breathing a nitrous oxide/oxygen mixture via a face-mask and Magill system and the volatile agents may be added to this in gradually increasing concentrations. The normal rule is to increase the concentration of the volatile agent after every three breaths until the safe maximum is obtained. This technique avoids the prolonged breath holding which occurs if the animal is suddenly introduced to high induction concentrations of the volatile anaesthetic agent. If the cat struggles it usually breathes rapidly and deeply so the induction of anaesthesia is more rapid; if breath holding is encountered care must be taken not to release the cat as it may be at the stage of narcotic excitement. This method of induction can be traumatic for both the cat and the anaesthetist and adrenaline release in the frightened animal may occasionally result in ventricular fibrillation and death unless acepromazine, which seems to exert some protective effect, has been given for premedication. However, it has been applied quite safely for very many years and the rapid postoperative recovery which results from not having given the cat any parenteral agents may often outweigh the disadvantages of the induction procedure. In heavily premedicated or very sick cats, induction of anaesthesia by volatile agents given by a face-mask can usually be carried out without invoking excitement or struggling, and is often the method of choice. Smooth induction can usually be anticipated with halothane or isoflurane in a nitrous oxide/oxygen, but even if they are very carefully introduced into nitrous oxide/oxygen, coughing, sneezing and breath holding may be encountered in vigorous, healthy cats.

Breathing circuits

Any breathing circuit used to administer inhalation anaesthetics to cats must have a very low resistance and small dead-space. In practice, this limits the possible circuits to non-rebreathing systems as the soda lime canister of rebreathing systems creates too much resistance to respiration.

The Ayre's T-piece system

This is the circuit of choice when the cat is intubated but it may also be used with a face-mask. It has minimal resistance and dead-space and IPPV can be carried out very efficiently by squeezing the partially filled bag of the Jackson–Rees modification of the T-piece system. Fresh gas flow rates of twice the minute volume of respiration (Table 16.1) are sufficient to prevent rebreathing.

Table 16.1 Average respiratory and cardiovascular data for anaesthetized normal adult cats

Respiratory rate	24–28 breaths/min
Tidal volume	12–24 ml
Minute volume	280–670 ml/min
Heart rate	160 beats/min
Arterial blood pressure	120–140 mmHg (16–18.7 kPa) systolic
	70–80 mmHg (9.3–11 kPa) diastolic
Arterial blood pH	7.34
P_aO_2	90–104 mmHg (12–13.9 kPa)
P_aCO_2	35 mmHg (4.7 kPa)

Measurements made at the Cambridge School between 1952 and 1990.

Coaxial circuits

In practice the Bain circuit does not behave like a T-piece system and appears to offer too much resistance for animals breathing spontaneously, but it seems that the performance of the modified Bain circuit is improved if the 'tail' of the bag is amputated! The Lack system behaves rather like a Magill system but the tubing is much stiffer and bulkier so that it tends to drag the face-mask away from the face or the endotracheal tube out of the trachea. The expiratory valve needs to be removed from the Lack circuit. The parallel circuits in these configurations (see p. 161) offer no advantage in feline anaesthesia.

The Magill system

Although the expiratory valve of the Magill system creates rather too much resistance for cats, the system is frequently used with a face-mask to administer

inhalation anaesthetics to these animals. If the mask is tightly applied to the cat's face most anaesthetists lift the valve plate off its setting by introducing a pin or needle beneath the plate. Other anaesthetists use a large face-mask which is not applied tightly to the cat's face so that free expiration can take place between the face and the mask. These modifications of the system result in considerable pollution of the atmosphere of the room by the anaesthetic agents.

Inhalation agents used

All the inhalation anaesthetics may be used in cats in a similar way to that in which they are used in dogs (Chapter 15). In cats the use of chloroform is usually regarded as being even more dangerous than in dogs and it has no place in feline anaesthesia.

Nitrous oxide

Nitrous oxide/oxygen mixtures (3/2) are useful after anaesthesia has been induced with Saffan, especially when it has been given by intramuscular injection, as they seem to suppress the muscle twitching often seen when the effects of Saffan are waning. However, nitrous oxide/oxygen mixtures are usually used in feline anaesthesia simply as the vehicle for the delivery of the volatile agents.

Ether

For well over 100 years ether has proved to be a particularly safe anaesthetic for cats. Today, however, it is being discarded in most of the developed countries in favour of more recently introduced agents. Nevertheless, although induction is slower, the margin for error is much greater than it is for more potent agents such as halothane. Many thousands of cats have been anaesthetized with ether and the number of deaths which can be attributed to its proper use is small. In man, anaesthetization with ether is often followed by nausea and this may occur in cats for many are reluctant to eat for the first 12–24 hours after operation. However, this is a small price to pay for the safety of the patient and the only real objection which can be made to the use of ether in feline anaesthesia is the risk of fires or explosions when it is mixed with air or oxygen. Anticholinergics are essential to reduce the copious secretions induced by the irritant nature of its vapour.

Halothane

Cardiac arrhythmias occur quite frequently in cats under halothane anaesthesia. When they occur they can usually be abolished and normal rhythm restored by the performance of artificial respiration (IPPV) to increase the gaseous exchange in the lungs. It appears that the respiratory depressant activity of halothane allows carbon dioxide to accumulate in the body and once the concentration of this gas exceeds a certain threshold value arrhythmias appear. Lowering the $P_a CO_2$ by IPPV is followed by a prompt return to normal cardiac rhythm. Very satisfactory anaesthesia results when an accurately calibrated vaporizer is used and halothane is administered in oxygen or a nitrous oxide/oxygen mixture through a non-rebreathing T-piece system. For cats the total fresh gas flow rate to the T-piece system need not exceed 1.5–2 l/min, little halothane is used and, consequently, the method is not expensive so, provided ducting of waste gases from the open end of the T-piece is practised, there is no justification for attempting to use closed methods of administration.

Methoxyflurane

In cats methoxyflurane is usually used to reinforce the effects of nitrous oxide/oxygen mixtures. A calibrated vaporizer offers some advantages but it is not essential, and the vapour is delivered in the gas mixture to a T-piece system as described above for halothane.

Enflurane

Although as yet there is little published information relating to the use of enflurane, it has been used quite successfully to produce anaesthesia with short induction and recovery periods. It may be volatilized, preferably from a calibrated vaporizer in a stream of oxygen or nitrous oxide/oxygen and delivered to the cat by any of the methods usually employed in feline anaesthesia. Evidence of central nervous irritation has not been observed, but myotonia is common during recovery.

Isoflurane

Isoflurane may eventually find a role in feline anaesthesia. Such limited trials as have been carried out in cats with isoflurane have shown it to be an apparently quite satisfactory agent although in cats not undergoing surgery respiratory depression is marked. Theoretically, for use in cats with cardiac disease isoflurane may have advantages over halothane but, in practice, this is not very obvious when halothane is given with care. In the UK the present high cost of isoflurane discourages its use in feline anaesthesia.

INTERMITTENT POSITIVE-PRESSURE VENTILATION (IPPV)

In the intubated cat, IPPV can be carried out by manual compression of the reservoir bag of the Jackson–Rees modification of the T-piece system, as described for small dogs (p. 335). It is perfectly possible to apply IPPV when an uncuffed endotracheal tube is in place and indeed the absence of a cuff acts as a safety device by preventing the application of too high a positive pressure and over-inflation of the lungs. When the cat is not intubated, IPPV can be applied through a tightly fitting face-mask attached to either an Ayre's T-piece or Magill system, but care must be taken to ensure that the airway is clear and that too much pressure is not applied or the stomach will be inflated. A clear airway is produced by avoiding over-flexion or extension of the head and applying forward pressure behind the vertical ramus of the mandible as the face is pushed into the mask. The Magill system is only used for emergencies because when IPPV is performed it gives rise to almost total rebreathing so that the mask has to be removed from the patient's face every few breaths to allow exhalation to the atmosphere and the mask to refill with fresh gas.

Most mechanical ventilators used in canine surgery produce tidal volumes which are too large for cats and if they are used in these animals a controlled leak has to be introduced into the circuit. Human paediatric ventilators are available which are quite suitable for use in feline anaesthesia but they are likely to be needed too infrequently to justify their purchase.

NEUROMUSCULAR BLOCKING AGENTS

In cats there is seldom any indication for the use of competitive neuromuscular blocking agents as muscle tone is insufficient to interfere with most feline surgery. However, when they are indicated they may be used at the same dose rates, and their action antagonized in the same way, as described for dogs (p. 314). The depolarizing agent suxamethonium is used to aid endotracheal intubation or endoscopy, and in adult cats doses of 3–5 mg by intravenous injection will, after the initial muscle fasciculation, give complete relaxation for some 4–6 minutes, depending on the anaesthetic agents in use. During the period of apnoea IPPV is, of course, necessary, and no difficulty is experienced in continuing this IPPV for much longer than the paralysis due to the relaxant lasts.

NEONATAL ANAESTHESIA

The small size of neonatal kittens make them particularly prone to develop hypothermia and to respiratory obstruction. Kittens should always be premedicated with an anticholinergic (0.005 mg of atropine is sufficient) and anaesthesia is best induced and maintained with volatile anaesthetics. Endotracheal intubation should be avoided unless absolutely essential — as it is if IPPV is needed. Very careful attention should be given to the maintenance of body temperature and to the replacement of blood or fluid losses.

POSTOPERATIVE CARE

Endotracheal tubes should be removed from cats when anaesthesia is still reasonably deep as their removal during light anaesthesia can give rise to troublesome laryngeal spasm. The quality of recovery in the cat depends to a great extent on the anaesthetic agents which have been employed. It is usually smooth and uneventful following the use of inhalation anaesthesia, but cats may be hypersensitive to noise and other stimulation after treatment with Saffan or ketamine. Whatever agent has been used, recovery will be improved by keeping the cat in a quiet and comfortable cage. It is particularly important for the cage to be of adequate size, as many of the 'seizures' seen during recovery are provoked by the cat being unable to stretch out fully without touching the sides of the cage. Cats are prone to develop hypothermia and the recovery area should be kept warm or the cage should be heated. It is difficult to keep cats warm with heated water pads or hot water bottles because their claws cause punctures if the cat moves as it regains consciousness.

Adequate pain relief is as essential in cats as in all other animals. Narcotic analgesics may be given safely by the intramuscular route as long as excessive doses are not employed. Davies and Donnelly [2] showed that morphine at a dose of 0.1 mg/kg did not cause excitement even in fit, healthy cats, and gave 3–4 hours of pain relief. Pethidine, given at a dose of 4 mg/kg gave analgesia for 2 hours but no effect was apparent after 4 hours and they recommend that the

use of this agent be restricted to preoperative use. In the authors' experience, pethidine in doses of 10–25 mg (depending on the size of the cat) given by intramuscular injection at 3–4-hourly intervals produced excellent pain relief in the postoperative period for the majority of animals. Buprenorphine (0.006 mg/kg) can also be effective.

As cats start to become conscious they may react violently to the presence of such things as chest drains and occasionally it is necessary to give drugs to control the animal at this time, even if they delay return to full consciousness. In such circumstances, provided that barbiturates have not been employed during anaesthesia, small incremental doses of Saffan given into an intravenous infusion by the nursing staff as required produce the necessary control of the animal, and the cat still awakens rapidly after the last dose [20].

It is often said that if local analgesics have been sprayed on the mucous membrane of the larynx to permit endotracheal intubation, the cat should not be allowed access to food or water for 4 hours afterwards in case the laryngeal reflexes are still blocked. In practice, the local analgesic solution is absorbed so rapidly from the laryngeal mucous membrane that it becomes ineffective about 15 minutes after administration. Cats may always be encouraged to eat and drink, provided that there are no surgical contraindications, as soon as they have fully regained consciousness.

LOCAL ANALGESIA

Local analgesia is seldom used in cats because of the problems involved in adequate restraint of the animal, but it can be valuable in very sick or moribund animals or when the animal is controlled by deep sedation or light anaesthesia. Whatever method of local analgesia is employed care must be taken that the total dose of the agent does not constitute a toxic dose. Extrapolating from the levels considered to be toxic in other species of animal, a dose of about 0.12 g, i.e. 12 ml, of 1% lignocaine should be the maximum employed in a 4 kg adult cat. In cats local

analgesia usually involves local infiltration of the operation site, but techniques such as intravenous regional analgesia or specific nerve blocks can be employed if restraint is adequate.

Epidural analgesia

The use of epidural analgesia in cats has been described [21]. The technique is identical to that used in dogs (p. 317) and, using 2% lignocaine, doses of 1 ml/4.5 kg given at the lumbosacral space will block cranially to the level of L1, while doses of 1 ml/3.4 kg extend the block to the fifth thoracic vertebra. Although the technique is claimed to be useful for caesarean section or laparotomy in the poor-risk patient, the abolition of sympathetic nervous control makes the cat more susceptible to hypotension and less able to compensate for surgical haemorrhage. Most anaesthetists consider that in view of the heavy sedation necessary to control the cat during operation, properly administered general anaesthesia is preferable in all circumstances when lumbar epidural block might be used.

REFERENCES

1. Clarke, K. W. and Hall, L. W. (1990) *Journal of the Association of Veterinary Anaesthetists of Great Britain and Ireland* **17**, 4.
2. Davies, L. E. and Donnelly, E. J. (1968) *Journal of the American Veterinary Medical Association* **153**, 1161.
3. Short, C. E. (1987) *Principles and Practice of Veterinary Anesthesia*, p. 550. Baltimore: Williams and Wilkins.
4. Amend, J. E. and Klavano, P. A. (1973) *Veterinary Medicine/Small Animal Clinician* **68**, 741.
5. Dunkle, N., Moise, S., Scarlett-Kranz, J. and Short, C. E. (1986) *American Journal of Veterinary Research* **47**, 2212.
6. Rex, M. A. E. (1980) *Anaesthesia and Intensive Care* **8**, 365.
7. Heavner, J. E. (1986) *Anesthesia and Analgesia* **65**, 133.
8. Price, D. A. (1961) *Journal of the American Veterinary Medical Association* **139**, 691.
9. Ernold, G. L. (1961) *Journal of the American Veterinary Medical Association* **140**, 795.
10. Cummings, B. C. (1963) *Small Animal Clinician* **3**, 539.
11. Strande, A. (1964) *Journal of Small Animal Practice* **5**, 153.
12. Hall, L. W. (1972) *Postgraduate Medical Journal* **48**, 55.
13. Evans, J. (1979) *Proceedings of the Association of Veterinary Anaesthetists of Great Britain and Ireland* **8**, 73.
14. Dyson, D. H., Allen, D. A., Ingwersen, W., Pascoe, P. J. and O'Grady, M. (1987) *Canadian Journal of Veterinary Research* **51**, 236.
15. Glen, J. B. (1973) *Veterinary Record* **92**, 65.
16. Chambers, J. P. and Dobson, J. M. (1989) *Journal of the Association of Veterinary Anaesthetists* **16**, 53.
17. Cullen, L. K. and Jones, R. S. (1977) *Veterinary Record* **101**, 115.
18. Arnbjerg, J. (1979) *Nordiske Veterinary Medicine* **31**, 145.
19. Verstegen, J., Fargetton, X. and Ectors, F. (1989) *Acta Veterinaria Scandinavica* **4** (Suppl. 85/1989), 117.
20. Hall, L. W. (1976) *Journal of Small Animal Practice* **17**, 661.
21. Klide, A. M. and Soma, L. R. (1968) *Journal of the American Veterinary Medical Association* **153**, 165.

CHAPTER 17

ANAESTHESIA OF BIRDS, LABORATORY ANIMALS AND WILD ANIMALS

The problems involved in anaesthetizing birds, laboratory animals and wild animals for clinical procedures are usually much less complicated than those encountered when these animals have to be anaesthetized for experimental purposes where it is important that the method of anaesthesia should have little or no influence on the result of the experiment. The techniques to be described in this chapter are those which the authors have found to be satisfactory for most clinical purposes in the various species of animals and, except in fish, do not require drugs not generally found in most veterinary practices.

ANAESTHESIA OF RODENTS AND OTHER SMALL MAMMALS

Although rodents and other small mammals are anaesthetized in large numbers for laboratory procedures with apparently few serious problems, when similar species are anaesthetized for clinical purposes the mortality is high. (In a recent survey by the Association of Anaesthetists of Great Britain and Ireland one in 32 small mammals or birds anaesthetized in small animal practices died.) The cause of the high clinical mortality probably results from unfamiliarity with the species and the generally less healthy state of the animals.

Many small mammals become very distressed by handling, increasing the risk of physical damage and of adrenaline release leading to problems under subsequent anaesthesia. The risk of physical damage is considerably reduced by proper handling [1] and animals may be weighed with minimal distress by placing them in a bag or small box hung from a suitable spring balance. Adequate preanaesthetic examination is often difficult but many have respiratory disease so oxygen should be available even if injectable agents are to be used. The high metabolic rate of these small mammals means that they require an almost constant supply of food, so preanaesthetic fasting should not exceed 3 hours. There is no need to curtail the water supply up to the time of induction of anaesthesia. During anaesthesia small mammals are particularly prone to hypothermia so precautions to avoid this should be taken. Removal of hair and wetting of the animal (particularly with alcohol-based preparations) should be kept to a minimum, and the animal should be placed on a heating pad during anaesthesia and in the recovery period. Heat loss can be considerably reduced by wrapping the animal in foil or bubble paper, although this reduces the access of both the surgeon and the anaesthetist to the patient. When inhalation agents are used, carrier gases also contribute to cooling effects, so gas flows should be adequate but not excessive. Adequate monitoring of the animal, including cardiac and respiratory function and ensuring it is not hypothermic, is essential until recovery is complete.

The commonest cause of death is respiratory failure. Ideally, oxygen and the ability to administer artificial ventilation of the lungs should always be available. However, intubation of rodents requires considerable practice as the narrow mouth makes visualization of the larynx difficult. Where relevant, suitable antagonists should be at hand and there may even be a place for the use of analeptic agents such as doxapram in circumstances where intubation is difficult. The other common cause of mortality is surgical blood loss so that care must be taken to minimize this and, wherever possible, to replace that which does occur.

The use of anticholinergic premedication is controversial as in other species but as small airways are easily blocked by saliva or mucus, its use is often recommended [1, 2]. Subcutaneous doses of 0.04–0.05 mg/kg of atropine are suitable for most rodents, but rabbits need much higher doses of the order of 1–2 mg/kg [3].

Small mammals are generally poor subjects for local analgesia since even if this is effective they still require restraint. If used, local analgesic drugs should be diluted and care taken not to overdose. General anaesthesia is preferred for most purposes and may be induced and maintained with volatile agents, induced with injectable drugs and maintained with volatile agents or maintained with injectable drugs alone.

Anaesthesia with volatile agents

In the opinion of the authors, the safest method of anaesthesia for the veterinarian who is inexperienced in anaesthetizing small mammals is that of induction and maintenance with volatile anaesthetics. The most popular agents are methoxyflurane, halothane and isoflurane. Ether, often used in the past, is not recommended as the excessive bronchial secretions it provokes may cause respiratory obstruction even if an anticholinergic premedication has been given. Methoxyflurane has the advantage of a high safety margin due to its low volatility while halothane and isoflurane allow for faster induction and recovery, but are easier to overdose.

Mask induction can lead to handling stress and the use of an induction chamber is to be preferred. Several such chambers are commercially available but they are very easy to construct and there is now little reason to use the much more dangerous method of simply putting the agent on cotton wool into a jar with the animal (this can result in very high concentrations of the anaesthetic agent in the jar). If this dangerous method has to be used it is safest with methoxyflurane, and the animal should be removed from the jar as soon as it becomes recumbent and care should be taken not to allow direct contact between the animal and the soaked cotton wool.

Once induced, anaesthesia should be maintained by volatilizing the agent in a stream of oxygen and administering the mixture through a T-piece or similar low-resistance breathing circuit. Suitable face-masks for small mammals can be made from syringes and should not be a tight fit around the muzzle, for allowing gas to escape in this way reduces the resistance to breathing. Such a leak of gas does, however, cause problems of atmospheric pollution and some form of active scavenging should be used.

Anaesthesia with injectable drugs

Theoretically, any injectable anaesthetic can be used in small mammals and usually the necessary doses are well known from the original development work in laboratory animals carried out by the drug company. However, practical limitations are set by the possible methods of administration. In some animals with easily accessible veins (e.g. rabbits) drugs such as propofol or thiopentone can be used in doses similar to those used in cats and dogs (although the duration of effect may be shorter). Where intravenous injection is more difficult, drugs which can be given by intraperitoneal, intramuscular or subcutaneous injection are generally used. The most popular combinations of drugs are the neuroleptanalgesics or incorporate ketamine. There are marked differences between species responses and even within one species of animal actions may be unreliable, a given drug producing deep anaesthesia in one animal whilst only providing some sedation in another.

Ketamine has the advantage that it is effective no matter what the route of administration. Doses required and efficacy vary greatly between the various species of animal (Table 17.1). Lower doses may be used for sedation and immobilization for non-surgical procedures. As in other species of animal, ketamine is used in combination with sedative drugs such as the benzodiazepines (diazepam or midazolam) and/or α_2-adrenoceptor agonists (xylazine or medetomidine) in order to reduce the dose of ketamine, improve muscle relaxation and to increase the effectiveness of the dissociative agent as an anaesthetic. It is worth noting that the formulations of ketamine at lower concentrations, which are available for use in children, can prove more convenient for use in very small animals than the standard veterinary preparation which needs to be diluted before use. Although most commercially available neuroleptanalgesic combinations can be used, the mixture of fentanyl and fluanisone sold as 'Hypnorm®' has proved to be most popular in the UK and this again can be administered by any route. The dose of fentanyl in Hypnorm® is high, resulting in a prolonged length of action and, occasionally, in respiratory arrest. The authors have encountered deaths using doses lower than those given in Table 17.1. Combinations of Hypnorm® with diazepam or midazolam give better muscle relaxation and allow a reduction of some 50% in the dose of Hypnorm® with consequent increase in safety. In an emergency fentanyl may be antagonized with naloxone (0.1 mg/kg) but in the UK this drug is expensive. Flecknell [1] has reported on the use of buprenorphine to antagonize fentanyl — the technique of sequential analgesia.

Alphaxalone/alphadolone (Saffan®) has proved useful in some species of animal when given intravenously (Table 17.1) and may also be given intramuscularly. *Propofol* and *thiopentone* should only be given intravenously. *Pentobarbitone* may be used by intraperitoneal injection in some animals but gives prolonged sedation and respiratory depression so that it cannot be recommended for clinical use.

Postoperative analgesia should not be neglected. Some suitable opioid drugs are listed in Table 17.1

Table 17.1 Some recommended doses of injectable anaesthetics and analgesics for small mammals

	Rabbits	Guinea pigs	Hamsters	Gerbils	Rats	Mice	Ferrets
Ketamine Combinations	Ketamine 25 mg/kg i.m. (sedation only) [1]	Not effective on its own	Not very effective	Always unreliable, not effective on its own	Ketamine 60 mg/kg i.m. (sedation)	Ketamine 100 mg/kg s.c. (sedation only)	Ketamine Ret 20–30 mg/ml i.m. (sedation only)
	Xylazine 3 mg/kg i.v. followed by 10 mins later by ketamine 3 mg/kg i.v.[2]	Ketamine 40 mg/kg Xylazine 5 mg/kg } s.c. (restraint only)[1]		Ketamine 50 mg/kg Xylazine 2 mg/kg } i.m. (still unreliable)			Ketamine 25 mg/kg Diazepam 2 mg/kg } i.m. (anaesthesia)
	Ketamine 20 mg/kg Medetomidine 300 µg/kg Diazepam 0.75–1.5 mg/kg[4]						
'Hypnorm' combinations NB 1 ml Hypnorm contains fentanyl 0.315 mg + fluanisone 10 mg. Reversal of Fentanyl if necessary with Naloxone 0.1 mg/kg	Hypnorm 0.3 ml/kg Diazepam 1–2 mg/kg[1] } i.m. Hypnorm 0.3 ml/kg Midazolam 1mg/kg } i.m.	Hypnorm 1 ml/kg Diazepam 2.5 mg/kg } i.m.	Hypnorm 1 ml/kg Diazepam 5 mg/kg i.p. or Midazolam 5 mg/kg i.m. or i.p.	Hypnorm 1 ml/kg Midazolam or Diazepam 5 mg/kg i.p.[2] Hypnorm 0.3 ml/kg Diazepam 5 mg/kg i.p.[1]	Hypnorm 0.3 ml/kg Midazolam 5 mg/kg	Hypnorm 0.01 ml/30 g Diazepam 5 mg/kg i.p.	
Alphaxalone/alphadolone	6–9 mg/kg i.v. (best used only for induction) 12 mg/kg i.m. (sedation only)						10–15 mg/kg i.m.
Postoperative analgesia [1]							
Buprenorphine	0.02–0.05 mg/kg s.c. 8–12 hours	0.05 mg/kg s.c. 8–12 hours			0.1–0.2 mg/kg s.c. 8–12 hours	2 mg/kg s.c. 12 hours	
Pethidine	10 mg/kg s.c. or i.m. 2–3 hours	20 mg/kg s.c. or i.m. 2–3 hours	20 mg/kg		20 mg/kg s.c. 2–3 hours	20 mg/kg s.c. 2–3 hours	

After Flecknell [1] and Cooper *et al.* [2].

and other methods utilizing such agents as the local analgesics should be considered. It is regrettable that the rat, which has probably contributed more than most animals to advances in medical and veterinary sciences, still seems to be neglected when postoperative analgesia is indicated.

Lagomorphs

Rabbits (*Oryctolagus cuniculus*) and hares (*Lepus europaeus*) need to be handled carefully; they tend to panic if placed on slippery surfaces and are best held for injection wrapped in a towel in the arms of an assistant or placed in a restraining box. A rabbit struggling against forcible restraint may fracture a vertebra, especially if restraint is applied to the neck, so any anaesthetic technique used should entail only the minimum of physical restraint. Intramuscular injections are made into the quadriceps or triceps muscles and intravenous injections are given into the marginal vein of the ear.

Although any intravenous anaesthetic agent may be used to induce anaesthesia in rabbits, they are not good subjects in which to maintain anaesthesia with injectable agents, even very small incremental doses causing death through respiratory arrest. Similarly, unexpected deaths may occur following ketamine or fentanyl combinations, but Mero *et al*. [4] reported no deaths in a series of 340 rabbits undergoing experimental surgery and anaesthetized by subcutaneous injections of a mixture of medetomidine (300 μg/kg), ketamine (20 mg/kg) and diazepam (0.75–1.5 mg/kg).

Induction with thiopentone (10–12 mg/kg), methohexitone (5–10 mg/kg) or Saffan (2–8 mg/kg), given intravenously to effect, is satisfactory, but it is doubtful whether methohexitone or Saffan have any real advantages over thiopentone. These agents are best given through a 0.8 mm (21 s.w.g.) butterfly needle strapped into the ear vein and may be followed with halothane/oxygen or isoflurane/oxygen to produce satisfactory anaesthesia for several hours should this prove necessary.

For an inhalation induction a 1:1 mixture of nitrous oxide/oxygen should be administered through a face-mask from a T-piece system at a flow rate of about 2 l/min for 1–2 minutes before halothane or isoflurane is cautiously added in small step concentrations up to 2–3%. Induction of anaesthesia is usually quiet when the volatile agents are vaporized in a nitrous oxide/oxygen mixture in this way and once anaesthetized the rabbit may be intubated with a 3–3.5 mm uncuffed endotracheal tube under direct vision using a laryngoscope with a small paediatric blade. An alternative method which is probably better if nitrous oxide is not available is to place the rabbit in a box and introduce a stream of halothane or isoflurane volatilized in oxygen into the box until the animal is unconscious. Anaesthesia is usually maintained with 1.5–2% halothane or 2–3% isoflurane vapour given by face-mask or through an endotracheal tube.

Judgement of the depth of anaesthesia is assessed by tickling the inside of the ear pinnae, since with many anaesthetic methods the pedal withdrawal reflex may remain strong until the animal is very close to death.

Rodents

There are very many ways of anaesthetizing *rats* and *mice* but simple halothane or isoflurane anaesthesia is very satisfactory for all clinical purposes. Anaesthesia may be induced in a box used as an induction chamber, or by a face-mask, with the agent volatilized in a stream of oxygen.

Ketamine is generally unsatisfactory in rats and mice (Table 17.1) and although a neuroleptic combination, given by subcutaneous injection, may be used, in experienced hands inhalation anaesthesia is safer.

It is most important to keep the rats and mice warm whilst they are anaesthetized and in the recovery period.

Guinea pigs are not good subjects for anaesthesia with injectable agents whether given by intravenous injection or by parenteral routes. Visible veins are fragile and venepuncture is often difficult, while the use of other routes necessitates an accurate estimation of body weight for computation of the dose. Since the gastrointestinal tract can contribute anything from 20–40% of the total weight of the animal, depending on its content of ingesta, it is not surprising that variable results follow from intraperitoneal or intramuscular injections of computed doses of injectable drugs. Moreover, respiratory disease is common.

Fortunately, halothane or isoflurane anaesthesia meets most of the needs of clinical practice. A mixture of the volatile agent with oxygen is supplied to an induction chamber (box) or to a face-mask at 1–2 l/min, starting with a minimal concentration of the vapour and gradually increasing it until the animal loses consciousness. Anaesthesia is usually produced in about 2–3 minutes and can be maintained with concentrations of halothane (0.5–1.5%) or isoflurane (1–2%), given through a face-mask from a T-piece system. Full recovery follows in less than 20–30 minutes after termination of anaesthesia.

Maintenance of a clear airway is not always easy in guinea pigs since nasal and oropharyngeal secretions tend to become viscid during anaesthesia and are liable to give rise to obstruction. The risk may be countered by frequent aspiration of the mouth and oropharynx using a fine rubber catheter attached to a 60 ml syringe. Endotracheal intubation is virtually impossible in these animals. As with all small mammals, conservation of body heat is important and a warm environment should be provided.

Ketamine, whether used alone or in combination with α_2-adrenoceptor agonists, immobilizes and produces anaesthesia in these animals.

Hamsters and *gerbils* are best anaesthetized by inhalation methods. They should be placed in an induction chamber such as a small cardboard box with a perforated lid and anaesthetized with isoflurane, halothane or methoxyflurane. These volatile agents can be introduced into the box in a stream of oxygen. The animal is removed from the box as soon as it becomes unconscious and anaesthesia is maintained using a face-mask. If injectable agents are obligatory, neurolept-analgesic techniques appear to give the most reliable results. Ketamine is again very variable in effect [2].

Mink are not domestic animals — they are nervous, fast and vicious. All mink are best anaesthetized in a mink carrying box with a volatile anaesthetic such as isoflurane, halothane or methoxyflurane. If necessary, the box may be covered with transparent plastic sheeting to make it more gas tight, and the animal is not removed from the box until it is unconscious.

Ferrets and *skunks* can be anaesthetized with isoflurane or halothane vapour passed into an induction box until they are unconscious and then through a face-mask from a T-piece circuit. Inhalation anaesthesia presents no special features in these animals.

Stoats and *weasels* can be dealt with in a similar manner, but it should be remembered that they are much more vicious than ferrets or skunks.

The preferred injectable agents are ketamine with xylazine or a benzodiazepine or Saffan (Table 17.1).

ANAESTHESIA OF CHELONIA

In tortoises, terrapins and turtles anaesthetic problems are posed by the very low metabolic rate which varies with environmental temperature, and the ability to retract the head into the protective shell. Some species present further problems due to their adaption to a semi-aquatic or aquatic mode of life. It should be remembered that some species of soft-shelled aquatic turtles can move quickly and handlers can be bitten or scratched.

The lungs are well developed and the respiratory movements are produced chiefly by muscles at each leg pocket beneath the viscera. Although these muscles have been described as diaphragms, they are too weak to drive gases around any anaesthetic system. Most chelonians have the ability to survive on a single ventilatory movement per hour, making attempts to induce anaesthesia with inhalation agents rather unsuccessful. Ketamine is probably the anaes-

thetic agent of choice although it does not produce muscle relaxation. It may be given in doses of 60–80 mg/kg into gluteal muscles and if the sedation produced is not adequate for surgery it may be deepened by the administration of isoflurane or halothane because the head will protrude from the shell and breathing will be reasonably rapid. Saffan may be used instead in doses of 12–18 mg/kg [2]. Loss of muscle tone in the neck and limb muscles is the best guide to the depth of central nervous depression. Chelonia are easily intubated.

Recovery from a dose of 60 mg/kg of ketamine takes up to 24 hours. Tortoises should be allowed to recover at normal room temperature, preferably in a straw-filled box. Terrapins and turtles should be kept at a slightly lower environmental temperature and have their bodies kept damp by the application of cold water at fairly frequent intervals.

ANAESTHESIA OF SNAKES

Snakes are difficult subjects for the anaesthetist. They have a low basal metabolic rate which is directly related to the environmental temperature so that if parenteral agents are used the induction and recovery times are very variable. Moreover, they are relatively resistant to hypoxia and can hold their breath for several minutes so that the induction of inhalation anaesthesia may be very prolonged.

Snakes also have peculiar anatomical features. The absence of an epiglottis and the position of the glottis makes it possible to intubate non-venomous snakes

under simple physical restraint and inhalation anaesthesia may then be induced by the use of IPPV. (Even so, non-venomous snakes can still inflict bite wounds which often become septic!) Most snakes have only one functional lung which consists of a thin-walled hollow tube terminating in an air sac extending to the level of the cloaca, the trachea being open along one side within the lung. There is no diaphragm and the three-chambered heart yields a slushing noise instead of the clear 'lub-dup' of the mammalian heart on ausculatation.

Snakes appear to be extremely sensitive to painful stimuli and strike or contract violently when an injection needle is inserted through the skin. It is, therefore, essential to have the snake properly restrained before attempting any injection. A simple aid to handling is to reduce the environmental temperature to below 10°C for this makes the poikilothermic snake very sluggish. If injectable agents are to be used only the lightest level of narcosis compatible with safe handling should be used, for deeper levels which require larger doses of drug may be followed by a recovery period extending over several days. Of the injectable central nervous depressants only ketamine is really useful and initial intramuscular doses of the order of 50 mg/kg produce moderate sedation which facilitates handling but muscle relaxation is poor and serpentine movements may occur. Ketamine anaesthesia can be supplemented by infiltration of the surgical site with 0.5–1% lignocaine, or by the administration of isoflurane or halothane after endotracheal intubation.

Snakes may also be anaesthetized with inhalation anaesthetics when a rapid recovery is important. Induction is best achieved by placing the snake in a clear plastic box, plastic bag or an aquarium tank into which 7–10% halothane or isoflurane vapour in oxygen or nitrous oxide/oxygen is piped. Induction may take as long as 15 minutes and the creature should not be removed until agitation or turning of the container demonstrates that the righting reflexes have been lost. It is then removed, intubated and anaesthesia maintained with about 3% of halothane or 4% of isoflurane vapour. Even when the anaesthetic is delivered through a T-piece system the expiratory movements of the snake will be too weak to expel gases and the lung must be ventilated artificially. Gases may be introduced into the lung by occlusion of the open limb of the T-piece and expelled by massaging the snake from the cloacal region towards the head. Induction of anaesthesia in a tank has the advantage that venomous snakes can be anaesthetized with the minimum of handling, but because the vapours are heavier than air they sink towards the bottom of the tank and snakes can raise their heads above the anaesthetic layer and delay the onset of anaesthesia so it is always wise to ascertain that the righting reflexes really have been abolished before removing the snake from the tank.

Most snakes exhibit a short period of excitement or agitation when first placed in a tank containing anaesthetic vapour but they quieten down and it is not always easy to determine the depth of anaesthesia. The first indication that the snake can be safely removed from the tank is certainly the loss of the righting reflexes but the tail withdrawal reflex is also valuable. Absence of response to pricking of the tail indicates that surgical anaesthesia is present. If the tip of the tongue is gently grasped with forceps there is a marked resistance to its withdrawal until the stage of surgical anaesthesia is reached.

When inhalation anaesthesia is employed it is important to ventilate at the respiratory rate observed in the previously conscious individual, and fluid balance should be maintained by giving 5 ml/kg of isotonic saline subcutaneously every 1–2 hours. Most snakes may be kept at normal ambient temperatures of around 20°C unless it is wished to cool them for the purpose of restraint.

ANAESTHESIA OF FISH

Fish are usually anaesthetized by allowing them to swim in a solution of the anaesthetic agent. The solution should be made up in some of the aerated water in which they normally swim (*not* in tap water) and various drugs are used:

1. Carbon dioxide may be used at a concentration of 200 ppm.
2. Diethyl ether 10–15 ml per litre of water is usual but 50 ml per litre has been used for large fish. In goldfish anaesthesia is induced in about 3–5 minutes; recovery takes 5–15 minutes.
3. Tricaine methanesulphonate is probably the best agent. It is a white powder which dissolves in both fresh- and sea water. Concentrations of 25–300 mg/l are employed, the more concentrated solutions being used for larger fish. Anaesthesia is induced in 1–2 minutes and fish recover in about 15 minutes.

When a fish is immersed in the anaesthetic solution there is initial excitement followed by erratic swimming. The fish then becomes inactive, sinking to the bottom of the tank to rest on its back. For surgery, the fish is removed from the tank and placed on a moist cloth. Complete recovery from the effects of the anaesthetic ensues when the fish is immersed in clean, aerated water (*not* tap water).

ANAESTHESIA OF BIRDS

In recent years interest in conservation of wild life appears to have led to an increased demand for anaesthesia for surgical purposes in wild or semi-wild birds as well as the more domesticated chicken, duck or goose. Cage birds have also become popular as companions, especially for elderly people living in urban districts, and as a result of these trends it is now commonplace for the veterinary anaesthetist to be confronted with avian patients requiring anaesthesia for a wide variety of conditions [5].

It is well known that birds do not react in the same way as mammals to stimuli which in man cause pain. For example, after a slight reaction to the skin incision, conscious birds do not show any response to the manipulations involved in caponization. Many operations on hens, such as the suturing of a torn crop or the removal of superficial neoplasm, cause little response and the heart rate, which might be expected to increase if pain was experienced, remains normal. In spite of these differences humane considerations seem to dictate that anaesthesia should be used for birds as it is for mammals.

The special problems presented by birds, especially wild ones, are related to their physiological, anatomical and metabolic differences from mammals. The problems of handling wild birds are often greatly exaggerated. Provided they are handled quietly and that the normal precautions are taken (such as the wearing of gauntlets when dealing with birds of prey), few difficulties or dangers are encountered.

The high metabolic rate has several implications for the anaesthetist. It implies a higher rate of utilization of foods so that starvation of 6–8 hours is often sufficient to produce fatal hypoglycaemia and ketosis. Metabolism of parenterally administered agents is also rapid.

The high avian body temperature means that excessive cooling occurs when the bird is exposed to a cool environment during or after anaesthesia, especially if many feathers are plucked around an operation site. Small birds such as budgerigars have very high, labile heart rates and heart failure is frequently encountered when these birds are frightened by handling. The blood volume of birds is such that small surgical haemorrhages may be sufficient to induce shock.

The avian respiratory tract is very different from that of mammals, one obvious difference being that inspiration in birds is normally passive whilst expiration is active. The respiratory system is constructed around a central 'core' of relatively fixed lung volume and its anatomy has been well described by Dunker [6] and Piiper and Scheid [7]. The trachea divides into two mesobronchi which in turn divide to give secon-dary bronchi, one group of which, the ventrobronchi, communicates with the cranial air sacs (cervical and interclavicular). The dorsal and lateral secondary bronchi arise from each mesobronchus before these terminate in caudal air sacs (abdominal and posterior thoracic air sacs). The dorsal and ventral bronchi are joined by narrow tubes, the parabronchi, which form the analogue to the mammalian lungs and are where gaseous exchange takes place between the air and the blood. Air passing through the parabronchi moves in only one direction during both inspiration and expiration; blood flows across the direction of gas flow. Thus, the gas composition must change from the inspiratory to the expiratory ends of the parabronchi so that the capillary blood must equilibrate with parabronchial gas at widely differing oxygen and carbon dioxide tensions. The arrangement is such that gas exchange takes place during both inspiration and expiration and its efficiency is dependent on an uninterrupted flow of air through the lungs. Tidal exchange is generated through the air sacs and fluid such as blood or injected solutions in these sacs will interfere with ventilation. Even short periods of apnoea are serious and will produce marked hypoxia.

Anaesthetic gases and vapours are rapidly absorbed into the blood stream so that induction is rapid when inhalation anaesthesia is used and, equally, recovery is also rapid. Most inhalation anaesthetics are less soluble in avian than in mammalian blood so that brain tensions equilibrate more rapidly with lung tensions and the clinical anaesthetist will often find induction and recovery disconcertingly abrupt.

After anaesthesia birds must be kept warm in a darkened, padded box and they should be supported in sternal recumbency. During recovery, vigorous flapping of the wings may occur and this should be prevented by wrapping the bird in a towel because a wing bone may be fractured if the wing beats against the cage or box wall.

Local analgesia

Because birds such as budgerigars are so small it is very easy to give a gross overdose of a local analgesic agent, but in larger birds local analgesia can be used without difficulties. Even so, in large birds it is wise to watch the total dose which is administered and to use very dilute solutions (e.g. 0.25–0.5% lignocaine) for injection because there is some evidence that birds are more sensitive to local analgesics than are mammals of the same body weight. Many workers consider that local analgesia has no place in avian anaesthesia because even when it is correctly used the bird still requires restraint and this may produce undue distress.

Injectable agents

Whenever possible birds should be weighed before any drug is given by injection. This is usually possible if the subject can be confined to a plastic box. Physical restraint should be kept to a minimum because small birds such as budgerigars and canaries are prone to become very distressed and large birds may fracture bones whilst trying to escape. Poultry should be grasped so that the wings are held along the thorax, turned on their backs and stroked on the abdomen to quieten them. Budgerigars and the like should be cradled in the palm of the hand with the neck between the index and middle fingers, taking great care not to apply pressure to the neck. Hawks usually present no problem after being hooded and parrots may be gripped around the neck and wings with a hand wrapped in thick towelling.

Intramuscular injection is made into the pectoral muscles on either side of the cariniform sternum or into the thigh muscles. Intravenous injections are made into the brachial vein where it passes over the ventral aspect of the elbow joint.

Although very many injectable agents have been used in birds of all kinds it is probable that ketamine is the one of choice in every case. When an injectable agent has to be used ketamine may be given intramuscularly in doses of 15 mg/kg. The bird should be confined in a warm, darkened box as soon as the injection has been made and the depth of anaesthesia produced is assessed by noting the response to pinching the wattle or the skin of the neck and although the eyelids often close the corneal reflex should persist throughout. Increments can be given to produce the desired degree of unconsciousness. There is a wide safety margin and doses of 25 mg/kg of ketamine may be safely given to all species of birds, although recovery may sometimes be prolonged.

Inhalation anaesthesia

Whenever possible anaesthesia should be induced and maintained with an inhalation agent. Birds may be restrained so that anaesthesia can be induced using a face-mask or they can be confined in a box made of transparent plastic material while anaesthetic gases or vapours are introduced into the box. Probably the best method is to induce anaesthesia by passing halothane and oxygen into the box in which the bird is confined and then to maintain anaesthesia by administering the same agent through a face-mask or endotracheal tube.

Endotracheal intubation is not difficult in birds and suitable tubes may be constructed from silicone rubber or PVC tubing. The tube should be long enough to reach the syrinx but dead-space must be kept to a minimum and the end should be cut at a bevel to facilitate passage into the trachea. Airway secretions may block the flow of gas in both intubated and non-intubated birds so it is always wise to have suction available for their removal by aspiration. Adequate suction can be provided from a 60 ml syringe fitted with a short length of fine catheter.

Most birds can be anaesthetized with 0.5–1% halothane vapour in oxygen delivered to the endotracheal tube or face-mask through an Ayre's T-piece but if it is available isoflurane should be used, for induction and recovery are more rapid and the safety margin appears greater. The air sacs should be flushed at about 5-minute intervals by occlusions of the open arm of the T-piece system, their overdistension being prevented by escape of gas around the loose-fitting endotracheal tube or by partial lifting of the face-mask. Total gas flow rates should be about two to three times the estimated minute volume of respiration of the bird, and as a guide Klide [10] suggests that an adult domestic hen has a minute volume of about 750 ml, a pigeon of about 250 ml and a budgerigar of about 25 ml.

Inhalation anaesthetics may also be administered through a needle introduced directly into an air sac, but this has little to commend it.

Recovery from anaesthesia is accelerated by administering oxygen and flushing the air sacs from time to time until the bird has regained its righting reflexes. Unless this is done the anaesthetic which passes into the air sacs may not be cleared by the depressed respiratory activity so that it wll be taken up again by the parabronchial capillary blood and recovery will be prolonged.

Combination of inhalation and injectable agents

Very satisfactory results are obtained by the combination of injectable and inhalation agents. Although many combinations have been used, the induction of unconsciousness with ketamine (10–15 mg/kg) followed by the inhalation of isoflurane/oxygen or halothane/oxygen is probably the simplest and the safest.

Measurement of the dose of ketamine for small birds such as canaries and budgerigars which may weigh from 30 to 60 g is not easy and these birds may be dosed with 1–2 mg per bird. The standard solution of ketamine for veterinary use contains 100 mg/ml and if 0.1 ml is diluted to 1 ml birds may be given 0.1–0.2 ml of the diluted solution by intramuscular injection into the pectoral muscles. The larger dose (0.2 ml of the diluted solution) will usually produce light anaesthesia in 2–3 minutes from the time of injection.

Saffan can be used in place of ketamine for most birds but when given by intramuscular injection it produces more variable results, probably due to the difficulty of ensuring that the dose is correctly administered into a muscle mass.

The aim should always be to give just enough of the injectable agent to make the bird unconscious and to use only as much isoflurane or halothane as is necessary for the maintenance of anaesthesia.

ANAESTHESIA OF WILD ANIMALS

Only species of wild animal which are likely to be encountered by those in veterinary practice in the UK will be considered here, but as a general rule the principles of anaesthesia as applied to domesticated or captive pet animals apply equally well in all wild animals and the main differences arise from the need to protect the anaesthetist and any assistants from injury by the unanaesthetized subjects. Semidomesticated species such as deer farmed for meat production can also be regarded as 'wild' for they may attack when approached.

Difficulty in getting close to the subject, either because of its timidity or aversion to mankind, and the obvious need to avoid being attacked, have led to two approaches to the problems of anaesthetizing wild animals. The first is the use of squeeze cages, the animal being enticed into the cage then squeezed between a fixed and movable wall so that it cannot turn around or move very far whilst being given an injection of a sedative or anaesthetic agent. These cages should be standard equipment at zoos, some research centres and similar establishments, and they have a role in the capture of farm deer, but they are unlikely to be available to the veterinarian in general practice. The second, which is, perhaps, more generally applicable, is the administration of agents from projectile syringes. These syringes may be projected from rifles, pistols, crossbows or blowpipes so that the administrator can remain a safe distance from the subject. They were originally developed for the capture of wild game animals but they are now finding a use in ordinary veterinary practice where, for example, current methods of farming (particularly of some European breeds of cattle) are producing virtually unhandled adult beasts which are often aggressive, especially if frightened. The use of projectile syringes for the capture and restraint of wild game animals present specialized problems which have been admirably reviewed by Harthoorn [8]. The problems related to the use of projectile syringes in general veterinary practice are somewhat different.

The projectile syringe is designed to inject its contents after the needle has penetrated the skin of the animal and its impact with the tissues can result in serious bruising. They should empty within seconds of penetration and the force of the injection should be adequate to push the plunger fully home even if the needle is partially obstructed by a skin-plug. To minimize tissue damage the syringe should strike the beast towards the end of the firing trajectory, although obviously this is less important when the projectile is propelled from a blowpipe. When fired from a gun or crossbow at too close range the syringe may enter the abdominal or thoracic cavities, and often when striking too hard, syringes bounce off without penetrating effectively in spite of barbs and collars on the needles. Extensive and fatal trauma may be caused by injection into the thoracic or abdominal cavities.

In all cases the shortest needle commensurate with penetration of the skin should be used and large-bore needles should terminate in a cone, with holes on the side of the shaft, for the ordinary open-ended needle may block with a core of skin. Collared needles are seldom satisfactory and tend to allow fluid to flow back out of the hole caused by penetration of the collar. To remove a barbed needle a small incision is made over the site of the barb.

Irritant solutions may not be used since their administration under the non-sterile conditions associated with the use of dart-guns may produce an abscess, but when simple precautions are routinely observed, untoward reactions at the site of injection are surprisingly rare. Valuable animals may be given a precautionary dose of antibiotic and in summer the wounds should be treated with fly repellants.

There are now many patterns of projectile syringe designed for use with rifles, pistols and crossbows but, in general, they usually inject their contents through the agency of an explosive cap and striker mechanism, or by gas evolved from a chemical reaction initiated in a capsule by a similar striker mechanism, incorporated behind the plunger. The projectiles used with blowpipes have needles with side holes which are covered with a short plastic sleeve and displacement of this sleeve as the needle penetrates the skin allows the pressure of air or gas previously injected behind the plunger to inject the syringe contents. Detonation of an explosive cap produces such a force that the ejected fluid penetrates far into the tissues and haematoma formation is common, so that the slower injection due to gas propulsion is usually to be preferred.

Projectile syringes usually have a capacity of up to

4 ml so that only relatively soluble drugs can be administered. If they are to be used on common land or in dense undergrowth any temptation to use Immobilon or etorphine should be resisted, for should the projectile bounce off the animals or the animal be missed completely, these projectiles are surprisingly difficult to locate in spite of their bright silver barrels and coloured flights, and their subsequent discovery by a child or even an adult could have fatal consequences for that individual. It must be appreciated that projection is very far from accurate. The weight of the projectile varies according to its capacity and degree of filling, and the wind velocity has a great influence at all but the shortest of ranges which can, in any case, only be estimated. Experience has shown that best results are obtained by getting as close to the animal as is possible or safe, and aiming for the neck or shoulder region.

It is always advisable to use doses of injectable agents which do no more than permit the animal to be approached with safety and so allow general anaesthesia to be produced with intravenous or inhalation agents. The recommendations made below for drugs and doses are from personal experience or gleaned from a number of articles [9–16].

Although a quick recovery is essential in the wild, as partially sedated animals are at risk from predators, it is not so important in captive animals. To date, the techniques most frequently used for immobilizing a wide variety of species (excluding the Felidae) have been based on the use of potent opioids such as etorphine or carfentanil coupled with sedatives, anaesthesia being terminated with antagonists such as diprenorphine. For Felidae, ketamine has long been the drug of choice, usually in combination with the α_2-adrenoceptor agonist xylazine or more recently with medetomidine. With the recent development of potent and effective α_2-adrenoceptor antagonists, such as idazoxan, RX82100A and atipamezole, the use of ketamine/α_2-adrenoceptor agonist combinations has become more popular in a wide range of species of animals since, providing low doses of ketamine are employed, immobilization can now be countered [17, 18]. A major advantage of ketamine-based combinations in ruminants is that regurgitation occurs less frequently than after the etorphine-based combination Immobilon has been used. The use of antagonists is not totally without risk, however. Often there is residual sedation from the non-reversed component of the drug combination (e.g. from ketamine or acepromazine). Also, recycling of drugs such as etorphine, or imbalance in duration of action of the agonist and antagonist, can lead to resedation.

The doses of drugs required by the various species

Table 17.2 Doses for some species of deer

Species	Drug combination	Dose in mg/kg			Notes
		Wild	Park	Farm or tame	
Red deer	Etorphine/ acepromazine as Immobilon	01.	0.04	0.02	Drug tolerant
					Tense
	or				
	Etorphine	0.06	0.02	0.01	More relaxed
	Xylazine	0.8	0.5	0.2	
	or				
	Xylazine	N/R	N/R	0.5–1.0	Need reversal
	or				
	Ketamine	N/R	4.0	1.0	Unpredictable
	Xylazine	N/R	3.0	1.0	
Sika deer	Etorphine/ acepromazine as Immobilon	0.05	0.035	0.03	Apnoea
	or				
	Etorphine	0.05	0.035	0.03	More relaxed
	Xylazine	0.4	0.3	0.1	Apnoea
	or				
	Xylazine	7.0	4.0	0.5	Need reversal
	or				
	Ketamine	N/R	3.0	2.5	Unpredictable
	Xylazine	N/R	4.0	1.0	Need reversal
	or				
	Ketamine	N/R	2.3	?	Unpredictable
	Medetomidine	N/R	0.23	?	
Fallow deer	Etorphine/ acepromazine as Immobilon Immobilon	0.06	0.05	—	Stress risk Hypoxia
	or				
	Etorphine	0.06	0.05	—	Stress risk
	Xylazine	0.85	0.65	—	Hypoxia
	or				
	Ketamine	8.0	6.0	4.0	Unpredictable
	Xylazine	10.0	8.0	5.0	
	or				
	Ketamine	2.0	1.0	—	Less reliable
	Medetomidine	0.125	0.08	—	but safer
	or				
	Tiletamine Zolazepam as Zolatil	?	?	19	Reliability undetermined
Muntjac	Ketamine	4.0	3.0	2.0	Excellent
	Xylazine	4.0	3.0	2.0	
	or				
	Etorphine/ acepromazine as Immobilon	0.1	0.06	—	Hypoxia
	or				
	Xylazine	3.5	2.5	1.0	Need reversal

N/R; not recommended
— ; no data available. ?; use debatable
Information supplied by Richard Kock, MA, Vet MB, MRCVS, Animal Manager/Veterinary Officer, Whipsnade Wild Animal Park, Dunstable, England. Reproduced with permission.

of animal and the breeds within a species varies enormously so that an extensive literature on the subject is now available.

Deer

There can be little doubt the xylazine/ketamine or medetomidine/ketamine mixtures are the drugs of choice for use in deer at the following doses, the smaller animals requiring proportionately larger amounts (Table 17.2).

Maximum effect is obtained in about 10 minutes from the time of injection and recovery usually follows in about 2 hours unless antagonists are given. More recently, medetomidine/ketamine has been used successfully.

Immobilon has been used successfully in sika, fallow and red deer (Hird, personal communication) for short periods of immobilization needed for blood sampling, faeces sampling and dosing for worms. Fallow deer seem to be particularly difficult and perhaps the safest combination for these is fentanyl (0.3–0.6 mg/kg) with xylazine (0.5–1.25 mg/kg).

All these agents are usually administered intramuscularly by projectile syringe and if the dose given does not produce surgical anaesthesia an inhalation agent should be administered as needed.

Wild cats

Large zoological Felidae can usually be trapped in squeeze or transport cages and when properly placed in a squeeze cage a limb can usually be roped and pulled through the bars so that an intravenous injection can be made without much difficulty. They may then be treated as large domestic cats and the procedures are not as difficult or hazardous as might be anticipated. If thiopentone is used the dose should be kept to a minimum since recovery from its effects can take up to 2 days in the larger animals such as lions and tigers. Many lions and tigers in zoological collections and circuses can be enticed up to the bars to have their backs scratched and, although some caution is needed, subcutaneous injections can often be made while they are apparently enjoying the scratching.

If the animal cannot be approached closely, xylazine/ketamine or medetomidine/ketamine can be administered intramuscularly by projectile syringe.

Bears

Bears do not have retractile claws and even a playful blow from a paw can inflict a severe injury; their faces are curiously expressionless and it is difficult to detect their mood. Grizzly and polar bears may deliberately attack human beings.

In zoos and circuses, bears can be confined in squeeze cages or airtight boxes where a number of drugs can be administered but if these facilities are not available, ketamine can be administered by a projectile syringe. The dose is not well established but various doses from 15 to 25 mg/kg have been administered with atropine to control salivation.

Venepuncture is not easy, even in sedated bears, because the limb veins are small and embedded in fat so that if sedation produced by ketamine does not allow surgery an inhalation agent such as isoflurane or halothane should be given. Endotracheal intubation is not difficult in the unconscious animal.

Non-human primates

Not only can monkeys inflict bites and scratches, they are also carriers of viruses which are extremely pathogenic to man as well as diseases such as tuberculosis, salmonellosis and shigellosis. For these reasons it is always undesirable to handle conscious monkeys and even domestic pets should be viewed with suspicion. Handling of the domestic pet monkey should be left to its owner.

If the owner of a small pet monkey can be induced to hold its arms behind its back the anaesthetist can usually make an intravenous injection of an anaesthetic such as thiopentone or Saffan into the recurrent tarsal vein on the dorsal surface of the gastrocnemius muscle. Caution is necessary for these monkeys often weigh much less than is estimated and it is seldom necessary to exceed 5 mg/kg of thiopentone or 2 mg/kg of Saffan. Once unconscious the monkey may be given a small dose of suxamethonium (i.e. 1 mg/kg) and intubated with an uncuffed tube. Anaesthesia may then be maintained by the administration of isoflurane or halothane in nitrous oxide/oxygen, or oxygen alone, from a T-piece system. When suxamethonium is to be given it is wise to inject atropine (0.15–0.3 mg) intravenously as soon as the induction agent has been given.

Alternatively, if the owner or an assistant can hold the monkey, again with its arms held behind its back, an inhalation agent can be used both for the induction and maintenance of anaesthesia. The use of nitrous oxide is a distinct advantage in these circumstances and halothane is probably the volatile agent of choice for, in the authors' experience, isoflurane often provokes breath holding. A suitable face-mask is held over, but not touching, the face and nitrous oxide/oxygen (3/1) is administered at a flow rate of 4 l/min for 1–2 minutes. Halothane is then introduced into the gas mixture, increasing the concentration of the vapour every 3–4 breaths to a maximum of about 3%.

The mask is applied to the face as soon as it is judged that the monkey is unconscious and induction is usually free from excitement and struggling. Anaesthesia is maintained with a 1.2–1.5% of halothane vapour in the nitrous oxide/oxygen mixture.

Larger or less cooperative monkeys may need sedating by intramuscular injection before an attempt is made to induce anaesthesia [19]. The use of projectile syringes is not to be recommended for monkeys are adept at dodging or even deflecting the projectile with their hands, and they usually pull the needle out before the injection is complete even when a hit is obtained! In the case of the smaller varieties it is usually possible to catch the monkey's arm and draw it out through the bars of the cage so that injection can be made into the deltoid muscle, but a squeeze cage may be needed for the larger, strong animals such as adult chimpanzees.

Ketamine is probably the agent of choice in all except squirrel monkeys and marmosets for chemical restraint or preanaesthetic sedation. At dose rates of 10–25 mg/kg, the volume of the veterinary preparation Vetalar which needs to be injected is small so that the drug can be given rapidly into the thigh muscles of even struggling animals. The peak effect is obtained 5–10 minutes after injection and the period of sedation is from 30 to 60 minutes. Recovery is complete in 1.5–4.5 hours depending on the dose and species of monkey. When the desired degree of sedation is not produced by the ketamine, further depression of the central nervous system is probably best produced by the administration of nitrous oxide/oxygen supplemented with 0.5–1% halothane delivered through a face-mask from a T-piece system.

For squirrel monkeys and marmosets Saffan is the sedative of choice and this preparation is also useful in other species of non-human primates. In squirrel monkeys and marmosets doses of 15–18 mg/kg produce light general anaesthesia some 5 minutes after injection into the thigh muscles. Anaesthesia lasts about 45 minutes and is followed by recovery to full consciousness 1–3 hours later. In baboons, doses of 12–18 mg/kg make the animal safe to handle about 10 minutes after injection and recovery is much quicker than in squirrel monkeys. In all monkeys anaesthesia may be deepened by giving increments of Saffan intravenously until the desired depth is obtained. The animals can then be intubated and maintained unconscious with inhalation agents such as halothane, or sequential incremental doses of Saffan can be given intravenously over several hours if need be. The main disadvantage of Saffan is the large volume of solution which has to be given intramuscularly, although such injections do not appear to result in pain at the injection site.

When it is impossible to give an intramuscular injection to a large monkey or ape the simplest thing is to entice the animal into the cage which can be made airtight by covering with a sheet of plastic material so that anaesthetic gases and vapour can be piped in. The animal must be observed carefully and removed from the cage as soon as it is unconscious and relaxed.

It is important to conserve body heat and the anaesthetized monkey should be placed on a warm water blanket maintained at 38°C. If sedation or anaesthesia is to last for more than about an hour, an intravenous drip infusion of N/5 saline or Hartmann's solution (Ringer's lactate) should be started as soon as the animal is anaesthetized or sufficiently sedated. The fluid should be given at the rate of 10 ml/kg and, for the smaller monkeys, it should be warmed to 38°C by passing it through a blood warmer before it reaches the animal. The use of atropine is somewhat controversial but it is probable that it should be given as soon as the monkey becomes anaesthetized, in a dose of 0.15–1.2 mg depending on the size of the animal.

Recovery from anaesthesia should take place in a warm environment and endotracheal tubes and intravenous cannulae should be removed while it is still safe to handle the animal. Postsurgical analgesia should be provided by the intramuscular injection of a suitable analgesic (e.g. pethidine at a dose of 2 mg/kg) as late as possible in the recovery period.

REFERENCES

1. Flecknell, P. A. (1988) *Laboratory Animal Anaesthesia.* Academic Press. London.
2. Cooper, J. E., Hutchinson, M. F., Jackson, O. F. and Maurice, R. J. (1985) *Manual of Exotic Pets.* Cheltenham: British Small Animal Veterinary Association.
3. Cooper, J. E. (1989) *Manual of Anaesthesia for Small Animal Practice,* chapt. 17. Cheltenham: British Small Animal Veterinary Association.
4. Mero, M., Vainionpaa, S., Vasenius, J., Vihkonen, K. and Rockkanen, P. (1989) *Acta Veterinaria Scandinavia,* Suppl. 85, p. 135.
5. Clarke, K. W. and Hall, L. W. (1990) *Journal of the Association of Veterinary Anaesthetists of Great Britain and Ireland* 17, 4.
6. Dunker, H. R. (1972) *Ergebnisse der Anatomie und Entwicklungsgeschichte* **45,** 1.

7. Piiper, J. and Scheid, P. (1973) *Comparative Physiology* (eds L. Bolis, K. Schmidt-Nielsen and S. H. P. Maddrell). Amsterdam: North Holland.
8. Harthoorn, A. M. (1971) *Veterinary Anaesthesia* (ed. L. R. Soma). Baltimore: Williams and Wilkins.
9. Bauditz, R. (1972) *Veterinary Medicine Reviews* 3, 204.
10. Klide, A. M. (1973) *Veterinary Clinics of North America* **3:** *Avian Anaesthesia*, p. 175.
11. Hime, J. M. (1974) *Veterinary Record* **95,** 193.
12. Manton, V. J. A. and Jones, D. M. (1974) *Journal of Zoology* **173,** 84.
13. Harthoorn, A. M. (1975) *Chemical Capture of Animals.* London: Baillière Tindall.
14. Jones, D. M. and Manton, V. J. A. (1976) *Journal of Zoology* **178,** 494.
15. Jones, D. M. (1977) *Veterinary Record* **101,** 340.
16. Jones, D. M. (1977) *Veterinary Record* **101,** 352.
17. Kock, R. A., Jago, M., Gulland, F. M. D. and Lewis, J. (1989) *Journal of the Association of Veterinary Anaesthetics of Great Britain and Ireland* **16,** 4.
18. Jalanka, H. (1989) *Acta Veterinaria Scandinavia* Suppl. 85, p. 193.
19. Green, C. J. (1979) *Animal Anaesthesia.* London: Laboratory Animals.

PART III

SPECIAL ANAESTHESIA

CHAPTER 18

ANAESTHESIA FOR OBSTETRICS

PHYSIOLOGICAL CHANGES AND THE ACTION OF DRUGS ADMINISTERED DURING PREGNANCY AND PARTURITION

There is no one anaesthetic agent or technique that is ideal for all parturient animals. In veterinary practice the choice of anaesthetic methods and drugs is often influenced by whether the offspring are alive and wanted or dead due to obstetrical problems. In any case the choice must be such as to ensure the safety of the mother and any living fetus(es), the comfort of the mother during parturition or hysterotomy and the convenience of the obstetrician/surgeon. To make a rational choice the anaesthetist must be familiar with the physiological alterations induced by pregnancy and labour, the pharmacology of the agents used, and the significance of obstetric complications necessitating assisted delivery of the offspring. Most of the studies of these have been carried out in ewes but the physiological alterations should be comparable in other species of animal even if their magnitude differs. The following brief account of the changes in physiology and in the actions of drugs administered during pregnancy and parturition is a summary of many published papers and accounts in standard textbooks and should apply to all species of domestic animals.

Physiological alterations induced by pregnancy

Cardiac output increases in pregnancy and there is an additional increase in cardiac output during all stages of labour. In third-stage labour it probably results from blood being expelled from the involuting uterus into the general circulation. Peripheral vascular resistance usually decreases during pregnancy so that arterial blood pressure does not change. Also during pregnancy blood volume is increased, the plasma volume expansion being greater than that of the red cell mass so that the haemoglobin content and haematocrit are decreased. A serious decrease in venous return can occur if the animal is restrained or positioned in the supine position due to compression of the vena cava and aorta by the enlarged uterus and its contents. This decrease in venous return will, of course, cause a fall in cardiac output for the heart cannot pump more than the blood being returned to it. Cardiac work is increased during pregnancy so that at parturition cardiac reserve is reduced and pulmonary congestion and heart failure may occur in animals that had previously well-compensated cardiac disease.

During pregnancy the sensitivity of the respiratory centre to carbon dioxide is increased, presumably due to changes in hormone levels, so that P_aCO_2 decreases although arterial pH is maintained due to long-term renal compensation. Oxygen consumption is increased by the demands of the developing fetus(es), placenta, uterine muscle and mammary glands. During labour ventilation may be increased further by apprehension or anxiety. Airway conductance is increased and total pulmonary resistance is decreased, apparently from hormone-induced relaxation of bronchial smooth muscle. FRC is decreased due to cranial displacement of the diaphragm and abdominal organs by the gravid uterus. The decrease in FRC means that it is possible for airway closure to occur at end-expiration.

Liver function is generally well maintained during pregnancy. Plasma protein concentration is decreased but the total plasma protein is increased due to the increase in blood volume.

Renal plasma flow (RPF) and glomerular filtration rate (GFR) are greatly increased in pregnant animals. As a result, blood urea and creatinine levels are lower than in non-pregnant animals.

Uterine blood flow is directly proportional to the perfusion pressure and inversely proportional to the uterine vascular resistance so that it can be compromised by vasoconstriction due to catecholamine release from fright or anxiety.

PHARMACOLOGY OF DRUGS ADMINISTERED DURING PREGNANCY

The effects of pregnancy on drug disposition, bio-transformation and excretion are largely unknown. The MAC of inhalation agents is decreased due to an unknown mechanism. The increase in RBF and GFR favours the renal excretion of drugs. Any drug administered to the mother is liable to cross the placenta to the fetus(es) and induce effects similar to those observed in the mother.

The placental transfer of drugs is governed by the physicochemical properties of the drug and the anatomical features of the placenta. Placental transfer of drugs can occur by simple diffusion, facilitated diffusion via transport systems, active transport and pinocytosis. Of these, simple diffusion is by far the most important and this will be affected by the surface area and thickness of the placenta. The larger farm animals have thick epitheliochorial placentae with relatively small areas for diffusion due to their cotyledonary or patchy diffuse distribution, whereas dogs and cats have thinner endotheliochorial placentae with larger zonular areas of implantation. Thus, the placental diffusion barrier is greatest in ruminants, pigs and horses and least in the dog and cat. However, the diffusion barrier does not appear to be of particularly great significance in the transfer of drugs from mother to fetus(es).

More important is the diffusion constant which is unique to each drug and determined by molecular weight, degree of protein binding in the maternal blood, lipid solubility and degree of ionization. Most drugs used in anaesthesia have large diffusion constants — low molecular weights, low degree of protein binding, high lipid solubility and poor ionization — and diffuse rapidly across the placenta. The exception are the neuromuscular blocking drugs which are highly ionized and of low lipid solubility.

Maternal blood concentrations of drug depend on the total dose administered, the site or route of administration, rate of distribution and uptake of it by maternal tissues and maternal detoxication and excretion. Thus drugs with rapidly declining plasma concentration after administration of a fixed dose (e.g. thiopentone) result in a short period of exposure of the placenta and hence fetus(es) to high maternal blood concentrations, whereas drugs administered continuously (e.g. inhalation anaesthetics) are associated with a continuous placental transfer to the fetus(es).

The concentration of drug in the umbilical vein of a fetus is not that to which the fetal target organs such as the heart and brain is exposed for most of the umbilical vein blood passes initially through the liver, where the drug may be metabolized or sequestrated. The remainder of the umbilical vein blood passes through the ductus venosus to the vena cava where it is diluted by drug-free blood from the hind end of the fetus. Thus, the fetal circulation protects vital tissues and organs from exposure to sudden high drug concentrations.

Clinical significance of changes during pregnancy and parturition

The circulatory changes of pregnancy and parturition can put a mother suffering from even normally well-compensated heart disease at risk unless care is taken to ensure a minimum of cardiac depression from anaesthetic drugs. Ecbolics used early on in labour can have an adverse effect on cardiovascular function. Oxytocin will induce vasodilatation and hypotension which will have an adverse effect on both mother and fetus(es) due to decreased tissue and placental perfusion. Ergometrine causes vasoconstriction and may give rise to an increase in systemic vascular resistance sufficient to produce heart failure in the immediate postpartum period when cardiac output is high from the increased circulating blood volume. Venous engorgement of the epidural space decreases the volume of local analgesic solutions needed to produce block to any given level.

The reduction in FRC means that any respiratory depression caused by drugs is more significant in pregnant than in non-pregnant animals and hypoventilation will lead to hypercapnia and hypoxaemia; the hypoxaemia is particularly undesirable during labour when oxygen consumption is increased. In small animals induction of anaesthesia with inhalational agents will be more rapid in pregnant than in non-pregnant animals due to the decrease in FRC and increased alveolar ventilation as well as the decrease in MAC, but in recumbent large animals shunting of pulmonary blood may make the induction and maintenance of inhalation anaesthesia more difficult.

There is an increased risk of both vomiting and silent regurgitation of gastric contents in parturient animals, for frequently the time of last feeding is unknown and the intragastric pressure is increased in the stomach displaced by the gravid uterus.

Drug actions

Opioids rapidly cross the placenta from the mother to the fetus(es) and can cause marked respiratory depression in the neonate as well as sleepiness with reluctance to feed. Opioid antagonists also readily cross the placenta and it has been suggested that they should be given to the mother immediately before delivery to counter neonatal depression but this deprives the mother of analgesia at the time when it is most needed. If they are used, the opioid antagonists such as naloxone should be given to the neonate. Because the action of naloxone is shorter than that of some opioids, depression may return when the naloxone is metabolized and careful observation is indicated to allow this to be detected and treated by the injection of more naloxone.

All the α_2-adrenoceptor agonists rapidly cross the placenta and can cause respiratory and cardiovascular depression in both mother and babies although this can be counteracted by the use of antagonists. The use of xylazine/ketamine or acepromazine/ketamine combinations is theoretically unwise but, in practice, provided only minimal doses are used little harm appears to result.

Low doses of thiopentone, methohexitone, propofol and Saffan produce minimal respiratory depression in the neonate. Neuromuscular blocking drugs do not readily cross the placenta and will not adversely affect the neonate. In obstetrical anaesthesia muscle relaxation is seldom a major problem. None is required for vaginal delivery and in caesarian section the only time it is needed is for suture of the abdominal wall but this is usually very relaxed following extraction of the bulky uterine contents. Use of neuromuscular blockers to decrease the quantity of the more depressant anaesthetic agents needed is, however, a legitimate indication for their use in balanced anaesthesia techniques.

Inhalation anaesthetics readily cross the placental barrier with rapid equilibration between the mother and fetus(es). The degree of depression they cause in the neonate is directly proportional to the depth of unconsciousness induced in the mother. Deep levels of maternal depression will cause maternal arterial hypotension, decreased uterine blood flow and fetal acidosis. Use of the less soluble agents, halothane, enflurane and isoflurane, will lead to more rapid recovery of the neonate than the use of the more soluble methoxyflurane. Nitrous oxide will often enable the concentration of the more potent but more soluble anaesthetic agent to be reduced and its use does not add to respiratory depression in the neonate.

Fetal haemoglobin can carry more oxygen for a given partial pressure than adult haemoglobin due to the low concentration of 2,3-diphosphoglycerate (2,3-DPG) in fetal red cells. This ensures a higher level of haemoglobin saturation at the normally low Po_2 of umbilical venous blood. Administration of oxygen to the mother results in a most significant increase in fetal oxygenation and inspired oxygen concentrations of over 50% during maternal general anaesthesia are associated with the delivery of more vigorous newborn.

Local analgesics are not as harmless as sometimes supposed. Amide derivatives (e.g. lignocaine, mepivacaine, bupivacaine) are broken down by hepatic microsomal enzymes. After absorption from the site of injection blood levels decrease slowly and can reach a significant level in the fetus(es), causing depression in the neonate. Sufficiently high concentrations seldom occur after epidural or paravertebral injections but can be found after the indiscriminate local infiltration of large volumes of solution. Epidural block may produce hypotension and this may be treated by infusing fluid to fill the dilated vascular bed or, better, by the injection of ephedrine. Ephedrine acts centrally to increase venous tone and thus cardiac preload; it has minimal vasoconstrictor effect on the arterial system.

Because glycopyrrolate does not readily cross the placental barrier it is probably the anticholinergic of choice for parturient animals. These agents are desirable to minimize the effects of traction on the uterus and broad ligaments during caesarian section.

ANAESTHESIA FOR OBSTETRICS IN HORSES

In horses, obstructed labour quickly leads to exhaustion of the mother and death of the foal. Prompt relief is necessary and for this anaesthesia may have to be provided for vaginal delivery of the foal or for caesarean section. The viability of the foal will depend on its state at the time of anaesthesia but the mother will invariably have a distended abdomen and may show signs of weakness from exhaustion or be in shock. The anaesthetic problems presented by the mare are very similar to those encountered in horses with bowel obstruction, although the degree of dehydration is generally much less severe. When the foal is alive, the effects of any drugs to be given to the mare on uterine blood flow and fetal oxygenation, as well as on the respiratory centre of the foal after delivery, must also be taken into consideration.

It can be assumed that any drug given to the mare will cross the placenta to the foal, but its actual level in the foal after delivery will, as indicated previously, depend on such factors as its fat solubility, degree of protein binding and ionization, the dose given and the time interval between its administration and delivery of the foal, and on the neonatal foal's ability to eliminate the drug from its body. Thus, narcotics such as pethidine given to the mare will produce respiratory depression in the foal, but low doses of thiobarbiturates will be tolerated because recovery from central nervous depression is more dependent on redistribution than on metabolism. The more insoluble inhalation anaesthetics given to the mare are readily excreted by the foal if it breathes properly after delivery. Although neuromuscular blocking drugs such as vecuromium, atracurium and pancuronium will not cross the placental barrier in significant amounts, guaiphenesin will, so for obstetrical anaesthesia it should be avoided if the foal is alive when anaesthesia is induced. Respiratory depression in the foal which results from the administration of narcotic analgesics to the mare can be antagonized by giving naloxone to the foal but, in general, stimulant drugs have only a minor role in the management of problems of the newborn animal although one of the authors (K.W.C.) considers that doxapram (0.5 mg/kg intravenously) is effective in provoking the first breath and aiding lung expansion.

The abdominal distension of the mare will probably be the problem which gives rise to most concern because many mares have great difficulty in breathing spontaneously once they are recumbent under general anaesthesia. Due to intrapulmonary shunting of blood they may also be difficult to keep asleep with inhalation anaesthetics. In the supine position which some surgeons prefer for caesarean section in mares, the weight of the uterus and its contents will compress the vena cava and aorta, reducing venous return and causing a marked reduction in cardiac output and arterial blood pressure. Once the foal is delivered, the condition of the mare shows a dramatic improvement — pulmonary ventilation increases and the arterial blood pressure rises towards normal levels. To minimize difficulties before delivery of the foal, the mare should be positioned so that she is lying inclined towards her left side and respiration may need to be controlled. As always in equine anaesthesia, the magnitude of the problems encountered is related to size and small pony mares present only relatively minor problems. It is important to re-

member this, for techniques which have been successful for elective caesarian section in small experimental pony mares operated on in lateral decubitus [1] are often inadequate for the large mares of the heavy breeds which may need emergency obstetric procedures in clinical situations.

In practice, vaginal repositioning and delivery of the foal can often be carried out in the sedated mare, using one of the drug combinations discussed earlier in this book, but if general anaesthesia is needed the α_2-adrenoceptor agonist/ketamine combination (see p. 218), in spite of some theoretical objections, can be recommended, for it has been used without giving rise to problems. Should a longer period of anaesthesia be required small intravenous doses of a thiobarbiturate may be given to prolong the effects of this combination of drugs. Caudal epidural block is not as useful as it is in cattle because in mares there is a rather long delay between injection and the full development of analgesia.

For caesarian section, if the foal is alive, induction with an α_2-adrenoceptor agonist before thiopentone or methohexitone followed by endotracheal halothane/oxygen seems to be satisfactory but ketamine is undoubtedly better than either of the barbiturates as the induction agent. Only the minimum amount of halothane should be used and IPPV may be necessary until the foal is delivered. Involution of the uterus is hastened when xylazine has been used and may be assisted by the intravenous injection of 2.5–10 units of oxytocin. Bleeding from the uterus is best controlled by the intravenous injection of 3–5 mg of ergometrine tartrate, but this may give rise to cardiac arrhythmias if given to a hypercapnic or hypertensive animal. If the foal is dead any technique of general anaesthesia suitable for laparotomy may be used and often vigorous supportive therapy with intravenous fluids will be necessary.

ANAESTHESIA FOR OBSTETRICS IN CATTLE

In cattle, caudal block (p. 249) is nearly always satisfactory for vaginal delivery of the fetus. Whenever possible sedation should be avoided but if needed to control the animal the intravenous injection of 0.05 mg/kg of xylazine will, in most cases, provide adequate maternal tranquillization to enable the block and delivery to be undertaken with minimal trouble.

Lumbar segmental epidural block (p. 252) may be useful for caesarian section carried out through the left flank of the standing animal but it is not easily performed and most veterinarians prefer to use paravertebral block of the thirteenth thoracic, first, second and third lumbar nerves (p. 244) on that side.

Local infiltration techniques can be employed but they do not relax the abdominal muscles and, if the fetus is alive, the injection of large volumes of the amide-type local analgesics may result in cardiopulmonary depression in the neonate.

Caesarian section via a ventral abdominal incision is usually carried out under general anaesthesia with endotracheal intubation. Anaesthesia may be induced by the intravenous injection of minimal doses of xylazine/ketamine, thiopentone or methohexitone and, after endotracheal intubation, maintained with a halothane/oxygen mixture. Alternatively, after xylazine or detomidine has been given to produce deep sedation, the animal may be intubated and anaesthesia completed by the administration of halothane. Guaiphenesin should be avoided since it crosses the placental barrier, while ketamine, enflurane and isoflurane may be too expensive for use in all except very valuable cattle.

Involution of the uterus after delivery may be assisted by the use of ecbolic drugs provided the animal is not hypercapnic or hypertensive. All cows subjected to caesarian section under general anaesthesia should be given a subcutaneous injection of calcium borogluconate to prevent the occurrence of hypocalcaemia which is otherwise frequently seen in the postoperative period. Postoperative analgesia is also important and 0.5–1.0 g of pethidine, depending on the size of the cow, repeated at 4–6-hourly intervals for the first 24 hours has proved to provide adequate analgesia as shown by the cow looking comfortable and cudding or eating.

Removal of a dead, putrefying normal-sized calf by hysterotomy should only be attempted after resuscitation of the cow with intravenous fluids; antibiotic cover is essential.

ANAESTHESIA FOR OBSTETRICS IN THE SHEEP AND GOAT

Sheep are seldom given any analgesia or anaesthesia for the vaginal delivery of lambs but in difficult cases requiring extensive repositioning of the lamb in the birth canal caudal block (p. 262) is very satisfactory.

For caesarian section, which is usually carried out through the left flank, epidural or paravertebral blocks (p. 262), local infiltration and general anaesthesia are all suitable. The ewe is easily restrained for operation and hence techniques of local analgesia are popular. Probably the technique of choice is paravertebral block of the thirteenth thoracic, first, second and third lumbar nerves for the ewe is then able to stand and nurse her lambs immediately the operation is completed and the wound area remains analgesic for one or more hours depending on the local analgesic drug used. If local infiltration is used care must be taken to restrict the dose of any amide-type local analgesic to minimize the likelihood of depression of the lambs.

Ewes carrying dead lambs or suffering from pregnancy toxaemia are often very toxic, dehydrated and dull or collapsed. Hysterotomy, if the expense of operation can be justified, should be preceded by resuscitation with intravenous fluids.

Postoperative analgesia is all too often neglected. The ewe, like any other animal, is entitled to adequate pain relief in the postoperative period and morphine, pethidine or epidural drugs should be used as freely as may be required to keep the animal comfortable.

ANAESTHESIA FOR OBSTETRICS IN PIGS

Anaesthesia for obstetrical procedures in sows is almost completely limited to the provision of anaesthesia for caesarian section. The general principles are similar to those in all other species of animal — it is necessary to provide adequate surgical conditions to prevent the sow from experiencing pain and to use a method which produces minimal depression of the piglets. Ideally, both the sow and piglets should recover from the effects of the anaesthetic in the minimum of time.

Caesarean section may be carried out under conditions which vary from those encountered on the farm to those provided in an operating theatre. Fortunately, the need for caesarean section to be performed on the farm is uncommon, due to the relatively small size of the piglets compared with that of the dam, making vaginal delivery relatively easy. Elective caesarean section, for the production of minimal disease herds of pigs, or gnotobiotic animals for research purposes, is much more common, but is usually performed in well-equipped operating theatres.

On the farm, caesarean section is probably best carried out under local or regional analgesia. Although paravertebral blocks are theoretically possible, they are difficult to perform because the thick layer of subcutaneous fat makes palpation of landmarks almost impossible, and infiltration of the line of incision is the method usually employed. Epidural block may also be used (see later).

The major problem is the restraint of the sow and today sedation with azaperone is usually used for this although the drug does cross the placental barrier and the piglets are sleepy when delivered. However, respiratory depression in the offspring is minimal and if kept warm they usually survive. The sedative effects of azaperone on the sow are rather prolonged; she may not be able to suckle the piglets for some hours; if left unattended with the piglets she may suffocate some by lying on them. If the sedation produced by azaperone is inadequate, intravenous thiopentone or metomidate may be given. This does not appear to add to the depression of the piglets and is preferable to increasing the dose of azaperone. If thiopentone or metomidate is used the sow loses control of her airway so care must be taken to see that respiratory obstruction does not develop. Local analgesia is usually still required.

Under conditions encountered in hospitals, techniques are not usually limited by availability of equipment and a wide variety of methods are in use. The piglets are not always returned to the dam and hence the speed of recovery of the sow is less important than under farm conditions. Surgical sterility is usually vital and the main task of the anaesthetist is to ensure that asepsis is not broken by movement of the sow during the operation. The staff and equipment needed for resuscitation of the piglets are usually available but in elective caesarean sections there is always a risk of delivery of premature young and the resuscitation of these may not be easy.

Probably the most viable piglets are obtained when anaesthesia is induced and maintained with a volatile inhalation agent given with a high concentration of oxygen. In the majority of sows anaesthesia is rapidly induced with agents such as halothane or enflurane, but if the sow is very large or difficult to handle, a minimal dose of a short-acting intravenous induction agent, e.g. methohexitone or propofol, can be employed.

Satisfactory results are also achieved by the use of ketamine, usually in combination with diazepam. Premedication with diazepam (2 mg/kg intravenously) and atropine is followed by the intravenous injection of ketamine given to effect. Usually about 5–10 mg/kg of ketamine is needed to produce a peculiar state in which the sow appears to be aware of the environment yet does not react to skin incision or other surgical stimulation. If necessary nitrous oxide can be used to control any slight restlessness which may occur towards the end of the operation.

Sedative premedication with azaperone, followed by induction with intravenous or inhalation agents, has been widely used for elective caesarean section with generally satisfactory results. However, in the authors' experience, there can be no doubt that piglets delivered after the use of this sedative drug are, for some hours, sleepier than if no sedation is employed. This may be acceptable under farm conditions where equipment and assistance are not plentiful, but there seems little point in using the drug where it is not necessary.

Methods of anaesthesia involving the use of neuromuscular blocking agents result in the delivery of lively piglets and rapid recovery of the sow; they can be used whenever endotracheal intubation and IPPV can be carried out. However, it is essential to ensure that the sow is completely unconscious and it is sometimes difficult to be sure of this without having to administer large doses of anaesthetic or other drugs which will give rise to marked respiratory depression in the piglets. Techniques of this nature are, therefore, best avoided except by the experienced veterinary anaesthetist.

Involution of the uterus after delivery of the piglets may, if the animal is not hypercapnic, be helped by the intravenous injection of 2–10 units of oxytocin or, if bleeding is a problem, 1–1.5 mg of ergometrine tartrate, but this latter drug may produce cardiac arrhythmias if the P_aCO_2 is elevated when it is given.

ANAESTHESIA FOR OBSTETRICS IN DOGS

Caesarean section, a procedure which is frequently carried out on bitches, presents certain problems to the anaesthetist who must be concerned with the welfare of both the bitch and her pups. It is essential that the minimum of depressant agents should have reached the pups by the time of their delivery, and that the bitch shall be conscious as soon as possible so that she will accept and be able to look after her offspring. It is also necessary, however, that the bitch shall not appreciate any pain during the operation and that the surgeon shall be provided with adequate operating conditions.

The bitch may be fit and healthy at the time of operation or she may be exhausted from a prolonged obstructed labour and even after several hours of starvation she often has a full stomach, so vomiting at induction of anaesthesia presents a major hazard. Premedication with a low dose of morphine or paraveretum (Omnopon) will usually provoke vomiting and ensure an empty stomach but will cause some degree of respiratory depression in the pups. However, as long as only low doses of these opioids are used this respiratory depression will rarely be serious. In any case, respiratory depression in the pups which results from opioid premedication of the bitch may be overcome by giving the pups naloxone. Similarly, the use of xylazine or medetomidine premedication for its emetic properties may cause prolonged and serious respiratory depression in the offspring but this can be overcome by the administration of atipamezole. Sleepiness of the pups caused by premedication of the bitch with acepromazine cannot, however, be counteracted for there is no specific antagonist to the phenothiazine derivatives.

Pressure on the major blood vessels from the gravid uterus causes circulatory disturbances in the supine animal and pressure on the posterior vena cava can interfere with venous return to the heart.

This pressure can be avoided by the use of a wedge of plastic foam material placed under the right side of the supine bitch. Major circulatory disturbances also occur once intra-abdominal pressure has been reduced by removal of the gravid uterus or the pups and the ability of the bitch to compensate for these disturbances may have been reduced by the drugs used for general anaesthesia or the sympathetic blockade induced by some techniques of local analgesia. It is, therefore, advisable to set up an intravenous infusion prior to the induction of anaesthesia, and this may be essential if the bitch is already toxic or very exhausted. Respiratory function usually improves greatly after delivery of the pups and the concentration of any inhalation agent being administered at this time may need to be reduced if overdose is to be avoided.

Some of the agents used during anaesthesia may interfere with the involution of the uterus after delivery of the pups. In women, halothane is particularly likely to lead to severe postoperative haemorrhage after caesarean section but the difference in placental attachment makes this complication much less common in bitches. Halothane, enflurane and isoflurane can all be used for caesarean section in bitches with very satisfactory results, but methoxyflurane usually produces marked depression of the pups for some time after their delivery. Provided the bitch is not hypercapnic an ecbolic (such as oxytocin, 2–10 units, or ergometrine up to 0.5 mg intravenously, depending on the size of the bitch) may be given after delivery of the pups to promote involution of the uterus.

Although there are considerable differences in the rate at which drugs cross the placenta, it is always safest to consider that any drug given to the mother will exert an influence on the pups in the postdelivery period. As long as respiratory depression is not severe, the pups will rapidly eliminate any of the less soluble inhalation agents which may have come to them from the mother but elimination of parenterally administered anaesthetic agents may be much more difficult due to the immaturity of the newborn pups' detoxicating mechanisms.

Anaesthetic-induced depression of the offspring can be avoided by the use of local analgesia. Epidural block (p. 318) is particularly suited to caesarean section but it should only be used in quiet bitches. If heavy sedation is needed for the performance of the operation the pups will be affected and the method will offer no advantage over a well-administered general anaesthetic.

In bitches of reasonable temperament, premedication may be limited to the use of an anticholinergic agent, but minimal doses of opioids may be used to cause vomiting and thereby ensure that the stomach is empty when anaesthesia is induced.

Induction of anaesthesia is best carried out with an inhalation agent given via a face-mask, and is usually rapid and excitement free in parturient bitches. The main disadvantage of inhalation induction is that vomiting may occur before endotracheal intubation is possible, so suction apparatus should be available to enable the anaesthetist to clear the airway rapidly should this complication be encountered.

In large or bad-tempered bitches it may be necessary to use an intravenous agent for induction of anaesthesia. Methohexitone, at a maximum dose of 2.5 mg/kg, or propofol in doses of 4–6 mg/kg are probably the drugs of choice, but thiopentone can be used in doses of up to 5 mg/kg without risk of serious depression of the pups. All that is required of the intravenous induction agent is to make the bitch lie down, and if intubation is not possible at this stage, anaesthesia may be deepened with an inhalation anaesthetic administered by the mask until it is. When intravenous agents are used it is advisable to wait a few minutes (about 15 minutes when propofol is used) before delivering the pups in order to let the blood levels of the parenterally administered agents decline. Dodman [2], when reviewing the literature on the subject, pointed out that there is often sufficient barbiturate remaining to cause considerable depression in the bitch at the time of delivery of the pups, yet the pups are surprisingly lively. He suggested that this is either through accumulation of the barbiturate in the fetal liver, as shown by Finster *et al.* [3], or by the further dilution of the drug before it reaches the fetal brain.

The volatile agents used, whether for induction or maintenance, should be those which are associated with a fast recovery from anaesthesia. Enflurane might seem to be the ideal anaesthetic, for the pups are born lively and the bitch is fully awake within a few minutes of the end of the operation. Halothane has been widely and successfully used, although it may delay involution of the uterus.

Techniques involving the use of neuromuscular blocking agents can be used very satisfactorily for caesarean section, as these drugs do not cross the placenta in sufficient quantities to paralyse the muscles of the offspring. However, the administration of the anaesthetic drugs necessary to ensure that the bitch is unconscious will result in slight depression of the pups and muscle relaxation for closure of the abdomen is quite adequate after delivery of the pups and involution of the uterus, so there is apparently no real advantage to be gained from the use of relaxants.

Where apparatus for the administration of inhalation anaesthesia is not available many veterinary anaesthetists use neuroleptanalgesic mixtures, such as Hypnorm (p. 71) or Small Animal Immobilon (p. 72) for caesarean section. Their use is associated with severe and prolonged respiratory depression of the pups and although the effects of the opioid agents may be countered with naloxone or diprenorphine, the sedative effects of the tranquillizer components cannot be antagonized so that the pups are exposed to the dangers of hypothermia and failure to feed. The neuroleptanalgesic techniques may be preferable to other methods of intravenous anaesthesia in these circumstances, but they must always be recognized as being considerably inferior to well-administered inhalation anaesthetics for the delivery of lively pups.

Enterohepatic recirculation of etorphine may result in the bitch and pups returning to a narcotized state even when diprenorphine has been used.

Postoperative pain relief for the bitch should be regarded as essential but care must be taken to ensure that any drugs used for this purpose are not excreted in the milk in concentrations which may affect the suckling pups. The provision of adequate pain relief may pose problems when opioid antagonists have been used to produce more rapid awakening of the bitch.

ANAESTHESIA FOR OBSTETRICS IN CATS

The requirements of anaesthesia for caesarean section in the cat, and the problems likely to be encountered, are similar to those already discussed above for dogs.

Although cats may vomit on induction of anaesthesia, inhalation of vomit is less likely than in dogs, for cats have more active laryngeal reflexes. Nevertheless, endotracheal intubation should be carried out as soon as anaesthesia is induced and a pharyngeal pack should be introduced around the tube.

Many cats presented for caesarian section or hysterectomy are carrying dead kittens and the uterus may be infected. Ideally, in such cases an intravenous drip infusion should be set up before anaesthesia but, unless the mother is exhausted or otherwise very ill, this is usually delayed until after anaesthesia has been induced.

Premedication before caesarian section is usually limited to the administration of anticholinergics, and induction with low-solubility volatile agents leads to the quickest recovery of both mother and kittens. With care, such an induction can be smooth, but many anaesthetists prefer to induce unconsciousness with small intravenous doses of thiopentone, propofol, methohexitone or Saffan, before going on to the inhalation anaesthetic. Only minimal quantities of any intravenous agent should be used, and volatile anaesthetics should be employed to maintain the lightest possible levels of anaesthesia.

If facilities for the administration of inhalation agents are not available and intravenous anaesthetics have to be used for caesarean section, Saffan is probably the best available. Although the Saffan steroids cross the placenta and will affect the kittens, no noticeable respiratory depression results. If it is necessary to use Saffan for this operation it is probable that it should be used in conjunction with local analgesic techniques so that the lightest level of general anaesthesia can be employed.

Neuroleptanalgesic methods are contraindicated in cats and after ketamine anaesthesia recovery is too prolonged for this drug to be used alone if the offspring are alive and need maternal care soon after delivery [2]. The advent of medetomidine, however, has changed this situation in that after its use for premedication (in doses of up to 80 µg/kg) the dose of ketamine can be reduced to low levels (e.g. 2 mg/kg), while the effects of the medetomidine itself can be antagonized with atipamezole.

Epidural analgesia can provide excellent analgesia and muscle relaxation for caesarean section, but in cats the need for deep sedation to control the head end of the animal severely limits its usefulness. All sedatives in current use will depress the kittens and their condition will be no better than after well-administered general anaesthesia.

Maternal postoperative analgesia may be provided by the use of small doses of morphine or pethidine, any suckling kittens being carefully watched for signs of undue sleepiness that indicate high drug levels in the milk.

REFERENCES

1. Edwards, G. B., Allen, W. E. and Newcombe, J. K. (1974) *Equine Veterinary Journal* 6, 122.
2. Dodman, N. H. (1979) *Journal of Small Animal Practice* 20, 449.
3. Finster, M., Morishima, H. O., Mark, L. C., Perel, J. M., Dayton, P., G. and James, L. S. (1972) *Anesthesiology* 36, 155.

CHAPTER 19

ANAESTHESIA FOR INTRATHORACIC AND CARDIAC SURGERY

The anaesthetic management of the pneumothorax created by the wide opening of the chest wall and/or diaphragm for surgical access to the contents of the thoracic cavity involves 'controlled respiration' or 'IPPV' (Chapter 8). Although in veterinary practice ventilation of the lungs by manual squeezing of the reservoir of the anaesthetic breathing circuit is still carried out in centres where little intrathoracic surgery is undertaken, the use of mechanical ventilators is becoming widespread. Surgeons find it easier to work with the regular movement produced by these machines and their use makes it possible to stabilize the tidal and minute volumes of respiration, the airway pressures and the duration of the inspiratory and expiratory periods in a way which cannot be achieved by manual 'bag squeezing'. Apart from the fact that IPPV is obligatory while the pleural cavity is open, the actual anaesthetic methods employed for intrathoracic surgery are largely governed by the personal preferences and experience of the anaesthetist. The main anaesthetic problems centre around the elimination of any pneumothorax remaining after closure of the thoracotomy incision and here close cooperation between the surgeon and anaesthetist is essential if they are to be satisfactorily resolved.

CLOSURE OF THE CHEST

The anaesthetic technique used while the chest is being closed varies with the nature of the operation but should always include drainage of the pleural cavity. In the past, after a limited operation not involving injury to the lung the chest was often closed without drainage. An attempt was made to achieve full re-expansion of any collapsed area of the lung tissue and to maintain full control of the breathing until the chest was airtight. However, the methods employed never succeeded in removing all the residual air from the pleural cavity, portions of the lung remained collapsed and often became a focus of infection. The air trapped in the pleural cavity caused movements of the chest wall to be transmitted to the lung by negative intrapleural pressure and pleural exudation occurred as a result of this. Proper drainage of the pleural cavity with removal of all the residual air overcomes all of these problems but if, on occasion, the chest has to be closed without drainage the amount of air trapped in the pleural cavity can be minimized by inserting a catheter through an intercostal space and applying suction after the chest wall is closed. The catheter is then pulled out with a sharp tug. Alternatively, when the thoracotomy wound has been closed a large-bore catheter connected to a suction apparatus is inserted into the pleural cavity and suction applied until there is a negative pressure present in the system. The catheter may become blocked by the lung and the method is therefore not very satisfactory. It is, however, commonly used in cats where after closure of the thorax a large (13 s.w.g.) intravenous catheter may be introduced into the pleural cavity, the needle part being withdrawn after penetration of the skin and the blunt plastic catheter forced through the intercostal muscles and parietal pleura.

When there is an injury to the lung which could cause an air leak, or there is any likelihood of continuing haemorrhage into the pleural cavity, the chest *must* be drained. Underwater drainage is undoubtedly the most reliable and informative procedure and for this the drain tube is connected to a bottle containing water or a weak aqueous solution of chlorhexidine. This acts as a non-return valve and allows air or fluid to be expelled from the pleural cavity but prevents the indrawing of air during inspiration. The drain tube dips about 2.5 cm below the surface of the water and should have an internal diameter of about 0.5 cm. The bottle must have an internal diameter of not less than 15 cm. When the closure of the chest is complete, inflation of the lung, or spontaneous respiratory movements of the animal, forces air out of the pleural cavity whenever the pressure within the pleural sac is greater than about 2.5 cmH$_2$O (0.25 kPa; i.e. the depth which the tube dips below the surface of the water). Provided that the bottle is kept at least 80 cm below the level of the animal's body, water cannot be aspirated into the chest, for no effort of the animal can lift the water up this distance. The larger diameter of the bottle ensures that no matter how high the level rises in the drainage tube the end of the tube will always be below the water surface (Fig. 19.1).

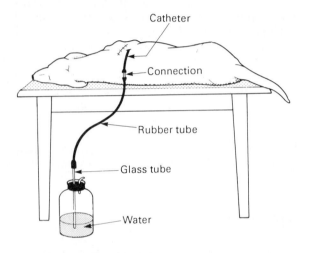

Fig. 19.1 Underwater chest drain. The water level should be at least 80 cm below the level of the animal's body.

When the animal breathes spontaneously the water level in the drainage tube rises on inspiration (as the cavity between the lung and chest wall increases) and falls on expiration. When the lung occupies the whole of the pleural space the pressure does not show marked fluctuations during the respiratory cycle. If, however, the lung is not completely expanded large variations of pressure occur. Observation of the behaviour of the water level in the glass tube thus provides useful information as to the state of expansion of the lung — the greater the amplitude of the swing of the water level, the poorer is the expansion of the lung. The drain should be allowed to remain in the pleural cavity until the lung is fully expanded. It is then pulled out, and a skin suture, which has been laid for the purpose, tied tightly to occlude the hole in the skin.

After any operation which has involved stripping of the visceral layer of pleura from the area of the lung there will be an air leak from the raw surface of the lung. In such circumstances suction may have to be applied to the far side of the underwater seal appara-

tus to control the pneumothorax. This suction must be maintained until there is no bubbling of air through the water, indicating that the leak has been sealed off by inflammatory reaction. It may not be possible to remove the drain tube for up to 48 hours after operation and during this time the animal must be kept well sedated. Experience has shown that in cats this sedation is best achieved by the use of Saffan given either as a continuous infusion or by intermittent injection, while in dogs combinations of morphine and diazepam give excellent results particularly when combined with the instillation of 2–5 ml (depending on the size of the dog) of 0.25% bupivacaine into the pleural cavity. Whatever sedation is used it is important that restlessness is overcome without at the same time producing respiratory depression. After any thoracotomy the animal must be examined both physically and radiologically for evidence of lung collapse. Collapse of a lung, or of a lobe of a lung, may necessitate immediate intrabronchial suction for the removal of any material which is occluding the bronchus to the lung or lobe. Whenever it is possible, an immediate postoperative chest radiograph should be taken to confirm full

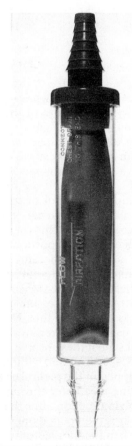

Fig. 19.2 Heimlich chest drain valve.

expansion of the lungs, the absence of pneumothorax and the position of any drainage tubes. It also serves as a reference against which later films can be assessed.

The underwater seal drain can be used in any animal but for horses, cattle, sheep, goats, pigs and ambulant large dogs it is sometimes more convenient to use a Heimlich valve (Fig. 19.2). This valve should be attached to the animal's chest wall by a skin suture and the drain tube tied securely to the valve inlet. It gives no indication as to the state of expansion of the lungs and regular, frequent inspection is necessary to check that it is working properly.

All drainage tubes introduced into the pleural cavity should be of adequate bore and made from a siliconized material which does not soften too much at body temperature. Small-bore chest drains are almost worse than useless — they occlude easily if they become slightly kinked around a rib and are readily blocked by the expanded lung or a small blood clot. For cats a 2.5 mm internal bore tube is the smallest which should be used, while for all but the smallest of dogs and puppies 7.5 mm bore tubing should be regarded as being the minimum size. In horses and cattle 10–12 mm internal diameter tubing should be used. Dogs and cats can be turned from side to side to promote drainage of either air or blood but in large animals such as horses it is often necessary to insert two chest drains — one ventrally for the drainage of blood and one dorsally for the drainage of air and these can be connected through a Y-tube to a Heimlich drain.

The time for removal of the drain should be a matter for consultation between the surgeon and anaesthetist. It is essential that it should be removed as soon as it is of no further use but should a pleural effusion or pneumothorax develop after it has been taken out, another intercostal drain should be introduced immediately under local infiltration analgesia.

THORACOTOMY FOR NON-PULMONARY LESIONS

Thoracotomies for non-pulmonary lesions present few special anaesthetic problems. Large neoplasms within the thorax can cause an animal considerable respiratory difficulty but removal of the space-occupying lesions eases the respiration at once. In removing some of the more extensive mediastinal tumours the surgeon may open both pleural cavities but with the maintenance of controlled respiration no trouble is encountered during operation. It may be necessary to drain both pleural cavities and the two intercostal drains can be connected to the same underwater seal by a Y-connector.

Oesophageal surgery

The problems in oesophageal surgery arise from the danger of regurgitation of food and saliva which have been retained in the oesophagus. Prompt intubation of the prone animal with the head raised will usually prevent this mishap from occurring. Thoracotomy for oesophageal surgery presents no special anaesthetic problems that have not already been discussed.

Repair of ruptures of the diaphragm

Although the majority of diaphragmatic ruptures are best repaired through an abdominal incision [1] the pleural cavity is, of course, opened to the atmosphere during the course of the operation. The anaesthetic management of these cases is not always easy.

Diaphragmatic rupture produces respiratory inefficiency which results both from reduced breathing capacity and from an unbalanced distribution of air and blood within the lungs. The presence of abdominal viscera and effusion within the chest reduces the vital capacity; the absence of effective diaphragmatic movement limits the enlargement of the thoracic cavity. Twisting or displacement of the lung lobes causes partial obstruction of the bronchi, leading to the uneven distribution of the inspired air. The blood passing through overventilated areas of lung will lose more carbon dioxide than it would under normal conditions, but it cannot become more fully oxygenated. In the underventilated areas of lung both oxygenation and carbon dioxide removal are impaired. Because of these effects the mixed blood returning from the lungs usually has a carbon dioxide tension near to normal, but its oxygen tension is low, i.e. the main threat to life of animal's suffering from rupture of the diaphragm is hypoxia. Anything which distresses the animal and thus increases its oxygen requirements may prove fatal. When most of the thoracic cavity is occupied by abdominal viscera and/or effusion, the animal can only survive by making maximal breathing efforts and the use of a respiratory depressant sedative or analgesic is most unwise. Heavy sedation for diagnostic radiography is particularly unwise. In dogs, phenothiazine ataractics such as acepromazine together with small doses of pethidine produce useful, safe sedation, and in cats small (10 mg) doses of pethidine are useful.

Anaesthesia for animals suffering from diaphragmatic rupture may be managed in a variety of ways. No hard and fast rules can be given and each individual case must be treated on its own merits. All cases must be handled very quietly and gently before anaesthesia is induced, and a smooth induction of anaesthesia with an intravenous agent is advisable. Some animals do not resent the application of a facemask and they may be given oxygen to inhale for 2–3 minutes before the induction of anaesthesia. In dogs, whenever it can be done without undue disturbance of the animal, an intravenous drip should be set up before anaesthesia, otherwise it is set up as soon as possible during the course of the operation. This drip is often needed to remedy the fall in blood pressure seen when re-expansion of the lungs alters the haemodynamic state of the body (presumably due to reopening of areas of the pulmonary vascular bed). Endotracheal intubation is, of course, essential in all cases.

At the end of the operation no attempt should be made to forcibly expand regions of lung tissue which have been in a collapsed state for some time, for this leads to pulmonary oedema. The use of a chest drain allows some overexpansion of healthy, non-collapsed lung to fill the pleural cavity and encourages the collapsed regions to re-expand over a period of time. Chest drainage also allows the removal from the pleural cavity of fluid which often appears in the postoperative period.

Postoperative pain, which limits breathing to rapid, very shallow movements of the chest wall, is best controlled by the injection of pethidine or morphine, in appropriate doses for the species of animal concerned, given as required. Infiltration of the abdominal incision with small quantities of 0.25% bupivacaine is also very effective in alleviating pain.

THORACOTOMY FOR PULMONARY SURGERY

One of the major problems in pulmonary surgery is the prevention of spillage or secretions or pus from the affected part to the remainder of the lung. In man this problem is overcome by drainage or isolation of the affected part of the lung with some form of blocker (usually employing a tube for drainage) or, alternatively, endobronchial tubes, either single or double lumen, provide a means of protecting the sound lung which can then be ventilated selectively. In animals, due to the shape of the chest and the anatomy of the bronchial tree, most of these techniques are impossible and reliance has to be placed on preoperative preparation with antibiotics and expectorants to make the lung relatively 'dry'. Non-irritating anaesthetic agents also play a part in reducing the volume of secretions produced during surgery, while any that remain can be removed by bronchoscopic aspiration carried out at frequent intervals through the endotracheal tube.

During lobectomy or pneumonectomy, ventilation after severance of the bronchus and prior to its closure presents surprisingly little difficulty and although IPPV results in some frothing of blood this does not usually obscure the surgeon's view of the bronchial stump. Should it prove to be impossible to obtain adequate lung expansion while the bronchus is wide open the surgeon may be asked to occlude the opening with a finger or thumb while the lung is inflated between the laying of sutures. Provided the minute volume is kept constant the removal of a lobe or even of one lung does not result in any significant rise in P_aCO_2 and indeed the P_aCO_2 may actually fall, indicating an improvement in the dead-space/tidal volume ratio. There is usually a fall in P_aCO_2 as soon as the chest is opened and measures which have been recommended to minimize patchy alveolar collapse during constant minute volume IPPV, such as intermittent manual hyperinflation and continuous manual inflation, are quite ineffective and may be harmful. The PaO_2 usually remains above 80 mmHg (10.6 kPa) when the inspired gases contain at least 50% of oxygen even when only one lung is available for ventilation.

Frequent suction is needed to clear the bronchial tree in bronchiectasis cases and the use of halothane/oxygen or isoflurane/oxygen without nitrous oxide has been found to be advantageous in avoiding hypoxaemia when ventilation of the lungs is interrupted for the passage of the suction catheter. Oxygenation by diffusion continues when ventilation is stopped but the P_aCO_2 rises until ventilation recommences.

In certain cases, such as operations for the removal of congenital cysts of the lung, it is advisable to allow spontaneous respiration to continue until the pleural cavity is opened. This avoids overdistension of the cysts with resulting collapse of lung tissue.

Replacement of blood loss during the operation and the maintenance of fluid balance should follow the usual practice for major surgery but after the removal of lung tissue animals seem to make better progress if they are slightly short of fluid. Overtransfusion with blood or the administration of excessive amounts of other fluids is associated with pulmonary oedema and this is particularly disastrous after resection of any significant amounts of lung tissue. It should be noted that, particularly in dogs, traction on the hilum of the lung can cause arterial hypotension; this is not an indication for the administration of fluids — blood pressure returns quickly to normal when traction ceases.

Postoperatively animals which have had a lung lobe resected should be nursed lying on the sound side until they are able to sit up; this encourages re-expansion of lung remaining on the side of operation and facilitates drainage of any pneumothorax. After pneumonectomy the animal should be nursed on the side of operation. The first dose of postoperative sedative analgesic should be given intravenously in order that the patient's needs may be more accurately assessed. A routine chest radiograph is advisable before removal of the intercostal drainage tube, but it must be recognized that the positioning for this may distress the animal and under these circumstances it may be necessary to rely upon auscultation of lung sounds to check that the lungs are fully expanded. Instillation of up to 5 ml of 0.25% bupivacaine into the pleural cavity on the operated side will provide most useful postoperative analgesia in dogs for up to 6 hours.

CARDIAC SURGERY

In considering anaesthesia for cardiac surgery it is essential to look beyond the problems associated with thoracotomy. The action of the anaesthetic drugs may affect the heart and alter the vascular tone generally. Equally, disorders of the circulatory system may modify the absorption and action of anaesthetic drugs. The problems that arise are often peculiar to each lesion but certain general principles of anaesthetic management can be enunciated.

All animals should be handled quietly to avoid excitement and reduce the load on the heart. In dogs a *small* dose of acepromazine is often valuable in reducing this load.

If an intravenous agent is to be used for induction of anaesthesia two points must be noted. First, slowing of the circulation due to the disease process causes a considerable lag between the administration of the drug and the development of its effect. This makes it very easy to give too much, for it may give the impression that the animal is resistant to the drug. Secondly, these drugs may depress the myocardium and produce peripheral vasodilatation. In animals where the cardiac output is fixed by valvular stenoses, the vasodilatation may produce a very marked fall in blood pressure. The drug should always be administered very slowly and in very dilute solutions. However, clinical experience indicates that the dangers of thiopentone in these cases have perhaps been overemphasized. The quiet, smooth induction of anaesthesia more than makes up for its supposed disadvantages which are, in any case, much less obvious with the small doses needed in properly premedicated animals.

Provided it does not excite the animal, oxygen should be administered through a face-mask before anaesthesia is induced, but in every case it should be administered as soon as consciousness is lost. A perfect airway is essential and a large-bore endotracheal tube must be introduced into the trachea as soon as possible.

Constrictive pericarditis and cardiac tamponade are very crippling conditions because they limit the cardiac output and depress tissue respiration by the widespread action of the raised venous pressure. Associated ascites and pleural effusions reduce the vital capacity and venous back pressure may damage the liver. Careful preanaesthetic preparation of these cases is necessary. Pleural and peritoneal effusions must be tapped and fluid retention reduced by the use of diuretics. Cardiac tamponade must be relieved by paracentesis under local infiltration analgesia.

Operations on the heart and great vessels which necessitate a short period of circulatory arrest are already being undertaken in canine surgery and it is likely that as diagnostic methods improve many more ambitious operations will be attempted in dogs and in other animals.

Much has been written concerning the anaesthesia of healthy animals and various species for experimental cardiac surgery but little of this is relevant to clinical veterinary practice. Clinical cases presented for cardiac surgery for the correction of acquired or congenital lesions almost invariably have circulatory disturbances which complicate their management and, in many, failure of medical treatment is the reason why operation is contemplated. It is extremely unlikely that any one veterinary centre will ever receive enough cases to enable the expertise necessary for their successful treatment to be developed. However, medical cardiac surgery teams are often willing to help by operating on these animals and the veterinary anaesthetist should be able to give expert assistance on these occasions. While medical cardiac surgery teams will usually be involved where cardiopulmonary bypass techniques are needed, some of the simpler lesions may be amenable to correction under moderate hypothermia by veterinary surgical teams. The veterinary anaesthetist should, therefore, be familiar with the principles of bypass techniques, and of moderate hypothermia, for circulatory arrest.

It is likely that most cardiac surgery will be carried out in dogs and the techniques of anaesthesia used in these animals will be described below but similar methods can be used in other species of animal should the need arise. It must be emphasized that surgery of this nature is never likely to be an economic proposition and it is usually undertaken out of an academic interest in the advancement of knowledge relating to circulatory disorders generally.

Ultrasonography

This technique of investigation can be carried out without risk to the animal provided it is handled quietly and the administration of drugs is usually quite unnecessary.

Cardiac catheterization

Most animals presented for cardiac surgery are first investigated by cardiac catheterization. Radiopaque catheters, visible by fluoroscopy, can be advanced from a peripheral vein into the right heart and pulmonary artery. By wedging the tip in a pulmonary artery, an indication of left atrial pressure can be obtained. In addition, a needle can be passed through the catheter when it is in the right atrium to pierce the atrial septum and measure the pressure in the left atrium directly. The left ventricle can be entered directly if a catheter is introduced from a peripheral artery. Information is obtained by pressure measurement, by measurement of cardiac output and by blood gas analysis on samples of blood taken from

known positions of the catheter tip. Angiography is usually carried out on the same occasion using large film rapid changers or cineradiography. Anaesthesia must not interfere with any of these diagnostic procedures. After full premedication it may be induced carefully by the intravenous injection of small doses of 2.5% thiopentone followed by 0.12 mg/kg of pancuronium and endotracheal intubation as soon as relaxation of the jaw muscles is obtained. To maintain the blood gases as near normal for the particular animal as possible, IPPV is carried out with gas mixtures containing 20% of oxygen in such a way as to maintain the P_aCO_2 between 35 and 40 mmHg (4.7 and 5.3 kPa). The use of IPPV overcomes alterations of P_aO_2 which may result in an uncontrolled way when the animal is breathing spontaneously. The procedure usually takes place in a darkened room and the wise anaesthetist withdraws briefly during radiation periods. Neuroleptanaesthesia which might be thought to offer an alternative to general anaesthesia with IPPV is generally not satisfactory as the animals remain sensitive to noise and may jump when the radiographic exposures are made.

Cardiac catheterization is not without risk. Severe arrhythmias and circulatory instability are relatively common. The anaesthetist must be prepared to deal with these as they arise.

HYPOTHERMIA

Provided that it has no work to do, the heart muscle itself is not harmed by short periods of circulatory arrest but the brain cells are extremely sensitive to oxygen lack and cannot survive if the circulation stops for more than 3–5 minutes. Reducing the temperature of the brain cell depresses their metabolism and enables them to withstand the effects of longer periods of circulatory arrest. For example, at 30°C the brain will survive and function after a circulatory arrest of 10 minutes.

Body temperature measurement

During the rapidly changing conditions of body cooling and rewarming associated with hypothermia techniques, a temperature measurement made in the mouth or rectum fails to provide an adequate index of temperature in other regions of the body. There is ample evidence, however, that the oesophageal temperature at heart level is a most reliable measure of the heart and blood temperature. For this reason a suitable calibrated thermometer probe introduced correctly into the oesophagus should always be used for temperature measurement.

Reactions to cold

In a conscious animal vasoconstriction in the skin is the first reaction of the body to a cold environment. Adrenaline is released from the adrenal glands and this, besides causing vasoconstriction, stimulates cellular metabolism mobilizing glycogen and increasing heat production. Other responses include the release of thyrotrophic hormone and adrenal corticoids both of which result in greater heat production. If these reactions are insufficient to maintain the normal body temperature shivering occurs and a tremendous increase in heat production results. Shivering is by far the most effective means of maintaining the body temperature.

Physiology of hypothermia

For an introduction to the voluminous literature on hypothermia reference should be made to *The Physiology of Induced Hypothermia* edited by R. D. Dripps (National Research Council, Washington, DC) [2] and to articles such as that by Cooper [3]. In the account which follows reference can only be made to a few of the physiological consequences of body cooling which are of practical interest in anaesthesia.

As the body cools, the heart rate falls and it is about halved when the body temperature reaches 25°C. This slowing is apparently due to cooling of the pacemaker and is accompanied by a prolongation of systole and isometric contraction. Changes in the electrocardiogram include prolongation of the P-R interval and a lengthening of the QRS complex. Elevation of the S-T segment or the appearance of a wave rising steeply from the S wave is said to herald the onset of ventricular fibrillation. The onset of ventricular fibrillation, when it occurs in hypothermia, is influenced by a number of factors:

1. *The type of anaesthesia.* Of the barbiturates, thiopentone sodium seems the least likely to cause fibrillation.
2. *Mechanical stimulation.* Stimulation of the heart by catheters in the ventricles or by surgical procedures may induce fibrillation.
3. *Underventilation.* Underventilation of the lungs, with a consequent rise in the carbon dioxide content of the blood and a fall in pH, predisposes to fibrillation.
4. *Changes in the ionic equilibrium.* The ionic equilibrium in the blood plays a part in the initiation of cardiac arrhythmias and the relative concentrations of potassium and calcium are particularly important.
5. *Sympathetic discharge* There is some evidence which suggests that blocking the sympathetic nerves to the heart protects this organ against fibrillation under hypothermia.
6. *Blood pressure.* Abrupt falls in blood pressure which give rise to a sharp drop in the coronary blood flow can, during hypothermia, precipitate ventricular fibrillation.

The blood flow in the brain, kidney and splanchnic region is reduced as the body temperature falls. The femoral vascular bed dilates down to oesophageal temperatures of about 34°C then vasoconstriction occurs and later at 20–25°C a second vasodilatation takes place. One of the common uses of hypothermia is in circumstances which require clamping of the aorta for a considerable time. The reactive hyperaemia which follows the release of the clamp is only reduced by hypothermia where the circulatory arrest is of short duration. After occlusions lasting more than about 30 minutes, the vasodilatation which follows the release of the clamp is large and lasts as long when the body is cold as when it is warm. This must be remembered as vasoconstrictor substances or blood transfusion may have to be used to counteract this effect during cardiac surgery.

A fall in the body and brain temperature results in a decrease in cerebral oxygen consumption. At 25°C the oxygen uptake of the brain is about one-third of that at 37°C and over this range the oxygen consumption is a linear function of temperature. A matter of major importance is the degree of protection afforded to nervous tissue from the effects of circulatory arrest by hypothermia. At 25°C the circulation can be stopped for 15 minutes without damage to the brain cells and for various reasons this time of 15 minutes seems to be the maximum which can be achieved by surface cooling (between 28 and 25°C the incidence of ventricular fibrillation rises steeply). The ECG begins to change as the body temperature falls to 36–34°C. The potential recorded shows a decreased amplitude and large delta waves appear, particularly in the frontal area, at about 30°C. The electrical activity then declines until between 18 and 20°C no activity is recorded on the ECG.

Technique for the production of hypothermia

Various methods including body surface cooling, body cavity cooling, intragastric cooling and bloodstream cooling have been used to induce hypothermia.

Body surface cooling

Before hypothermia can be produced by surface cooling the animal's natural defence action to cold must be obtunded. Otherwise, attempts at reducing the body temperature are likely to increase, rather than decrease, the cellular metabolism. The efficacy of surface cooling therefore depends on maintaining a coincident vasodilatation of the superficial blood vessels and preventing shivering. Fortunately, the anaesthetic drugs which affect one reaction generally modify the other. Many systems of anaesthesia may be used quite satisfactorily but the one to be described below has proved to be quite adequate. It not only facilitates the induction of hypothermia but also ensures a rapid return to consciousness at the end of operation.

Provided there are no contraindications to its use atropine (0.3–0.6 mg) may be given, and 0.2 mg/kg chlorpromazine hydrochloride with 0.006 mg/kg of buprenorphine should be administered about 1 hour before anaesthesia is to be induced. Chlorpromazine appears to be still the best drug to produce vasodilatation and prevent shivering. Acepromazine may be used in place of the chlorpromazine but it does not seem to result in the production of as marked cutaneous vasodilatation.

Anaesthesia is induced with thiopentone sodium given by slow intravenous injection until the jaw muscles are relaxed. In animals where it is needed for endotracheal intubation a relaxant may be administered at this stage. After intubation with the largest possible cuffed tube, anaesthesia is maintained with nitrous oxide and oxygen and 0.5% halothane. The nitrous oxide helps to prevent shivering during the cooling process, and the halothane assists in the production of cutaneous vasodilatation. Next, 0.15 mg/kg pancuronium is administered to make shivering impossible and IPPV is commenced as soon as spontaneous respiration ceases. An indwelling intravenous cannula is inserted into a suitable vein and a very slow infusion of 5% dextrose is made through it.

The temperature probe is introduced into the oesophagus and the animal's body is immersed in a bath of water at 15–20°C. The head is not immersed but no harm results if it is accidentally submerged at any time. It is important that the water should be circulated over the body and manual stirring of the water has not been found to be very effective. Agitation of the water is best performed by using a jet of water from a hose connected to a cold water tap. The jet of water is moved slowly over the submerged part of the animal's body. Cooling is rapid and there is no need to use ice to lower the temperature of the water. The body temperature falls to 30–25°C within about 30 minutes.

The animal is removed from the bath when the oesophageal temperature is about 30°C and dried with towels. One of the principal dangers of surface cooling is the 'after-drop' which occurs when the animal has been removed from the bath. The 'after-drop' reduces the oesophageal temperature by up to 2°C and it is important to allow for this, for ventricular fibrillation is common at temperatures below 28°C. Between 28 and 25°C the incidence of ventricular fibrillation rises steeply. The reason why the after-drop occurs is that when the animal is removed from the bath the skin and neighbouring tissues are extremely cold. In fact they are much colder than the temperature of the circulating blood and as the blood reaches these parts it continues to cool long after the active cooling measures have been stopped.

In many cases the animal has rewarmed sufficiently by the end of the operation but if it has not done so it may be partially immersed in a bath of warm water. The anaesthetic gases are turned off when the animal's temperature reaches 35°C and it is allowed to inhale pure oxygen. The recovery of consciousness should be almost immediate. Only rarely is it necessary to use atropine and neostigmine to reverse the paralysis produced by the relaxant, but these drugs should not be withheld if there is any evidence of residual curarization.

The method described above is a messy, inconvenient one, but it does not involve the use of any complicated apparatus and it can be applied by even inexperienced personnel with a fair degree of safety to animals of most species below about 70 kg body weight. Obviously, the best results will only be obtained by an experienced surgical team using suitable devices to monitor the process. Absence of such monitoring equipment will, of course, increase the risks involved but if the condition of the animal is such that it will die unless operation is performed and operation necessitates the production of temporary circulatory arrest, then the risks associated with unmonitored hypothermia may be accepted as being reasonable.

Intragastric cooling

Intragastric cooling is a slower but much more sophisticated process. A very good, relatively inexpensive apparatus for use in dogs has been described [4]. Cold water is circulated through an intragastric balloon which is introduced into the stomach via the oesophagus after the induction of anaesthesia. The average length of time required to lower the rectal temperature of dogs weighing about 30 kg to 25°C is about 2 hours. This may seem to be rather a long time, but during the cooling process monitoring devices such as electrocardiographic leads and blood pressure transducers can easily be attached, vascular cannulations can be made and surgical procedures started. Rewarming can be started at any time during surgery (without interrupting its progress) by circulating warm water through the balloon, and rewarming is more rapid than can be achieved by any other method.

Bloodstream cooling

Bloodstream cooling is normally regarded as being part of cardiopulmonary bypass procedures but hypothermia can be produced in this way with relatively simple equipment.

An external circuit containing a transfusion warming coil and a roller peristaltic pump is primed with a plasma substitute such as Haemaccel and the coil is immersed in a bath of water maintained at 4–5°C. Cannulae are introduced into the animal's femoral or carotid artery and the femoral or jugular vein and it is given 3 mg/kg of heparin (using heparin without a preservative). The cannulae are then connected to the external circuit so that arterial blood is run through the coil and pumped back into the vein. The animal cools quite rapidly and the external circulation is stopped when the desired oesophageal temperature has been reached.

Heparin has a half-life of about 1 hour and to

maintain the heparinization of the animal it is necessary to give half the initial dose for each hour of operation.

Rewarming can be achieved by recommencing the external circulation with the water in the water bath maintained at 40°C. Once the animal has been rewarmed the external circulation is stopped and the heparinization reversed by the administration of protamine sulphate at the rate of one and one-half to two times the initial dose of heparin.

CARDIOPULMONARY BYPASS

Cardiopulmonary bypass enables the heart and lungs to be excluded from the circulation while an adequate blood supply to the rest of the body is maintained. In order to exclude the heart and lungs from the circulation, the vena cavae or the right atrium are cannulated and blood is allowed to flow through these cannulae to the pump-oxygenator or 'heart–lung' machine. Having passed through the oxygenator it is pumped back into the circulation via a cannula inserted into the aorta or one of its main branches. The heart–lung machine is provided with a means of altering the temperature of the perfusing blood (and hence of the patient) as required. It is also provided with a number of suction pumps which are used to aspirate blood from the heart cavities and pericardium during the bypass procedure for return to the patient's circulation via the oxygenator.

The pumps used for heart–lung machines are usually roller peristaltic pumps which occlude and milk siliconized rubber tubing against the track and thus cause the blood contained in the tubing to flow along it. The mechanical part of the pump does not come into contact with the blood and this minimizes haemolysis.

Oxygenators are designed to expose a thin film of blood to a gas mixture in order to allow oxygenation to take place and carbon dioxide to be removed. Those used today are disposable and produce minimal blood damage. Whatever the actual design, gas input is adjusted to maintain satisfactory levels of gaseous exchange. Usually oxygen with added carbon dioxide is used and the flow rates are adjusted to keep the blood gas tensions of the patient near to normal.

Heart–lung machines must of necessity have a large surface area for gaseous exchange and this leads to considerable heat loss. It is also desirable to achieve levels of hypothermia during bypass procedures and, therefore, all these machines incorporate some form of heat exchanger.

In order that blood may be pumped through the heart–lung machine without clotting, the patient must receive anticoagulants before being subjected to bypass. Heparin in the anticoagulant used and various procedures for heparinization are adopted. At the end of the procedure heparinization is reversed by the use of protamine sulphate which has to be given carefully to avoid undesirable side-effects such as hypotension.

Before a patient can be connected to a heart–lung machine, the apparatus must be filled with fluid and air must be excluded from the system. In the early days of cardiopulmonary bypass the apparatus was primed with freshly drawn heparinized blood but today a typical prime allows for the administration of 30–50 ml/kg of 5% dextrose or Ringer lactate solution. The haemodilution produced by this prime when the bypass commences reduces the viscosity of the blood and enables better body perfusion to be achieved. At the end of perfusion sodium bicarbonate may be added to the pump-oxygenator to correct any metabolic acidosis which may have resulted from poor perfusion of some tissues and massive blood replacement.

Anaesthetic management for cardiopulmonary bypass

Anaesthesia for open heart surgery must be administered so as to cause as little disturbance to the circulation as possible and agents causing changes in heart rate or blood pressure, or having a direct depressant effect on the myocardium, should be avoided. To ensure a good tissue blood flow during bypass an agent which causes vasodilatation (e.g. halothane) may be added to the gases fed to the oxygenator.

Premedication

Effective doses of sedative drugs are safe in cardiac disease and full premedication is usual. Drugs such as diazepam, midazolam, morphine, hyoscine and papaveretum may be used in full doses and most anaesthetists include a small dose of atropine with them. Sedation helps to allay fear, induction is smoother and the total drug dosage used during anaesthesia are reduced.

Induction of anaesthesia

It is probable that sodium thiopentone is the best induction agent for dogs. A 2.5% solution is injected slowly until the eyelash reflex is just abolished. Total doses lie between 5 and 7 mg/kg after effective premedication has been given and their injection from a 20 ml syringe through a 23 s.w.g. needle ensures that the rate of administration is not excessive. Some small reduction in blood pressure occurs but is seldom of significance. IPPV is commenced after the injection of a relaxant, usually pancuronium (0.15 mg/kg), has abolished spontaneous breathing.

An intraoesophageal thermometer probe is placed in the middle of the thoracic oesophagus and other temperature probes are placed in the nasopharynx and on the tympanic membrane. An intravenous infusion is established and closed bladder drainage is set up with a self-retaining urinary catheter or, in male animals, with a catheter retained in position with a stitch through the penis.

A catheter for arterial pressure monitoring is introduced and another for central venous pressure measurement is passed through a jugular vein. ECG leads are attached using needle electrodes, and the electrocardiogram is monitored continously thereafter. The arterial and venous catheters are attached to their respective manometer lines, including three-way taps in the set-up for the easy withdrawal of blood samples.

Maintenance of anaesthesia

IPPV is usually carried out with nitrous oxide/oxygen (50/50) supplemented with minimal concentrations of halothane (0.5%), or by the intravenous injection of small doses of fentanyl. The ventilation is adjusted to maintain the P_aCO_2 at about 35 mmHg (4.6 kPa). During the period of total bypass, ventilation is stopped and the lungs held at an airway pressure of about 10 cmH$_2$O (1 kPa) to avoid the development of collapse. Since the pulmonary blood flow is interrupted during total bypass, anaesthesia can only be maintained by drug added directly to the systemic circulation — usually into the pump-oxygenator system.

If supplementary drugs are not added to the priming fluid in the pump-oxygenator, there is an abrupt fall in the relevant tissue levels of these drugs when bypass begins. It is, therefore, necessary to add relaxant (usually pancuronium) to the prime fluids. Nitrous oxide cannot be given via oxygenators because they only work satisfactorily at high P_{O_2}s. Typically, the oxygenator gas consists of 97% oxygen with 3% carbon dioxide with an added volatile anaesthetic agent (usually halothane, 1%). Nitrous oxide is reintroduced for IPPV after coming off bypass as soon as an arterial blood sample shows that the P_aO_2 is satisfactory. No more relaxants are given as the end of the operation approaches.

In addition to the management of anaesthesia, the anaesthetist plays an important role in the monitoring of respiratory and circulatory function and the correction of any departures from optimum as may occur.

The preperfusion period is often the most hazardous. The heart lesion is uncorrected and the induction of anaesthesia may have produced a further deterioration in the animal's condition. When the mediastinum is opened and the heart and great vessels are manipulated by the surgeon the effectiveness of the heart's action may be temporarily impaired. Arrhythmias are easily provoked by contact between the heart and suction catheters, and swabs or retractors may obstruct the venous return or the flow in the pulmonary artery. Constant observation of the arterial pressure waveforms as displayed on an oscilloscope, and of the ECG are, therefore, essential. The surgeon may have to be asked to stop activities until the heart has recovered normal rhythm.

Arrhythmias of all kinds may be seen, but are often only transient, resolving spontaneously when the cause is removed. Bradycardia may be due to hypoxia, which must be eliminated as a cause before atropine is given. In the absence of sinus rhythm isoprenaline may be needed; an incomplete heart block is also treated with this drug. Myocardial irritability may be due to hypokalaemia and is often corrected by the very slow intravenous injection of potassium chloride, but if this does not produce the desired result lignocaine may have to be given. It is most important to have facilities for the rapid estimation of blood electrolytes readily available. Very rarely, cardiac irritability may be the result of a metabolic acidosis needing treatment with intravenous sodium bicarbonate.

During perfusion the haematocrit falls because of the diluting effect of the pump prime and the aim is to keep it between 20 and 25% by the addition of blood to the pump circuit as needed. Some redistribution of body fluids occurs and urinary output usually increases so that additional priming fluid has to be added during the perfusion. Diuretics (e.g. frusemide) are used if the urinary output is unsatisfactory and potassium is given to replace that lost in the urine.

Ventilation of the lungs is recommended immediately before perfusion is stopped. Caval snares are released and blood fills the heart and enters the lungs. The surgeon uses this blood to ensure that air is displaced from the left heart before allowing the systemic circulation to depend on the left ventricular contraction. Proper cardiac filling is, of course, essential and blood is transfused from the pump circuit or by intravenous infusion until atrial pressures are adequate. Initially, atrial filling pressures may have to be increased slowly to 15 mmHg (2 kPa) or until no further improvement in arterial pressure occurs, and inotropic support (adrenaline) may be needed, but usually over a period of about 30 minutes a much lower atrial filling pressure of 5–6 mmHg (0.7–0.8 kPa) becomes effective.

Perfusion technique

Perfusion is usually controlled by a highly skilled perfusionist and the aim is to produce adequate tissue perfusion without the use of excessive flow rates which result in blood destruction and may thus cause a greater incidence of postoperative bleeding problems. It is possible to reduce the perfusion flow rate needed by inducing hypothermia and, consequently, nearly all centres in the UK combine cardiopulmonary bypass with general body moderate hypothermia and many use additional profound hypothermia of the heart for cardioplegia. Although there are many variations the technique of perfusion used for the surgical correction of Fallot's tetralogy in a dog [5] is typical of modern methods.

After heparinization (3 mg/kg) cardiopulmonary bypass is begun without arrest of the patient's own circulation and systemic cooling to 32°C is instituted as soon as bypass is established. Once the desired body temperature is reached IPPV is discontinued and a left ventricular vent is placed through the apex of the ventricle. The caval snares are then drawn tight and the aorta cross-clamped to institute total bypass. The heart is electrically fibrillated with low voltage alternating current shock and perfusion of the aortic root with a cold cardioplegic solution causes rapid arrest of the heart in diastole. At the same time external cardiac cooling is commenced via a recirculation cooling system using cold saline. The cardioplegic solution contains potassium, calcium, magnesium, bicarbonate, heparin and procaine, and is administered at 15°C. The cardiac muscle usually cools to about 18°C and is then completely flaccid. This gives at least 30 minutes' operating time.

Rewarming is accomplished by removing the clamp from the aorta and allowing blood, warmed in the pump-oxygenator, to perfuse the animal, including, of course, the coronary circulation. The myocardium recovers in 10–20 minutes, coarse fibrillation being observed. This fibrillation is converted to normal activity by the application of a direct current shock of about 45 J applied directly to the heart, and the caval snares are released. Supportive bypass is maintained while sodium bicarbonate (1 mmol/kg) is given and attempts are made to adjust the right atrial pressure to about 5 mmHg (0.7 kPa). Supportive bypass is then discontinued and protamine sulphate is given over a 10 minute period while blood is tranfused from the heart–lung machine into the animal to maintain

the right atrial pressure, and further bicarbonate is given as necessary to correct acidosis. Any tendency to hypotension in spite of an adequate right atrial pressure is treated by the infusion of a weak solution of adrenaline (1:50 000 in Hartmann's solution) given at the rate of two to three drops per minute, or administered by an infusion pump.

Oxygenators

The most common type of oxygenator is the bubble oxygenator and damage to blood cells can occur at the blood–gas interface. Membrane oxygenators are similar to the physiological arrangements in the lungs as the prefusion fluid and gases are separated by a membrane. Membrane oxygenators cause less haemolysis and higher platelet and white cell counts are obtained than when bubble oxygenators are used and although they are more expensive they offer advantages for lengthy procedures.

Postoperative care

All animals subjected to open heart surgery with cardiopulmonary bypass should be treated in an intensive care unit with continuous nursing attention for at least the first 24 hours. During this time the arterial and venous pressures, the heart and respiratory rates, and the P_aO_2 and P_aCO_2 should be measured and recorded at 30 minute intervals and a continuous watch should be kept on the ECG and the urinary output.

Surgical bleeding is not uncommon and treatment may require reopening of the chest. Although the pericardium is seldom sutured, cardiac tamponade should be suspected when the arterial pressure is low, the central venous pressure is high and the urinary output poor. If clotting studies produce normal results, any animals which continue to bleed from the skin wound or into the chest require surgical re-exploration.

Poor tissue perfusion, low output states and massive blood replacement together with lung collapse may all lead to acid–base changes necessitating the administration of sodium bicarbonate.

Emboli may be introduced into the circulation at any time during bypass and surgery. They may be particles of silicone antifoam from the oxygenator, air or oxygen, or tissue debris. The most important results of such embolism are neurological and it can produce anything from transient monoplegia to total brain death.

Sedation and pain relief are particularly important for the facilitation of nursing care in the first 24 hours after surgery and intravenous frusemide (1 mg/kg) may have to be given to prompt a satisfactory urinary output. Chest drains are usually removed some 24–36 hours after operation and it may be necessary to administer concentrated plasma to counteract the effects of haemodilution at the time of bypass if oedema develops in the postoperative period.

INSERTION OF PACEMAKERS

Pacemakers are devices which ensure that the heart beats sufficient times per minute, regardless of the intrinsic rhythmic activity. They are inserted for different types of conduction deficit and usually only when the animal is showing symptoms.

Temporary pacemakers have wires passed through the veins to rest in the right ventricle. There are some needle electrodes which can be inserted into the myocardium via the chest wall but these are for emergency use only. Oesophageal pacing is also possible. Permanent pacemakers are frequently inserted under general anaesthesia. The pacing wire passes via the jugular vein and tricuspid valve to the right ventricle where it is anchored to the trabeculae by some kind of hook. A subcutaneous pocket is then constructed for the 'pacemaker box' or it is placed in the abdomen. They are powered by various types of battery. Less commonly, permanent pacemakers are implanted into the epicardium via a mini-thoracotomy.

Pacemakers have one of three modes of operation. They may be fixed rate and have the advantage of simplicity but are now seldom used (Fig. 19.3). Demand pacemakers have the ability to suppress pacemaker activity if the heart rate is adequate but cut in if the rate falls below a pre-set minimum; they are the most common kind. Sequential pacemakers are complex with atrial and ventricular electrodes, usually fired by the P wave of the electrocardiogram; they have not been used in veterinary medicine.

Anaesthesia for the fitting of pacemakers usually presents no difficulty but the surgeon should avoid the use of diathermy and the pulse should be monitored by a precordial or oesophageal stethoscope, or a peripheral pulse monitor which is not obliterated by electrical interference. It is advisable to have an isoprenaline infusion ready for use should bradycardia develop in the anaesthetized animal before the pacemaker can be made operational.

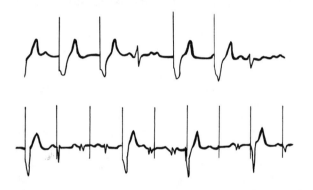

Fig. 19.3 Top: ECG with demand pacemaker. These have an internal ability to suppress pacemaker activity if there is an adequate heart rate but 'cut in' if the rate falls below a preset minimum. Bottom: ECG with fixed rate pacemaker — these are seldom used today. ECG complexes are usually abnormal during pacemaker function because of depolarization commencing from an ectopic site.

REFERENCES

1. Walker, R. G. and Hall, L. W. (1965) *Veterinary Record* **77**, 830.
2. Dripps, R. D. (1956) *The Physiology of Induced Hypothermia*, National Research Council Publication No. 451. Washington, DC: National Research Council.
3. Cooper, K. E. (1959) *British Journal of Anaesthesia* **31**, 96.
4. Schneider, H. P. and Pyenson, J. I. (1945) *Journal of the American Veterinary Medical Association* **147**, 828.
5. Hall, L. W. (1981) *Proceedings, Association of Veterinary Anaesthetists of Great Britain and Ireland* **9**, 36.

CHAPTER 20

ACCIDENTS AND EMERGENCIES ASSOCIATED WITH ANAESTHESIA

When the profound physiological changes initiated by drugs used in anaesthesia are considered it is surprising that serious accidents and emergencies are not more common. Familiarity with these drugs can lead to an attitude which may be described as nonchalant and it is easy to forget that the anaesthetic may be a greater hazard to the animal than the operation. During anaesthesia many accidents occur suddenly and the reason for the mishap must be recognized immediately so that the appropriate remedy can be applied at once. Other accidents are less dramatic and their results may only become apparent during the postoperative period. Moreover, one kind of emergency may lead to another. Few serious emergencies are truly sudden in onset; they are the result of the summation of various problems which may have been overlooked. Most disasters can be avoided by critical assessment of the potential hazards of the particular situation and by careful monitoring which enables problems to be detected at an early stage. Nevertheless, prevention is not always possible and serious problems can ensue if the anaesthetist is not always ready to apply the appropriate remedy in any difficult situation which may arise. Anaesthesia is still an art, and there is no substitute for experience, but even the inexperienced anaesthetist can deal successfully with most mishaps if aware of the nature of the more common accidents and emergencies.

The final result of most serious or fatal anaesthetic accidents is that of tissue hypoxia. The brain cells are particularly easily damaged, and even mild hypoxia may result in a loss of intelligence and change in temperament following anaesthesia, whilst a more prolonged insult results in coma, and possibly death. Circulatory arrest is, in North America, termed the '3 minute emergency' signifying that unless (at normal body temperature), cerebral circulation is restored within 3 minutes irreversible brain damage is likely to occur. Hypoxia of the myocardium will reduce myocardial contractility and may, particularly if coupled with hypercapnia, sensitize the heart to other stimuli and result in cardiac arrest. Lack of oxygen will also damage the liver, kidneys and even somatic muscle, both directly and by increasing the particular toxic effects of any anaesthetic used, although the results of such damage will not become obvious until the postoperative period.

In order to ensure that the tissues are adequately oxygenated it is essential that:

1. The blood carries adequate available oxygen
2. An adequate circulation carries this blood to and from the tissues

Most monitoring procedures are directed towards ensuring that this is occurring, and resuscitation is aimed at reinstating the adequate oxygenation and removal of waste products from the tissues. Simple resuscitative measures to ensure this are usually considered under the headings *A* for airway, *B* for breathing and *C* for circulation. Although this categorization is an oversimplification, it provides a basis for establishing a routine for both monitoring and for resuscitation, and is particularly useful for training nursing staff to cope with emergencies until veterinary aid becomes available.

AIRWAY

Respiratory obstruction is generally considered to mean prevention of the free flow of gases within the patient's airway. However, obstruction or excessive resistance within the patient circuit of the anaesthetic machine will have the same result. A conscious or lightly anaesthetized animal responds to obstruction by making frequent violent attempts to breathe, but the short vigorous inspiratory efforts make the situation worse as they increase the resistance created by the obstruction. The response to obstruction in a deeply anaesthetized animal is usually quieter — ventilation simply becoming inadequate. If a patient circuit including a reservoir bag is in use, the best guide to the patency of the airways is the excursion of the reservoir bag, but if it is not, diagnosis of airway obstruction may be difficult. Although complete obstruction is usually obvious, a partial obstruction is more difficult to detect and may result in the insidious onset of hypoxia and hypercapnia.

Causes of respiratory obstruction

In the non-intubated animal respiratory obstruction is usually due to the base of the tongue or the epiglottis coming into contact with the posterior wall of the pharynx. This type of obstruction may be overcome by extending the head and drawing the tongue forwards out of the mouth. In pigs overextension of the head will also cause respiratory obstruction and in these animals care should be taken to keep the head in a normal position in relation to the neck.

Brachycephalic dogs may develop respiratory obstruction due to the ventral border of the soft palate coming into contact with the base of the tongue, for many of these animals are almost unable to breathe through their nostrils. This type of obstruction can only be overcome by endotracheal intubation. The main problem in these breeds occurs during recovery, from the time when the dog will no longer tolerate the endotracheal tube until it is fully conscious and able to maintain its airway. Ideally, anaesthetic agents which ensure a very rapid return to consciousness should be used to reduce this danger time, but spraying of the larynx with local analgesic at the end of the anaesthetic may enable the endotracheal tube to be tolerated for an adequate period.

Large blood clots may accumulate in the pharynx after tonsillectomy, tooth extraction or endotracheal intubation when the tube has been passed through the nostril. These blood clots must be found and removed at the end of the operation. Animals unconscious after mouth, nose and throat operations should be placed in a position of lateral decubitus during the recovery period and kept under observation until fully conscious.

The fact that an endotracheal tube is in the trachea does not necessarily mean that the airway is clear. Endotracheal tubes may kink (particularly if the head is flexed) (Fig. 20.1), they may become blocked with mucous and in the case of cuffed tubes a faulty cuff may actually occlude the end of the tube, or its pressure obliterate the lumen of the tube (Fig. 20.2). An overlong endotracheal tube may pass down one bronchus (usually the right), effectively obstructing the airway to the other lung. Obstruction may also be caused by the animal biting on the tube.

An uncommon but serious cause of respiratory obstruction is impaction of the epiglottis in the glottic opening. This may occur during 'blind' intubation in young horses and sheep, when a soft, flexible

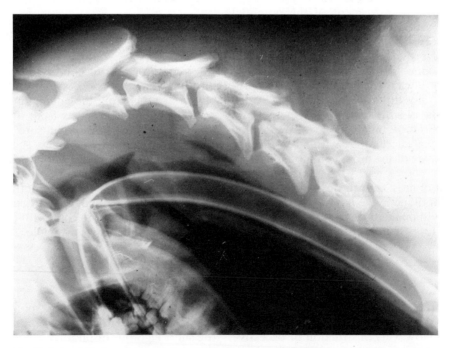

Fig. 20.1 Acute flexion of the neck for radiography leading to kinking of the endotracheal tube with complete obstruction of the airway.

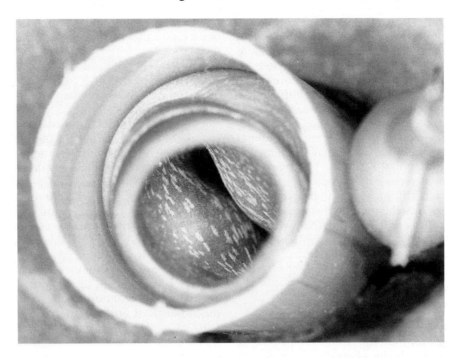

Fig. 20.2 Occlusion of a soft-walled endotracheal tube by overinflation of the cuff forcing the wall inwards until the lumen is almost obliterated. (This picture was obtained by inflating the cuff with the tube inside the barrel of a plastic syringe.)

epiglottis is forced backwards into the laryngeal opening by the forcible passage of an endotracheal tube. Unless the epiglottis is dislodged by the withdrawal of the tube at the end of anaesthesia, it can give rise to serious respiratory obstruction in the recovery period until either coughing occurs, or the cause of the obstruction is diagnosed and overcome by the anaesthetist hooking the epiglottis out of the airway.

In horses, oedema of the upper respiratory passages develops during general anaesthesia if the head is in a dependent position or if the jugular veins are partially occluded for any length of time. This can result in serious respiratory obstruction in the recovery period that can only be relieved by endotracheal intubation, preferably with a tube passed through one nostril.

Animals suffering from laryngeal paralysis or tracheal collapse may obstruct during the recovery period when the increased effort of breathing tends to draw the sides of the larynx and/or the trachea together. As with the brachycephalic breeds, it may be necessary to leave an endotracheal tube in place for longer than would otherwise be done.

Laryngeal and bronchial spasm

Laryngeal spasm appears to be seen more commonly than bronchial spasm, but both conditions can occur together during general anaesthesia. Laryngeal spasm can occur in all kinds of animals but it is perhaps most frequently encountered in cats when attempts are made to force them to breathe high concentrations of an inhalation agent before the protective laryngeal reflexes have been subdued. Another common complication of anaesthesia in cats is laryngeal 'crowing' — the crowing noise being caused by a partial spasm of the vocal cords due to irritation by a blob of mucous, saliva, blood or vomit.

When laryngeal spasm is troublesome the best treatment is to administer a relaxant, in order to relax the spasm, and then to intubate with an endotracheal tube. Attempts at intubation without the aid of relaxants will usually be unsuccessful and will prolong the spasm. Forcible intubation through a closed glottis may result in oedema of the mucous membrane of the larynx and necessitate tracheotomy.

Constriction of the bronchioles or 'bronchial spasm' is uncommon but occasionally seen in all kinds of animal. Ruminants appear to be particularly liable to develop this complication of general anaesthesia. This may well be due to unsuspected regurgitation and inhalation of fluid from the rumen. Bronchial spasm may also be initiated reflexly during light anaesthesia by stimuli from the site of operation and there is some evidence which suggests that the passage through the brain of blood deficient in oxygen and rich in carbon dioxide causes bronchoconstriction.

The first warning sign that bronchial spasm is imminent is a bout of coughing and if an endotracheal tube is not in use the larynx closes. Complete respiratory arrest follows. The chest is rigid and the lungs cannot be inflated by pressure on a rebreathing bag, nor can they be deflated by pressure applied to the chest wall. Cyanosis sets in and is soon replaced by a grey pallor. If ill, the animal may die, but usually the severe hypoxia releases the spasm and the animal gasps. The gasp is followed by normal spontaneous respiration and the animal recovers. Unfortunately bronchial spasm may recur if the stimulus responsible for the first attack is still present. In all cases where bronchial spasm occurs the anaesthetist must ensure that the upper airway is clear and that whenever possible the first gasp of the animal will be of an oxygen-enriched atmosphere.

Aspiration of material from the oesophagus and stomach

This accident probably occurs more frequently than is commonly realized for material from the oesophagus and stomach may reach the pharynx as a result of vomiting or passive regurgitation. In either case the primary problem caused is one of respiratory obstruction, possibly accompanied by bronchospasm if foreign material has penetrated deeply enough into the lungs. Inhalation pneumonia may follow over the next few days.

Vomiting is an active process which occurs in light anaesthesia either during induction or recovery. It is often preceded by swallowing or 'gagging' movements.

When vomiting occurs, the protective mechanisms of laryngeal closure, coughing and breath holding are present, and the accident should not have serious consequences. All that is necessary is for the anaesthetist to clear the pharynx of the vomited material, by swabbing or suction, and to allow the animal to cough vigorously before proceeding with further administration of the anaesthetic. The dog, however, has very weak protective reflexes and in a few cases, particularly where vomiting occurs during the recovery period and the dog is still sleepy, these reflexes fail and the food material is inhaled. In such a case it may even prove necessary to reanaesthetize the animal in order to use vigorous suction to clear the tracheobronchial tree.

It is obvious that if anaesthetics are not given to animals whose stomachs might contain food then aspiration is unlikely to occur, but this is counsel of perfection which cannot always be realized in veterinary practice. Clearly it can never be achieved in ruminants and in simple stomached animals the stomach may contain material many hours after the eating of a meal, particularly if an accident has occurred in the meanwhile or if the animal has gone into labour.

Passive regurgitation is most commonly seen in ruminant animals but it also occurs in horses, pigs, dogs and cats. It usually happens when the animal is in a head-down position, or lying horizontally on its side, and relaxation is induced by deep anaesthesia or the use of relaxant drugs. In these circumstances the protective reflexes are not active and aspiration occurs all too readily. In deeply anaesthetized ruminants any increase in intra-abdominal pressure will force fluid ingesta up the oesophagus into the pharynx, and this regurgitation is frequently seen in adult cattle when anaesthesia is induced with a small, rapidly injected dose of thiopentone sodium. To prevent regurgitation in cases of equine surgical colic the stomach should be decompressed by the passage of a stomach tube prior to the induction of anaesthesia. It is almost impossible to pass a tube into the stomach of an anaesthetized horse (p. 210).

In cases of oesophageal dilation or obstruction there may be an accumulation of fluid on the oesophagus, while the stomach may contain fluid material if there is an obstruction of the pylorus or small intestine.

The most certain practical way of preventing the aspiration of material from the oesophagus and stomach is to perform endotracheal intubation with a cuffed tube immediately anaesthesia has been induced. In the case of small animals, keeping the head raised after induction of anaesthesia until the trachea is intubated and the cuff inflated will completely prevent the danger of inhalation from passive regurgitation, but this is obviously not practicable in the ruminant.

Often, the first sign that aspiration has occurred is the unexpected appearance of cyanosis, dyspnoea and tachycardia. Obviously the severity of the condition depends on the quantity of fluid aspirated and the extent of the lung area involved.

Immediate treatment consists of thorough aspiration of the tracheobronchial tree — although this is more easily advised than performed. Oxygen should be administered and attention directed towards the relief of bronchiolar spasm. If, after operation, the animal develops bronchopneumonia the appropriate treatment must be instituted (antibiotics, etc.).

Emergency tracheostomy

The obvious treatment of respiratory obstruction is to locate the obstruction and remove it, but this is not always possible and occasionally an emergency tracheostomy is required to save the animal's life. In a cat, a 14 gauge needle or catheter, placed

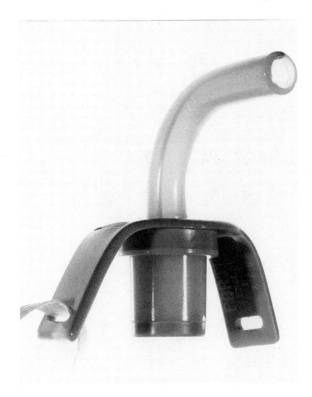

Fig. 20.3 'Portex' disposable tracheostomy tube. This type of tube is suitable for dogs, cats, sheep, goats and small calves.

percutaneously directly into the trachea, provides an adequate airway in the short term, and 10 gauge catheters may be used in a similar manner in dogs up to medium size. In all but small dogs the size of such an airway is totally inadequate for any length of time, but may be sufficient to sustain life whilst a tracheostomy is carried out. Curved plastic tracheostomy tubes or cannulae (Fig. 20.3) are available in sizes suitable for most dogs, and are inserted through the cricothyroid membrane, between two tracheal rings, or by slitting a tracheal ring longitudinally. Once such a tracheostomy tube is in place in a dog, the patient should be under constant observation as the tube may become dislodged or blocked by folds of skin, secretions, or the dog flexing its neck.

In the horse, tracheostomy is much easier to carry out, and if necessary can provide a safe airway for a long period of time. In emergency, or for short-term use, narrow curved tubes are used (Fig. 20.4). On superficial examination these tubes appear to provide far too small an airway, but they are fully effective in such situations.

For more prolonged use a tracheostomy tube which can be removed and cleaned is employed.

It must be pointed out that the need for an emergency tracheostomy is rare. In the cat it is required because of severe, persistent laryngeal spasm, but in most other species it is made necessary by pathological obstructions of the airway which prevent endotracheal intubation. In many cases, therefore, the requirement can be foreseen and equipment for tracheostomy kept readily available.

BREATHING

Respiratory insufficiency and arrest

Apnoea during anaesthesia is very common, and its successful treatment depends on the original cause. Although respiratory arrest is obvious, it is often preceded by respiratory insufficiency, which is much more difficult to assess. In either case, the immediate requirement is that oxygenation of the tissues should be maintained, so that as soon as the problem is noted the anaesthetist should carry out the following routine:

1. Check the airway and, if necessary, take steps to clear it
2. Apply artificial respiration (ensuring there is no anaesthetic in the inspired gas)
3. Check the pulse

Assuming that the circulation is adequate, in the majority of cases these measures should prevent further hypoxia and hypercarbia, and give the anaesthetist time to assess the problem and apply further measures accordingly. The reports from veterinary practices to the Association of Veterinary Anaesthetists of Great Britain and Ireland of anaesthetic emergencies encountered have shown that in the UK the commonest reason for the failure to resuscitate an apnoeic animal is delay in instituting artificial ventilation and it must be emphasized that there are no circumstances in which such ventilation is contraindicated in the treatment of this condition.

Methods of ventilation

The efficiency of artificial ventilation in emergency situations depends on the apparatus available and the size of the patient. Where anaesthetic circuits utilizing reservoir bags are being employed it is possible to ventilate by squeezing the bag, but otherwise resuscitation is more difficult. Self-filling bag/valve units such as the Ambu bag (Fig. 20.5)

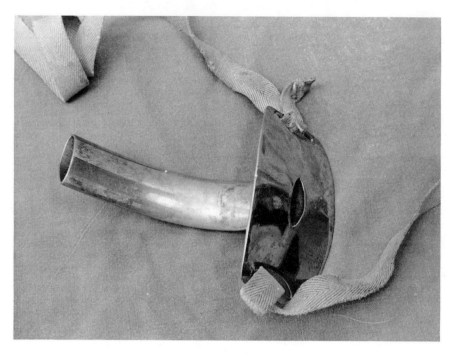

Fig. 20.4 A laryngotomy tube for a horse. These tubes are intended for insertion through the incision should respiratory obstruction develop after a laryngoventriculectomy, but they may be used as emergency tracheostomy tubes because they can be easily slipped through an incision between the tracheal rings.

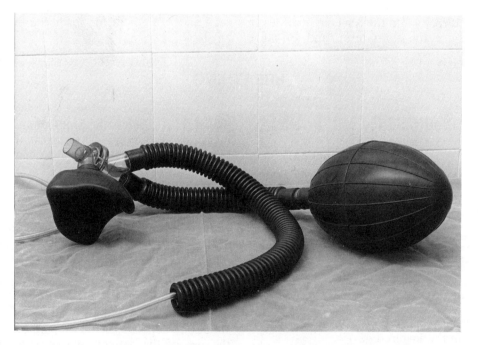

Fig. 20.5 Ambu self-inflating bag for IPPV. If available, oxygen can be given to enrich the inspired air by delivering it through the small-bore plastic tubing.

are useful to ventilate small animals via a non-rebreathing valve attached to a face-mask or an endotracheal tube. Ventilation is with room air but, if it is available, extra oxygen may be added to the inspired gas. Such units are excellent in emergencies away from the operating theatre, and should be part of any portable resuscitation kit for small animals. Outside the operating theatre where only an endotracheal tube may be available, a dog or cat can, in an emergency, be ventilated by a person blowing gently down the tube. With this method, however, inspired oxygen levels are only just adequate (expired air contains about 15% oxygen) and this method is very tiring to perform.

In the absence of any apparatus, small animals can be ventilated by blowing down the nostrils while the mouth is held closed, but the person performing this must produce a seal with his or her lips around the nostrils. In these circumstances the only other method of artificial ventilation, i.e. intermittent pressure on the animal's chest wall, may be preferred. This is totally inadequate in providing adequate respiration for any length of time, but may keep the animal alive for a few minutes. Often, compressing the chest triggers a reflex spontaneous respiration, which is more effective than the original attempt to ventilate.

Reflex stimulation of respiration

Stimulation of the animal in various ways may result in a reflex spontaneous respiration. Such reflex is the 'chest deflation reflex' described above. Movement of the tube in the trachea may also make the animal breathe. Most reflexes, however, are associated with painful input, the most obvious one being the respiratory response to the commencement of surgery. Janssens *et al.* [1] suggest the use of acupuncture to stimulate respiration, and recommends the placing of a needle in the nasal septum. Certainly in cats and dogs that area is extremely sensitive, and its stimulation may trigger reflex respiration, but in lightly anaesthetized animals it may also trigger cardiac arrest. In horses stimulation of respiration by twisting the ear appears more effective. It must be emphasized that adequate artificial respiration must be continued whilst attempts to stimulate respiration are being made.

The common causes of apnoea are listed in Table 20.1. As treatment further to initial immediate artificial ventilation is dependent on the cause of failure, it is essential that the anaesthetist is capable of making the diagnosis.

The most common cause of apnoea is respiratory obstruction or (commonly in horses) too great resistance within the patient circuit. Once the resistance is

Table 20.1 Some causes of respiratory arrest

Common
Obstruction of airway
Resistance in patient breathing circuit
Central depression:
1. from drug overdose
2. from hypoxia and hypercapnia
Breath holding in light anaesthesia

Less common
Hypocapnia from hyperventilation
Mechanical prevention of lung expansion (pathological)
Neuromuscular block
Pain
High spinal or epidural block

removed, spontaneous ventilation resumes. On induction and recovery from anaesthesia the animal may hold its breath for a few seconds, particularly if an endotracheal tube is in place. Examination of the level of consciousness shows very light anaesthesia, and spontaneous respiration resumes rapidly once the endotracheal tube is removed.

Depression of the central nervous system is the most serious common cause of apnoea under anaesthesia. It is particularly serious as it may be accompanied by circulatory inadequacies, so that the pulse must be carefully monitored until recovery occurs. Such depression may be caused by overdoses of anaesthetic agents or by hypoxia of the brain. In either case the animal will be deeply anaesthetized, but estimation of the depth of unconsciousness can be very difficult for the inexperienced anaesthetist. Hypoxia and hypercapnia, from whatever cause, can lead to a jerky form of respiration which may result in jaw and limb movement, leading the unwary into thinking that anaesthesia is light. Gasping respirations of the Cheyne–Stokes last-gasp type may precede apnoea, and again the overall movement of the animal which accompanies these may be misleading. Despite movement, there is, at this stage, no tone in the muscles, and all reflexes show that anaesthesia is, in fact, deep.

Treatment of drug overdoses are best treated by maintaining artificial ventilation until the drug can be eliminated. Where volatile agents have been employed this is simple, as they are removed from the circulation by ventilation, and rapid recovery occurs. Parental agents, however, are more difficult to remove from the circulation. Where the drug has been given by intravenous injection, anaesthesia usually lightens as redistribution of the agent occurs, but where a relative or gross overdose has been administered the only method of increasing excretion may be to increase renal output by means of an intravenous infusion.

Where respiratory depression is due to opioid drugs such as morphine, it may be reversed by the use of specific antagonists. Diprenorphine (Revivon) is the specific antagonist to etorphine, whilst naloxone (Narcan) is the drug in current use to reverse the effect of the other opioid agonists. Naloxone is a pure antagonist, and should have no effects of its own on the animal. The dose required depends on the depth of narcosis to be reversed, and as naloxone is very short acting further doses may be required. Naloxone is most effective against the pure opioid agonists, and is less effective against partial agonists such as buprenorphine. However, in anaesthesia naloxone may be given whenever respiratory failure occurs in an animal which has been given a morphine-like drug either for premedication or during anaesthesia, and to pups born from a bitch given one of these drugs during labour. Overdoses of the α_2-adrenoceptor agonists can, similarly, be treated with antagonists such as yohimbine or atipamezole.

The place of analeptic drugs in the treatment of respiratory failure during anaesthesia is debatable and it is undoubtedly true that an experienced anaesthetist finds it necessary to use such drugs only on rare occasions. However, no anaesthetic drug is perfect and the use of analeptics to counteract the effects of an unintentional overdose, or certain undesirable properties of the anaesthetic drugs, may be regarded as being reasonable once other methods of resuscitation have failed. When overdosage is small, treatment with an analeptic will restore respiratory function and a single dose may overcome all danger. When, however, overdosage has been large, the duration of action of the analeptic may be too transient to restore completely the respiratory activity and respiratory failure may occur. Thus it becomes necessary to maintain a careful watch on the animal until signs of recovering consciousness are evident and should breathing again become alarmingly shallow or cease, repeated doses should be given.

Doxapram hydrochloride (Dopram V) has replaced most of the earlier analeptic drugs. It increases the respiratory minute volume by acting on the respiratory centre and, in general, doses considerably larger than those used clinically must be used before general stimulation results in convulsions. There are reports of its safe and successful use at intravenous doses of 2 mg/kg in a wide range of species [2]. For clinical purposes an initial intravenous dose of 1 mg/kg is usually employed and further doses given if required. Doxapram may also be used by the sublingual route to stimulate respiration in the newborn. Despite the claims as to the specificity of the action on the respiratory centre, in practice, clinical doses are usually found to decrease the levels of unconsciousness of the anaesthetized animal. Whilst this is useful if apnoea is due to central depression, this drug must be used with care in large animals such as horses, where the awakening may be violent.

Normal levels of carbon dioxide in the blood are necessary to maintain spontaneous respiration. However, the role of carbon dioxide in resuscitation in veterinary anaesthesia has been grossly abused. Although a slight increase in carbon dioxide stimulates respiration in the conscious animal, this reflex is considerably reduced under anaesthesia. Further increases in carbon dioxide tension in the blood causing increasing central nervous depression, which will itself eventually result in apnoea. Hypercapnia also sensitizes the heart to arrhythmias and may precipitate cardiac arrest. In the majority of cases apnoea is preceded by respiratory insufficiency and by the time that respiration ceases, hypercapnia already exists. The only circumstances where carbon dioxide is required to stimulate respiration is following hyperventilation, usually after vigorous IPPV. If carbon dioxide is required to correct hypocapnia it is best added to the inspired gas either from cylinders on the anaesthetic machine, or by increasing the deadspace of the patient circuit, as in this way it is possible to continue ventilation and prevent hypoxia from occurring. Artificial ventilation should never be stopped to allow accumulation of carbon dioxide.

Failure to reverse the effects of muscle relaxants used during the anaesthetic technique will result in respiratory failure. Treatment consists of the continuation of artificial ventilation until the relaxant's effects have worn off or been adequately antagonized. Pain, particularly involving the thorax and abdominal regions, may cause hypoventilation in the postoperative period. If opioid analgesics in limited doses are used in such circumstances, the increased ventilation through pain relief is usually greater than any respiratory depression as a direct result of the drug. Other causes of inadequate ventilation include pathological changes in the lung which prevent its aeration, such as space-occupying lesions of the lung or pleural cavity, and bleeding into the substance of the lung.

Normal carbon dioxide tensions are essential for the maintenance of normal tissue perfusion and hypocapnia leads to a decrease in cerebral blood flow. However, severe hypocapnia does not occur in spontaneously breathing animals and the cerebral circulation is only likely to be affected when IPPV is carried out in such a way as to remove excessive amounts of carbon dioxide.

Hypoxaemia

Hypoxaemia can be very difficult to detect as cyanosis, usually considered the commonest sign, may be masked by pigmentation of the skin and mucous membranes, and may not be seen at all in anaemic or shocked animals. Hypoxaemia may result from any of the airway or breathing problems already discussed, or through problems preventing oxygen transfer into the blood. However, assuming ventilation to be adequate, the commonest cause in anaesthesia is an inadequate level of oxygen in the inspired gas as the result of apparatus failure (sometimes to an empty cylinder), an inadequate oxygen input, an accumulation of nitrogen or nitrous oxide in a low-flow circuit, or faulty valves preventing the correct gas circulation around a circle absorber system. Such accidents occur far too commonly, and should be suspected if an animal becomes cyanotic despite an adequate respiratory minute volume and an apparently adequate circulation. Treatment consists of the administration of oxygen, preferably utilizing a simple non-rebreathing patient circuit. However, as long as the animal is breathing spontaneously, simply disconnecting it from the machine and allowing it to breathe room air will usually provide adequate oxygen whilst the fault in the apparatus is located.

Respiratory acidosis

Serious consequences are seen when the minute volume of respiration is decreased since this causes a diminished excretion of carbon dioxide from the lungs and therefore results in the development of respiratory acidosis. This state is commonly seen when the total gas flow rate in a non-rebreathing circuit is too low, or when the soda lime in an absorber is exhausted. It also occurs when the airway is obstructed, or when the respiratory movements are hampered by the position of the animal's body on the bed or operating table. Usually this disturbance of the acid–base balance of the blood results in very little harm when the duration of anaesthesia is short, but it may have serious effects if the anaesthetic period is prolonged. Death occurs when the pH of the blood falls below about 6.7.

The signs of respiratory acidosis are not always obvious. Hypoxaemia may have been avoided by an increase in the inspired oxygen tension so that the animal's mucous membranes remain pink and its pulse slow and of good volume. It is important to note that, although in the normal animal an increase in the alveolar carbon dioxide tension causes a frank increase in the tidal volume, in the anaesthetized animal this may not be seen. The blood pressure first rises, then returns to normal and finally falls. Circulatory failure, when it occurs, is rapid and is due to heart failure. When respiratory acidosis has developed, the animal may collapse at the end of the operation, for the excess carbon dioxide is rapidly excreted as respiratory depression decreases and the circulatory reflexes are not active enough to compensate for the sudden change in the acid–base status of the blood. The condition may be diagnosed as shock, but unlike shock, is characterized by a slow pulse and, in otherwise fit animals, by rapid spontaneous recovery.

CIRCULATION

Failure of the circulation may be due to an inadequate circulatory volume or to primary cardiac insufficiency.

Inadequacy of the circulating fluid volume

Inadequacy of the circulating fluid volume to fill the existing vascular bed may be due to an absolute reduction in blood or body fluid volumes, or to an increase in the vascular space as a result of peripheral vasodilatation. In either case the immediate treatment is to ensure that the animal is lying flat out or in a head-down position to improve venous return and the cerebral circulation, and to administer fluids intravenously as rapidly as possible.

A common cause of circulatory failure under anaesthesia is surgical haemorrhage. There may be a sudden effusion of blood or, more commonly, an almost imperceptible loss over the course of a long operation. Unless blood loss is actually measured by swab weighing or some other technique, it is very difficult to estimate the amount of haemorrhage occurring, and most surgeons tend to underestimate grossly the blood loss they cause. Many of the drugs used in anaesthesia abolish the normal physiological response to haemorrhage, and cardiovascular collapse can occur following even moderate blood loss. For practical clinical purposes an animal can be considered to have a blood volume of 88 ml/kg and when a loss of 10% of this (i.e. 8–9 ml/kg) has occurred infusion of fluid should be commenced.

Where blood loss is not too severe, infusion of crystalloid solutions (in four times the volume needed for a solution which is retained within the circulation) may be adequate until the homeostatic mechanisms come into effect, but when gross and/or rapid loss occurs, compatible whole blood, plasma or a plasma substitute such as one of the gelatine solutions should be given; the quantity and speed of replacement are the factors which determine the fate of the patient. Dextran solutions which are often used in veterinary practice as plasma substitutes should always be used with caution, because the infusion of large quantities of dextran results in failure of the blood-clotting mechanism, and bleeding may be increased.

Fluid deficits which may have arisen in the pre-operative period may lead to circulatory failure under anaesthesia. When the fluid loss is primarily an electrolyte loss, such as seen in vomiting dogs or equine colic cases, circulatory changes are severe and the animal appears shocked. However, in cases where the depletion is primarily of water, the deficit is more difficult to recognize and assess but unless this is done such animals will develop cardiovascular failure following the administration of vasodilator anaesthetic drugs, or following an apparently small blood loss. Also, elderly animals often do not tolerate haemorrhage well. In all these cases deficits should, whenever possible, be corrected before anaesthesia is induced, the only exceptions being cases of intestinal obstruction where it is sufficient to restore only the circulating fluid volume prior to anaesthesia.

Peripheral vasodilatation due to drugs administered during anaesthesia or, more serious, due to endotoxins may lead to circulatory failure but in their absence major changes in the peripheral circulation and the volume of the vascular bed can occur in response to autonomic reflex activity. For example, a sudden fall in blood pressure during an operation sometimes occurs without warning in an animal whose cardiovascular system is apparently healthy and where there has been little loss of blood. The pulse becomes imperceptible, respiration ceases and the veins (noticeably in the tongue) are dilated. The pupils remain normal in size and this may be the only indication that the heart has not stopped beating. This rather alarming reaction appears to be initiated by certain surgical manipulations. For example, it may be seen during caesarean hysterotomies in cattle and sheep when traction is exerted on the mesovarium or on the broad ligament of the uterus. It may also be seen in dogs and cats when swabs or retractors are allowed to press upon the coeliac plexus, or when the stomach and liver are handled by the surgeon. When it arises the surgeon should stop and not recommence operating until recovery has occurred. The reaction may be avoided by gentle surgery and the anaesthetist should note that gentle surgery is only possible when the patient's muscles are adequately relaxed.

Shock

Shock is a caricature of the physiological responses to haemorrhage; the outline of the defensive features remains recognizable but it is exaggerated and distorted to a degree which becomes both absurd and damaging. The major factors in its initiation and maintenance are decreased cardiac output, increased vascular resistance and decreased effective circulating blood volume. Each of these feeds back, either directly or through the sympathetic nervous system, to perpetuate the condition of shock. Reduction in cardiac output leads to increased sympathoadrenal activity which leads in turn to a selective reduction of blood flow in the splanchnic and cutaneous circulations, thereby producing the clinical signs of shock. Hypotension is not a primary manifestation or feature, and only occurs when the increased sympathoadrenal activity fails to compensate for losses in effective circulating blood volume and decreased myocardial contractile force.

The most common and dramatic cause of shock is sudden external haemorrhage, but a similar state can arise if blood is lost internally or if large quantities of electrolytes and water are lost to the body through vomiting and diarrhoea or intestinal obstruction. Nearly all cases of surgical or traumatic shock respond to prompt transfusion and a fatal outcome is usually due to undiagnosed complications such as pneumothorax, fulminating cerebral fat embolism, cardiac tamponade, bilateral adrenal haemorrhage, air embolism or pre-existing cardiac, pulmonary or other diseases, such as diabetes mellitus.

Sometimes, however, shock is unresponsive to treatment and the condition is said to be 'irreversible'. This state is not uncommon in animals suffering from systemic bacterial infection or peritonitis. It can also arise from undertransfusion or too long a delay before replacing fluid losses. Dogs bled until they have become severely hypotensive recover if the blood is replaced within a certain time but after a delay of 2–4 hours transfusion has little or no effect. The animals die and their intestinal mucosa, especially in the ileum, is found to be haemorrhagic and haemorrhages are found under the endocardium and elsewhere.

The processes which lead to irreversibility are complex and difficult to unravel, but if peripheral circulatory failure is the mechanism, then the final common pathway should be found in the microcirculation. It has been suggested that irreversibility begins when ischaemic anoxia changes to stagnant anoxia in certain tissues, and prolonged vasoconstriction is thought to be a key factor. After severe haemorrhage, sympathetic activity and catecholamine secretion produce vasoconstriction and ischaemia anoxia in the splanchnic bed, liver and kidneys. This regional vasoconstriction enables the circulation to be maintained through the unconstricted cerebral and coronary vessels in spite of any reduction in cardiac output. Transfusion at this stage improves cardiac output, relieves hypotension and much of the vasoconstriction, allowing tissue perfusion to be restored. If transfusion is delayed, the constricted arterioles become less and less responsive to adrenaline, apparently due to accumulation of metabolites in the tissues. Eventually the capillaries become engorged and flow stagnates because it is suggested [3] that venules remain constricted. The reason for the persistence of venular spasm when the arterioles become paralysed is not at all clear, however. Capillary engorgement then raises the hydrostatic pressure so that fluid exudes from the capillary beds and oligaemia becomes more severe. Anoxic changes become serious, local haemorrhages appear and the cycle to death begins. Transfusion is now of no avail, because it merely engorges further the stagnant capillary bed. The venous return and the cardiac output continue to fall and the heart stops or fibrillates as the coronary flow is reduced.

Changes in the abdominal viscera and sympathetic activity are of importance in irreversibility as is the endotoxin of Gram-negative bacilli. This toxin is absorbed from the damaged (anoxic) bowel, acts on the nervous system, produces a relentless abdominal sympathetic-induced vasoconstriction, and then cannot be detoxicated because of failure of a reticuloendothelial enzyme in the hypoxic spleen and liver. Endotoxin action certainly has an important adrenergic component; its lethal effect is counteracted by adrenolytic compounds and it potentiates the pressor responses to catecholamines [4, 5].

Vasopressors are much more likely to be harmful than beneficial in shocked animals. The only measures which consistently reduce mortality are those which increase blood volume or reduce vasoconstriction [6] and this leads to the inference that vasodilators may have a place in the treatment of shock. Although not to be used when the blood volume is already reduced and no substitute for correct fluid therapy, there are some encouraging reports that antiadrenergic drugs and other methods of inhibiting sympathetic activity improve survival after haemorrhage or trauma [6], provided further transfusion is also given to cover the increased capacity of the vascular system. It is extremely doubtful if the adrenal cortex plays any part although hydrocortisone (itself a vasodilator) given in massive doses of 50 mg/kg has been used [3]. Such massive doses are impracticable for large animals, but phenylbutazone, in doses of 15 mg/kg, were as effective as corticosteroids in the treatment of endotoxic shock [7]. Unfortunately, the best results are only obtained when these drugs are given before shock actually develops. Flunixin (1 mg/kg, intravenously) is claimed to have a beneficial effect by countering endotoxaemia in equine colic cases. During shock the endogenous opioid β-endorphine is released from the pituitary and it has been suggested that it may contribute to hypotension since this is alleviated by the administration of naloxone. Although the use of naloxone may be efficacious it might also restore pain sensitivity which is usually reduced in shock.

Currently, there are indications that the infusion of small volumes of hypertonic saline may be beneficial in shocked animals. This approach is quite distinct from volume replacement therapy and may be useful in veterinary practice since it necessitates the use of only small volumes of solution. More research is needed to evaluate its real worth.

Much work has been done to establish the best methods of estimating the state of the circulation. Undoubtedly the most useful determinations are measurement of the arterial blood pressure, the central venous pressure and the urinary output. Capillary refilling time and the state of distension of the peripheral veins may also be of assistance.

Obviously, the best treatment for shock is to prevent it from occurring. Early transfusion to restore the blood volume and expeditious operation to arrest bleeding, remove damaged tissue and, if necessary, fix broken bones, will prevent shock from becoming irreversible.

Disturbances of cardiac rhythm

Tachycardia is usual in young animals, but in adults the pulse rate increases in shock or after the administration of anticholinergics. It must be emphasized, too, that in cases where relaxants are being used tachycardia may indicate an insufficient depth of anaesthesia.

Cardiac arrhythmias are common in all kinds of animal under all forms of anaesthesia but they are frequently unrecognized since unless the ECG is continuously displayed the anaesthetist is unlikely to become aware of them.

The origin of these disturbances of cardiac rhythm is still uncertain. If the anaesthetic agent is known to depress the functional capacity of the heart muscle it is natural to assume that the direct action of the drug on the myocardium is the cause, but it is more probable that serious arrhythmias are caused by the action of autonomic nerves to the heart. The nervous system is often hyperactive immediately before operation, especially if the animal is frightened, and stimulation of sympathetic nerves to the heart may cause ventricular ectopic beats or even ventricular fibrillation if the heart muscle is sensitized by anaesthetic agents. Carbon dioxide may accumulate in the body, and mild degrees of hypoxia may cause stimulation of the sympathetic nervous system, so arrhythmias are common when respiration is depressed or obstructed.

Treatment of cardiac arrhythmias will depend on

their cause and an accurate diagnosis can only be made when an electrocardiograph is available. The use of drugs for the treatment of cardiac irregularities is not justified in the absence of an accurate diagnosis. However, during general anaesthesia most cardiac arrhythmias disappear once an adequate respiratory exchange has been established. An unobstructed airway must be ensured and pulmonary ventilation assisted by IPPV whenever respiratory depression is encountered.

Heart failure

There are two distinct types of heart failure: the first is ventricular fibrillation, the second is ventricular asystole, frequently termed 'arrest of the heart'.

The causes of heart failure are numerous and in any one case it is likely that several factors may be implicated but in the majority of cases hypoxia and hypercapnia contribute significantly to its occurrence. Fibrillation is more common under conditions of oxygen lack (e.g. in shocked or anaemic animals). Cardiac arrest or asystole is the type of heart failure associated with overdosage of anaesthetic agents. Gross overdosage is probably rare, but relative overdosage is more frequent (e.g. the use of normal doses or concentrations of anaesthetic agents in old or debilitated animals).

Cardiac arrest of neurogenic origin, usually stimulation of the vagus nerves, is the exception to the general rule of multiple causation. Where the surgeon stimulates the vagus nerve, either directly or by initiating a reflex such as the oculocardiac, the heart may stop with no prior warning. Such a cardiac arrest can only be detected by continuous palpation of the pulse, or with an electrocardiograph, as the suddenness of the cessation of circulation means that the tissues are initially well oxygenated, the mucous membranes remain pink, and spontaneous respiration may continue for 2–3 minutes until the respiratory centres become anoxic. By the time respiration has ceased and the pupil has dilated, cerebral hypoxia makes successful resuscitation much more difficult. The horse and the cat are the species of animal most sensitive to vagal arrest of the heart and they should be protected by the administration of anticholinergics prior to surgery in the head and neck regions.

If counter-measures are to be successful, diagnosis of heart failure must be rapid. Where, as may happen during anaesthesia, circulatory arrest has been preceded by respiratory or circulatory insufficiency, the brain may already be hypoxic when the crisis occurs and in these circumstances even less time is available in which to restore an effective cerebral circulation.

Diagnosis of circulatory arrest

Diagnosis of circulatory arrest is based on the absence of a peripheral pulse, absence of heart sounds, and ashen-coloured mucous membranes. The surgeon will notice an absence of bleeding from the wound but the anaesthetist should have diagnosed the condition before this is obvious. These signs are closely followed by wide dilatation of the pupil and either agonal gasping or apnoea. It must be remembered that respiration does not cease immediately the circulation fails, but continues until the respiratory centres become anoxic.

Treatment

Conservative treatment is not only useless but also wastes valuable time. The only way of restoring an effective circulation is the immediate institution of resuscitative measures. Once an effective circulation has been produced, the immediate danger is over.

There are two ways of attempting to provide an effective circulation to the brain and myocardium. One, and the first that should be tried, is chest compression; the second is direct compression of the surgically exposed heart. The use of cardiac stimulant drugs should not be considered until the myocardium is once more well oxygenated and, therefore, they have no place in the initial treatment.

The veterinary anaesthetist should have a simple, set routine for the treatment of circulatory arrest,

Table 20.2 Cardiac resuscitation routine

Stage 1: *establishment of an artificial circulation*
1. Notify surgeon and note time
2. Clear and maintain airway
3. Ventilate (if possible with O_2)
4. External compression; if ineffective, internal massage
5. Where possible, maintain in head-down position

Stage 2: (this is sometimes left until after Stage 3)
Infuse fluid to restore or maintain circulating volume

Stage 3: *restoration of normal cardiac rhythm*

Heart in	
Asystole	*Ventricular fibrillation*
Adrenaline i.v., i.t.	Electrical defibrillation or Lignocaine i.v.

Stage 4: *post-resuscitation*
1. Continue pulmonary ventilation
2. Counteract acidosis — hyperventilate or give sodium bicarbonate
3. Prevent cerebral oedema — corticosteroids, diuretics
4. Circulatory support as needed — adrenaline
   dopexamine
   dopamine
   dobutamine

which is known to all those working in the theatre or recovery unit. Table 20.2 sets out such a routine.

As soon as circulatory arrest is detected, the anaesthetist should inform the surgeon and stop the administration of any anaesthetic; a clear airway must be ensured and IPPV instituted, preferably with oxygen. At the same time external chest compression (see below) should be commenced in order to improve the venous return to the heart; whenever possible the animal should be placed in a head-down position. The effectiveness of chest compression may be judged by the presence of a palpable carotid pulse caused by each compression and a reduction in the diameter of the pupil. If chest compression does not prove to be effective, then direct cardiac compression via a thoracotomy must be considered.

Effective external chest compression is possible in most animals although it is probable that except in cats and other small animals this will not compress the heart itself (see below). In cats and small dogs the chest walls over the region of the heart are compressed between the fingers and the thumb of one hand. Larger animals are quickly placed on their side on a hard, unyielding surface. The upper chest wall over the region of the heart is then forced inward and allowed to recoil outwards, movement of the lower chest wall being restricted by the hard surface on which the animal is lying. It is an advantage if the lower chest wall can be supported. In dogs and other small animals pressure on the uppermost chest wall with the hand is adequate, but in adult horses and cattle the knee or foot is used. The rate of compression should be about 60 compressions/min in dogs, or 30 compressions/min in adult horses and cattle. A remarkably effective circulation can be maintained in this way (Fig. 20.6). Regular respiratory movements

may return, although they are usually inadequate to provide proper gaseous exchange and it is inadvisable to cease IPPV. The size of the pupils should decrease and the level of unconsciousness should lighten. The authors have seen a horse start to recover consciousness and to move its limbs while thoracic compression was being performed.

The way in which external chest compression produces blood flow in the body is somewhat debatable. It was initially thought that when the chest was compressed the heart was squeezed, so ejecting blood into the aorta. This may be so in small animals, particularly in cats and narrow-chested dogs where it is usually possible to feel the resistance to compression of the ventricles through the compliant chest wall but it is unlikely to occur in larger animals. Recent evidence [8] suggests that blood flow is induced by intrathoracic pressure changes, pushing blood in a retrograde and forward fashion, but due to the presence of the valves and the collapse of veins, retrograde flow is stopped early on and blood is allowed to flow into the aorta. The flow of blood through the lungs is thought to be due to a cascade effect between the right and left sides of the heart but emptying of the lungs is also augmented by pulmonary ventilation.

Several techniques have been advocated for improving the pulmonary pump mechanism. The first is to bind the abdomen with an Esmarch bandage to limit the caudal displacement of the diaphragm and hence increase the intrathoracic pressure during chest compression. The second is to alternate compression of the chest and abdomen but this gives rise to risk of damage to abdominal viscera such as the liver. A third technique is to limit the collapse of the lungs during compression by ventilating as the compression is applied. None of these techniques have been shown to improve survival in veterinary clinical practice.

Fibrillation may be present when circulatory arrest occurs or may be precipitated in an asystolic heart by the effects of drugs or even chest compression. The best and most specific treatment is to pass an electric shock through the myocardium so that when the contraction which this causes passes off the whole muscle remains in a relaxed state of asystole. Then, it is hoped, normal contractions will start spontaneously. Electrical defibrillation attempts will do no harm to a heart that is in asystole and may even induce it to start beating, so applying a shock, or shocks, is now regarded as one of the first measures to be undertaken in cases of cardiac failure during anaesthesia and time should not be wasted in applying ECG leads for diagnostic purposes.

Electrical defibrillation should, however, only be attempted with properly constructed apparatus;

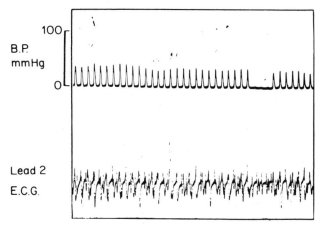

Fig. 20.6 Tracing showing the carotid arterial pressure produced by chest compression in a dog suffering from coarse ventricular fibrillation.

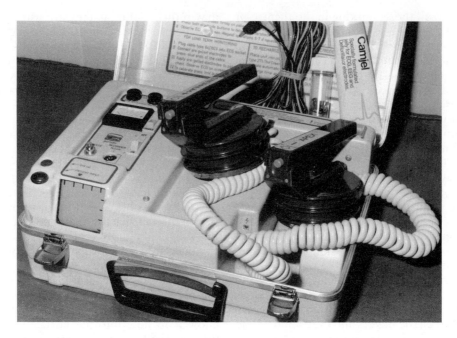

Fig. 20.7 Typical defibrillator for external use. Note that for reasons of safety both of the electrodes have switches in their insulated handles. These switches need to be pressed simultaneously to deliver the shock. This particular model of defibrillator has its own monitor ECG.

improvised apparatus connected to the mains supply of electricity is most dangerous.

Compact and relatively inexpensive apparatus is now available for external defibrillation (electrodes placed on the chest wall (Fig. 20.7)) and internal use (electrodes placed on the myocardium itself). All these pieces of apparatus are designed for man and they are suitable for use in small animals but their output may be inadequate for large animal use unless repeated shocks are given.

For defibrillation through an intact chest wall, with good electrode contact assured by conducting gel, shocks of about 1 J are necessary in cats, from 1 to 8 J in dogs and 400 J (repeated shocks at 15 second intervals) in horses and cattle. When the electrodes are applied over saline-soaked pads directly on the myocardium shocks of about 0.2 J/kg appear effective in most cases. Attempts at electrical defibrillation are much more likely to be successful if the myocardium is coarsely fibrillating and well oxygenated before the shock is applied.

If an effective circulation cannot be produced by external chest compression coupled with electrical defibrillation, then the heart must be exposed by a thoracotomy incision. Obviously, facilities for IPPV must be available before this can be done.

No time should be lost in 'scrubbing up' or in preparing the site before making an intercostal incision and when the heart is exposed the ventricles

must be squeezed rhythmically. The squeezing should be carried out with a motion from the apex towards the base of the heart (rather like the reverse of hand milking of a cow's teat). The rate of compression should not be too rapid for the chambers must have time to fill with blood between compressions and a slight head-down inclination of the body aids the filling of the heart. In small animals the ventricles can be compressed by the grasp of one hand but in larger animals both hands must be used. In every case care must be taken to avoid rupture of the heart by the fingertips. The effectiveness of artificial circulation produced by the massage may be gauged by the maintenance of a small pupil size indicating that the cerebral circulation is adequate.

Often, when the chest is opened because external compression is proving to be ineffective it is found that the venous return is not sufficient to fill the heart between compressions, indicating that the reason for the cardiac failure was hypovolaemia, and in these circumstances direct cardiac compression is also ineffective until an infusion has corrected the deficit in the blood volume.

Once an artificial circulation has been established there is no longer any necessity for haste and there is time for a considered approach. Ideally, as soon as the primary resuscitative measures have been commenced intravenous fluids should be given to expand the circulatory volume. Where cardiac failure is of unknown origin, 5% dextrose is used, but if haemorrhage caused the problem, then a plasma volume expander such as a gelatine solution is to be preferred. However, in veterinary anaesthesia there may be no venous line in place and so this may be a counsel of perfection as venepuncture is usually very difficult at this time. Attempts to set up an intravenous infusion should not interfere with resuscitation and, if impracticable, should be left to later on when the situation is more stable.

In the past bicarbonate was often administered at this stage to counteract the acidosis which occurs as a result of hypoxia. However, its use is controversial and, today, the consensus of opinion appears to be that acidosis should be counteracted by deliberate hyperventilation of the lungs. This avoids the risk of alkalosis due to too much bicarbonate provoking arrhythmias and resulting in intractible ventricular fibrillation.

Although calcium chloride was formerly often used, adrenaline is now generally considered to be the cardiac stimulant of choice. Treatment with adrenaline will do no further harm to a fibrillating heart and indeed Safar [9] reports that, against all theoretical considerations, it may even be successful in restoring normal rhythm. It acts at the α- and β-sympathetic receptors, not only stimulating the myocardium but also increasing peripheral resistance and hence improving coronary perfusion. An initial dose of 10 μg/kg should be given and the action of the drug is short lived so that further doses are often required every 3–4 minutes. It may be given intravenously or into the trachea (although it is less effective when given in this way). Attempts to inject directly into the ventricles are inadvisable since coronary vessels may be damaged.

When an electrical defibrillator is not available lignocaine hydrochloride in doses of 1 mg/kg may be injected intravenously and massage continued to force it into the coronary vessels. At this dose lignocaine depresses cardiac excitability and prolongs the refractory period of heart muscle, but it also decreases myocardial contractility. Although worth trying, experience has shown that its use is only seldom successful in stopping ventricular fibrillation.

Ventilation of the lungs with oxygen should be continued until all evidence of circulatory failure has vanished. At this stage, there will be a metabolic acidosis due to the products of anaerobic metabolism in the peripheral tissues being returned to the circulation.

Bradycardia with heart block is common following restoration of the circulation after prolonged myocardial hypoxia. This bradycardia is usually refractory to treatment with atropine and many cases do not respond to sympathomimetic drugs so electrical pac-

ing of the heart may offer the only hope of successful treatment. In veterinary practice electrical pacemakers are unlikely to be readily available but even if they are it is always worth trying the effects of a slow infusion of 1:50 000 adrenaline before considering their use. External pacing of the heart uses voltages of 100–150 V and frequently leads to skin burns at the site of the electrodes, so that internal pacing using 3–5 V from a wire electrode passed from the jugular vein into the right ventricular chamber is to be much preferred.

If, in spite of transfusion to a satisfactory right atrial filling pressure (as shown by a central venous pressure of 6–7 mmHg, and distension of peripheral veins), the spontaneous heart beat is incapable of maintaining an adequate cardiac output and arterial blood pressure, inotropic support should be given. Dopamine is claimed to have the advantage that it improves renal blood flow by stimulation of renal dopamine receptors and is a relatively safe inotropic drug. Dobutamine, on the other hand, is a pure β_1 agonist which is said to work primarily by improving stroke volume rather than heart rate. Isoprenaline, another β agonist, also improves cardiac output but causes a marked tachycardia. Adrenaline (1:50 000 in Hartmann's solution) given at the rate of 0.02 ml/kg/min or as necessary to maintain systolic arterial pressure of about 120 mmHg, is probably the drug of choice. Once inotropic support has been started it cannot be withdrawn abruptly and careful weaning is necessary, usually over a period of several hours.

Cerebral oedema is not uncommon due to hypoxia during the circulatory arrest and animals which have apparently been successfully resuscitated may lapse into unconsciousness some hours later. To limit this oedema, the resuscitated animal should be given large intravenous doses of corticosteroids (e.g. 1 mg/kg methylprednisolone, every 6 hours for four doses) and diuretics such as sucrose, mannitol or frusemide. If the animal is in normal fluid balance frusemide is to be preferred since it reduces cerebral oedema both by causing a decrease in cerebrospinal fluid production and an increase in its clearance [9].

The greater the time necessary to restore spontaneous circulation, the poorer the prognosis, but at Cambridge there have been a few animals successfully resuscitated after efforts lasting over 40 minutes. The heart is more resistant to the effects of hypoxia than is the brain so that if the heart does not respond to resuscitative measures it is likely that cerebral function will be severely compromised. Usually, it is not worth attempting resuscitation on an animal that has had no effective circulation for more 5 minutes unless it is very hypothermic or has become so during general anaesthesia.

EMERGENCY RESUSCITATION EQUIPMENT

In the operating theatre, most animals are routinely intubated and facilities for airway and ventilation control are available on the anaesthetic machine. An emergency trolley for use in the operating theatre should carry syringes and needles; a fluid administration set and intravenous cannulae; several bags of infusion fluids, and the drugs necessary for the treatment of cardiac arrest. Whenever possible the kit should include a cardiac defibrillator and electrocardioscope. All drugs ampoules and bottles should be clearly labelled with the doses, in terms of volumes of solution, required for the size of animal — in an emergency there is no time to calculate the doses from those given on the data sheets in milligrams per kilogram. Where a drug such as adrenaline needs to be diluted this should also be clearly indicated. In general, drugs on the emergency trolley should be kept to a minimum, e.g. adrenaline, lignocaine, atropine and naloxone. Other drugs such as vaso-pressors, cardiac stimulants, β-blocking agents and diuretics, are best kept on a second shelf or in a drawer of the trolley so that identification problems do not arise at the time of greatest emergency.

Because the success of resuscitation depends greatly on the speed and efficiency with which it is applied it is advisable to have a basic resuscitation kit available wherever animals are recovering from anaesthesia. The actual requirements depend on the species of animal concerned and on the particular circumstances. Airway problems are likely to be important and the kit should contain endotracheal tubes, laryngoscope and a self-inflating bag (e.g. an Ambu bag, Fig. 20.5). Some drugs such as adrenaline and naloxone should be included with a suitable range of needles and syringes, and a bag of intravenous infusion fluid together with an administration set may be thought to be worthwhile.

HYPOTHERMIA AND HYPERTHERMIA

Although body temperature may rise during anaesthesia, hypothermia is much more commonly encountered. Whenever return to consciousness is unexpectedly delayed hypothermia should be suspected and to detect its development the oesophageal temperature should be monitored (p. 33). Waterman [10] has reviewed the causes, effects and prevention of hypothermia. Basically, the causes consist of a reduction in heat production by the animal coupled with an increased heat loss. It is very difficult to influence the heat production, but Waterman recommends several methods of reducing heat loss. She suggests that care should be taken not to wet the animal excessively to reduce evaporative heat losses, placing the animal on a warm surface, preferably a water blanket heated to 38°C (Fig. 20.8), and keeping the drapes over the animal as dry as possible. Ambient room temperature should be kept high but not so high as to make for impossible working conditions (20–22°C is usually satisfactory). Respiratory heat losses are increased when the animal breathes cold dry gas from non-rebreathing systems. Although such losses are reduced by the use of rebreathing circuits, the use of these circuits offers too much resistance to breathing for the small animals which are most at risk from hypothermia. In these small animals a suitable humidifier can be used to reduce heat losses [11]. Particularly in small animals, all infusion fluids should be heated to 38°C using an electric fluid warmer or by letting them flow through a coil of tubing immersed in a basin of warm water.

With the smallest of animals hypothermia is a very serious problem, but it may be the cause of slow recovery from anaesthesia in any dog or cat. Should it occur, it is easily treated by warming the patient, but many hypothermic animals will shiver violently in the recovery period and this causes a considerable increase in oxygen consumption so that the administration of oxygen should be considered in addition to the provision of warmth.

Hyperthermia, or heat stroke, is an unusual complication of anaesthesia. It may, however, occur in a warm environment if small animals are anaesthetized using a low-flow system with absorption of carbon dioxide, thus preventing them from losing heat by panting and the evaporation of water from the respiratory tract. Treatment is to change the system to one which delivers cold dry gases, to cool the animal with ice-packs and cold water applications and, if necessary, to administer drugs which cause vasodilatation. Active treatment should be discontinued when the body temperature is still 1°C above normal or it may overshoot in a most disconcerting way. Hyperthermia will, of course, also occur in pathological sensitivity reactions such as porcine malignant hyperthermia.

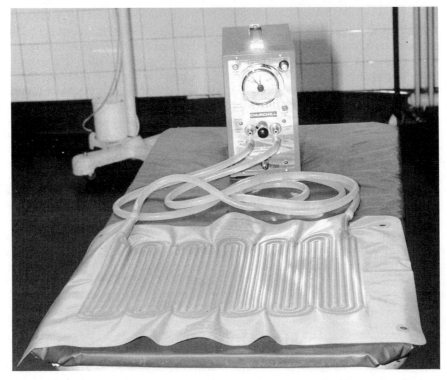

Fig. 20.8 Circulating pump and water blanket for use in small animal patients.

ACCIDENTS ASSOCIATED WITH POSTURE

All anaesthetized animals should be moved with great care to ensure that they are adequately supported at all times. In small animals, mishandling of the patient can, for example, result in the protrusion of a calcified invertebral disc. The arthritic patient, if mishandled, may appear to be in considerable pain for several days following anaesthesia for purposes unassociated with its joints. The problems in large animals may be even more serious. If the hind-legs of horses and cattle are abducted during anaesthesia obturator paralysis may result so that the animal is unable to regain the standing position on recovery. The facial nerve of the horse is easily damaged by pressure on the face from the buckle of a head-collar or the edge of an operating table, with consequent facial paralysis. Ischaemic muscle damage in horses has already been considered (p. 204) and these animals appear to suffer intense pain from this condition.

The position of the animal during operation must always be given careful consideration; pressure points may need to be protected by suitable padding, and limbs should never be held abducted but always restrained forward or backwards.

ANAESTHETIC EXPLOSIONS AND FIRES

Probably the main cause of explosions in operating rooms used to be static electricity, and it is very difficult to ensure that conditions are always such that a dangerous discharge of static electricity is absolutely impossible. However, other more obvious causes, such as smoking and the use of gas and electric fires in locations where flammable anaesthetics are used, can easily be eliminated. Today, with the almost universal use of non-flammable and non-explosive anaesthetic agents, fires in the operating theatre are generally associated with the use of diathermy and alcoholic skin disinfectants by surgeons. It must be remembered that many substances will burn in oxygen and, therefore, that no oil or grease must be used on oxygen cylinder connections.

ACCIDENTS ASSOCIATED WITH INTRAVENOUS INJECTIONS

The commonest mishap associated with the performance of an intravenous injection is the accidental injection of an irritant solution such as guaiphenesin or thiopentone sodium into the perivascular tissues. When this happens the injected irritant solution should be diluted by the immediate injection of a large volume of saline into the site. Hyaluronidase may be dissolved in the saline and this enzyme will hasten the absorption of the irritant drug. No other treatment is required. It is often suggested that a local analgesic such as lignocaine should be injected into the site of extravasation because solutions of these drugs have a low pH that counteracts the high pH of solutions of thiopentone, but it is likely that any beneficial effect noted is due to the vasodilation they produce. The injection of solutions of them containing vasoconstrictors such as adrenaline does not have any beneficial effect.

Venous thrombosis is common after the injection of 5% solutions of thiopentone sodium but, as it does not appear for 5–10 days, it may be missed unless the anaesthetist has occasion to give another injection after that time. Whenever possible, thiopentone should be used as a 2.5% solution and care should be taken to see that the venous return is not obstructed when the injection is made. Venous obstruction caused by acute flexion of the elbow or unnatural positions of the limbs will result in thiopentone being retained in the limb veins and this may give rise to thrombosis. In horses similar consideration apply to guaiphenesin and care should be taken to ensure that it is not retained in the jugular vein due to obstruction of this vein.

Permanent obliteration of vessels results from repeated, clumsy attempts at venepuncture, the use of unnecessarily large needles, and from allowing large haematomata to form at the site. In animals superficial veins are not too plentiful and their preservation is important.

LOCAL ANALGESIA

Toxic reactions to local analgesic drugs arise when the drugs are absorbed into the general circulation at a rate greater than that at which they can be broken down by the body. Rapid absorption occurs from any hyperaemic or inflamed tissue and the rate of absorption is increased by the use of solutions which contain spreading agents such as hyaluronidase. Accidental intravascular injection may occur even though no blood can be aspirated into the syringe. The rate of absorption is decreased by the addition of vasoconstrictor drugs to the solution.

Local analgesic drugs both stimulate and depress the activity of the central nervous system. Often the toxic effects are manifested by stimulation of one part of the brain while another part is depressed. Obviously the effects will vary according to the area of the brain affected. Cortical stimulation produces generalized clonic convulsions, while stimulatory effects on the medulla cause an increase in the rate and depth of respiration, tachycardia and vomiting. Typical general anaesthesia with respiratory and vasomotor depression usually follows. It is uncertain whether death is due to cardiac or to respiratory failure, but it seems probable that intravascular injection causes sudden primary cardiac failure, while rapid absorption from the tissues results in depression of the central nervous system and respiratory failure (p. 178).

The minimum lethal doses of various agents for the different species of animal encountered in veterinary practice are apparently unknown and it is probable that insufficient attention is given to the quantities of local analgesics used in clinical anaesthesia.

In every case where collapse has occurred after the use of a local analgesic drug artificial respiration must be commenced at once. Analeptic drugs increase the oxygen requirement of the brain and should be withheld. Convulsions should be controlled by the injection of hypnotic doses of short- or ultrashort-acting barbiturates. Any fall in blood pressure due to peripheral or central vasomotor failure may be treated by the intravenous injection of vasopressor drugs such as methoxamine. Primary cardiac failure must be treated by cardiac massage.

COMPLICATIONS ASSOCIATED WITH SPINAL AND EPIDURAL ANALGESIA

Drugs used to produce spinal analgesia may cause a reaction which affects the meninges and nerves. Clinical signs resulting from damage to nerves appear rather rapidly after the effects of the nerve block should have passed off and the nerves and the region of the spinal cord subjected to the greatest concentration of the drug show the most marked pathological changes. Where the main change is to the meninges, clinical signs appear later and the reaction to the drug takes the form of an aseptic meningitis which may be mild or severe. These complications do not appear to be due to faults in technique. Injections of solutions of local analgesic drugs into the substance of the spinal cord produces a severe myelitis and neuritis.

In man, postlumbar puncture headache is a well-known complication and it has been observed that sheep which have been subjected to spinal analgesia behave in a manner which suggests that they too suffer from headache. The headache is believed to be due to a low cerebrospinal fluid pressure caused by leakage of the fluid through the needle puncture in the dura mater. It does not occur after epidural analgesia.

Infection of the epidural space is fortunately rare, but has been reported after caudal epidural block in cattle. The prognosis appears to be better than in those cases in which the infection is within the dura for it usually remains localized. Strict aseptic precautions should be employed whenever a spinal or epidural block is attempted. The rapid injection of a large volume of fluid into the epidural space may cause arching of the back and opisthotonus. This reaction is presumably due to a rapid increase in the pressure in the epidural space and is usually of short duration. No treatment is required.

DANGERS TO THE ANAESTHETIST

Modern drugs are very potent and it is most important that the anaesthetist does not come under their influence. Drugs such as ketamine, the α_2-adrenoceptor agonists or their antagonists, which are normally injected into animals, may be absorbed through the skin or mucous membranes and care should be taken when handling them. Splashing on to the skin, the lips or eyes should be avoided but, if it does occur, immediate, copious irrigation of the site with water is essential to avoid their effects. Gloves should be worn when handling some of the α_2-adrenoceptor antagonists and Immobilon. Syringes and needle cases should *never* be held in the mouth (which appears to be a common practice under field conditions) because their exterior surface may have been contaminated with the drug while it was being drawn up and any air expelled from the syringe.

Although not constituting an emergency or accident the dangers of exposure of the anaesthetist and operating room personnel to trace concentrations of the inhalation anaesthetics should be noted. In the UK, the Department of Health [12] has advised that reasonable measures should be taken both to reduce the risk of serious contamination of the atmosphere with inhalation anaesthetics and to remind operating theatre staff of possible hazards. Scavenging devices should be provided and any female who is or who plans to become pregnant should not work in areas where inhalation anaesthetics are used. Similar, but much more elaborate, recommendations have been published in the USA (National Institute of Occupational Safety and Health, 1977) [13] and upper limits of acceptable contamination have been suggested, although these seem to be quite arbitrary.

The control of atmospheric pollution in veterinary practice has been well reviewed by Jones [14] and few would disagree with his conclusion that room ventilation is *not* the answer to the problem.

Sensible, simple measures which can be taken in veterinary practice to minimize atmospheric pollution include:

1. Vaporizers should always be filled outside the operating theatre and, whenever possible, out-of-doors. When available, proper filling apparatus should be used but if this is not possible funnels should be used to avoid spillage of the liquid anaesthetic.
2. Vaporizers should be turned off when not in use.
3. Strict care should be taken in handling anaesthetic agents and they should not be used for cleaning purposes (especially of clothes!) or skin disinfection.
4. Whenever it is safe and convenient to do so, low-flow systems of administration should be used.
5. Scavenging of waste gases and vapours should be encouraged.
6. Whenever practicable, endotracheal intubation should be practised to prevent atmospheric contamination due to ill-fitting face-masks.
7. Breathing circuits should be checked, regularly, for leaks.

Detailed descriptions of scavenging techniques have been given by Smith [15] and a number of devices are suitable for veterinary purposes but care must be taken to ensure their use does not have an adverse effect on the patient. Passive systems allow the expired gases to be driven by the animal's own breathing efforts and should not involve long pipe runs because of the resistance to gas flow which may arise. Active systems suck the gas out along a pipe by the use of flow inducers such as fans, pumps and injectors. Activated-charcoal containers are also available for removing vapours such as halothane from the exhaled gases and they can be useful in practices where nitrous oxide, which they do not absorb, is not used.

REFERENCES

1. Janssens, L., Altman, S. and Rogers, P. A. M. (1979) *Veterinary Record* **105,** 273.
2. Beretta, C., Faustini, R. and Gallini, G. (1973) *Veterinary Record* **92,** 217.
3. Lillehei, R. C., Longerbeam, J. K., Bloch, J. H. and Manox, W. G. (1964) *Annals of Surgery* **160,** 682.
4. Gourzis, J. T., Nollenberg, W. and Nickerson, M. (1961) *Journal of Experimental Medicine* **114,** 593.
5. Nickerson, M. (1955) *Journal of the Michigan State Medical Society* **34,** 45.
6. Wiggers, H. C., Ingraham, R. C., Roemhild, F. and Goldberg, H. (1948) *American Journal of Physiology* **152,** 571.
7. Burrows, G. E. (1981) *Equine Veterinary Journal,* **13,** 89.
8. Schleien, C. L., Berkowitz, I. D., Traystman, R. and Rogers, M. C. (1989) *Anesthesiology* **71,** 133.
9. Safar, P. (1982) *Cardiopulmonary and Cerebral Resuscitation.* World Federation Society of Anesthesiologists.
10. Waterman, A. E. (1981) *Proceedings of the Association of Veterinary Anaesthetists of Great Britain and Ireland* **9,** 73.
11. Dodman, N. H. and Brito-Babapulle, L. A. (1979) *Proceedings of the Association of Veterinary Anaesthetists of Great Britain and Ireland* **8,** 141.
12. Department of Health (1976) *HC(76)38 or SHHD/DS (76). 65.* Department of Health and Social Security: London.
13. National Institute of Occupational Safety and Health (1977) Department of Health, Education and Welfare, Publication No. 77–140, Washington, DC: US Government Printing Office.
14. Jones, R. S. (1977) *Proceedings of the Association of Veterinary Anaesthetists of Great Britain and Ireland* **7,** 54.
15. Smith, W. D. A. (1978) *British Journal of Clinical Equipment* **3,** 49.

APPENDICES

DUTIES OF AN ANAESTHETIST

The practice of veterinary medicine and surgery in the UK is governed by the Veterinary Surgeons Act 1966, and under that Act (with certain quite minor exceptions) no one may practise veterinary surgery unless he or she is registered with the Royal College of Veterinary Surgeons. The following guidelines relating to the duties of the anaesthetist in the UK have been set out by the Registrar of the Royal College of Veterinary Surgeons, Mr A. R. W. Porter MA:

'Halsbury's Laws of England state that — [1]

"A person who holds himself out as ready to give medical advice or treatment impliedly undertakes that he is possessed of skill and knowledge for the purpose. Whether or not he is a registered practitioner, such a person who is consulted by a patient owes him certain duties, namely a duty of care in deciding whether to undertake the case; a duty of care in deciding what treatment to give; a duty of care in answering a question put to him by a patient in circumstances in which he knows that the patient intends to rely on his answer. A breach of any of these duties will support an action for negligence by the patient."

These principles apply equally to a veterinarian — save that his duty of care is owed to his client, who is normally the owner of the animal. When the veterinarian is an anaesthetist one can, therefore, say that he has a duty of care towards the client in deciding whether anaesthesia can be safely undertaken; a duty of care in deciding on the appropriate form of anaesthetization; a duty of care in the administration of anaesthetic and a duty of care in consultation with any other veterinarians involved in the case of ensuring that the client is properly advised regarding the course to be followed and any special notes involved.

The anaesthetist must, like any other veterinary or medical practitioner, "bring to his task a reasonable degree of skill and knowledge, and must exercise a reasonable degree of care" [2]. Whether reasonable skill and care have been exercised in any particular case where something has gone amiss is a matter which has to be decided in relation to the facts of the case, but it is clear that failure to exercise the necessary degree of skill and care which results in the death of or injury to an animal will give the owner the right to bring a legal action for the recovery of damages.

In general terms, a veterinarian in general practice, assuming responsibility for the anaesthetization of a patient, will be judged against the standard of the good, careful and competent general practitioner but a veterinarian of consultant status within the field of anaesthesia must expect to be judged against the standards set and observed by his peers.

It has sometimes been said that a mere error of judgement does not amount to negligence, but a medical case which went all the way to the House of Lords [3], indicates that a more accurate statement would be that an error of judgement does not necessarily amount to negligence. Whether or not the requisite degree of competence, skill and knowledge has been exercised in a particular case is normally tested against evidence which seeks to demonstrate what is normal, currently acceptable practice.

There is a further question to be considered and that is the responsibility of the veterinary anaesthetist for any negligence by any person assisting him in the anaesthetization of the animal. Halsbury [4] states that:

"The liability of a practitioner for the negligence of other persons depends upon the relationship between him and them. The relationship between a practitioner and a nurse in a hospital is not, as a general rule, such that the practitioner is liable for the negligence of the nurse in carrying out, or failing to carry out his instructions."

That statement relates to the position of doctor and nurse in a hospital for human patients, since the doctor is not the employer of the nurse. The doctor may, therefore, avoid personal liability for the nurse's negligence, which may be the responsibility of the hospital authorities instead.

The statement might apply also to the veterinary surgeon and veterinary nurse in, say, a veterinary school or animal welfare society where, again, the veterinary surgeon and nurse would not be in an employer/employee situation. However, in situations in which the veterinary surgeon, and his nurse or other lay assistant have an employer/employee relationship (such as in general practice) it is almost certain that the veterinary surgeon would have to bear responsibility for the negligence of his employee.

In assessing any action for negligence involving a lay assistant (whether the employer is the veterinary surgeon or an institution) the courts will have regard to his or her qualifications and training. Accordingly, veterinary anaesthetists should always make sure that anyone they ask to assist them is competent to perform the tasks assigned to that person.'

During the course of veterinary practice it is frequently necessary to use drugs which in the UK are controlled by the Misuse of Drugs Act 1971 and the Misuse of Drugs Regulations. The legislation covers a much more diverse range of drugs than those previously described as 'dangerous drugs'. Over 100 compounds are controlled under the Act but relatively few are in regular use in the UK. In the Regulations they are placed in four schedules for the purpose of the controls to be applied to their legitimate use. This classification scheme is based mainly on the extent of their use in medicine, dentistry and veterinary medicine, and on the need to prevent misuse.

The regulations impose on all practitioners important legal obligations in the prescribing and administration of controlled drugs. Separate registers must be kept of all controlled drugs obtained and supplied or used. Veterinarians as individuals are required by the regulations to keep the controlled drugs which they are authorized to employ 'in a locked receptacle which can be opened only by him or by a person authorized by him' and every precaution must be taken to prevent their falling into the hands of unauthorized persons. A locked motorcar has been held not to be a locked receptacle for the purpose of the regulations and it follows, therefore, that controlled drugs left in a motorcar in the practitioner's absence from the vehicle must be in a separately locked receptacle. Thefts of controlled drugs should be reported at once to the police. The contravention of any of the various provisions of the Misuse of Drugs Act or Regulations by a veterinary practitioner may be made subject to criminal proceedings and all practitioners should ensure that they are conversant with statutory regulations.

Veterinary anaesthetists in the UK will find the booklet *Legislation Affecting the Veterinary Profession in Great Britain,* 5th edn, 1987, published by the Royal College of Veterinary Surgeons, a useful guide to these regulations.

NOTES

1. *Halsbury's Laws of England,* 4th edn, vol. 30, para. 35.
2. *Halsbury's Laws of England,* 4th edn, vol. 30, para. 36.
3. Whitehouse v. Jordan and another (1981) All ER 267.
4. *Halsbury's Laws of England,* 4th edn, vol. 30, para. 39.

GLOSSARY OF ABBREVIATIONS

A	Amp
$(A–a)P_{O_2}$	Alveolar–arterial oxygen tension difference
atm	Atmosphere
cmH_2O	Centimetres of water
CPAP	Continuous positive airway pressure
ECG	Electrocardiogram/electrocardiograph
ED_{50}	Median effective dose
EEG	Electroencephalogram/electroencephalograph
FRC	Functional residual capacity
g	gram
Hz	Hertz
i.c.	Intracardiac
i.m.	Intramuscular
IPPV	Intermittent positive-pressure ventilation (of the lungs)
i.t.	Intratracheal
i.v.	Intravenous(ly)
J	Joule
kg	Kilogram
kPa	Kilopascal ($\approx$ 7.5 mmHg or 10 cmH_2O)
l	Litre (= 1000 ml)
MAC	Minimum alveolar concentration
μg	Microgram
mg	Milligram
ml	Millilitre
mm	Millimeter
mmHg	Millimeters of mercury
mmol	millimole
mol	Mole
mOsm	Milliosmole
P_{CO_2}	Carbon dioxide tension
PEEP	Positive end-expiratory pressure
P_{O_2}	Oxygen tension
P_aCO_2	Arterial carbon dioxide tension
P_ACO_2	Alveolar carbon dioxide tension
P_aO_2	Arterial oxygen tension
P_AO_2	Alveolar oxygen tension
s.c.	Subcutaneous(ly)
SD	Standard deviation
SEM	Standard error of the mean
s.w.g.	Standard wire gauge
V	Volt

UK AND US APPROVED NAMES OF SOME DRUGS USED IN ANAESTHESIA

US approved name	UK approved name
Acetominophen	Paracetamol
Alfadolone	Alphadolone
Alfaxalone	Alphaxalone
Cromylin sodium	Sodium cromoglycate
Dibucaine	Cinchocaine
Epinephrine	Adrenaline
Ergonovine	Ergometrine
Flunixine	Flunixine
Furosemide	Frusemide
Isoproterenol	Isoprenaline
Lidocaine	Lignocaine
Meperidine	Pethidine
Pentobarbital	Pentobarbitone
Phenobarbital	Phenobarbitone
Quinalbarbitone	Secobarbital
Salbutamol	Salbutamol
Scopolamine	Hyoscine
Succinylcholine	Suxamethonium
Tetracaine	Amethocaine
Thiopental	Thiopentone

UK approved name	US approved name
Adrenaline	Epinephrine
Alphadolone	Alfadolone
Alphaxalone	Alfaxalone
Amethocaine	Tetracaine
Cinchocaine	Dibucaine
Ergometrine	Ergonovine
Frusemide	Furosemide
Hyoscine	Scopolamine
Isoprenaline	Isoproterenol
Lignocaine	Lidocaine
Methohexitone	Methohexital
Paracetamol	Acetominophen
Pentobarbitone	Pentobarbital
Pethidine	Meperidine
Phenobarbitone	Phenobarbital
Salbutamol	Salbutamol
Secobarbital	Quinalbarbitone
Sodium chromglycate	Cromolyn sodium
Suxamethonium	Succinylcholine
Thiopentone	Thiopental

INDEX